Design of Experiments and Advanced Statistical Techniques in Clinical Research

Basavarajaiah D. M.
Bhamidipati Narasimha Murthy

Design of Experiments and Advanced Statistical Techniques in Clinical Research

Springer

Basavarajaiah D. M.
Karnataka Veterinary, Animal and
Fisheries Sciences University
Karnataka
India

Bhamidipati Narasimha Murthy
National Health Mission, Govt. of India
National Institute of Epidemiology
Chennai
India

ISBN 978-981-15-8209-7 ISBN 978-981-15-8210-3 (eBook)
https://doi.org/10.1007/978-981-15-8210-3

This Springer imprint is published by the registered company Springer Nature Singapore Pte Ltd.
The registered company address is: 152 Beach Road, #21-01/04 Gateway East, Singapore 189721, Singapore

Dedicated to the front line COVID19
Health-care Professionals and workers

Preface

Statistics is the grammar of science and unique among the academic disciplines, and statistical thought is needed at every stages of research study almost all research investigations including planning, selecting the sample, managing the massive research data sets, and interpreting the resulted findings. Statistics is the science of learning from data and of measuring, controlling, and communicating uncertainty, providing a scientific navigational tools essential for taking appropriate clinical decisions at crucial times. Both clinical and statistical reasonings are very important to progress in medical research. The clinical research must infer from a few to many and combine evidence with several theory. Scientific discipline and study of empirical knowledge is generated from practical observations and ramification with research interest. Medical and statistical theories are based on established and existing hypotheses radically derived from mathematical intervention and real probability. Always Medical research requires both a theoretical basis in science and statistical support for testing real hypothetical statements about any kind of research based on the observed data sets, the theoretical and applied statistical methods layout is formally accounting for known sources of controlling random state of clinical variables and various attributes, (even so we shall estimate patients response rate to treatment and efficacy). In addition, the use of statistics in clinical trial allows the clinical researcher to form reasonable inference at sample and larger population level. Infact, the banquet of new statistical approach can be used to delineate various patterns present in the medical science, indicate various simulation methods absolutely report for checking randomness and uncertainties in the varied research setup, and as such used to draw the effective inference about the research being studied. The pragmatic knowledge of statistics will be derived necessary tools and overall conceptual analytical foundation for qualitative and quantitative reasoning, to extract the true research evidence from experimental area (infer new findings from the massive data sets of clinical and medical researches); this is often supported for testing the null hypothesis (H_0) effectively. Practically now, we have observed that health is an important quotient for individual species, especially the days when health domains show negative trend in developing and developed countries, for example, the recent spikes of COVID19 in 215 countries, and the remaining countries are also not free from this deadly disease. As far as human life is concerned, all governments and private agencies seek prevention and control measures such as treatment with existing drugs and development of vaccine or new drugs at population level. In this overall research frame, advanced statistical methods are needed to understand the complex phenomenon of COVID 19 with real-life data sets on patient selection, early screening of infected patients from machine learning tools, evaluation of cases based on clinical perspectives, etc. Still, for prophylaxis, development of vaccine is very essential for prevention of COVID 19. The FDA and WHO have already initiated steps in this direction, and clinical trials in different epidemic sites by using quality-by-design approach are in progress. Advanced design of experiments and statistical methods are needed to develop new vaccines and understand the entire process of drug or vaccine development (until the approval of FDA) for the health benefits of human beings. More advancement for developing a drug or vaccine through trials especially for COVID 19, one has to consider genetic complexity in the population and its interaction with environmental factors. For this purpose, advanced statistical and genetic models are to be developed and tested with real-life data sets. Similarly, pharmacokinetic models to study drug metabolism, its duration, and its effectiveness are also needed to be considered. In the present classic book, we are inspired and motivated to explore various new analytical choices to escalate advanced statistical methods and its mechanisms, new methods that help us to know the relation between different clinical attributes, to describe real data sets and formulation of necessary design of experiments (DOE) for conducting drug or new vaccine trials at global level. Eventually, advanced statistical methods and design of experiments (DOE) tools are in a close association between the researcher to understand and anticipate new clinical findings and to know the relationship between causative factors and its associated variables; in turn these variables will be tested for credibility and real probabilities. Many statistical techniques developed earlier by scientists/researchers so far used for clinical or drug trials in various kinds of diseases are fundamental and derived from frequentistic approach for handling new clinical and medical research datum for evaluating and applying prior research interventions. With these postulates, the present book discusses distinct methods for building predictive and probability distribution models in clinical situations and recent ways to assess the stability of these models to draw qualitative conclusion using real-life experimental data sets. Post hoc tests are used for comparing treatment effects and precision of the experimentation at greater accuracy. Initially, the book starts with basic ingredients for design of experiments in clinical and medical research and statistical methods for analysis. Then, step-by-step various complex design of experiments and necessary advanced statistical methods or models are developed using intellectual conceptualization of clinical existence, natural histories, clinical response with likelihood and illustrated with real-life data sets. Selection of suitable or appropriate designs, sample selection for clinical trials, use of neural networks, adoption of genetic and environmental factors, pharmacokinetic mechanism, advanced imputation methods for usually occurring missing observations, and above all ethical considerations are some of the challenges that are faced while writing this book. The present book covers 12 chapters, all chapters briefly describe new intervention of design of experiments and advanced statistical methods. Chapter 1 deals with the design of clinical research and its practical approach; Chap. 2 briefly describes advanced design of experiment approach to clinical and medical research; Chap. 3 brings newer techniques of random forest and concept of decision tree model association with clinical and medical research and how to construct different trees based on the observed data sets; Chap. 4 demonstrates different applications of machine learning in medical research; Chaps. 5 and 6 briefly describe advanced statistical genetics and its application in drug trail and theoretical implications for estimation of genetic traits in human vaccine trials; Chap. 7 focuses on foundation of statistical implications and its practical approach to research methodology; Chaps. 8 and 9 deal with various statistical models in relation with life-threatening diseases demonstrated with real-life data sets and meta-analysis; Chap. 10 describes in depth pharmacokinetic and statistical modeling; Chaps. 11 and 12 describe advanced tools of imputation methods for deriving missing observations and ethical perspective approach to clinical and medical research, etc. All chapters are derived with theoretical formulations and their applications and necessary conclusions with eye catching illustrations and fashionable diagrams. The reader should easily understand all the concepts of analysis with practical intuition. Though, we conceived the idea of writing this book in calendar year 2016, the actual process started 2 years ago, and the true impulse is happened after the COVID 19 lockdown period. On a more applied level, clinicians and researchers need basic understanding and good apprehension toward statistics well enough to follow and evaluate the real empirical studies (e.g., formulation of randomized control trail) that provide insight and evidence base for clinical practices. We hope that this book will be very useful for clinical trial investigators or researchers, applied statisticians, planners, and policymakers, especially on health and environment, research scholars, and academicians for furthering their skills on design of experiments and variou recent applications of advanced statistical methods.

Karnataka, India — Basavarajaiah D. M.
New Delhi, India — Bhamidipati Narasimha Murthy

Acknowledgments

This book is based on real-life research data sets collected from different health institutes and academic universities. We are grateful to the Karnataka Veterinary Animal and Fisheries Sciences University authority, Bidar, National Institute of Epidemiology of Indian Council of Medical Research and National Health Mission, Ministry of Health and Family Welfare, Government of India, for giving permission to publish this book. Firstly, we would like to extend our sincere thanks to Prof. H.D. Narayanaswamy, Hon'ble Vice Chancellor, KVAFSU (B), Director, National Health Mission (NHM) and Secretary (DHR) and Director General, ICMR, for their moral support and guidance, and also we extend our whole hearted thanks to all the key officers and teachers of KVAFSU(B), Prof. H.M. Jayaprakasha, Dean, Dairy Science College, Hebbal, Bengaluru; Prof. KC Veeranna, Registrar; Prof. NA Patil, Director of Extension; Prof Sri BV Shiva Prakash, Director of Research; Prof. Manik Kishan Tandle, Director of Instruction, Postgraduation Studies; Prof. Narayan Bhat, Dean Veterinary College, Bengaluru; Prof. Mohamed Nadeem Fairoze, Former PG Dean, KVAFSU(B); Prof. H.N. Narasimhamurthy, Former Dean, VCH (B); Prof. Jayanaik; and Prof. Dr. Mrs. Bharathi (Sociology), Former Dean, Dr. M D Surangi PPMC head for their constant encouragement. We would like to acknowledge Mrs. Netra Rajpurohit for her technical support on proof reading. Finally our sincere thanks and highest gratitude to our beloved family members for their constant encouragement and support toward completion of the entire work. This book would not have been possible to be brought out without them. We feel immensely proud for extending our heartiest thanks to the various health institutes for providing research data for embedding this beautiful book.

Contents

About the Authors

Basavarajaiah D. M. is working as an Associate Professor and Head, Department of Statistics and Computer Science, Karnataka Veterinary Animal and Fisheries Sciences University (B), Hebbal, Bangalore. He obtained PhD from National Institute of Epidemiology (NIE), ICMR, Chennai (affiliated to University of Madras). His area of research heeds statistical theory, statistical modeling on high-dimensional data sets of agriculture, medicine, veterinary, and animal sciences. He penned 70 research articles and 7 academic books published in national and reputed international publishers (Springer Nature group). He is serving as an Editorial Board Member and Scientific Board Advisor of various international indexed journals. Life Member of various academic organizations and scientific societies. He had honored several accolades for his academic and research excellency, "Chartered Scientist" award stalwart by Science Council, United Kingdom, in Collaboration with Royal Statistical Society. Best Reviewer award 2016 from "TRANS STELLAR" Journal Publications and Research Consultancy, TJPRC Ltd. (NAAS rated Journals), Fellow of Royal Statistical Society, UK (London), Fellow of Mathematical Society, UK (London), Bharathshikshratana and Indo-Dubai Achiever's Pacific award honored by Global Society for Health and Educational Growth, New Delhi, Best Reviewer 2015, Best Scientific Board Advisor 2016, and Best Editorial and Researcher award bestowed by International Academy of Engineering Science and Technology, USA. He has delegated as an active member of Board of Studies and Academic Council of various universities.

Bhamidipati Narasimha Murthy is a well-known academician and researcher, Former Scientist "G" (Director Grade cadre), National Institute of Epidemiology of ICMR, Chennai. At present, he is a National Level Monitor, National Health Mission, MOH&FW, Government of India. He obtained PhD from International Institute for Population Science (IIPS), affiliated to Bombay University (1985). His areas of research are mainly Mathematical Statistics, Operational Research, Clinical Research, Public Health, Demography and Vital Statistics, Mathematical Modeling with respect to Medical Science and Public Health. He penned more than 100 research articles published in reputed National and International journals. He is serving as an editorial Board Member and Scientific Board Advisor of various international indexed MCI and UGC recognized journals. He is a Life Member of various academic organizations and professional societies. He honored several accolades for his academic and research excellency, viz. Prof. R. N. Srivastava Gold Medal award, "Bharat Jyothi Award," and "Best Citizens of India Award." He serves as a member of Board of Studies of various National universities (University of Madras, Acharya Nagarjuna University, and University of Kerala) and also a visiting emeritus Professor of Johns Hopkins University, Bloomberg School of Public Health, Baltimore, Maryland, North Carolina University, USA, etc. He is a reviewer of National and International journals.

List of Figures

List of Tables

1 Designs of Clinical Research and Its Practical Approach

1.1 Introduction

The statistical method is a backbone of clinical research and surmises the sound knowledge of drug formulation, Pharmacokinetic (PK) effects, drug delivery process, etc., while the final experimental decision will be drawn based on various advanced statistical techniques and design of experimentation (DOE) (Aggarwal and Ranganathan 2019). The design of experimentation (DOE) is a very important analytical tool to prove or disprove the null hypothesis (H_0) at desired levels of significance α and power of the test (β) with varying population size. Conversely, the researcher drewan effective conclusion or inference about the population or sample on the experimental findings with various attributes and real experience. Besides that, the design of experimentation (DOE) tools infer effective research information to clinicians, drug development quality controlling officers (DDQC), and clinical researchers for the implementation of new randomized control trail (RCT) guidelines and hands-on training program for drug developers, specialists, and research beginners at larger extent (Ademex 2002). Numerous clinicians and researchers are failing to adopt the recent statistical and DOE tools in their research work due to lack of statistical literature and suitable reference books. In this book we have discussed various types of statistical methods according to clinical research, study design, sample size determination, Power of the test, testing of Null Hypothesis (H_0) and formulation of drug development process by using several advanced statistical methods and various mathematical models that were demonstrated by the real data sets (Bello et al. 2008).

The practical insight of clinical or medical research states that, clinical trial is a type of research study that helps us to know the effect of drugs on human subjects, in which the treatment (intervention) can be initiated specially for new therapy evaluation. Altogether, we can define "clinical trial" as a type of research study for comparing the effect and value of intervention (cases) against a control group (placebo) on human subjects (Bello et al. 2008). Further, the clinical trial is an experimental testing of medical treatment on human subjects (Ademex 2002). The researcher can elucidate and define the clinical trial in so many ways; for example, the comparison of Stavudine fixed (STV) drug dose versus no treatment (Placebo) to know (estimation) the length of survivability of people living with HIV/AIDS (PLHIVs) and also evaluate side effect of administered drug (weakness, numbness, tingling or burning pain in hands or feet, rashes and headache during the treatment follow-up of people living with HIV (PLHIV)). Since one more intervention of DOE is to evaluate the effectiveness of new antifungal medication on Athlete's foot in defined time intervals, the above

B. D. M., B. Narasimha Murthy, *Design of Experiments and Advanced Statistical Techniques in Clinical Research*, https://doi.org/10.1007/978-981-15-8210-3_1

said cited research inculcate to know the prognostic effect of treatment on human subject for the reduction of hazard rate among PLHIV's and Athlete's foot patients. Absolutely, the clinical trial is more important perspective to save sick patients over extensive time period (Ademex 2002). It seems to be noted that, many clinicians obtained evidence-based results and admittedly valid conclusion from their research findings based on the practical and theoretical approach, overwhelmingly the DOE is very easy to provide anecdotal information about the benefit of new therapy to be accepted and provide health services for critically care patients wearisome. In day-to-day life, the pediatric health care specialists or health care workers are solely experienced on the intervention of supplementation of high level concentration of oxygen (O_2) among children who are suffering from pneumonia at neonatal stage. It is a very useful therapy for surviving premature infants until a clinical trial demonstrated its harmfulness. Aggarwal and Ranganathan (2019) reported that with the prolonged use of hormonal replacement therapy for women suffering from menopause problems, the intervention of menopause will be prevented when administering Neurontin against estrogen. This supplemented drug showed deleterious effects on the bodily changes of a person who is suffering from menopause problems (age group between 46 and 55 years), and the results were significantly associated with psychological domain and drug dosage. In this vein, the Statistics and DOE play a key role in any clinical trial (micro or macro) from design, conduct, compilation, and reporting in terms of controlling biological and environmental variations (minimizing biases). The advanced statistical method is very useful for a researcher in extracting confounding factors and measuring random errors at sample and population level with desired level of significance. And also it will provide formal accounting for unknown source of variability in patients, treatment, and dosage and drug response. The knowledge in statistics is important in conducting a clinical research from setting up the research topic to drawing a valid conclusion and disseminating the effectiveness of research. Researcher wish to learn from the statistical methods how we look at the data from a statistical point of view, which is essential for us to mitigate more advanced statistical knowledge and choose the correct tests in the future line of research at micro- and macrolevel. Before a drug is approved by FDA for use, it has to undergo clinical trials to test its efficacy and safety. Especially clinical research involves investigating proposed medical treatments, assessing the relative benefits of competing therapies and establishing optimal treatment combinations. All types of clinical research attempts to answer our salient questions such as should a man with prostate cancer undergo radical prostatectomy or radiation or wait and see? And is the incidence of serious adverse effects among patients receiving a new pain relieving therapy greater than the incidences of serious adverse effects in patients receiving the standard therapy. In this regime, the statistical tools are very essential for clinicians and drug manufacturer for taking right decision at the right time. As the field of evidence-based medicine, the theoretical statistics driven in the form of inferential process, especially the planning and analysis of massive electronic data sets, survey and observational studies (Aggarwal and Ranganathan 2019) has developed in the twentieth century. The clinical research has fully utilized statistical methods and provide formal accounting for unknown sources of variability in recruited patients and response of the treatment. The statistics will allow the clinical researchers to draw reasonable and accurate inferences from collected information and to make sound decisions in the presence of uncertainty. Mastery of statistics and DOE concepts can prevent numerous errors and biases in medical and clinical research. The statistical reasoning is characterized by the following key points.

1. Selection of research topics with salient objectives our of interest for conducting clinical investigations
2. Placing data and theory on an equal scientific ethos
3. Designing data sets production through experimentation

4. Quantifying the influence of chance factor
5. Estimating systematic and random effects by fixed and random effect models.
6. Combining theory and collected data using formal methods (formulation of new models)

The clinicians will examine and intervene individual cases at an early stage. The understanding of the clinical challenges they will need to address and of the likely past and future courses of the clinical conditions they are seeing and evaluation of the effectiveness and risks of their clinical actions and strategies are all based on considerations of the various attributes and historical data sets of clients similar to the one they are now visualizing and with whom they may be about to intervene. The design of experimentation is a fundamental tool linking the multiplicity of potential observations of every client with more illustrative concepts of clinical and biological entities, natural histories, clinical response and risks, etc. These more conclusive parameters construct the foundation on which clinical decisions rest. On a more applied level, clinicians need to understand statistics well enough to follow and evaluate the base for clinical practices. Many studies conducted decades ago found major lacunae in physicians knowledge of statistics. This is a problem more recent studies have found to be only somewhat reduced in magnitudinal differences between research and ethical considerations. It leads clinicians to mistrust, misunderstand, and ignore the statistics and study design at inception of study and also final reporting. Clinical research approach to statistical application is often viewed as the corner stone of scientific progress at global level. It is a systematic process based on scientific methods that consists of testing null hypothesis considering too many clinical and biological attributes, careful observations and measurements, systematic evaluation of clinical data sets, and drawing valid statistical conclusion. The prospective of clinical research methods is shown in the following flow chart (Fig. 1.1).

1.1.1 Identification of Research Problem

It is the first statement made in any research. An example of research problem, which may be of a

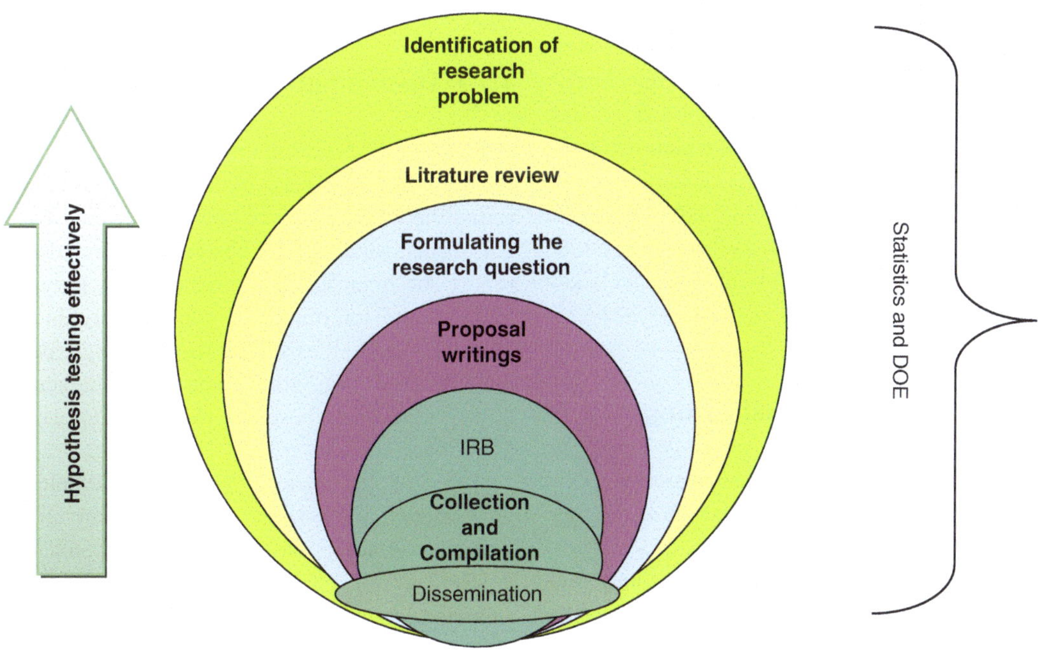

Fig. 1.1 Flow chart of clinical research

local concern for the community, is violence among children. This is the problem to be investigated. At this stage, the identified problem is still too broad in scope. Therefore, the scope of the study needs to be narrowed down, which can only be done after a thorough literature review.

1.1.2 Literature Survey

A literature survey encompasses the process of surveying for information related to the research topic across multiple databases, and information related to reading, evaluating, and analyzing them helps refine the topic and objective of our research and overview to be written. A good literature review helps in finding research gaps, asking good questions, and accurately defining problems, as well as identifying a proper methodological aspects.

1.1.3 Formulating the Research Question

The next step in the research process after the objective refining on the objective basis thorough literature survey will be done after identification of research problem, which involves translating that research idea into an answerable question. A research question is a question that a researcher wishes to study or a hypothesis which he or she wishes to test. The most important part of the questions is to be researchable and answerable using established scientific methods and procedures. It should attempt to fill a research gap extensively.

1.1.4 Research Proposal Writing

The main purpose of writing a research proposal is to obtain an ethical approval, as well as funding. A well-written proposal provides a structured outline guiding the researcher throughout each step of the research process. It is written to justify the postulated research questions and to present a detailed methodology in which the research should be best conducted.

1.1.5 Institutional Review Board (IRB)

IRB is specific human subjects committee that review and determine the ethicality of research. IRB exists in research institutions and consists of academicians, researchers, clinicians, and a representative from the community. The main task of the IRB is to protect the rights of participants in research being conducted. IRBs have the authority to require modification on the proposal pertaining to all aspects of the research, as well as to disapprove a proposal.

1.1.6 Data Collection and Compilation

Data collection is a process of collecting the information that will be used to answer the research question. Its most important aspect is to select the relevant information needed to answer research questions. Compilation is the process of analyzing data sets using suitable statistical tools in order to draw valid conclusions that support or reject the null hypothesis or answer the research questions.

1.1.7 Dissemination

Publishing the research findings is the final step of the research process, which entails summarizing the whole research key findings in different forms, such as an abstract, presentation, report, or manuscript published in a reputed national and International indexed journals for end-users. The research questions always focus on PICO criteria; good example of research questions selected based on the PICO criteria is as follows:

Topic of our interest: Sex worker Women's HIV status

Narrowed topic: Women and sexual contact

Focused topics: Women to be HIV tested (infected or not infected)

P = Women (Prostitute work >10 years); **I** = Sexual contact history (1–6 Person per day)

C = without condoms' **O** = Status of HIV

PICO stands for four letters **P**: Exposed population; **I**: Intervention to be tested; **C**: Comparison used in the research topic; and **O**: Outcome to be measured as a result of the intervention

1.2 Practical Implication of Study Design in Clinical Research

In many ways the design of a study is more important than the analysis. A badly designed study can never be retrieved, whereas a poorly analyzed one can usually be reanalyzed, viz. consideration of design is also important because the design of a study will govern how the data is to be analyzed. Most medical and clinical research considered input, which may be human intervention or exposure to a potentially toxic compounds, and an output, which is some measure of health that the intervention is supposed to affect. The simplest way to categorize studies is with reference to the time sequence in which the input and output are studied and the most powerful study design discussed in latter part of the section. One of the most commonly asked questions to a statistician is about the design of the number of patients to include; it is an important question, because if a study is too small it will not be able to answer the questions posed and would be a waste of time and economy. It would also be deemed unethical because patients may be put at risk with no apparent benefit. However, studies should not be too large because resources would be wasted if fewer patients would have sufficed. The sample size depends on four critical quantities namely type I and II errors, power of the test, desired level of significance, and design effect. In this paradigm, entire theoretical and practical application of DOE and advanced statistical methods are discussed in the separate forthcoming sections.

1.2.1 Objectives of the Book

The design of experiment is a tool and very extensively used in the field of Medical, Clinical, Agricultural, and Engineering science research. The experiment can be time consuming, particularly if the researcher is interested in measuring the long-term effects. Any kind of (Quantitative and qualitative) research is very difficult to layout or inception at an early stage without proper designing of experiment. If the design has not been formulated properly in prior, the whole research findings will give unrealistic conclusion about the population because due to faulty selection of sample, study subjects, duration, etc. In latter part of the study, it is too difficult task to control extraneous effect of the different variables or attributes. Overwhelmingly entire resulted part will become false positives and not to produce any further research hypothetical statement at population or sample level. Particularly in the field of medical, clinical, and agricultural research, many confounders would be aroused from the research; the effect of confounders will be greatly increasing the standard error (SE) in the experimental results and also researcher may deliberately contaminate the results part. In this practical situation, we attempt to demonstrate various types of advanced study design (particularly more applicable to medical, animal and agricultural research) by using real data sets and also we explore the newer techniques for designing the various types of design of experiment (DOE) to be capable of examining the casual relationship between the different factors at various levels. The present book saliently attributed high degree of control of extraneous and exogenous variables explicitly with direct and indirect control of errors. The following salient objectives were considered for demonstrating various types of design of experimentation.

1. To explore new technologies for constructing the various design of experiment approach to advanced statistical measures to prove analytical intervention of clinical, Medical, Agricultural, and Animal Sciences research.
2. To develop a basic understanding of the various study subjects or factors each at different levels that control sampling and nonsampling errors for producing very good results from the experimental groups.

3. To develop recent or advanced Statistical methods or measures that are superior to existing technologies for improvement of drug trail (clinical research), Medical and Agricultural science various attributes to be tested at greater accuracy with highest precision.
4. To demonstrate the various treatment effects at desired level of significance and also we extrapolate any significant association between the selected factors in the experimental groups and identify the optimal or acceptance level of research at microlevel.
5. To derive the different analytical intervention of design of experimentation (DOE) and its modelling techniques for the development of cascade of research study at various levels or end users (clinicians, research beginners, drug developers, academicians, etc.)

1.3 Statistical Historical Perspectives of Clinical Trail

The first clinical trial was escalated from Scurvy experiment conducted way back in 1747 by James F. Lind, a physician onboard of the "Salisbury." In the year 1920 onwards, Prof. R. A. Fisher introduced randomization as a core principle in the statistical theory of the design of experiments (DOE). In the year 1947–1948 Streptomycin in tuberculosis (TB) was the first randomized controlled clinical trial conducted by tuberculosis team, USA, and it was (RCT) published in the British Medical Journal. Another study was reported by Byron and Kenward (2003); a total of 1.80 million children participated in the largest trial to assess the effectiveness of the Salk vaccine for preventing paralysis and death from poliomyelitis. Such massive odd number was selected for the above-cited experimental trail just because the higher incidence rate of polio was noticed in the affected area (1/2000). As an experimental insight, the researcher has attempted to minimize standard errors (SE) from utilizing treatment evidence, efficacy, and tolerance level. All the clinical parameters were extracted from the historical data of selected subject. As per the research trail findings, the Salk vaccine showed to be more effective (> 95% efficacy) when compared to naïve group ($p = 0.0001$) and also it was routinely administered from the physician. Similar study was reported by (Biberstein and Parker 1985) who noticed that, the formulated vaccine showed significantly good control and comorbid condition of cancer patients when compared to naïve or control group ($p < 0.001$). Statistically there were two components (randomized and non-randomized) that were considered for extrapolation of the results and testing of hypothesis in RCT trail. Many researchers have formulated the randomized control trail (RCT) for conducting clinical, agricultural, and Biological experimentation in varied settings. The randomized control trail (RCT) is uniquely adopted to demonstrate vaccine trail at global level, during the study period, the subject of RCT was categorized into two types, namely, (1) randomized component-study subject and (2) non-randomized component-study subject without randomness. Hopewell et al. (2010) conducted randomized control trail on children. A total of one million children in the first through third grades participated. The second grade was offered a vaccine whereas first and third grades were formed as control groups (naive). An approximate of 0.81 million children were randomized in double-blind placebo-controlled trial. The incidence of polio in the randomized vaccinated group was less than half of that in the control group and even larger differences were seen in the reduction of paralytic polio (Casagrande et al. 1978). Ostensibly as well as observably several attempts were made to formulate the regularity conditions of clinical trial based on the mathematical and statistical simulation modelling techniques. Campbell and Machin (1999); Byron and Kenward (2003), Choi and Noseworthy (1992), Chavalarias and Ioannidis (2010), Chambers and Fairbarn (1998), and Dupont (1988) have fitted various statistical models to draw the clinical decision about the population and sampled observation on drug trail experimentation. As per the cited results, the hierarchical model was fitted by Choi and Noseworthy (1992) and the formulated model is very useful for testing of hypothesis when the observations subject to smaller numbers (in the context of small clinical trials for assessing the efficacy and potency of the drug). Further study was done by DuPont et al. (1990, 2008) captivating the hierarchical mathematical models, and the model result signifies a natural framework for combining various clinical information on a series of small randomized clinical trial (RCT) data sets extrapolated within the ecological sites (e.g., space missions or clinics). In the above experimental subjects, scientifically the data sets are completed in the same way to preclude good treatment response; it was measured by suitable mathematical simulation modelling techniques (available for each individual cases);similar analytical intervention was done by DuPont et al. (1990, 2008); he opined that the fitted hierarchical regression model will provide a more valid and rigorous solution for randomized control trail (RCT) when compared to traditional statistical models (meta-analysis naive model); as per the summary of the above-cited results, Ademex (2002) conclude that there is no reason for the further usage of the above models to draw a valid conclusion and summarization just because of the lesser amount of precision (R^2 = 0.65, akaike information is lesser than average). However, a confidence must be paid in the manner of time and economy (i.e., the total sample size should be increased) to formulate or design a larger trial out of a series of smaller RCT trials (Ademex 2002). Secondly, the hierarchical models were fitted by Ademex (2002) and the model results have furnished full-blown or cutting edge foundation for the analysis of longitudinal clinical studies; fitted models are necessary for increasing the power and precision of research involving small RCT clinical trials (Durack et al. 1981; Detsky and Naglie 1995). In addition to that, the researchers Ademex (2002) have obtained clinical data sets from the same subject in the similar objective of the interest with defined time intervals; extracted data sets were showed to be a truncation; as part of this intervention (overlapping) the researcher has added additional subjects to conduct the experiment to curb standard error (SE). In spite of these above problems, Ademex (2002) fitted new hierarchical mixed effect model to extrapolate the salient research findings and re-designed the entire experimental unit or subject based on the different attributes with the addition of new subjects; summing of the results indicates that all parameters were found to be positively associated with objective of the interest (R^2 = 0.65, p = 0.0001). A similar study was reported by Durack et al. (1981) and Detsky and Naglie (1995) at global level; he opined that a in single treatment with varied time interval, the design can yield more consistent results; by addition of new subjects (not over lapping) the design will be re-designated as a crossover study. In case of Univariate model (correlation between age versus treatment effect), the researcher has assumed certain hypotheses, viz. observations are independent and identical in nature, collected data is normally distributed (normalcy), and error is associated with mean and common variance, $\epsilon_{ij} \sim N(\mu, \sigma^2)$. For building Univariate model (e.g., regression model) an important criteria was mainly associated with certain salient assumptions (a subset of the regression parameters is normally distributed with mean and common variance). However, the population variance and model residual effects are linearly distributed. On the other hand, the distribution of sampled observation in the heterogeneous population (different age and gender matched frequency) the response of the drug within population showed more deviation, and also in the population that belongs to the different class or heterogeneous (ethnic and race), the binary logistic linear regression mixed effect model is more suitable for describing resulted findings. Different clinical models were fitted by Dalma et al. (2019); Ebrahim and Sullivan (1999); Fleiss (1981); Freedman and Osicka (2006), namely, regression with randomly dispersed parameters (Chambers and Fairbarn 1998), exchangeability between multiple regressions ((Durack et al. 1981; Detsky and Naglie 1995); two-stage stochastic regression (Gottlieb et al. 1981; Grimes and Schulz 2002), variance component models (Gabbe et al. 2003); random coefficient models (Hulley et al. 2001); hierarchical linear models (Jorgensen et al. 1999); multilevel models (Kaerlev et al. 2004), and random-effect regression models

(Lilienfeld and Lilienfeld 1980). Survival model approach is used in people living with HIV/AIDS.

1.4 Global Milestone

1747-James Lind is the originator of modern clinical research because he was the first to introduce the use of as control group. He conducted the trail group of sailors suffering from scurvy.

1800-Arrival of placebo, first used in clinical trial and emerged as important tools in medical research. Placebo is noneffective medical treatment given to control group and to compare the resulted findings with those from the novel drug or regimen

1923-Randomization or blind clinical trials were introduced. This involves giving random treatment to participant, one being a placebo and another a new drug; it is called blind trail because neither group knew which treatment was received

1944-This period saw the introduction of multicenter clinical trials, where multiple studies were conducted at various sites (geographical location), but used the same protocol to get wider testing and better statistical data

1947-The Nuremberg code was developed, that outlined ten basic statements for safety of human participants in clinical trials

1964-The declaration of Helsinki was developed that outlines ethical codes for physicians and safety of participants trials worldwide

1988-The US FDA was given more authority and accountability over the approval of novel drugs and treatments

1988-Assembly of the International Conference on Harmonization (ICH) to provide help and eliminate differences in drug development requirements for three global pharmaceutical markets, the USA, Europe, and Japan. The ICH initiates promoting increased efficiency in the development of novel drugs and making them more available to patients and the public

2000-A common technical document (CTD) was developed. The CTD acts as a standard case book used in Europe, Japan, and the USA for proposing data gathered in clinical trials to respective Governing authorities.

1.4.1 Indian Milestone

1832–1890-Sporadic research in various setups for the development of small pox vaccine lymph in India

1890-Laboratory in Shillong started producing small pox vaccine lymph

1897-Plague vaccine produced by Dr. Haffkine in makeshift of 20 rooms in Grants Medical College, Mumbai

1899-Plague laboratory, Bombay, later on named as Haffkine Institute (1925), Mumbai

1904–1905 Central Research Institute, Kasauli, Himachal Pradesh

1907-Pasteur Institute of India, Coonoor, Tamil Nadu

1910–1930 Additional vaccine institute established in India, producing majority of small pox vaccine

1948-BCGLaboratory, Guindy, Madras

1952-Zydus Cadila

1953-Biological ELtd

1966-Serum Institute of India Ltd.

1985-Indian Immunological limited

1988-Panacea Biotec

1989-IVOL and BIBCOL

1992-Shantha Biotechnic Ltd.

1996-Bharath Biotech Ltd.,

2008-Green Biopharma Ltd.

1.5 Clinical Research

On a broader perspective, clinical research may be defined as an investigation done on human subjects intended to discover or verify the clinical, pharmacological, and/or other pharmacodynamic effects of investigational products or drugs, and/or to identify the adverse reactions, absorption, distribution, metabolism, and excretion of the investigational products or drugs with the salient objective of safety and efficacy interest (Lazarus et al. 2018). Generally, all the clinical research has been approached to evaluate the human and animal health-related diseases in terms of prevention, diagnosis, and treatment on the human subjects or animal subjects, etc. The clinical research may be broadly classified into two groups, namely with and without intervention (intervention and nonintervention).

1.5.1 Intervention

Intervention is a type of clinical study in which participants were assigned to groups that receive one or more intervention or treatment group, so that, the researcher can evaluate the effect of the intervention on Biomedical or health-related outcomes; e.g., Abemaciclib, abiraterone acetate tablets 250 mg was administered for cancer patients to evaluate the health outcome of patients at defined time intervals; this type of experiment is called as experimental insight study (randomized control trial double- and single-blind approach).

1.5.2 Nonintervention

It is a type of observational study; in general a nonintervention objective was affixed for obtaining observations from different cases or subjects at defined time interval; the patients received regular medicines prescribed in accordance with the structured label; the researcher can evaluate the subjects to inhibit and influence as little as possible on the subjective condition, while studying the effectiveness of the medicine with respect to safety, efficacy, and tolerability under real-life condition. The nonintervention (NIS) design will provide an opportunity to evaluate how a drug controls diseases or procedure to perform in a real-life situation, e.g., case–control study, cohort with or without drug intervention (Fig. 1.2).

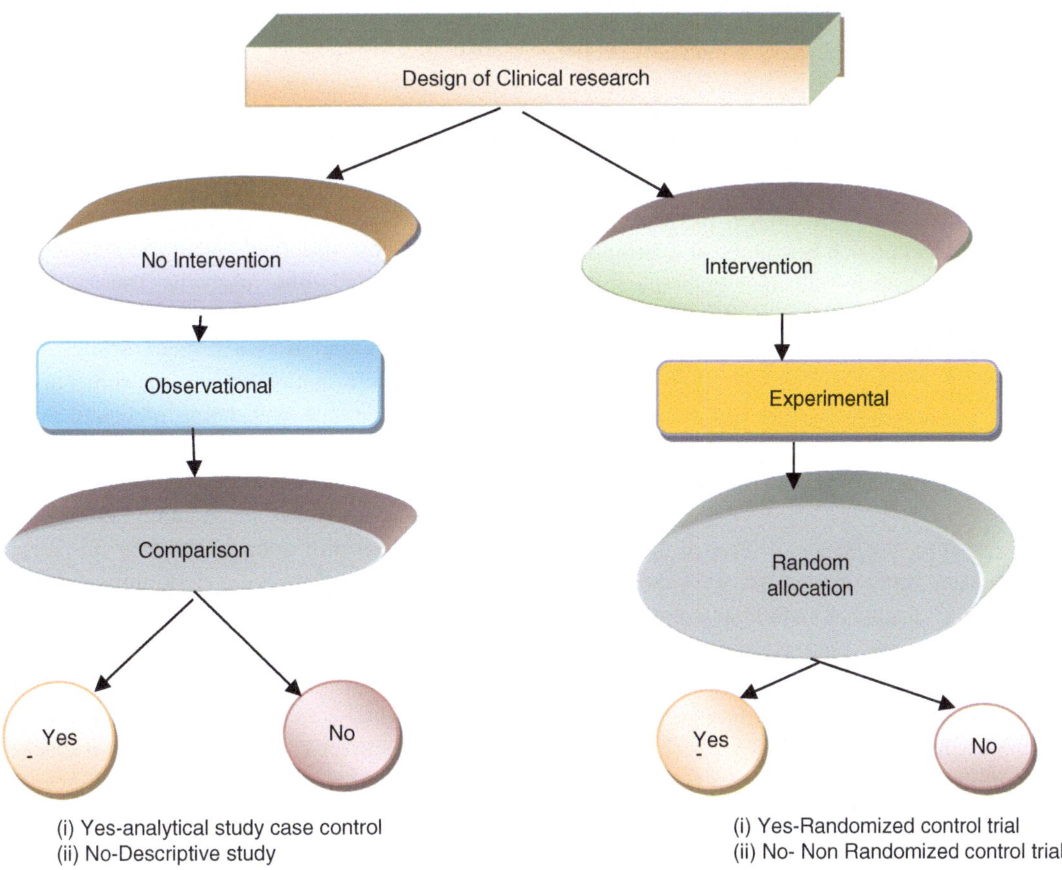

Fig. 1.2 Flow diagram of design of clinical research

1.6 Types of Clinical Research

As per the scientific ethos and FDA regularity, the clinical research has been classified in the following manner.

1.6.1 Patient-Oriented Research

It involves a particular person or use of materials from human to prevent broad mechanism of human diseases; this study pertaining to the treatment invention is to develop newer technology related to exposed diseases, e.g., a new drug administered for patient suffering from HIV (PLHIVs) and life-threatening diseases like cancer and artery disease. Masur et al. (1981) considered that for a patient-oriented research. In many developing countries like India, Sri Lanka, and South Africa, the patient-oriented research (POR) has been conducted systematically (POR), which endorsed the active partnership of patients, researchers, health care professionals, and policy decision makers in research so as to build a sustainable and accessible health care system that optimizes the health of citizen. In other words, this research approach has intended to promote a better health system and their outcomes of the individuals, alternatively which can promote health index at global level.

1.6.2 Epidemiological and Behavioral Studies

Looking at the incidence or level of distribution of disease at different sites, so many factors will be affecting health of individuals and also this above intervention can assess the affected people's quality of life (QOL) and health status to make relief from the diseases through therapeutic option. Simultneously we experienced that the health-related decisions like Zika fever at global level (also known as Zika virus disease) is an illness caused by Zika virus (Africa), and the disease has been sporadically distributed worldwide during 2015–2016. Most of the Zika cases have showed no symptoms, but when presenting the symptoms it was showed to be very mild that exhibits a symptom similar as dengue fever. The symptoms may include fever, red eyes, joint pain, headache, and appearance of maculopapular rashes on the skin. Eventually, this type of intervention alerts for an early screening and diagnosis of the exposed population. In this proximity, the epidemiological and behavioral studies will help the researcher to take right decisions at the right time (all incumbent behavioral and disease outbreak was incarcerated in the selected sites).

1.6.3 Outcome and Health-Related Services Research

Generally we have seen national and global public health system; the public health care specialists have to identify the most effective and efficient interventions like treatment and services. A majority of the research emphasize to identify the health outcome by different health-related indicators, e.g., patients administrated new drug on selected population, prospectively researcher has observed health-related outcomes at defined time intervals. The field of health services (HSR) is relayed upon decision-making theory and it is a primary source for gathering of information on how the subjects or individuals maintain well-being of health system at global level and in other developing countries. Moseley et al. (2002) studied the goal of HSR and opined that the research findings or outcome of health-related services is very important domain for taking right clinical decision and in solving real health problems at early stage and also it has provided many scientific information that menace well-being of public, eventually which can lead to the improvements of health of citizens. The HSR is a multidisciplinary field that moves beyond basic and applied research; each research hypothesis was drawn from the health professionals and many academicians with various medical disciplines, including Biostatistics, epidemiology, health economics, medicine, nursing, operational research, psychology and sociology, etc.

1.7 Risk in Clinical Research

There are always certain risks or side effects that drew up in clinical trials; the risk factors may be unpleasant, serious, or even life threatening side effects to the experimental subjects. The experimental subjects may not be given full-blown or versatile information to the researcher for experimental trail; therefore a separate protocol will be necessary for induction of research at population or sample level. Nevertheless, a consistent time and attention will be assigned for non-protocol treatment inclusion with certain visits done to the study sites for gathering full information (more treatments, hospital stays, complex dosage requirements, etc.). If the side effect was found to be undesired actions or negative impact on the experimental drugs, the absolute treatment will be necessary for the subjects, which can help the researcher to know the risk of an individual subject (Mapes et al. 2003). During the study period negative or adverse effects may also include headache, nausea, hair loss, skin-irritation, or other physical problems that aroused from the selected subjects. In the insight of clinical research we may assess many risk factors driven at the population as well as sample level; e.g., if the probability on threat damage, injury, liability loss, or any other negative occurrence was noticed during the study period and also it was caused by the internal or external vulnerability, the researcher should address the above intervention at early stage and resolve the problems before conducting the research or else it may be avoided by the following preemptive actions: (1) Proper drug assignment, (2) Site accountability, (3) Dose management, etc., and (4) Migration—A systematic reduction in the extent of exposure to a risk or the likelihood of its occurrence, viz. EDC, randomization, drug inventory management, metric reporting, electronic reported patients outcomes, etc.

1.8 Clinical Trial

The clinical trial is a type of experimentation done on human subjects (prospective, behavioral research studies). In another terminology, the clinical research is an architectural design to preclude the answer to the specific questions about biomedical and behavioral interventions, including new treatment aspects (such as novel vaccines, drugs, dietary choices, and medical device). Medical or clinical research intervention triggered by various attributes to assess the treatment evaluation or comparison. As such being the case, the clinical research is a versatile research and will generate human life data sets on safety and efficacy on the human subjects; there is no provision to generate an overlapping information or data sets (datum) from single and multiple series of experimentations. The concept of clinical trial was described in the way back 1796–1797 by Edward Jenner; he has failed to use control group (naïve) to evaluate the efficacy and safety of the administered drug intervention. The first proper clinical trial was conducted by the Physician James Lind; he adopted study and naive group concept and also demonstrated on disease scurvy, which is caused by vitamin C deficiency, often to be terrible effects on the welfare crew of long distance ocean voyages. Different types of clinical designs were described in the later part of the chapters. The important types of clinical trial are described in the following section.

1.8.1 Treatment Trial

All clinical trial research was performed on people that are aimed at evaluating medical, surgical, and behavioral interventions. These are the primary ways that researchers find new research gap or outcome of the trial. In practical insight, the physicians have administered Abacavir 200 mg drug to the people living with HIV/AIDS for evaluating the efficacy or potency of the drug for the improvement of cluster differential cells or longer survival (CD_4 counts) at cohort of 6-month and 1-year period and so on. If the treatment is not being effective, the new drug has been administered by the caregivers to know the efficacy and safety of people living with HIV/AIDS (PLHIVs). Often many clinical trials adopted statistical model or DOE to describe the longevity and tolerability of novel regimen. As per the trail, the researcher has demonstrated various treatment aspects at single point considering study and naïve population. After completion of trail he has attempted to evaluate the drug on safety, tolerability, and efficacy; further he has derived the various aspects on the treatment; since the new treatment was more effective and/or was less harmful with lesser side effects than the standard one, this intervention is called parallel study design. A clinical trial may also look at how to make life better for people living with HIV/AIDS or cancer (life-threatening diseases). The clinical trial sometimes demonstrates the role of caregivers/support groups. Before the US Food and Drug Administration (FDA) approves a clinical trial to derive certain modalities in this move, the scientist performed various laboratory test and studies on animal subjects to test the potency of the drug (potential therapy). If these studies showed formidable and favorable results, then FDA shall give approval for intervention to be tested on the human subjects. Further, the treatment trial was done in all stages of the clinical trials (phase I, II, III, IV). The early phase of clinical trial aims to demonstrate the safety and side effects of a new treatment, later phases aim to evaluate the tolerability and comparative trail on time performance; if the new treatment works better than the current treatment, then the design was called as off time performance trail. For trial that compares two or more treatments, the people at the receiving part are put into a treatment group at random. In this above context, randomized trial is the best way to get reliable information about how well a new treatment works.

1.8.2 Prevention Trial

The prevention trial involves different tests to find a new way to prevent a particular medical condition, or if people are already exposed to the disease conditions, the researcher should prevent them from reoccurring. The emphasis of these studies might be done on the medicines, vitamins, and minerals or life style changes. Underlying the prevention trial as model for evidence, one expect to observe a reduction in incidence in a relatively short time frame. The duration of prevention may accord to 5 or 10 years of the RCT (Mantel and Haenszel 1959) strong evidence of Cox_2 inhibitors reducing genetic changes in the progression of normal colonic epithelium to adenomatous polyp and process and then observes a reduction in the incidence of cancer. The design consideration for such a trial, with polyp or invasive colon cancer as the endpoint, must reflect the temporal relation between exposure and onset of disease. As prevention trials screening of patient is a primary indicator and is more complex than some other interventions. The combination of early detection together with effective treatment underpins effective screening. The salient principles are summarized below:

1. The condition sought should be an important health problem.
2. There should be an accepted treatment for patient with recognized disease.
3. Facilities for diagnosis and treatment should be available.
4. There should be recognized latent or early symptomatic stage.
5. There should be suitable test or examination.
6. The test should be acceptable to the population.
7. The natural history of the condition, including development from latent to declared disease, should be adequately understood.
8. There should be an agreed policy on whom to treat as patients.

9. The cost of case findings should be economically balanced in relation to the possible expenditure on medical care as a whole.
10. Written consents obtained from the patients or caretakers.

1.8.3 Quality of Life Trial

Health quality of life (HQOL) is enormously increasing now a days and it has driven comfort zone for patients or subjects. The quality of life is a (QOL) very essential tool for each individual patient to know the overall well-beings. The trail finaloutcome is an endpoint in clinical research, particularity in diseases assessment and health condition of individual cases; e.g., Prognosis was assessed in 50 cases of colon cancer (metastatic stage); the QOL domain is the major concern or factor for the assessment of health status of colon cancer patients. However, the clinicians are still reluctant to accept quality of life (QOL) as an endpoint equivalent to more objective of interest. The endpoint considered by physician metastatic stage, level of independence, physical, clinical and psychological well-beings, etc. The above factor was assessed by the statistical modelling and image processing techniques; thus disease-free survival of patients with cancer was monitored by certain world health organisation (WHO) norms. The quality of life (QOL) mainly deals with practical insight and time-consuming issues such as randomization, selection of sample, collection of data sets, simulation, and informed consent obtained from the patients or caretakers. Finally, the characterization of study medication was done by the health care specialists while enrolling patients into the clinical trials, meanwhile the clinician or health care specialists have considered the assessment of "QOL" as an additional burden to national economy. Basavarajaiah studied quality of life (QOL) of people living with HIV/AIDS in Indian context. As per his findings, the QOL of people living with HIV/AIDS (PLHIVs) have received Zidovudine and Efaverenz (EFV) drugs that were administered by the physician for the period of 3 years; majority of the people living with HIV/AIDS patients were suffering from drug reaction and their overall quality life (QOL) was found to be worsened. From the past four decades we have seen that the development of a new technology in medicine was posed entirely on data sets; the driven data was obtained from PLHIVs self-reports and historical record; after the compilation of data sets, the results were found to be of longer duration for the treatment and have rigorously affected the quality life of PLHIVs, and will also affect the functional and mental status. Since health care specialists administered that drug based on the different attributes as a result of self-report of PLHIVs, the QOL assessment was made at defined time intervals. Especially, QOL is very useful tool for elucidating the effects of various drugs administered by the health care specialists (I and II Line highly active antiretraviral therapy-(HAART) treatment) and also it is very important health quality domain to describe the overall well-being of PLHIVs. The QOL has provided additional information to the researcher, health care specialist, and policy makers to know the HIV endpoint and policy intervention at right time.

1.8.4 Diagnostic Trial

Diagnostic trials usually include people who exhibit signs or symptoms of the diseases or conditions or stages of diseases that were studied during the study period. Therefore, the diagnostic trail solely refers to sign and symptoms; this trail was adopted to know or explore better tests or procedures for diagnosing a particular disease. The clinician relies heavily on diagnostic procedures to decide whether patients are exposed or not exposed to disease conditions. Despite these interventions, clinicians, patients, governments, third party payers, and the public take for granted such diagnostic tests being accurate, safe, and effective intervention. If robust study, the experimental design is the yardstick for randomization, the clinician or researcher may be seriously mislead by the study design to explore newer tools. In case the study will be conducted at population level, the diagnostic trail would be properly designed by the statistician before conducting the experimentation, since randamized control trail (RCT) are the gold stan-

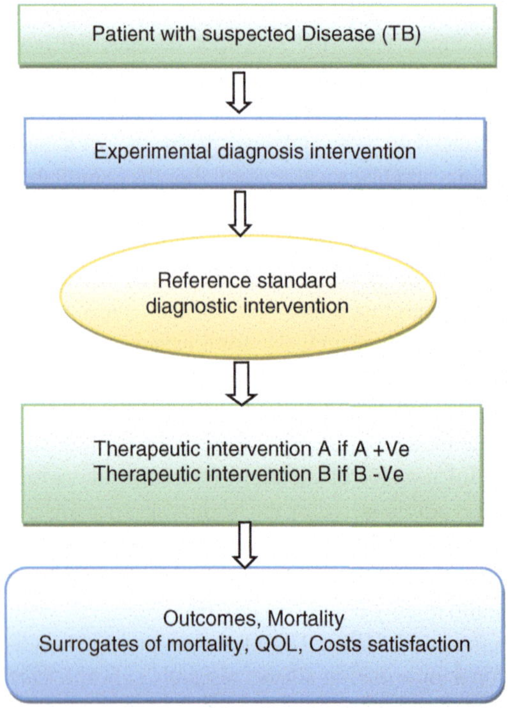

Fig. 1.3 Diagnostic procedure for Tuberculosis (TB) cases

dard for assessing the effectiveness and safety intervention in diagnostic trail (Pearson and Hartley 1970). While the study is conducted at sample level without RCT and nontherapeutic interventions, the design must ensure the level of significance and precision of experiment. For example, in case of surgical procedures and behavioral interventions to stay those of drugsadminstered by the clinician in number and also subjects were maintained good drug adherence, the RCT procedures are even rarer tool for diagnosis of the patient. Further, the clinician knowledge is very important until the experiment was completed; the reason for this intervention is lack of time, cost, and accuracy of the experimentation (Fig. 1.3).

1.9 Glossary

Subjects—The people who volunteer to take part in the study (sometimes called participants or patients)

Randomized—Subjects are randomly assigned to different groups

Open label—Subjects and researchers are all aware of the drug being given

Blind—The subjects do not know which group they are in, e.g., whether they are in the treatment group or the placebo group

Double blind—neither the researcher nor the subjects know to which group the subjects belong until it is revealed at the end of the study.

Placebo—A substance which does not contain the active ingredients of the experimental drug but looks the same (sometimes called a dummy drug)

Add-on—All subjects receive an existing treatment but some then receive the additional experimental drug while others do not or are given a placebo

Single center—The study carried out at one location

Multicenter—The study is carried out in several locations (i.e., different towns or even different countries)

1.10 Brief Concept of Study Design

Study design is defined as a framework of methods and techniques chosen by a researcher to pool various attributes or components of research in a well logical architectural manner, so that the research problem is efficiently handled by the researcher. Different study design has been classified based on the usage and accessibility (Fig. 1.4).

1.11 Experimental Study

An experimental study design is a prime method for measuring the potency of new drug therapies and other related interventions, including innovation of new drugs, etc. By the 1930s, the pharmaceutical industry has used spouse fact finding methods and other research interventions for solving the realistic problems of drug trail; they created study designs to rely upon the innovation

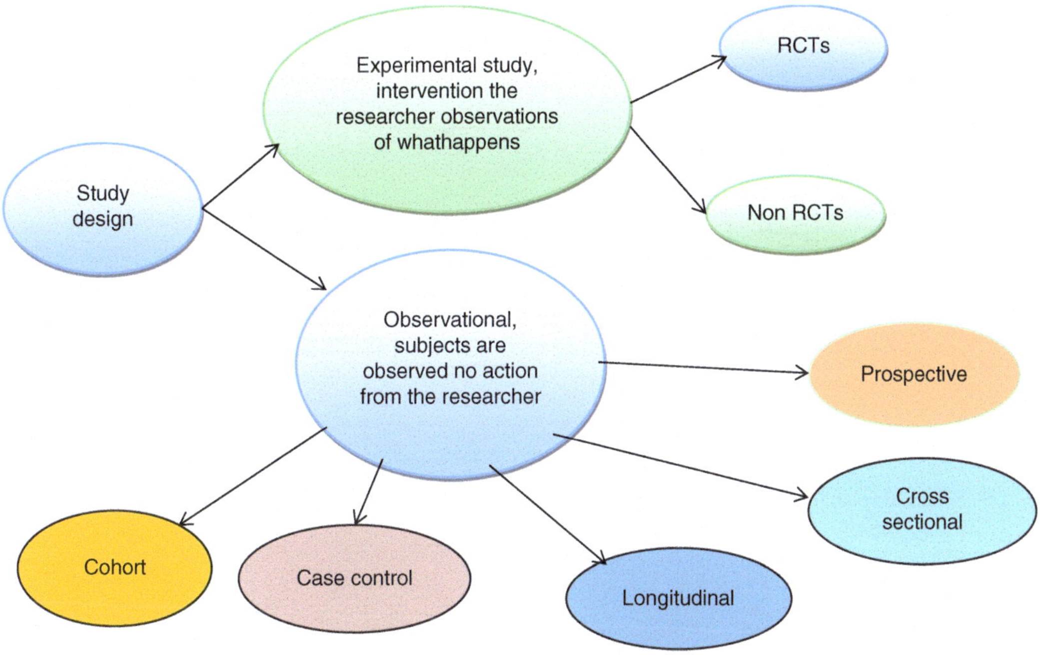

Fig. 1.4 Classification of study design

of new compounds, develop or to improve the production performance and tested the new drugs for treatment or therapeutic benefits. The full potential layout of the experimental methods in drug research was realized way back in the 1940s and 1950s besides with the growth and scientific knowledge of medical or industrial technology. In drug trail experimentation, the study was designed to compare full-blown benefits of the intervention on standard treatments when compared to no treatment (new drug therapy objective to know the cause and effect). The experimental study design will be performed prospectively, cross sectional, and subjects on case–control methods; each sample was selected from a study population, assigned to the various study groups and monitored in defined time interval to determine the final outcomes that concurred.

1.11.1 Randomized Controlled Trail (RCT)

It is the unique method of experimental design, and this is a trial in which subjects are randomly assigned to one of the two groups, viz. One (the experimental group) receiving the intervention, i.e., being tested, and the other (the comparison group or control) receiving an alternative (conventional) treatment. The two groups are then followed up to evaluate any significant differences between them in the final outcome. The results and subsequent analysis of the trail were used to assess the effectiveness of the intervention, which is to an extent a treatment, procedure, or service that benefits the patients more than harming. RCTs are the most stringent way of determining whether a cause and effect relation exists between the intervention and the outcome of the trail (Fig. 1.5).

1.11.2 Non-randomized Controlled Trail (RCT)

It is another type of comparative study with an intervention and control groups that were subjected; each group was approximated at the same time. The subjects were assigned on the various attributes, and treatment assignment has not been done by a random process; generally the subjects were selected based on the different

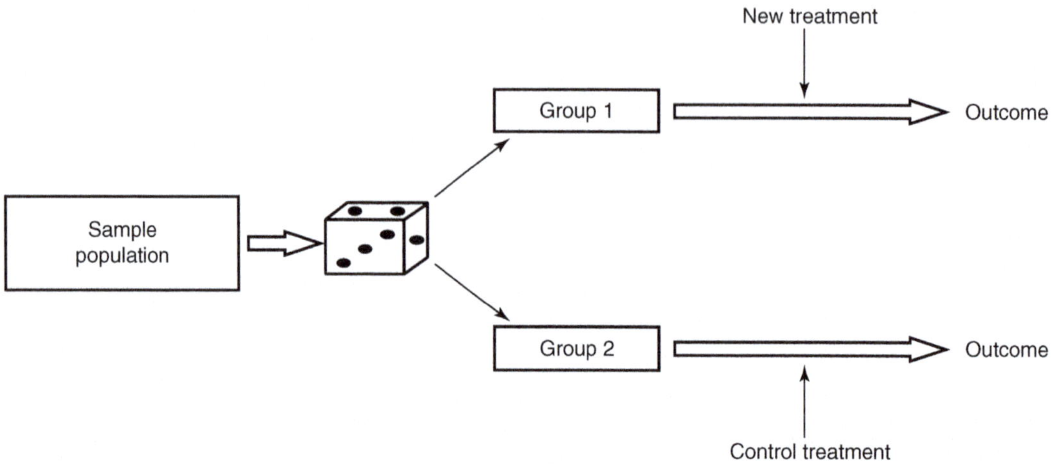

Fig. 1.5 Schematic plan for RCTs

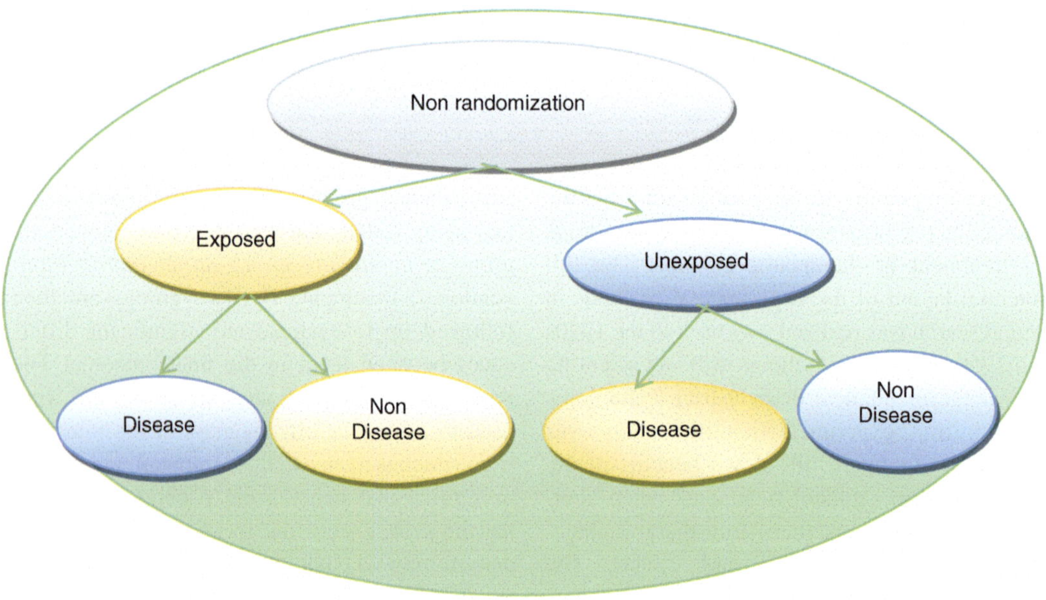

Fig. 1.6 Non-randomized controlled trail (RCT)

objectives of the interest. In this study design, researcher has benefited more for time saving; usually the assignments have not been done by a random process and there is no complexity of design at preliminary stage of the experimentation, one important limitation of non-RCT is that it consumes more time and is associated with lower precision for obtaining reliable results. Whereas, the researcher has been conjecture to make potential bias that the study groups were strictly comparable to other subjects (Price et al. 2008) (Fig. 1.6).

1.12 Randomization Study

The randomization is a prior method for the assignment of subject on human or animals, since randomization schemes were allocated to one of the two risk factors or more. The random mechanism will ensure to control standard error (SE) of the population or sample; each individual has been given an equal chance for selection. The randomization was done based on the pipette random number (four digits random number table); the number could be used for allocating individual treatments to one or more groups based on the appearance of last two digits is an example of such process. For further intervention, in studying the efficacy or potency of new drug relative to standard one, the names of patients could be entered sequentially, label by label in book, and a number from a table of pipette random number could be assigned to each label or line. However, the cases were assigned in even numbers and were allocated to the new medication and those with odd numbers to standard one. A more sophisticated procedure was used for allotment of treatment to the experimental unit, since the randomization procedure should be used for allocation of experimental subject to experimental unit. For example, the randomization will be done on human subject, the experimental unit requires an equal number of patients in the two arms of drug trail (groups), and each arm trail shall follow randomization procedures simultaneously. After the intervention of randomization process (RP), an incumbent study intervention was determined on a particular subject; treatment would be assigned in a particular group equally. However, the researcher must have encompass to control the standard error (SE). It is clearly depicted that there is no way to conduct a randomized study intervention without randomization mechanism, if the researcher must accept the assignment of the therapy or comparison of various groups on study subjects has been solely determined by the nature or by some ethical process. The primary aim of the randomization is to demonstrate the experimentation effectively and curb standard error (SE). The error will be aroused from sampling and nonsampling methods; the sampling error profusely bears high probability significance when compared to nonsampling error. Since the two groups will be similar in nature (assignment), the sampling error was found to be positively associated with precision and accuracy ($p < 0.001$). Truly, we have described on the research induction method, the standard error (SE) differences were seen in higher rate as compared with non-induction method (treatment between the two groups will be received on the odds number). Therefore, if the treatment has no effect, the distribution of the final outcome among the two groups would be quite similar in nature. Relayed on the succeeding sections, we described more extensive information and properties of the randomization. Further, the randomization addressed too many ménages, e.g., the researcher would like to consider randomized allocations canceled with achieved greater accuracy, randomized method were found to be consistently expressed with certain modalities of the research program. For example, randomization procedure will be used in systematic processes of drug trail experimentation; the allocations were chosen randomly without any bias, and such type of allocation would be varied with every second subject or all the subjects with more precision; e.g., an odd age of the respondent to one of the two groups is similar when compared to other group, and such processes may be seen in human and plant kingdom (varied in nature). Generally, these systematic processes will be extensively used in medical, agriculture, and engineering research; the rationality of randomization procedure is unique in nature and provide intuitive information to the research at the time of inception and interim research. Nevertheless, randomization procedure will always be triggered by the various risk factors, e.g., drawing the sampling from the finite population driven by breeding trail and drug trail experiment; every bit of information is equally important for the researcher for selecting the above said intervention. Therefore, the characteristics or attributes on which the allocation will be done on prior objectives of investigations (order of arrival, birth year, etc.) is related to the final outcome laid down by certain basic principles of the study objectives, so that its effects cannot be delineated from that of the treatment aspects. This practical method can be used for conduction research on exclusive setup, where there is no well-defined method that will be used to form the groups; the randomization process may clearly depict the overall novelty of the subjects which are driven by the various attributed data sets in addition to serious or emergency implications that are imposed from the research. The investigators may allocate the treatments often unconsciously; such being the case randomization procedure will be overlapped and obviously the standard error becomes more in that particular instances. Thus, finally an assignment of each subject to the treatment allocations is under the control of the researcher and randomization procedure; it is safest to use for preventing or controlling the standard error (SE).

1.12.1 Salient Properties of Randomization

1. Implied equal distribution of subject attributes in each group and thereby facilitates on causal conclusion or inference

On the realistic approach, the number of subjects will become very large in clinical research (Group A and Group B); researcher unlikely selects two groups, the two groups have showed a larger deviation with respect to multiple characteristics that has affected the final outcome under study hypothesis (whether or not these characteristics are known to the researchers). To intervene this above prior hypothesis, the researcher wishes to compare the A and B drug for reducing blood pressure in hypertensive patient; significantly he has assumed certain hypothetical statement about the population and sample, also he has determined that whether the drug A is more effective when compared with drug B for reducing blood pressure with hypertensive exposed population. Long ago, the researcher has identified the number of hypertensive patients (n_{11},n_{12}...n_{1k}) for study intervention. After determination of sampled number he has perceived the randomization techniques for the allocation of treatment groups in experimental subjects (allotment of intervention). The number of patients were considered as a replication and treatment subjects was drug A and B, respectively; consequently, the researcher will attempt to assess the response of randomization not only in precision but also he can evaluate drug trail total potency. The procedure for conducting randamized trail will be depends on many criteria viz, the researcher can assure them; each individual group is more likely to have similar distributions of the variables which can affect the blood pressure. Most precisely, the probability on confounded variables like risk factors, food habits, and physical exercises will have markable influence on blood pressure (BP). Since, the probability is very larger, the potential confounded variables will be differing extensively in the two groups by a large amount. If the drug A group is found to be significantly ($p < 0.01$) associated with lower average blood pressure than does the drug B group, the randomization will make it clear and unlikely distribute and show a marginal error (ME) differences in the resulted findings. The marginal error is caused by various risk factors rather than the trail. For example, we have seen that HIV Stavudine drug group was found to lower the blood pressure and it was highly associated with lower morbidity ($p < 0.01$) when compared with efaverenz (EFV) drug; the reason behind this is that the intervention is mainly subject to food habit, physical exercise, and mental status of the people living with HIV/AIDS.

1.12.2 Elimination of Selection Effects

Many studies vouchsafe the issues of randomization. If individuals or subjects are found to be eligible for randomized experimentation (randomized into groups), at an early stage or induction of experiment, the researcher is not to be assumed relative likelihood parameters; the bias was done during the randomization process. Sometimes an error aroused from the experimental materials or subjects from the non-randomized scheme. Further we argued that the undifferentiable standard errors were associated with selected subjects because for many confounding and non-confounding effects triggered the standard error. However, we need to take extra precautionary measures to prevent standard error of estimates for testing the null hypothesis (H_0) at reliable precision (α). For example, blood pressure (BP) will be estimated from the hypertensive patients considering with confounders and non-confounders, the logical paradigm of the researcher will be extrapolated confounding effect before measurement of blood pressure. Since the patient he or she would not be randomized properly, the error of estimates were found to be significantly subsidized at the time of treatment.

1.12.3 Preclude for Effective Statistical Inference

An overall scheme of randomization procedure will allow us to assign the various probabilities to observed subjective differences on the final outcome under the hypothetical assumption, that the treatments has not been correlated cause and effect relation and we can perform significance tests. If the significance level (alpha = 0.001, 0.05) was hedged on the sample or population level, if the sampled observation lead to fewer number, therefore an overall observed difference was very large, it is unlikely that the differences was driven due to chance factors and sampled data. The purpose of a statistical significance test is to rule out the random explanation at population and sample level. If it is used in contrary with randomization, it rules out every explanation rather than the experimental material, etc.

Note: When the number of cases in experimental study is small, the probability of imbalance on important background factor between the groups may be substantial. The prior measures should be taken at the design induction stage to reduce this probability and to decrease the random variation around the difference in outcome.

1.12.4 Subject Assignment-Randomly Assigned Subject to Treatment Groups

Each column shows the assignments for a block. For example, the third column for the second row (not counting headings) shows the group assignment of the second subject of the third block.

Subject no	Block 1	Block 2
1	B	A
2	A	A
3	B	B
4	B	B
5	C	B
6	C	B
7	B	C
8	A	C
9	C	B
10	A	B
11	A	C
12	A	C
13	B	A
14	C	A
15	A	C
16	C	A
17	C	A
18	B	C

The random number generator is seeded with the time of day, so it works differently each time you use it. Each subject is first assigned to a group none randomly. Then the assignment of each subject is swapped with the group assignment of randomly chosen subjects. This should suffix the entire process is repeated twice to make sure it is really random.

Randomly shuffle order of subjects within groups.

Sequence number	Group-1	Group-2
1	5	4
2	3	3
3	4	2
4	1	6
5	2	5
6	6	1

1.13 Non-randomization

If the treatment or intervention group is potentially harmful, it is generally unethical for a researcher to assign people to this treatment. An example study knows the effects of severe acute malnutrition (SAM) in children, where we simply cannot assign subjects to intolerable diets. Thus, we compare malnourished populations with those on adequate diets. Certain investigations require the implementation of treatment that may affect children's lives. In a democratic society non-randomized study implementation of such treatments is not always feasible. Consider with example, the question of fluorinated dating towns' water supply. Let us assume that the voters in any town or their elected representatives have the final say about whether the water supply is fluioriated. No experimenter can make this decision. We would then have a series of towns, some of which have elected fluorination and others which have not. An advantage of non-randomized study is that they usually cost less per subject and may not require the extensive planning and control that are needed for randomized studies. This makes non-randomized studies particularly attractive in the early stages of any research efforts. Preliminary estimates of the relative importance of many background variables and their variation may be developed at a reasonable cost. These data may be important for designing future randomized experiments. Non-randomized studies may be closer to real-life situations. To the extent that randomization differs from natural selection mechanisms, the conditions of a randomized study might be quite different from those in which the treatment would ordinarily be applied (Pocock 1983).

1.13.1 Cohort Study

The cohort study was undertaken to support the existence of association between suspected case and disease. The presence of relative risk factor (RF) is determined before the outcome occurs, e.g., a group of people who share common characteristics/attributes or experience with defined time period/interval (birth cohort, marriage cohort, exposure cohort, and synthetic cohort) (Fig. 1.7).

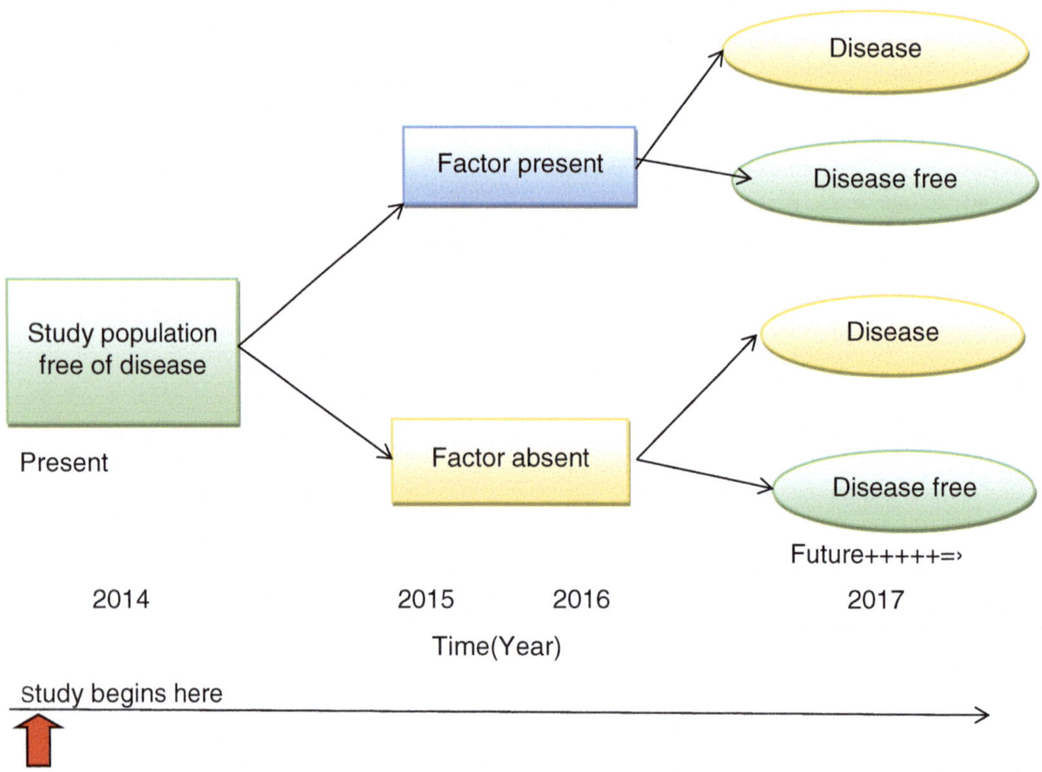

Fig. 1.7 Schematic flow diagram of cohort study

1.13.1.1 Elements of Cohort Study Design

The elements are very important indicators for conducting cohort study in biological, medical, and animal science entity. The following elements are being enlisted for the study purposes:

1. Selection of study subjects
2. Obtaining data sets on exposure
3. Selection of relative comparison groups
4. Follow-up record
5. Compilation and inference

1.13.2 Selection of Study Subjects

The selection of appropriate and suitable participant group plays a major role in the design of experiment before conducting experiment or research. The researcher should be selected and dealt with two basic principles, viz. the size of the population and duration, the researcher intend to select whole population or a representative of sample must be clear before onset of experiment conducted. A special group of population (occupation or professional group) exposure (person having exposure to same physical or chemical or biological) is carefully selected based on FDA regularity. Since the sample or population would be selected based on three criteria, viz. human research, autonomy, beneficence and Justice. However, autonomy is understood to mean that becoming a research subject is totally a legal act on human subjects. An individual must be solicited to the research work without coercive factors or even implied coercion rules. An individual must be fully informed and understood about what they are signing up for the document is mandatory criteria.

1.13.3 Carrying Out Research on Special Populations

It is an essential parameter to conduct drug trail at micro- and macrolevel on human subjects. The people who are willing to accept your research hypothesis and outcomes for one reason or another are vulnerable. This includes sample or population who react differently to drugs than adults and for whom too little research is carried out (Quinn et al. 2009). The beneficence that means an intention of the research is done for goodwill and human mankind. Broadly beneficence has been demonstrated in the risk analysis (SWOT) carried out by the researcher laid down by the FDA regularity guidelines. Of course many studies offer no personal benefit to the participants, and for these, great care must be taken that the risks are minimized.

1.13.4 Justice

The legal aspects and Justice relates to access the research of all relevant recruited populations specifically including with age, ethnicity, gender, preexisting conditions, etc. The FDA clearly envisages that the studies should try to include homogeneous ethnic groups and gender equality proportion in the community unless there is a good scientific reason not to subjects (for example, studying hypertension in African Americans). Issues that must be considered in justice determinations include Socioeconomic Status, Gender, Race, Age, existing medical conditions, etc. The following factors are to be considered for justice:

Vulnerable populations (as noted above)

6. Determining ability to consent
7. Ensuring understanding of protocol
8. Appropriate surrogate for consent
9. Coercive nature of relationship (prisoners)
10. The need to use such populations must be justified

1.13.5 Obtaining Data Sets on Exposure

The goal is to turn data into information, and information into insight, the driven data sets are very useful for compilation and draw effective conclusion and inference. The datum or clinical data sets are collected from different methods.

Personal interview

a) Review of records (dose of drug, radiation, type of sharing)
b) Medical examination/special test (BP, Serum Cholesterol)
c) Environmental survey (water, air, sanitation status)
d) By obtaining the data sets on exposure we can classify cohort exposed or unexposed and by the degree of exposure we can classify the cohort.

1.13.6 Selection of Comparison

Internal comparison—Only one cohort involved in the study process, researcher has compared the subjects internal sites based on the objective of the interest and also subclassification was done with internal components or variations (Ranganathan and Aggarwal 2018).

External comparison—More than one cohort in the study for the purpose of comparison (e.g., cohort of radiologist compared with ophthalmological intervention). Further HIV complications will be compared with same exposed population, etc.

Comparison with general population rate—The study group does not have relative comparative group (comparison group is available); researcher can compare the rates of study cohort with general population (Cancer rate of uranium miners with cancer in general population).

1.13.7 Follow-Up Record

In medical or clinical science today's health care system, follow-up action with patients is not only critical compliance and outcomes but also a proactive approach for reducing risk and improving safety and efficacy of the drug. According to WHO, the study protocol is one of the key factors for actively engaging to extrapolate the patients follow-up record; it is very important domain to demonstrate various health complications and treatment subjects. For example, we obtained data sets from the experimental area; the following methodological interventions were used for the compilation of research novelty (Ranganathan and Aggarwal 2019):

1. Mailed questionnaires, telephonic calls, personal interview
2. Periodical examination data collected from electronic data base
3. Reviewing records from past literature
4. Surveillance of death records
5. Follow-up is the most critical part of study subjects.

1.13.8 Compilation and Inference

The quality of a patient record (data base) or a patient data record system solemnly depends on its full-blown ability to fulfill the urge and requirements of those who use it. As discussed by many authors (Spilker 1996; Stel et al. 2007; Schlesselman 1982), effective data compilation inculcate the various aspects and novelty of the objective of the research gap. Many authors have cited the following parameters; it would be authenticated at the time of data compilation and data base management (DBMS), viz. (1) identify the customers; (2) understand their requirements; and (3) translate those requirements into functional characteristics of the system.

1.13.9 Strength of Cohort Study

1. Researcher can establish population-based incidence
2. Determine the accurate relative risk (risk ratio) estimation
3. Researcher will often examine a rare exposures
4. To establish cause and effect relationship between the variables
5. To know the magnitude of risk factors would be quantified
6. Demonstrate likelihoods of more than one disease related to single exposure

7. Statistically derived multiple outcomes in the interest of the study subjects (smoking, lung cancer COPD, Larynx cancer)

1.13.10 Weakness of Cohort Study Design

1. Cohort study Often to require larger sample size (population level)
2. It will take long time for completion on the study intervention
3. It is more expensive when compared to other studies
4. Facilitate laborious ethical issues, nonresponse, and migration and lost to follow-up (LOF)
5. Establish good environmental condition (envois) to change perception of the researcher

1.14 Cross-Sectional Study

In cross-sectional study, the data sets were obtained from a random sample of the population at one point of time. Thus, it gives a snapshot of an entire population. Since the classification was done based on the single survey approach at specific population or a random sample thereof, wherefore we determined the proportion of an individuals with heart disease in tertiary care hospitals, the entire risk data sets were collected at one point of time systematically. This is referred to as the prevalence of disease. We may also collect demographic and other information which would allow us to break down to estimation of prevalence by age, race, sex, socioeconomic status, geographic location or region, etc. Importantly a special case was also considered for the incidence estimation (cross-sectional data were obtained); when the exposure and diseases are dichotomous, data was collected systematically. Cross-sectional study can be represented by the following 2 × 2 contingency table.

Population	Disease	No disease	Total
Exposed	A	B	$(A + B)$
Unexposed	C	D	$(C + D)$
Total	$(A + C)$	$(B + D)$	GT

Prevalence of disease (%) $= \frac{A+C}{GT}$, Probability of exposure $= \frac{A+B}{GT}$, Prevalence of disease among exposed population $= \frac{A}{A+B}$, Prevalence of diseases among unexposed population $= \frac{C}{C+D}$. We can also assess the association between the exposure and disease using data from a cross-sectional study. One such measure is relative risk was estimated by the following ratio

$$\omega = \frac{\text{Prevalence of disease among exposed population}}{\text{Prevalence of disease among un exposed population}}$$

It is very easy to conclude that, the relative risk ω had following properties:

$\omega > 1 \Longrightarrow$ positive association, i.e., the exposed population has higher disease probability than the unexposed population.

$\omega = 1 \Longrightarrow$ no association, i.e., the exposed population has the same disease probability as the unexposed population.

$\omega < 1 \Longrightarrow$ negative association, i.e., the exposed population has lower disease probability than the unexposed population.

It is compared one at a time; different samples are used for formulation of cross-sectional study and also snap shot is given at one point in time. The intervention of cross-sectional study design has summarized statistically with different headings of analytical formula

$$\text{Specificity}\,(\%) = \frac{d}{b+d} \times 100$$

$$\text{Sensitivity}\,(\%) = \frac{a}{a+c} \times 100$$

$$\text{PPV} = \frac{b}{a+b};\ \text{NPV} = \frac{d}{c+d}$$

$$\text{PAF} = \frac{P(RR-1)}{1+P(RR-1)}$$

$$\text{Relative risk} = (a/a+b) \div (c/c+d)$$

$$\text{Risk difference}(\text{RD}) = (a/a+c) - (c/c+d)$$

$$\text{Number needed} = \left(\frac{1}{RD}\right);\ \text{NNG} = (\text{NNT}/P)$$

1.15 Longitudinal Study

In a longitudinal study, subjects are followed over time and single or multiple measurements of the variables of interest are obtained. Longitudinal epidemiological studies generally fall into two categories prospective, i.e., moving forward in time or retrospective, going backward in time. We will focus on the case where single measurement was taken. Longitudinal study has been described in many ways; the mechanism of longitudinal study has been changed at individual level and also we have taken as several points at a time.

The stress level of students is the best example for longitudinal study; Longitudinal cohort was conducted in the year 2008–2018; the stress that was found to be significantly affecting student's academic level (Fig. 1.8) clearly depicted that, the average stress level was very low (20th percentile) in 2008; stress level recorded at the end of the 2018 (41st percentile) was found to be statistically significant (chi square 56.33, $p < 0.01$). Stress scoring was obtained at 0–100 scale, i.e., 0–9 minimal score; 10–18 mild stress, 19–27 moderate stress, 28–36 severe stress.

1.16 Prospective Study

In a prospective study, a cohort of individuals are obtained who are free of a particular disease under the intervention and life data sets are collected on certain risk factors, i.e., children were exposed to contaminants with respect to age, sex, race, etc. The individuals are then followed over for some specified period of time, to determine whether they get the disease or not. The relationship between the probabilities of getting disease during certain time period is called as incidence of the disease.

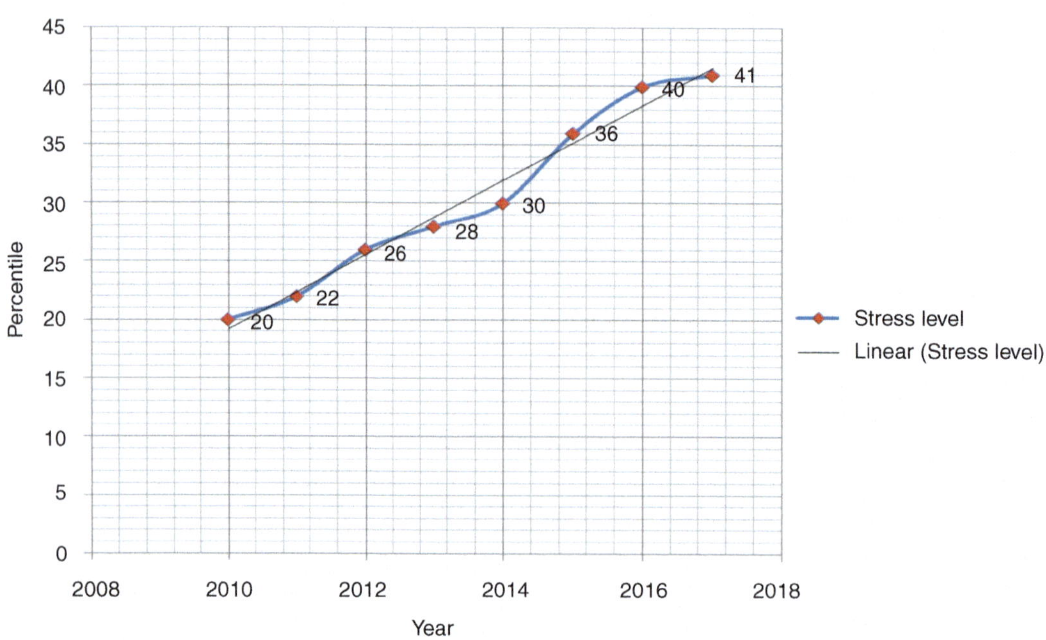

Fig. 1.8 Assessment of Stress level of Students at defined time intervals

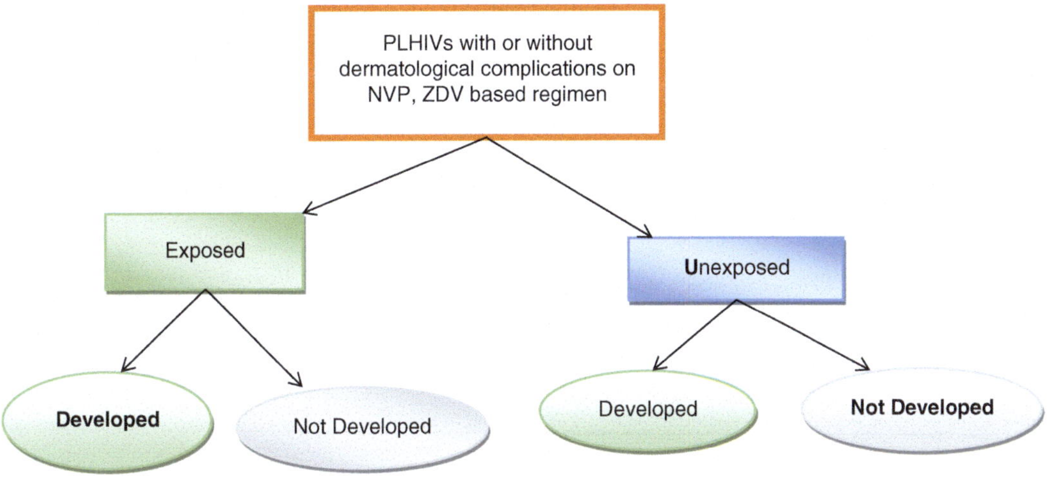

Fig. 1.9 Flow diagram of prospective design

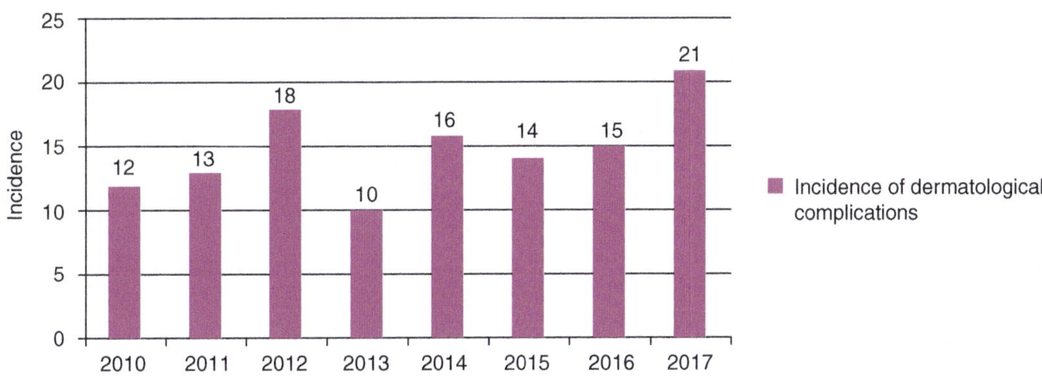

Fig. 1.10 Incidence of dermatological complications in HIV-infected patients

Prospectively we have compared the incidence of dermatological complications in HIV-infected patients during 2010–2017, (Fig. 1.9) and results revealed that the incidence of dermatological complications was significantly associated with treatment of NVP and Zidovudine based regimen $p < 0.01$ (Fig. 1.10).

1.17 Retrospective Study: Case-Control

It is very popular design and many epidemiological and RCT studies were conducted on cross sectional basis. In case of retrospective study: case–control study, individuals with disease (called cases) and the individuals without disease (called controls) were identified. Using records or questionnaires the investigators go back in time and ascertain the exposure status and risk factors from their past. Such data are used to estimate relative risk (Fig. 1.11).

Sensitivity (%) = $\frac{A+C}{GT}$, Specificity (%) = $\frac{A+B}{GT}$, Drug responded among cases = $\frac{A}{A+B}$, Drug not responded among cases = $\frac{C}{C+D}$, relative risk was estimated in accordance with the abovementioned formula.

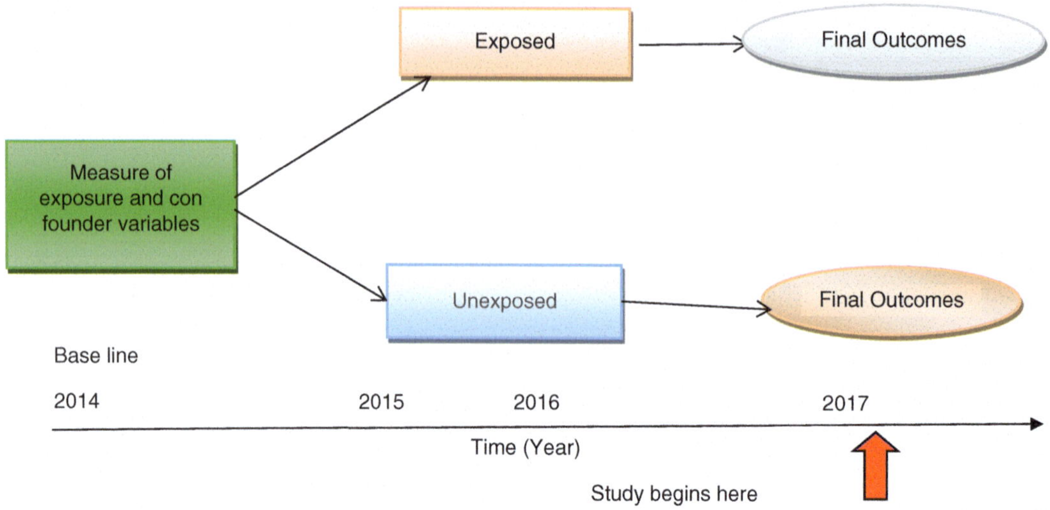

Fig. 1.11 Retrospective study: case–control

Drug response	Cases	Controls	Total
Responded	*A*	*B*	(*A* + *B*)
Not responded	*C*	*D*	(*C* + *D*)
Total	(*A* + *C*)	(*B* + *D*)	*GT*

1.18 Case-Control Study

In a case–control study, we assemble the groups of various subjects on the basis of their outcomes or events and then collect data on their historical exposure to the risk factors (RF). Schoenfeld and Richter (1982) conducted experimentation on case–control group; They preclude the case–control conducted on their own way; e.g., case–control study assembled fifty pedestrians fatally injured by motor vehicles to form the case group and 200 live pedestrians to form the control group, respectively. Schoenfeld and Richter (1982) were immensely interested to know the relation between various risk factors such as age, heavy drinking, and so on with pedestrian deaths, etc. To ensure comparability between the two groups, they forced comparability on background variables (other than the risk factors) that they thought related to both the outcome and the risk factors, by assigning to each case four controls with the same gender, found at the same accident site, at the same time of day, and on the same day of week of accident. That is, they "matched" cases and controls on four background variables (Schoenfeld and Richter 1982); they compared the age distribution on both groups, the blood alcohol content, and other risk factor distributions in the two groups. By using a case–control approach, the researcher/investigators are able to visualize the influence of several risk factors by means of a single study intervention. The cited study is rather economical since they are needed to assimilate the entire data sets on 250 recruited people; if they had used a cohort study, tens of thousands of people would have been needed to get a few pedestrian deaths in each risk factor group (Tuccinardi et al. 2019).

Population	With lung cancer	Without lung cancer
Smoker	*a*	*b*
Nonsmoker	*c*	*d*

The difference in lung cancer rates in the smoking and nonsmoking groups. The relative risks of developing lung cancer for smokers as compared to nonsmokers. The odds ratio, that is, the ratio of the odds of developing lung cancer in the smoking group to that of developing lung cancer in the nonsmoking group. The association of smoker and lung cancer has been determined based on the chi square goodness of fit and some descriptive statistics.

$$\text{Chi square} = \frac{n(ad - bc) * 2}{(a+c)(b+d)(a+b)(c+d)}$$

$$\text{CI95\%} = A \pm 1.96\sqrt{\frac{1}{A}+\frac{1}{B}+\frac{1}{C}+\frac{1}{D}}$$

$$\text{Sensitivity}\left(\%\right) = \frac{a}{a+c} \times 100$$

$$\text{Specificity}\left(\%\right) = \frac{d}{b+d} \times 100$$

$$\text{Over all incidence} = \frac{b}{a+b+c+d} \times 100$$

$$\text{Under incidence} = \frac{c}{a+b+c+d} \times 100$$

1.19 Open and Double-Blind Trials

Any novel regimen has ultimately been assessed in human's subjects, irrespective of how successful it is in the test-tube and in experimental animal groups. In other words, it must be subjected to clinical trial of some sort of research findings. A clinical trial is a planned experiment designed to assess the efficacy of treatment in human and comparing the outcomes from a group of selected patients treated with the test treatment (cases) with those observed in a comparable group of patients receiving a control treatment (placebo), where patients in both the groups are enrolled, treated, and follow-up action was taken over the same time and also under similar conditions. The groups were established through randomization techniques. The final outcome was measured (death or survival, a nonfatal clinical event, or a laboratory test). The period of observation being short or long depends upon the outcome measures. Thus, the basis of requirement of clinical trials is unbiased when comparing a tested treatment (e.g., new drug) with control group or placebo (intervention is Standard drug or Placebo or both).

1.20 Open Trial

Generally in clinical trials, the treatment a particular patient receiving is known both to the doctor and the patient. Such trials are known as Open trials. But open trials have some kind of merits, especially if the assessment parameter is subjective in nature (e.g., nausea), all the interventions of the therapy should be known by doctors and patients. In another example, the research worker wish to know the incidence of giddiness among tuberculosis patients (TB) treated with a regimen containing streptomycin and refamycin single dose. It is well known that the streptomycin cause giddiness. Hence, if we are assessing the physician has to know that a particular patient is being treated with streptomycin, he would be looking for the signs of giddiness and label a patient as having giddiness no sooner the patient complains of it. Thus, his assessment would be biased and subconsciously if a patient knows that he is being treated with streptomycin, he will be tempted to report giddiness may be a biased personal assessment. To avoid such biases, trials are often made in a double-blind process.

1.21 Double-Blind Trials

A clinical trial in which both the doctor and the patient are unaware of the treatment and the patient receives a therapy known as double-blind trial. Double-blind trials are easier. The drugs under trial (e.g., test drug and Control drug) should be made identical and similar in size, shape, color, taste, etc. Also, the dosage, time of administration, and duration of treatment should be the same for both the groups. This is very difficult to achieve for obtaining pertained clinical history. To overcome this problem we employed indigenous methods to conduct double-blind study. Here we indicated some of the problems we encountered while conducting double-blind trials using Traditional Remedies and we have also explained the methods adopted to overcome these problems in the later part of the chapter.

1.22 Some Special Problems of Double-Blind Trials

The cases and control drugs may be of different colors (e.g., Black and White), the dosages also differ from one individual group to another (e.g., 500 and 250 mg), the duration of treatment has not been the same (e.g., 40 and 12 days) or the time of administration will differ or dissimilar (e.g., before food and after food). Let us see how the researcher wishes to compile and overcome these above problems in designing double-blind trial.

1.23 Color Matching

Suppose the test drug is black in color while the Control group is white. We added a coloring agent (e.g., charcoal) to the white colored control drug and we prepared identical test and control drug capsules, so that the researcher can easily distinguish.

1.23.1 Dosage Matching

Another problem we enlisted from the snapshot techniques from clinical study is that, the test and Control group drugs are different dosages. For example, the dosage of the test drug is 500 mg while that of the Control drug is 250 mg. The Test drug is capsulated by using empty capsules of 500 mg capacity. We can use similar size capsules for the control drug by adding 250 mg of some substance (e.g., lactose) to 250 mg of control drug and capsulate the mixture using similar size empty capsules.

1.23.2 Duration Matching

Yet another problem we noticed during trail period is, viz. planning, the planning of double-blinded study had different duration of treatment for the test and Control drugs. The duration of treatment with the test drug is 40 days and that with the Control drug is 12 days. We had one method to overcome this problem, we shall pack the test drug for 12 days in pink bottle and remaining 28 days in white bottle. Similarly, pack the control drug for 12 days in pink bottle and a placebo for 28 days in white bottle. The researcher should instruct recruited study patients to consume the content of the pink bottle first and then that of the white bottle.

1.23.3 Time of Administration and Matching

The test drug has to be taken before food and the Control drug after food. To overcome this intervention, we shall follow the methodological flow chart given for the benefit of researcher, the simple chart is as follows.

Capsulate	Color of the capsule	Prescribe
Test drug	Green capsules	Green capsules before food and Red capsules after food
Control	Red capsules	
Placebo	Placebo in Green and in Red capsules	

We ensure that the test drug is taken before food and the Control drug is consumed after food, the matrix of the table is as follows

Timings	Test series	Control Series
Before food	Test drug (Green)	Placebo (Green)
After food	Placebo (Red)	Control drug (Red)

If the assessment parameter is based on the objective (e.g., blood sugar), an open trial is being undertaken at sample or population level, we have to carefully design the research at an early stage.

1.23.4 Data Collection and Quality Assurance

The decisions regarding the data collection, the schedule time and data-related formats are the most important in clinical trial. It will determine both the amount and quality of data generated in the trial. We must decide the schedule at which patients are seen, both before and after entry into the trial and on the specific items of information to be collected at each point of time. Once this is decided, then the process of development of data forms should be started. This should be done by a personnel who is experienced in dully format construction, familiar with methods of data collections and data processing on prospective basis.

A review of sample formats used in other trials should be considered for finalization, especially those from the trials with design and operating features similar to the one in question, useful in the development of study formats. The sample format would be obtained through published literature or by writing directly to the investigators. The data format was developed and tested before conducting clinical trails and if any suggestions made by experts should be corrected at an early stage (received from the clinic personnel and should be taken into account before finalizing them)

1.23.5 Baseline Visit

Every clinical trial must provide data collection at a minimum of two time points; at or just before randomization and the initiation of treatment to provide a baseline data, and at least once after randomization for collection of follow-up data sets.

Baseline visits

1. Determine patient's eligibility for enrollment.
2. Provide baseless data for assessing changes occurring after the treatment.
3. Explain the purpose of the study to the patient and to obtain consent for participation in the trial.
4. Issue the treatment assignment.

It is very useful to a researcher and a patient to make at least two visits to the clinic before enrollment. The report visits make it possible to replicate certain key baseline measurements. A time separation (days/weeks/months) between visits is necessary to Perform screening and diagnostic procedures for determining patient's eligibility criteria. Further, allow adequate time for clinical staff to evaluate the collected data evaluation on the patient before enrollment.

The required diagnostics and data collection procedures should be designed to minimize patient inconvenience and try to overcome the problems of expose to unnecessary risky procedures. Hence, whenever the event is feasible, the simplest procedures were employed to mitigate the risk and perform accordingly and also then prove ineligible who can be spared of risk oriented parameters, it is more complex and time-consuming procedures for evaluation of cases.

1.23.6 Follow-Up Visit

A follow-up visit is a prime parameter in clinical research; FUV is either required or non-required is the decision taken by the researcher based on the objective of interest. We study individual patients in specified clinic who enrolled into the trial that takes place after the randomization visit. The required visits should be scheduled to take place at specified time period after the randomization visit.

1.23.7 Follow-Up Visits Key Points

1. Carry out procedures specified in the study protocol, including treatment administration.
2. Evaluate the patient's response to treatment.
3. Assess patient adherence to the assigned treatment.
4. Collect data needed for evaluation of the treatments.
5. The time-table for required follow-up visits will be dictated by various factors, including.
6. Requirements for treatment administration and for assessing adherence to treatment.
7. Rate of occurrence of the outcome(s) of interest.
8. Patient health care needs.
9. Cost of patient visit.
10. Patient convenience considerations.

The schedule for required follow-up visits is designed to allow more frequent visits immediately after enrollment (e.g., weekly) to permit clinic personnel to initiate and administer the assigned treatment. The interval between visits may be increased to some maximum (e.g., monthly) and held constant thereafter. Follow-up visits that are made on an ad hoc basis because of special problems experienced by the study patients after enrollment are referred to as non-required follow-up visits. Provision should be made in the data format to distinguish between required and non-required follow-up visits. The differences among the treatment groups in the number of non-required follow-up visits can lead to biases in the diagnoses and reports of clinical events used to evaluate the study treatment.

1.23.8 Visit Time Limits

Ideally, the entire set of baseline and follow-up visits for a patient should be done at precise time points relative to time of randomization. However, such precision is generally not possible, nor is it necessary for most of the observations required in the typical clinical trial. The usual approach is to consider a visit and relevant data collection as valid, if the visit took place within a defined interval (e.g., a week).

1.23.9 Quality Assurance

The quality assurance is a fundamental parameter for assessing the clinical trial, which is applied to clinical trials at all levels, in any method or procedure for collecting, processing, or analyzing study data that amid to maintain or enhance their reliability or validity of study intervention. The following key information dealt with quality assurance:

1. Visual checking for completion of data set formats for noneligible responses and for unanswered or incorrectly answered items.
2. Re-capsulation of data as a check for errors in the data entry process.
3. Edit procedures to check on the accuracy of items on completed data formats.
4. Repeat the laboratory determination to check on reproducibility.

1.23.10 Visual Check

Visual check is the process in which a member of the research team (e.g., statistical assistant) shall scrutinize the complete data format for completeness and correctness. It is a good practice to have a visual check done immediately, after a format is fully completed, as far as possible, so that corrections, if any, can be carried out then and there. By this process illegibly answered items, unanswered or incorrectly answered items would be picked up and corrected simultaneously.

1.23.11 Data Entry and Verification

The ideal data intake system is one in which data is edited and entered on the day of generation, or very shortly afterwards. However, this is usually not practical. One viable approach is to complete the study format during patient examination and then enter the data as soon as possible. In multicentric trials, the completed format may be sent periodically (e.g., once a month) to data center for data entry and retrieval. Once the data in a completed format is fed to the computer, rekeying of the same by a different person to detect errors in the data entry process (known as data verification) and any Errors aroused from the collected data is removed from the unwanted data sets in the master chart.

1.23.12 Data Edit

The term data editing refers to the process of detecting, querying, and, when appropriate, correcting values in a data set that are invalid. The normal editing process involves a series of edit checks and edits queries. An edit check is an operation carried out on an item or series of items on a completed data form for the purpose of identifying possible errors. For instance, check of information supplied in one section (e.g., anemia) against another section (e.g., Hb) on the same form for inconsistencies and check for identifying items with values that exceed specified ranges (e.g., age range: 15–45). An edit query is a question generated form review of a completed form that concerns the accuracy or adequacy of some items of information and that requires someone at the generation site to review the information in order to respond to the query.

1.23.13 Replication

1. Replication of an observation or reading is often used as a check on the quality of the data obtained.
2. Comparison of two independent measurements, such as a lab test, to determine if the difference observed is outside a specified range.
3. Use two independent readings of ECG to identify items of disagreement for adjudication by a third reader.
4. Averaging two or more consecutive blood pressure readings made on a patient during a given clinic visit in order to have a more reliable estimate of the patient's true BP.

1.23.14 Quality Control of Lab Data

As bias can creep into lab investigations, it is important to devise systems in which there is not even scope for bias. For example, when smears are examined or urine tests are undertaken, it should be arranged such that the lab technicians are unaware of the source of individual specimens. Also standards in the lab should be monitored by slipping in controls without prior warning.

1.23.15 Site Visits

A site-visit may be defined "as a visit to a center in a trial made by personnel from outside that center for the purpose of assessing its performance." It may be done by just one person or group of people. The activities of the visiting team may include (a) meeting with the clinic director, (b) meeting with the members of the clinic staff, (c) observation of clinic personnel carrying out specific procedures, (d) check of forms, etc., at the clinic to assess whether they are up to date, (e) conversations with study patients as a check on the informed consent process, etc. To conclude, all efforts should be made to collect quality data so that valid conclusions may be drawn at the end of a clinical trial. No amount of sophisticated statistical methodology can compensate for poor quality data.

1.23.15.1 Patient Follow-Up

A process involving periodic contact with the patient after enrollment into the trial for the purpose of administering the assigned treatment, observing effects of treatment, modifying the course of treatment, and collecting data to evaluate the treatment.

1.23.15.2 Patient Close-Out

A process carried out to separate a patient from the trial, involving cessation of treatment and termination of regular follow-up.

1.23.15.3 Patient Post-trial Follow-Up

A process that involves patient follow-up after completion of the close-out stage of the trial and that is designed to yield information on the primary or a secondary outcome measure.

1.24 Management of Investigator and Patient Interest

1.24.1 During Follow-Up

The follow-up process requires a dedicated and committed staff to schedule and carry out the required examinations and a willing patient population. Both are needed if the trial is to succeed.

1.24.2 Investigator Interest

Investigator commitment to the trial and interest in its activities must be high throughout if it has to be succeeded. An interest will be easy to maintain in a short-term trial, where the initial enthusiasm that usually accompanies the start of any new activity is enough to carry it through the completion. However, even in such cases, spirits can sag before the data analyses have been done and the final document has been written. They can sag long before that point in long-term trials. The following list describes some of the aids that can be used to maintain investigator interest.

1. The periodic meetings of all study personnel.
2. Distribution of periodic progress reports on patient recruitment and follow-up, data collection and other performance characteristics of the trial for review by all members of the investigative group.
3. The periodic newsletters distributed to study personnel designed to inform them of study progress, protocol changes, and so forth.
4. Investigator participation in the analyses of results and in writing or presenting papers concerning the trial.
5. Preparation of reports and papers during the course of trial summarizing the design, organizational and operating features of the trial.
6. Execution of concurrent ancillary studies.
7. Certificates of appreciation from the sponsor.

The above list is written with long-term multicenter trials in mind. However, morale problems are not unique to multicenter trials. They can be just as great as in single-center trials also.

1.24.3 Patient Interest

A patient's interest in the trial and willingness to continue can be expected to diminish with the passage of time. The longer the period of follow-up, the greater is the need for measures to counteract the loss of interest and to improve participation levels. Factors and approaches that can help sustain patient's interest in the trial are given below.

The most important factor is the attitude of the clinical staff. The clinical staff should treat patients with courtesy and dignity and should develop interest in fulfilling their needs all-round the clock.

1. Clinic should be located in pleasant physical surroundings and in a secure environment.
2. Payment of clinic registration fees and costs for procedures required in the trial.
3. Special clinics in which patients are able to avoid the confusion and turmoil of a regular out-patient clinic.
4. Scheduled appointments designed to minimize waiting time.
5. Clinic hours designed for patient's convenience.
6. Written or telephone contacts between clinic visits.

1.24.4 Lost to Follow-Up

A lost to follow-up occurs whenever an item of information is required as part of a schedule follow-up examination, not obtained in the permissible time window. The lost to follow–up is due to

1. Failure of the clinical staff to complete an item on an otherwise properly completed data form.
2. Failure of the patient to agree to certain procedures during an examination.
3. Failure of the patient to return to the clinic for an examination within the time window specified for it.

Losses due to missed examinations or examinations that are not done within the specified time window, and hence are counted as missed, are more worrisome than the losses resulting from failure to complete specific items or procedures during an examination. Further, an occasional missed examination for a patient has different implications than a sequence of missed examinations. The longer the sequence, the greater the uncertainty regarding the outcome status of the patient.

Patients who are no longer able to or willing to return to the clinic for schedule follow-up examinations are dropouts. This declaration may be made by the patient (e.g., by announcing an intent to leave the study because of a lack of interest or because of a forthcoming move to another place) or by clinic staff. A clinic declaration should not be made until (1) clinic staff has made a concerted effort to locate the patient if he has disappeared, and to try to convince him to return to the clinic for a follow-up examination and (2) the patient has missed a specified number of follow-up clinic visits. The data of the patient's last completed follow-up examination should be used as the date of dropout. The patient should remain classified as a dropout until or unless he returns to the clinic for a follow-up examination.

1. The willingness of a patient to remain under active follow-up depends on variety of factors including the followings.
2. The amount of time and inconvenience involved in making follow-up visits to the clinic.
3. The importance of the procedures performed at follow-up visits from a health maintenance point of view. The potential health benefits associated with treatment versus potential risks.
4. The amount of trauma and discomfort produced by the study treatment or procedures performed.
5. The number and type of side effects associated with treatment.

Certain number of dropouts in long-term trials will occur simply because of patient relocations. Dropouts should be contacted at periodic intervals. The contacts may be made via home visits or by mail.

1.24.5 Close-Out of Patient Follow-Up

The process of disengaging patients from a trial may require much skill and care as the enrollment process. The following is a summary list of considerations that should be addressed in planning for close-out

1. Time Schedule.
2. Information to be collected.
3. Phased treatment disengagement (applicable to drug trials).
4. Nature of recommendations given to patients regarding subsequent treatment.
5. Method of ensuring proper transfer of patient care responsibilities to alternate clinic or physician when appropriate.
6. Ensuring patients have ample opportunity to make alternative arrangements for care and to have any questions answered regarding the trial and its outcome before separation.
7. Method of summarizing baseline and follow-up data for subsequent use by the patient's private physician.

The separation can be an emotional experience for both patients and clinical staff. It should be based on a detailed plan that has been constructed and reviewed before the start of close-out. The details of the separation should be discussed with patients well before separation occurs. Clinic staff must spend whatever time is necessary to answer questions and help to find suitable alternative sources of care. This is essential in any trial that has been providing patients routine medical care. Close-out provides an opportunity to assess the adequacy of the mask in masked trials. Theoretically, such checks could be made at various time-points throughout the trial. However, they are not usually carried out because of a desire to discourage speculation concerning the treatment assignments since the assessment involves asking the masked individuals to state a guess regarding treatment assignment. A key consideration at close-out has to be done with whether to carry out added data collection on patients as they are separated from the trial. The wisdom of making such provisions depends on the importance of the data generated in relation to the aims of the trial. Results were obtained on the tests or procedures for which there are no corresponding base line values and is limited for the use of making treatment comparisons. The method of terminating therapy in masked drug trials must be given special consideration. A dosage step-down scheme may be necessary, if an abrupt cessation of one or more of the drugs is considered unsafe. In addition, a patient wish to know the treatment he was on. Hence, study physicians must be supplied with treatment codes well in advance of close-out visits. Patients should be told at close-outs if the clinic plans to keep in touch with them and, if so, then the reason for doing so has to be told and the way in which a contact will be maintained (e.g., via mail, telephone, or home visits). They may be asked to sign a consent authorizing the contacts and to provide updated location information if contacts are planned. In fact, it is a good idea to alert patients to the possibility of future contacts and obtain consents from them even if the subsequent contacts are not planned.

1.25 Post-trial Patient Follow-Up

There should be a sound rationale for any post-trial follow-up involving direct patient contact. The prime motivation for most post-trial follow-ups stems from a desire to extend the period of observation for death or some other nonfatal event. Another reason may be to observe patients for a disease or condition that may be caused or aggravated by treatments administered during the trial. The usefulness of the information obtained depends on the completeness of the follow-up and the nature of intervening treatments administered after close-out. Interpretation of the results will be easiest if patients have not been exposed to any additional treatment after separation from the trial. It will be problematic if they have been exposed to do so.

1.25.1 Design of Proformae

The design of proformae is the translation of a protocol into the form of a well-defined, unambiguous questions, acceptable to all those associated with the conduct of the study. If the questions are incomplete or ill-conceived or inadequately answered, no statistical analysis can compensate for the resulting defects and produce the answers that the investigator had hoped to get. Hence, it is worth spending considerable time on this aspect of proformae design as better the design, easier and efficient will be the subsequent analysis.

1.25.2 Steps in Proformae Design

1. Keep the study objectives in mind.
2. Make a detailed list of information needed and the study variables.
3. Decide on the main subdivisions of information needed and select a logical order of types of information.
4. For each piece of information or variable in each subdivision as decided earlier, write a question as it will be conversed.
5. Assess each and every question to ensure that it is simple, clear, short, unambiguous, and whether it can be answered well.
6. Do pre-testing and revise, if need be.

Assessment of each question to verify whether it is clear, short, unambiguous, simple, or whether it could be answered well has to be done rigorously. This can be done by posing the following questions to each and every question.

1. What will I discover from the answer?
2. Will the answer be meaningful?
3. Will the answer be relevant?
4. Can I leave it out completely?

These questions make sure that we will fetch the required answer and take care of the content part of the question.

The following two questions, namely,

1. Is the question unambiguous?
2. Are the words simple?

Will help us in framing the questions properly, i.e., the wording aspect of the question.

Then we must decide whether to have an open-ended question or a closed (pre-coded) question (i.e., Form). This depends on the situation and also on the nature of variables. Finally, the logical positioning of the questions in the proformae is to be determined, i.e., ordering of the questions has to be done.

1.25.3 Question Content

In our anxiety we can include many questions. We should not add irrelevant questions in our proformae as irrelevant questions are costly, since it uses time which is precious and may reduce efficiency. Responders get tired and bored. Also, the investigators sense the irrelevant questions and will ask them carelessly. This will have a carry-over effect to subsequent more important questions. Next aspect is even if it is relevant, is it possible to collect the required information preciously. The responder may not remember the answer, as memory may fade away with the passage of time or in some instances the responder may not reveal the correct answer due to fear or prestige. This is especially true in the case of sensitive issues like income, history of abortions, etc., as questions on these issues or aspects may arouse fear, emotions, etc.

1.25.4 Question Wording

The wording should be sufficiently specific and the language should be simple, i.e., they must be very specific to the point (crystal clear). We must avoid ambiguity and also vagueness and finally we must not lead the respondent. This is most important. Therefore, we must avoid putting leading questions which will imply spontaneous approval/disapproval of the issue being investigated.

1.25.5 Open-Ended Question

Advantages

1. Allow the respondent to give more complete answer.
2. Will not constrain the respondent to precise responses, and thus we may obtain answers that were not anticipated at all and had not been studied earlier.
3. Most suitable for exploratory studies.

Disadvantages

1. Interviews may be too long and difficult to keep to point.
2. More difficult to code and analyze responses as we may get a wide variety of responses.
3. The respondent may forget to mention the important points.

Closed question-Advantages

1. Responses can be obtained and registered quickly.
2. Respondent is helped to concentrate on important issues/points.
3. As response is structured, the data processing and analysis are made easy.
4. Grading of subjective response can be done.

Disadvantages

1. Options are limited by previous knowledge.
2. There is a tendency by the respondent to select the middle option/alternative of a list of options/alternatives given.
3. The interviewer may lead the respondent with the alternatives provided in the proformae.
4. May be less useful for exploratory studies.

1.25.6 Question Order

It is important that opening questions should be easy to gain the confidence of the respondent and highly sensitive questions should be left as late as possible in case they cause refusals. The sequence of questions to specific answers often seems to be appropriate. We must set a logical sequence in ordering the questions.

1.25.7 Number of Questions

Attention should be given to this aspect. Obviously, the number of questions need to be asked vary widely with circumstances. But the designer of the proformae should ask for himself the following three questions for each question to be included in the proformae:

- Is this question very essential?
- Can I obtain a useful answer to it?
- Can I analyze them usefully at the end?

Such a self-discipline is likely to reduce the size of any proformae. But in our desire to reduce the size of the proformae, we should not arbitrarily cut short the number of questions. We must strike a balance.

1.25.8 Number of Proformae

Consider a clinical trial in which patients are to be treated for a period of 1 year with monthly follow-ups. Can we just have a single form to collect the data for the entire 1 year period. No, as it is operationally convenient and also efficient to have several forms for each patient. Also, multiple forms per patient ensure compliance of patients. Errors can be detected by periodical scrutiny of the data collected and necessary mid-course corrections, if need be, can be taken. Also, we can have an up-to-date, database which will facilitate quick interim analysis.

1.25.9 Practical Aspects—Document Lay Out

(a) The items should not be crowded.
(b) No more than one question in a line.
(c) Adequate space should be provided for open-ended questions.
(d) Provide boxes for coding open-ended questions.
(e) The unit of measurement should be specified along with each item.
(f) In case of questions with many alternatives, provide a box next to each alternative to mark the answer with a tick ( )
(g) Skip instructions should depend only on the answer to the question immediately preceding the instruction.
(h) Provide a separate box for coding each numeral.
(i) Size of each box for recording numbers should be sufficiently large.
(j) Boxes should be arranged serially and vertically.
(k) Layout should permit the data entry personnel to proceed in an orderly fashion.
(l) The use of capitals, letters of different types, italics and lines of varying thickness that appeals to the eye makes the schedule agreeable as well as easily understood.

Allot a running serial number of each item to be filled-up

1.25.10 Physical Characteristics

1. Use good quality and standard size paper.
2. Use clear fonts in printing.
3. Print on one side only.
4. As few sheets as possible.

1.26 Preparation of Protocol

A protocol may be described as a document that sets out, in great details, the aims and objective of the investigation, the design of the experiment including the sample size, and the procedures involved in the execution. It serves many purposes. First of all, it compels the investigator to set out in writing all the relevant facts and procedures. There is, fortunately, a healthy fear in most minds for putting things down in writing, and consequently the process of writing will usually ensure that the investigator has spent a reasonable amount of time in the planning of the study, in consultation with other experts including a statistician. Secondly, in situations where many persons are involved in investigations, for example, a cooperative study involving a number of centers, a written protocol is the most satisfactory way of ensuring that all the coinvestigators understand the purpose of the study and the method of conducting it. Finally, for individuals or institutions seeking financial support for their investigations, a good protocol can go a long way in influencing the decision of technical committees that allot funds for various projects. The ingredients of a comprehensive and satisfactory protocol are given below.

1.27 Background or Preamble

To begin with, a brief explanation regarding the background to the proposed investigation should be given. This must make appropriate references to previous work on the subject by the investigator as well as by others, and might also indicate the value of the proposed investigation.

1.28 Clear Statement of the Aims

Often, investigations have more than one aim. It is therefore important to mention clearly about the various aims, and also indicate their relative importance as there can sometimes be a clash of interests. For instance, if the proposed investigation is a controlled clinical trial to investigate a new regimen, the main aim of the investigation could be to determine the therapeutic efficacy of the new regimen in comparison with a standard regimen, and evaluation of toxicity and acceptability could be subsidiary objectives. To take another example, the main aim of a laboratory study could be to determine the effect of storage of sputum specimens at room temperature on the viability of the tubercle bacilli in them; a subsidiary objective could be to examine the implications on the susceptibility of the bacilli to anti-tuberculosis drugs.

1.29 Population

Next, the population for study must be clearly defined. This could be (a) all residents in a specified geographic area,(b) all patients with a particular disease in a specified group of hospitals, (c) all women in the child-bearing age in a specified urban community, (d) all diagnostic specimens of sputum received in a laboratory over a specified period of time, etc. In order to avoid ambiguity and with a view of making meaningful generalizations, terms like residents, disease, child-bearing age, and diagnostic should be defined. One of the studies at our center is an investigation of the efficacy of isoniazid chemoprophylaxis in close family contacts of tuberculosis patients. The words "close family contacts" and "tuberculosis patients" may mean different things to different people. The former meant "persons related to the patient by blood or marriage and who have been living in the same house and using the same kitchen as the patient for at least the 3 months immediately preceding the start of treatment for the patient," and the latter meant "persons with radiographic and bacteriological evidence of pulmonary tuberculosis."

1.30 Sampling Procedure

For economy in time, labor, and money, investigations are usually undertaken on a sample of the total defined population. The technique adopted for selecting the sample is extremely important and usually has a great bearing on the confidence that can be placed on the findings of the investigation. For one thing, the procedure must be free of bias. There are several methods of sampling from a population, for instance, purposive sampling, simple random sampling, stratified random sampling, multistage sampling, and cluster sampling. These methods vary considerably in their complexity and efficiency and much thought must therefore be given to the subject of selecting the optimal sampling design.

1.31 Number of Subjects

The number of subjects to be included in an investigation must always be determined in consultation with a statistician and depends on various assumptions. For instance, in a study of vaccine, the assumptions made could be that the incidence of disease in non-vaccinated subject would be 10% and that the vaccine would be at least 50% effective. While fixing the sample size, allowances must be made for loss of information due to various causes, for instance, absconding by patients in clinical trials and nonresponse by subjects in surveys. It must be emphasized that if the proportion of such losses is large, the sample may no longer be representative.

1.31.1 Specification of Investigations to Be Undertaken

The nature of investigations that are to be undertaken must be specified clearly, so that some degree of uniformity is preserved during the study. The techniques employed for laboratory tests or clinical assessments must be described extensively, unless they are standard methods.

1.31.2 Conduct of the Investigation

For investigations that involve one-time assessments, the main problem is one of "nonresponse." The procedures to be employed for tackling this problem should be included in the protocol. For instance, a revisit may be made at a convenient time to the respondent. For investigations that involve repeated observations on subjects (e.g., guinea-pigs, patients, contacts) over a period of time, the assessments and the periods at which they are to be undertaken must be specified. For example, in a diabetes trial blood sugar and HbA_{1c} estimations may be made monthly and once in 3 months, respectively. Also, the full details of management and methods for coping with non-cooperation during the course of the study must be spelt out. Finally, the circumstances under which a subject can be withdrawn from the study should also be stated (e.g., a diabetes trial patient may be withdrawn from the trial if the postprandial blood sugar is above 300 mg, at any time during the trial treatment period, and confirmed by another assessment made 1 week later).

1.31.3 Formats

A copy of forms that are proposed to be used in the study must be included in the protocol, since the mode of recording the data is as important as that of collecting it. In the case of a clinical trial, copy of the consent form should also be enclosed.

1.31.4 Planned Analyses

Although it may not always be necessary, it would nevertheless be valuable to state the various analyses contemplated on the data to be collected. This would have the advantage that analyses which are considered important at the time of planning the study are not forgotten at a later date, especially in studies of chronic diseases which are spread over several years. In the diabetes trial for instance, the criteria for the control of diabetes may be stated as "fasting blood sugar less than 120 mg%, postprandial blood sugar less than 180 mg%, and HbA_{1c} less than 8.5%."

1.31.5 Remarks

A protocol must be treated as a sacrosanct document, departures from which are not permissible. This being the case, it would be prudent to consider initially itself all aspects of the study, including possible complications that may arise later. Such a step would usually ensure that he study is completed strictly in accordance with the initial protocol. Despite the greatest care, however, situations may sometimes arise in which a departure from the protocol may become necessary, probably due to ethical considerations or due to some new facts that have come to light since the time the protocol was prepared. In such situations the original protocol should be amended and copies of the amendment circulated to all those connected with the study.

1.32 Need for Control

What is a "control" treatment?

The drug, device, test, or procedure administered in a clinical trial that serves as the standard against which "test treatments" are evaluated is called a "control treatment." The control treatment may consist of a placebo, sham procedure, a standard treatment regimen, or no treatment of any kind, depending on the study design. The table below gives remarkable examples of entirely inaccurate conclusions that an investigator might draw in the absence of a control group of patients.

Cured or improved	Anti-histamine	68% of 579
Common cold	Placebo	65% of 577
Relapse rate	3 years treatment	1% of 77
Pulmonary tuberculosis	2 years treatment	0% of 74
Incidence of giddiness	Streptomycin + INH PAS + INH	35% of 78 11% of 70

Considering the first example, which deals with the common cold, a British Medical Research Council trial showed that 68% of patients receiving an anti-histamine preparation had a complete cure or improvement in their condition within 2 days, a highly encouraging finding for the use of anti-histamines. However, practically the same proportion, namely 65%, of the placebo patients also had a cure or improvement within 2 days. In reality, therefore, the antihistamine had no effect, and the improvement noted was probably the natural course of the disease. The next example is from the Tuberculosis Research Centre, Madras, and refers to relapse rates in patients with bacteriological quiescent tuberculosis. In patients who received chemotherapy for 3 years, the total relapse rate in the third, fourth, and fifth years was only 1.0%. This shows low proportion; it could allow the recommendation that 3 years of chemotherapy is necessary to keep the relapse rate low (Indeed, similar recommendations have been made in the literature on the basis of findings like above). Such a recommendation is very necessary; however, in patients who received only 2 years of chemotherapy, the relapse rate was 0%. The third example is also from the Tuberculosis Research Centre, Madras, and gives the incidence of giddiness among patients while on treatment. The incidence of giddiness was 35% in 78 patients who were treated with streptomycin and isoniazid compared to 11% in 70 patients who were treated with PAS and isoniazid. In the absence of the second group (i.e., PAS + INH), one may have concluded that the incidence due to streptomycin was 35%, but by considering the finding in the second group, the incidence attributable to streptomycin is more accurately estimated (35 − 11% = 24%). After accepting the need for a control group receiving standard treatment, many researchers are still reluctant to assign patients randomly to new or standard treatment. Such reluctance often stems from the investigator's desire to enter all future patients on the new treatment because of his wish to gain as much experience of it as possible and his inclination to believe it is better anyway. The most common way of avoiding randomization is to compare retrospectively one's current patients on the new treatment with previous patients who had received standard treatment, this latter group of patients being commonly known as historical controls. Such an approach has one major flaw: how can one ensure that the comparison is fair. That is, if the treatment and control groups differ with respect to any feature other than the treatment itself, how can one guarantee that any apparent improvement in patient response is actually due to the new treatment. Due to the "potential incompatibility," we divided the group on the basis of two broader areas, patient selection and the experimental environment, each of which may give rise to several sources of biasness.

1.32.1 Patient Selection

In historical control group it is very less likely to have clearly defined criteria for patient inclusion, since such patients on standard treatment were not known to be in the clinical trial when their treatment began. Since historical controls were recruited earlier and possibly from a different source, there may be a change in the type of patient available for selection.

There is a danger that the investigator may be more restrictive, either deliberately or subconsciously in his choice of patients for a new treatment.

1.32.2 Experimental Environment

An experimental environment has included the following rationality:

1. Quality of recorded data for historical controls may be inferior.
2. The criteria of response may differ between the two groups of patients.
3. Ancillary patient care may improve on the new treatment.

The study was conducted on the historical controls that would be exaggerate the value of a new treatment, most satisfactory way out of these dangers is to have a control group that is concurrent, i.e., a control based on data collected over the same period of time as that used to generate all other data in the study.

Even when the investigators have agreed to conduct a prospective clinical trial in which future patients are to be assigned to the various treatments, there may still be some reservations about whether such assignments should be categorized based on a random mechanism. Instead, it was decided to use some predetermined systematic methods (assign patient according to date of birth, date of presentation, etc.) or worse still degree of judgment by investigator and or patient may be adopted. Both these methods could introduce considerable bias. For instance, a trial of anti-coagulant therapy for myocardial infarction whereby patients admitted on odd days of the month received anti-coagulant and patients admitted on even days did not. There were 589 treated and 442 control patients, a sizeable imbalance indicating a preference towards admitting patients onto anti-coagulant. In general, randomized controlled trials, with concurrent controls, are an essential tool for testing the efficacy of therapeutic innovations. The proper use of randomization guarantees that there is no bias in the selection of patients for the different treatments and also helps us to considerably reduce the risk of differences in experimental environment. Randomized allocation is not difficult to implement and enables trial conclusions to be more believable than other forms of treatment allocation.

1.33 Randomization in Clinical Trails

In a controlled trial, the mode of deciding the regimen for any individual patient must not only be free of bias, but also appear to be free of bias. One can readily see the danger in entrusting the choice of the treatment for individual patients to the clinician. To take a simple example, if patients were to be treated at home or in sanatorium at the clinician's discretion, it is almost certain that the more ill patients would tend to be admitted to sanatorium while the less ill patients would be treated at home. Another undesirable procedure is the method of alternation, whereby the first patient is prescribed treatment A, the second treatment B, the third treatment A, the fourth treatment B, and so on. A variant of this is to admit all patients on odd days to treatment A and those on even days to treatment B. Such procedures are, however, capable of bias because the order in which patients are admitted to a study can be manipulated without much difficulty. The best protection against all accusations of bias is random allocation. Apart from validating statistical tests of significance, the purpose of random allocation is to avoid personal preferences in the choice of treatment for individual patients. It must be emphasized that these personal preferences can be conscious or, more often, subconscious. The great advantage of random allocation is that it is highly likely to result in the construction of two groups which are similar in all aspects. The baseline characteristics of the test treated and control group must be more or less similar in order to provide a valid basis for comparison. The ideal experimental model for comparing two treatments is one in which the base line characteristics of the two study groups are identical in all aspects. This requires a homogeneous group of patients who are arbitrarily assigned to the test and control treatments. Once an eligible patient has agreed to be enrolled, it is essential that the treatment assignment be made free of influence from both the patient and clinic personnel so as to avoid selection bias. The general conditions that should be satisfied in order to have a sound allocation scheme are detailed below

1. Assignment remains masked to the patient, physician, and all other clinic personal until it is needed for initiation of treatment.
2. Future assignments cannot be predicted from past assignments.
3. The order of allocations is reproducible.
4. Methods of generation and administration of the schedule are documented.
5. The process used for generation has known mathematical properties.
6. Departures from the established sequence of assignments can be detected.

1.33.1 Patient Registration

In practice, it is advisable to adopt a more formal, well-defined routine for registering and randomizing patients. For each patient who might be considered suitable for inclusion in a clinical trial, the following formal sequence of events should take place

1.33.2 Patient Recruitment

The identification of appropriate patients may seem an obvious step, but it is important to ensure that the patients entered in the trial are representative of all patients with the disease under investigation so that the trial's conclusion can be readily applied to the entire population of such patients. The clinician should avoid being unduly selective in his choice of patients.

1.33.3 Checking Eligibility

The eligibility of each possible patient should be checked. The clinician should go through the list of eligibility criteria in the protocol and exclude the patient automatically if any criterion is not fulfilled. Of course, some eligible patients may slip through the net only to be identified later and such patients may be excluded from the analysis. A more serious problem is the ineligible patient who goes undetected due to poor supervision.

1.33.4 Agreement to Randomize

It is vital to ensure that the clinician should agree to accept any of the random treatment assignments before he formally enters the patients into the trial. Otherwise, one may have the problem that after the treatment is assigned the clinician opts to use some other treatment instead. Such action is totally unacceptable and could seriously invalidate the trial. It is preferable that each clinician must be willing to enter and randomize all his eligible patients, but in practice one must allow a clinician to exclude the occasional patient he considers unsuitable.

1.33.5 Patient Consent

In general, there is an ethical need to inform each patient about his entry into a clinical trial and obtain his agreement before proceeding further. In the United States it is a legal requirement that fully informed patient consent should be obtained in writing prior to randomization whereas in some countries there is a more informal attitude to patient consent.

1.33.6 Formal Entry to Trial

It is essential that each patient entering the trial be formally identified before random assignment of treatment is made. This can be achieved by having the patient's name, and possibly a few other details such as date of birth and date of entry. There is a value in keeping a separate log of eligible patients who are not entered into the trial, since this provides insight into the representativeness of patients who are in the trial.

1.34 Random Treatment Assignment

Only after the above steps have been successfully completed does the doctor learn which treatment the patient has been assigned. In most clinical trials, a randomization list of consecutive random treatment assignments has been prepared in advance. One essential feature is that the clinician does not know the order of this list and is unable to predict what the next assignment will be. To achieve this aim the list should be prepared by an independent person, possibly a statistician.

The randomization list could be transferred to a sequence of sealed envelopes each containing the name of the allotted treatment on a card. The clinician opens the envelope in a sequence when the patient has formally entered into the trial. Sealed envelopes are well-tried methods of randomization but are not totally fool proof. If the trial is a double-blind evaluation of drug therapy, then the pharmacist preparing the drugs should be involved. He need to be given the randomization list in order to produce a corresponding sequence of drug packets containing the appropriate treatments but identical in appearance, etc. These packets are then presented to the clinician and the treatment assignment proceeds as for sealed envelope randomization except that the clinician still does not know which treatment the patient is on even after randomization. An unsuitable alternative is to supply each clinician with sufficient of each drug, coded A or B, so that he does not know which drug is which, and then to use one of the other methods for randomization to assign A or B to each patient. This procedure is ill-advised since if the clinician "breaks the code" for any single patient either by necessity or by chance, then the actual treatment is revealed for all his patients and blindness is destroyed.

1.35 Preparing the Randomization List

First, we shall consider a simple unrestricted method of randomization which is essentially equivalent to repeated coin tossing. Then, various methods are described for restricting randomization to ensure approximately equal numbers of patients on each treatment. There are also various "stratified" randomization methods which can be taken into account for a few patient characteristics in order to ensure that the treatment groups are not dissimilar.

1.36 Simple Randomization

For a randomized trial with two treatments (say A and B) the basic concept of tossing a coin (head = A, tail = B) over and over again is quite reasonable, but it is rather clumsy and time consuming. Thus, people find it more convenient to use table of random numbers instead. For instance, Table shows (Annexure) such a table of random digits 0–9. Each digit occurs on an average the same number of times. The table presents digits in pairs merely to help the user in scanning across the page. A randomization list may be generated by using the digits, one per treatment assignment, starting with the top row and working downwards

For two treatments, assign A for digits 0–4	
and B for digits 5–9	
Hence, the numbers in the top row of Table	
	0 5 2 7 8 4 3 7 4 1 6 etc.
Produce a list starting	A B A B B A A B A A B etc.
For three treatments, say A, B, and C,	
assign A for digits 1–3	
B for digits 4–6	
C for digits 7–9	
and ignore 0	
so that numbers	0 5 2 7 8 4 3 7 4 1 6 etc.

Produce a list starting	A B A B B A A B A A B etc.
For four treatments, say A, B, C, and D,	
assign A for digits 1–2	
B for digits 3-4	
C for digits 5-6	
D for digits 7–8	
and ignore 0&9	
so that numbers	0 5 2 7 8 4 3 7 4 1 etc.
Produce a list starting	C A D D B B D B A etc.

Such randomization lists can be made as long as necessary and since the process is so easy that one should make a list before the trial starts and make it long enough to complete the whole trial. The advantage of such a simple method is that each treatment assignment is completely unpredictable, and probability theory guarantees that in the long run the numbers of patients on each treatment will not be radically different. However, clinical trials are of finite size and one should consider the possibility that the treatment numbers may end up unequal. For instance, using the above list for two treatments and 20 patients one may end up with eight patients on A compared with 12 patients on B: not a huge difference but somewhat inconvenient and inefficient especially if “A” happens to the new treatment and “B” the standard. Clearly, it would be catastrophic if a trial with 20 patients had four on one treatment and 16 on the other. Only in large trials, say with over 200 patients, does the chance of severe imbalance becomes so remote that simple randomization may be recommended, but a problem could still arise if one intends to analyze early results while the trial is in progress. Thus, it is often desirable to restrict randomization to ensure similar treatment numbers throughout a trial.

1.37 Replacement Randomization

After preparing a randomization list as described above one can check if there is any serious inequality in treatment numbers. If it is unsatisfactory, then one can generate an entirely new simple randomization list to replace the first one. It is unlikely that one will need to repeat this more than once to achieve reasonably equal sized treatment groups throughout the trial. The decision to replace a randomization list should be based on objective criteria. For instance, for a trial with two treatments and around 100 patients, one could specify that a simple randomization with inequality of 10 or more at any point should be replaced.

1.37.1 Random Permuted Blocks

A more conventional method of restricted randomization is to ensure exactly equal treatment numbers at certain equally spaced points in the sequence of patient assignments. For blocks of relatively small size one can use a table of random numbers (Table) to produce the randomization list.

For two treatments and blocks of two patients,			
Assign AB for digits 0-4			
And BA for digits 5-9			
C for digits 5-6			
Then the numbers	0 5 2 7 8 4 3 7 etc.		
Produce a list starting	AB BA AB BA BA AB AB BA etc.		
For three treatments and blocks of three patients			
assign	ABC	for digit	1
	ACB	for digit	2
	BAC	for digit	3
	BCA	for digit	4

	CAB	for digit	5
	CBA	for digit	6
			And ignore 0 & 7–9
Then, the numbers	0 5 2 7 8 4 3 etc.		
Produce a list starting—CAB ACB BCA BAC etc.			
For two treatments and blocks of four patients,			
Assign	AABB	for digit	1
	ABAB	for digit2	
	ABBA	for digit	3
	BBAA	for digit	4
	BABA	for digit	5
	BAAB	for digit	6
			and ignore 0 & 7–9
Then the numbers	0 5 2 7 8 4 etc.		
produce a list starting—BABA ABAB BBAA etc.			

One problem here is that at the end of each block a clinician who keeps track of previous assignment could predict what the next treatment would be. Evidently, the smaller the block size, the greater is the risk of randomization becoming predictable so that one should particularly avoid a block size of two. Thus, in general a trial should have a reasonable large block size so as to reduce predictability but, if interim analysis is intended, not so large that serious imbalance might occur.

For example, a trial with say 100 or more patients could have a block size of 20. Appendix gives a list of random permutations of numbers 0–19 to be used as follows:

For two treatments, and blocks of 20 patients,		
Assign A	for digits	0–9
and B	for digits	10–19
Then starting with the top permutation and working downwards we obtain the following list		
Block 1		
11 19 15 5 9 0	8 3 4	
B B B A A A	A A A	
Block 2		
14 12 0 1 19 8	6 13 3	
B B A A B A	A B A	
For three treatments, and blocks of 15 patients,		
Assign A	for digits	1–59
B	for digits	6–10
C	for digits	11–15
and ignore 0 & 16–19		
Block 1		
11 19 15 5 9 0	8 3 4	
C - C A B -	B A A	
Block 2		
14 12 0 1 19 8	6 13 3	
C C - A - B	C C A	

If one prefers to use random permuted blocks of size 10 or less, one can still use Table (annexure) by simply ignoring numbers 10–19 in each block. To help reduce the predictability of random permuted blocks one could vary the block size at random from one block to the next.

1.38 Stratified Randomization

In any randomized trial it is desirable that the treatment groups should be similar as regards certain relevant patient characteristics. For instance, in a breast cancer trial, it would be unfortunate if the proportion of premenopausal patients was very different between treatments. It would affect the credibility of any treatment comparisons: although there exits methods of statistical analysis to allow for such lack of comparability, readers are more likely to be convinced when valid conclusions can be achieved from a simple presentation of results for comparable treatment groups. Stratified randomization is like an insurance policy in that its primary aim is to guard against the unlikely event of the treatment groups ending up with some major difference in patient characteristics. The first issue is to decide which patient factors one should stratify by. This is best achieved by studying the outcome of previous patients, preferably in earlier trials. One should be quite convinced about a factor's potential for making an impact on outcome before it is included in stratification. If investigators have only a vague idea about which factor may affect the outcome, then they may be wise to proceed with un-stratified randomization. For example, consider a breast cancer trial, in which there were two patient factors considered to be of major prognostic importance, i.e., nodal status (number of positive auxiliary nodes) and age. As regards the former, one expects a poorer prognosis for patients with a larger number of positive notes and the importance of age is that older patients tend to have a shorter survival. After choosing the relevant patient factors, the next step is to categorize each one into two or more levels. Accordingly age was split into under or over 50 while nodal status was split into 1–3 or ≥4 positive nodes. The choice of split is inevitably somewhat arbitrary but should take into account the numbers of patients likely to be in each category. Also, in this case age 50 provides an approximate division into premenopausal and postmenopausal status. The purpose of categorizing each factor is to end up with several patient types or strata. In this case the four (=2 × 2) strata are

Age < 50 and 1–3 positive nodes
Age ≥ 50 and 1–3 positive nodes
Age < 50 and ≥4 positive nodes
Age ≥ 50 and ≥4 positive nodes

Then, before the trial begins, a separate restricted randomization list is prepared for each of the patient strata, random permuted blocks being the usual approach.

1.39 Essential Design Features of RCT

Attempts to evaluate the use of therapeutic procedures in the past had been very haphazard and often they were inconclusive. During the last 30 years scientific principles of experimentation have been followed for evaluating the efficacy and safety of new treatments. The purpose of this lecture is to explain the main scientific and statistical principles which are important in measuring the treatment effectiveness at the end of a clinical trial.

1.40 Research Design Features: Choice of the Test and Control Treatments

The test treatment must be different from the control treatment. Both treatments must be justifiable on medical grounds to allow investigators to allocate patients to either treatment. The general requirements to be satisfied by the test and control treatments are:

1) They must be distinguishable from one another.
2) They must be medically justifiable.
3) There must be an ethical base for use of either treatment.
4) Use of the treatments must be compatible with the health care needs of study patients.
5) Either treatment must be acceptable to study patients and to physicians administering them.
6) There must be a reasonable doubt regarding the efficacy of the test treatment.
7) There should be reason to believe that the benefits will outweigh the risks of treatment.

The method of treatment administration must be compatible with the design needs of the trial (e.g., method of administration must be the same for all the treatments in a double-masked trial) and should be as similar to real-world use as practical. The choice of the control treatment has important bearing for the size of the treatment difference that can be expected. The more effective control treatment, the more difficult it will be to establish the superiority of the test treatment. The control treatment in a drug trial will be a standard form of drug therapy, a placebo, or no treatment at all, depending on the nature of the disease. Treatment cannot be withheld from control patients if it is unethical to do so. Some form of medical care must be provided if a patient has a condition that requires treatment.

The classical trial design comparing two treatments A and B can be depicted as

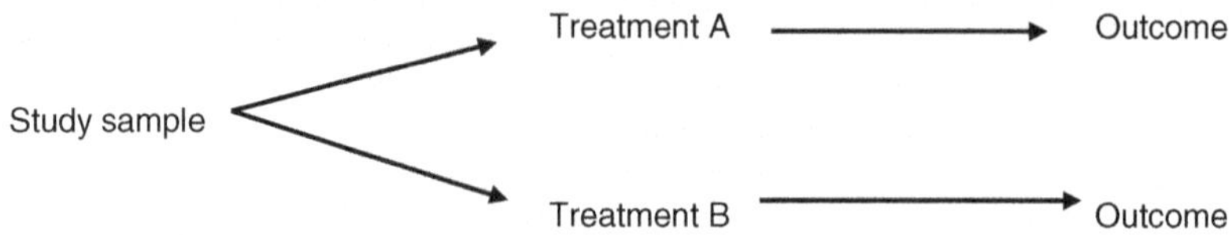

The asterisk indicates the randomization or other mode of treatment assignment.

1.41 Outcome Measure

The outcome measure used for treatment comparisons will be a clinical event (e.g., death, myocardial infarction, significant loss of vision, recurrence of a disease) or a surrogate outcome measure (e.g., blood pressure change, serum lipid level). The desired characteristics for the primary outcome measure are:

1. Easy to diagnose or observe
2. Free of measurement or ascertainment errors
3. Capable of being observed independent of treatment assignment
4. Clinically relevant
5. Chosen before the start of data collection

The investigator has the usual difficult choice between "hard" (objective, easily measurable) and "soft" (subjective, not so easily measurable) outcomes. The latter may lead to differential information bias in favor of a new experimental treatment, and suitable blinding of both study subjects and observers of the outcome is necessary to protect such bias.

1.42 Establishing Comparable Study Groups

The baseline characteristics of the test and control-treated groups must be more or less similar in order to provide a valid basis for comparison. The ideal experimentation mode for comparing two treatments is one in which the baseline characteristics of the two study groups are identical in all aspects. This requires a homogeneous group of patients who are arbitrarily assigned to the test and control treatments. An alternative design involves enrolling pairs of patients into the trial, with each pair matched on all important baseless characteristics, and where one member of the pair is assigned to the test treatment and the other to the control treatment. However, matching is not practical in real life. The comparability of the study groups for a few key baseline characteristics may be assumed by first classifying patients into sub-groups defined by those characteristics, and then assigning members of each sub-group to the test or control treatment in the same proportion as for all other sub-groups. However, this approach known as stratification at best can control the distribution of only a few variables. The need for comparability can be partially satisfied by suitable patient selection. The eligibility and exclusion criteria in most trials are designed to reduce the variability of the study populations. However, the desire for patient homogeneity and the resultant improvement in study precision must be balanced against reduced opportunities for generalizations when a highly homogeneous population is studied. Once an eligible patient has agreed to be enrolled, it is essential that treatment assignment be made free of influence from both the patient and the clinic personnel to avoid selection biases in the way study groups are formed. The general conditions that should be satisfied to have a sound allocation scheme are presented below.

Assignment remains masked to the patient, physician, and all other clinic personnel until it is needed for initiation of treatment.

(a) Future assignments cannot be predicted from past assignments.
(b) The order of allocations is reproducible.
(c) Methods for generation and administration of the schedule are documented.

(d) The process used for generation has known mathematical properties.
(e) The process provides a clear audit trial.
(f) Departures from the established sequence of assignments can be detected.

The accepted standard for creating treatment groups is randomization. There is still a good deal of misunderstanding regarding the reasons for randomizing. While the process does provide a basis for certain types of statistical analysis, it is far more useful as a method of making bias-free treatment assignment. The term random is often misused in medical circles by investigators who equate haphazard and random process (as in referring to a random blood sugar determination, or in characterizing a group of arbitrarily selected individuals as a random sample). The details of randomization procedure will be separately dealt with.

1.43 Parallel Versus Crossover Design

In the clinical trial designs we have considered a group of patients receiving a test treatment being compared with control treatment. Such a design is called parallel design, because the study groups receive their respective treatment simultaneously, i.e., in parallel. In a crossover design, however, each study patient receives each treatment in series by "crossing over" in sequence from one to the other. For example, patients with asthma might each receive in sequence two different treatment regimens to see which of the two treatments is more efficacious among the group as a whole. Crossover trials have a major advantage over parallel trials in statistical efficiency, in that a given treatment difference is demonstrable with fewer patients. There are two reasons for this:(a) each patient receives both treatment (in a two treatment comparisons) and thus counts twice, and (b) variability in treatment response due to individual patient characteristics is eliminated. Proper conduct of crossover trials, however, requires randomization of treatment sequence (A, B vs. B, A), time-dependent (rather than outcome-dependent) crossover treatments, and elimination of (or control for) carry-over effects from the first treatment. More about crossover trials will be dealt separately.

1.44 Blinding and Bias Control

The aim of any trial should be to collect data that are free of bias, particularly treatment-related bias. This has the potential for obscuring a treatment difference or creating the impression that one exists when in fact it does not. The usual practice to protect against treatment-related bias is blinding or masking. Blinding of study patients is needed to protect against contamination (confounding) of the true treatment effect by the so-called placebo effect. The placebo effect is the nonspecific effect that any treatment can have on the outcome, especially when the patient believes it to be efficacious. The main reason for providing look-alike, feel-alike, smell-alike, taste-alike placebo treatments when comparing an experimental treatment with no treatment is to facilitate patient blinding. Blinding of observers is also necessary to prevent the information bias that would occur if the outcomes are determined by observers who are aware of the treatment received. Such awareness can influence the outcome assessment, either consciously or unconsciously, especially if the outcome is subjective. It is conventional to refer the trials as un-blinded, single-blinded, or double-blinded. A double-blinded trial is one in which neither the patient nor the physician responsible for treatment is informed of the patient's treatment assignment; a single-blinded trial is one in which the patient is not informed of the treatment assignment but the treating physician is, and an un-blinded trial is one in which both the patient and the physician are informed of the treatment assignment. The logistics of blinding are not easy. They are discussed separately. Unfortunately, blinding may be infeasible for some treatments. This is obviously true for most of the surgical procedures but also pertains to many behavioral and health care interventions. Furthermore, un-blinding can arise owing to differences inside effects that occur with different treatments, even if those treatments originally seem indistinguishable. A double-blinded trial, as defined above, is characterized by masked data collection. However, even single-blinded or un-blinded trials may be designed so that data collection is done in a masked fashion, that is, treatment information is withheld from personnel responsible for data collection. This requires one set of personnel to administer the study treatments and another to collect the data needed for assessing the study treatments. Laboratory tests should be performed, recorded, and reported by personnel who are masked to treatment assignment, regardless of the level of treatment masking in the rest of the trial. The only exceptions are cases in which treatment assignment is needed to determine the tests to be performed. Also, data processing should be performed by personnel who are masked.

1.45 Efficacy vs. Effectiveness in Clinical Trials

One of the major problems likely to arise during a clinical trial is that patients either may have received or complied with the treatment to which they were assigned or, having received it initially, may have switched to another. Another problem is that subjects may withdraw from participation in the trial before treatment or follow-up are complete. Such problems have led to two different ways of analyzing the results of a clinical trial and, consequently, to two different interpretations; which of the two approaches is taken depends on whether one is interested in treatment efficacy or treatment effectiveness. Efficacy refers to the potential effect of treatment under optimal circumstances, i.e., whether treatment can have an effect on outcome. Effectiveness refers to the actual effect of treatment in the "real world" of people who comply poorly, change treatment or become lost to follow-up, i.e., whether treatment does have an effect on outcome. Both efficacy and effectiveness may be important. Efficacy is of primary interest for those who are interested in the biological potency and mechanism of action. Clinical trials remain the "gold standard" for evaluating treatments. They have contributed enormously to the evolution of more effective therapeutic and preventive measures for a variety of clinical conditions and are represented by an increasing proportion of articles published in the leading medical journals, although use of a clinical trial design, even with randomized treatment assignment, does not offer certainty on the conclusions of the study. The RCT is the research design of choice whenever randomized assignment is feasible and ethical.

1.46 Different Phases of Clinical Trial

The process of drug development is broadly classified into preclinical and clinical. Preclinical refers to experimentation that occurs before governing on human subjects, whereas clinical trials refer to experimentation conducted on human's subjects. This course of procedure will be considered only in clinical research; the research was assumed that any significant variation in drug efficacy and any side effects shall affect the subjects. If the drug has been already developed by the chemist or biologist without any trail, the suoumoto legal action would be imposed on the above intervention. The trail should be tested by using standard protocol (SOP) of FDA; all laboratory and biological activity (*in vivo*) procedure will be conducted at Institutional level; later part interim analysis was done on the particular subjects to know the drug efficacy and tolerability. As per the interim analysis researcher shall draw the conclusion about the trail. The new drug or therapy is found to be classified in different generic names and intervened tested drug is sufficiently promising to be introduced at population level (humans). Within the paradigm, we have classified the clinical trial into following four phases.

Phase I—To explore possible toxic effects of drugs and determine a tolerated dose for further experimentation. Also, during this phase the pharmacology of the drug may be explored.

Phase II—Screening and feasibility by initial assessment for therapeutic effects and further assessment of toxicities.

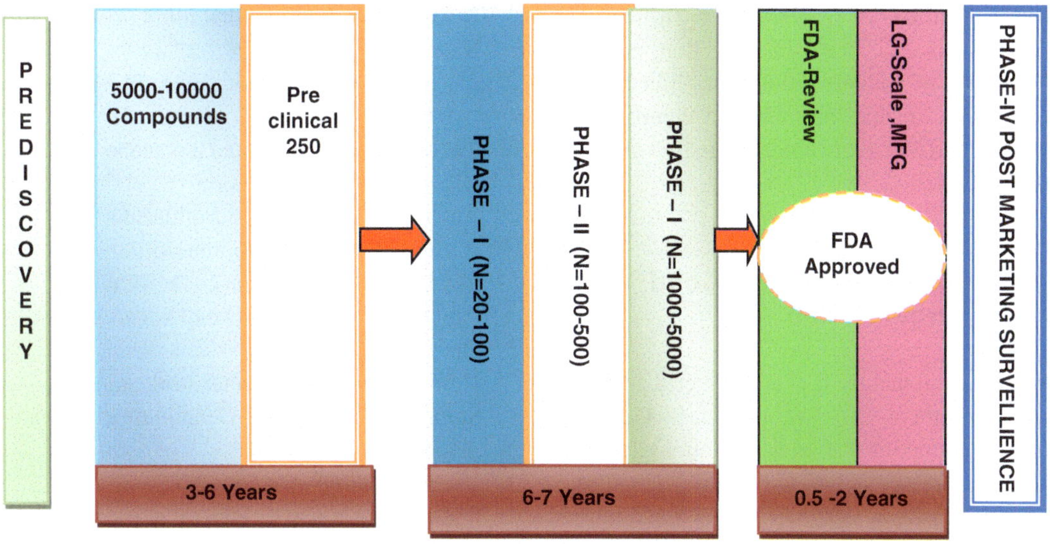

Fig. 1.12 Schematic diagram of Clinical trial experimentation

Phase III—Comparison of new intervention (drug or therapy) to the current standard of treatment, both with respect to efficacy and toxicity.

Phase IV—Observational study of morbidity/adverse effects on human intervention (Fig. 1.12).

1.47 Rationale of Randomized Controlled Trials (RCTs)

Now let us see the scientific rational of full-scale (Phase II) controlled clinical trials. The first priority for clinical research is to come up with a good idea for improving treatment. Naturally, the proponents of any new therapy are liable to be enthusiastic about its potential: preclinical studies and phase I/II trials may indicate considerable promise. Unfortunately, many new treatments turn out not to be as effective as was expected once they are subjected to the rigorous test of a properly designed phase III trial. One fundamental rule is that phase III trials are comparative. That is, one needs to compare the experience of a group of patients on the new treatment with a control group of similar patients receiving a standard treatment. If there is no standard treatment, then it is often appropriate to have a control group of untreated patients (placebo group). Also, in order to obtain an unbiased evaluation of the new treatment's value on usually needs to assign each patient randomly to either new or standard treatment. Hence, it is now generally accepted that the randomized controlled trial is the most reliable method of conducting clinical research.

1.48 Define the Purpose of the Trial: State Specific Hypothesis

From an initial idea about a possible improvement in therapy one needs to produce a more precise definition of trial aims in terms of specific hypothesis regarding treatment efficacy and safety. That is, one must define exactly the type of patient, the treatments to be compared, and the methods of evaluating each patient's response to treatment.

1.49 Design the Trial; A Written Protocol

The next step is to develop a detailed design for a randomized trial and document one's plan in a study protocol. The design needs to fulfill scientific, ethical, and organizational requirements so that the trial may be conducted efficiently. Two important issues are: (a) Size—the trial must recruit enough patients to obtain a reasonably precise estimate of response on each treatment. (b) Avoidance of bias—the selection, care, and evaluation of patients should not differ between treatments, so that the treatment comparison is not affected by factors unrelated to the treatments themselves.

1.50 Conduct the Trial; Good Organization

It is essential that the trial is conducted according to the protocol, in letter and spirit. Generally, while conducting the trial, deviations from the protocol are not allowed. However, unexpected deviations may be carried out after amending the protocol accordingly.

1.50.1 Analyze the Date; Descriptive Statistics, Tests of Hypotheses

Statistical methods should be applied to the results in order to test the prespecified study hypotheses. In particular, one may use significance tests to assess how strong the evidence is for a genuine difference in response to treatment.

1.50.2 Draw Conclusions; Publish Results

Finally, one needs to draw conclusions regarding the treatment's relative merits and publish the results so that other clinicians may apply the findings in their clinical practice.

1.50.3 Illustrative Examples of RCTs Conducted at Global Level

1. New treatment vs. standard treatment
   Disease: Anal fistula
   New treatment: Kshaarasootra (Ayurvedic medicated thread)
   Standard treatment: Surgery (ICMR 1991)
2. New treatment versus placebo
   Disease: Acute myocardial infarction
   New treatment: Anturan
   Placebo: Inactive tablets resembling Antura (ARTRG 1980)
3. Two active treatments and a placebo
   Disease: Mild hypertension
   Active treatment: 1. Bendrofluazide
   Active treatment: 2. Propranolol
   Placebo: Inactive substance (MRCWP 1977)
4. Patient management: Special versus general
   Disease: Acute stroke
   New management: Special stroke unit
   Standard management: General medical ward
5. Two standard treatments
   Disease: Operable breast cancer
   Standard treatment 1: Radical mastectomy
   Standard treatment 2: Simple mastectomy + Radiotherapy

The aim of any clinical trial should be to obtain a truthful answer to a relevant medical issue. This requires that the conclusions be based on an unbiased assessment of objective evidence rather than on a subjective compilation of clinical opinion. Hence, randomized controlled trial is the most reliable method of assessing the true efficacy of a treatment/management for any particular disease condition.

1.51 Study Population

Population is universe. The target population of the study must be defined in advance with unambiguous inclusion and exclusion criteria and the impact of these criteria on study design will be visualized on the basis of location. Individual population group or sample will be able to generalize the recruitment procedure and it will be considered in accordance with human ethical guidelines.

1.51.1 Statistical Issues and Methods

Our goal in clinical trial is to estimate an endpoint related to the treatment efficacy and sufficient precision to aid the investigations for determining whether the proposed treatment should be studied for further period or following endpoints should be correlated:

1. The proportion of patient responding to the treatment arm [response has to be unambiguously defined].
2. The proportion with side effects known.
3. Average decreased level of serological markers over a period of time.

Statistical methods have been correlated on perspective basis generally time taken for estimation and level of precision, i.e., the problem is often posed through a probability distribution modeling with population parameters. For example, we consider the patients with esophageal cancer, who were treated with chemotherapy prior to surgical resection. A complete response is defined as an absence of macroscopic tumor at that time of surgery; we suspect that this may occur with 35% probability using a drug under investigation in phase-ii. The 35% is just a guess, possibly based on similar acting drugs used in the past and the goal is to estimate the actual response rate with sufficient precision, in this case we want 95% confidence interval to be within 15% of the true or positive values.

As researchers, we view the world as follows: we start by positioning a statistical model; i.e., let "*p*" denote the complete population response rate. We conduct an experiment, η patients with esophageal cancer were treated with the chemotherapy prior to surgical resection and we will be collecting the data with respect to the number of patients with the chemotherapy, who have complete response. The result of this experiment yields a random variable "*X*," the number of patients in a sample of size "*η*" that have a complete response. A popular discrete probability model for this scenario is to assume that

$$p(X = x) = nc_x p^x \left(1 - p\right)^{n-x}), X \sim \text{Binomial}(\eta, p) \quad (1.1)$$

where n = number of cancer patients, p = probability of treatment success, (1 − p) = probability of treatment failure, and "*x*" is random variable with different time period. We assume that, the probability of treatment success is equal to the probability of failure. The treatment effect should be dichotomous and the probability of success and failure is always equal to one, the mean of the probability was "*np*" and standard deviation was "*npq*." If the number of patients increased in treatment arm, the binomial distribution tends to be poison distribution. When "*n*" is sufficiently large, the distribution of the sample proportion $p = \frac{X}{n}$ is well approximated by a normal distribution with mean "*np*" and variance p (1 − p)/n, $p \sim N\left(p, \frac{p(1-p)}{n}\right)$. This approximation is useful for inference regarding the population parameter "*np*." Because of the approximate normality, the estimator "*p*" will be within 1.96 standard deviations of "*np*," approximately 95% of the time (Approximation gets better with increasing sample size). Therefore, the population parameter "*np*" will be within the interval ±1.96 {p(1 − p)} 1/2, with approximately 95% probability. Since, the value "*p*" is unknown to us, we approximately use "*p*" to obtain the approximate 95% confidence interval. Switch back to abovementioned example, where best guess for the response rate is about 35%, if we want the precision of our estimator to be such that of the 95% confidence interval within the 15% of true "*p*," then we need to calculate sample size.

$$n = \frac{\left\{(1.96)^2\right)(0.35)(0.65)\right\} 1/2}{\left(0.15^2\right)} = 39 \text{ patients were needed for our experimentation.}$$

If the number of patients increased in phase II and III trial, the binomial distribution tends to be poison approximation $n \to \infty$, the probability of success is very small or nearer to zero. Binomial distribution showed to be poison approximation, the density function is given by:

$P(X = x) = \frac{e^{-\lambda}\lambda^{x}}{x!}$, so that the binomial distribution tends to the Poisson distribution with mean λ'. It was showed that the expected number of patients x' is equal to λ and that variance of x is also λ. This distribution tends to the normal distribution as λ gets large in essentially the same sense as the binomial distribution tends to normality. The Poisson law is useful in getting quick approximation to binomial probabilities.

1.52 Application of Multinomial Distribution in Clinical Trial

Let us consider the simple situation of clinical trial conducted in different geographical locations and obtaining the data as per the norms. We assumed "*n*" clinical trials and there were "*t*" possible results, *viz.* a_1, a_2, $a_{3,}$......at with probability that we shall get n_1a_1's n_2a_2's..an. Again the matter was solved by permutation and combination for any possible arrangements of n_1a_1's, n_2a_2's ...and so on, the probability of trial is equal to:

$$p_1^{n1}, p_2^{n2}, p_3^{n3} \ldots\ldots p_n^{nt}$$

Then, the cumulative probability for pooled trial is calculated by the following density function:

$$p(Xi = x) = \frac{n!}{n_1!n_2!n_3!n_4!}(p_1)^{n1}(p_2)^{n2}(p_3)^{n3}(p_4)^{n4}\ldots(p_n)^{nt} \tag{1.2}$$

For example, the new-clinical trials were conducted in the following geographical location, the resulted observations are mentioned below:

Location	No. of patients	Sample number	Probability values
Northern region	14	n_1	0.23
Southern region	15	n_2	0.22
Middle region	19	n_3	0.36
Eastern region	28	n_4	0.44
Western region	32	n_5	0.52
Total	108		

$$p(Xi = x) = \frac{n!}{n_1!n_2!n_3!n_4!}(p_1)^{n1}(p_2)^{n2}(p_3)^{n3}(p_4)^{n4}\ldots(p_n)^{nt}\; p(Xi = x)$$
$$= \frac{108!}{14!15!19!28!32!}(0.23)^{14}(0.22)^{15}(0.36)^{19}(044)^{28}(0.52)^{32}$$

1.53 Gehan's Two-Stage Design

If it is unlikely that a treatment will achieve some minimal level of response or efficacy, we may want to stop the trial as early as possible. For example, suppose that 20% response rate is the lowest response rate, i.e., we have considered acceptable for new treatment experiment. Suppose, we get no responses in "*n*" patients and if "*n*" is sufficiently large, then we may feel confident that the treatment is ineffective. Statistically this may be posed as follows; how large must "*n*" be drawn, so that if there are zero responses among "*n*" patients, we are relatively confident that the response rate will not be achieved even 20% or better if $X \sim b(n, p)$ and $p \geq 0.20$.

$$p_i(x_i = 0) = (1-p)^n \leq (1-0.2)^n = (0.8)^n \tag{1.3}$$

Choose "*n*" so that $(0.8)^n = 0.05$ or $n \ln 8 = \ln(0.50)$. This leads to ≈ 15 (rounding up), thus with the patient is unlikely (≤ 0.50) that no one could response, if the treatmentesponse rate

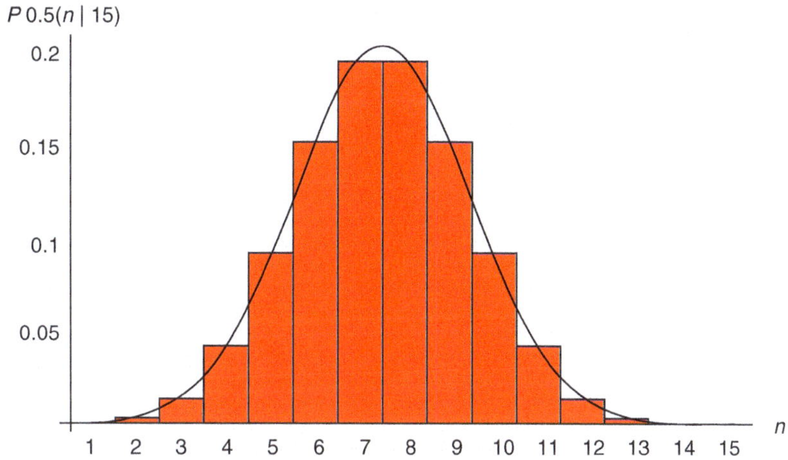

Fig. 1.13 Normal distribution simulated curve from Gehan's two-stage design with 99% confidence interval. From (Fig. 1.12) Gehan's design was treated 15 patients initially. If none responded, the treatment would be declared as failure and the study stopped

was greater than 20%. Thus, zero patients responding among 15 might be used as evidence to stop the clinical trial and declare the treatment failure. This was the logic behind Gleans two-stage design and he also suggested the following strategy: if minimal acceptable response rate is p_o, then we choose the first stage with n_o patients such that:

$$\left(1-p_o\right)^{n0} = 0.5; n_o = \frac{\ln(0.50)}{\ln(1-p_o)} \quad (1.4)$$

If there is zero response among the first n_0 patients, then the treatment has to be stopped and can be declared as failure. Otherwise, continue with recruiting additional patients that will ensure certain degrees of freedom of predetermined accuracy in 95% confidence interval (Fig. 1.13).

1.54 Two-Stage Simon's Experimental Design

Another way of using two-stage designs was proposed by Richard Simon. Here, the investigators must decide on value P_0 and P_1 with $P_0 < P_1$ for the probability of response so that if $p \leq p_0$, then we want to declare the drug ineffective with high probability, say $(1 - \alpha)$, where $\alpha$was taken to be small. If $p \leq p_1$, we want to consider this drug for further investigation with high probability say $(1 - \beta)$, where β was taken to be small. The values of α and β are generally taken between 0.05 and 0.20, the region of the parameter space $p_0 < p < p_1$ was the indifference region

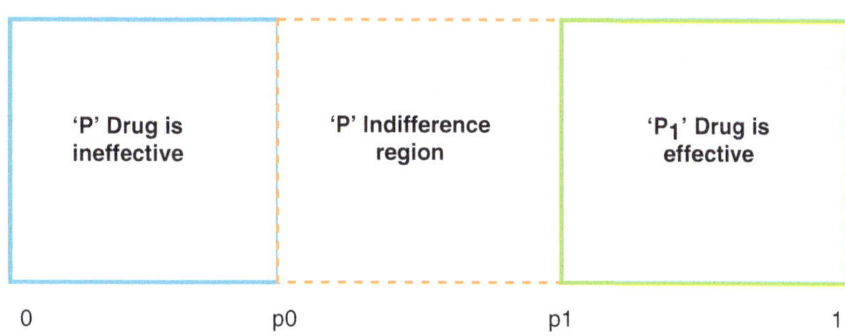

A two-stage design have been dealt with the following characteristics, we consider the integer n_1, n, r_1, r with $n_1 < n$, $r_1 < n_1$ and $r < n$ were chosen and n_1 patient were given treatment in the first stage. If r_1 or less responds, then declare the treatment as failure and stop the process. If more than r_1 respond, then add $(n - n_1)$ additional patients for a total of n patients. At the second stage, if the total number that respond among all n patients is greater r, then declare the treatment as success;

otherwise it could be declared as a treatment failure and can stop the entire process of clinical trial. The following statistical method was used to test the null hypothesis

$$t_{\text{Cal}(\alpha=0.01)} = \frac{\left|\overline{P_0} - \overline{P_1}\right|}{sp^2\sqrt{\frac{1}{n_1} + \frac{1}{n_2}}}$$

$$\text{Pooled variance}\left(sp^2\right) = \frac{S^2{}_1\left(n_1 - 1\right) + s^2{}_2\left(n_2 - 1\right)}{n_1 + n_n - 2}$$

$$S^2{}_1 = \frac{1}{n_1 - 1}\sqrt{\sum_{i=1}^{n}\left(P_0 - \overline{P}_0\right)^2}, S^2{}_2 = \frac{1}{n_2 - 1}\sqrt{\sum_{i=1}^{n}\left(P_1 - \overline{P}_1\right)^2}$$

$$\overline{P}_0 = \frac{\sum_{i=1}^{n} P_o}{n}, \overline{P}_1 = \frac{\sum_{i=1}^{n} P_1}{n}$$

$$t_{\text{Cal}(\alpha=0.01)} > t_{\text{tab}(\alpha=0.01)\text{ at }(n1+n2-2)df\text{ reject }H_O}$$

Maximum likelihood estimation of "*t*" test for the above illustration

$$H_0 : \theta \epsilon P_0; H_1 : \theta\epsilon$$

$$L(\theta) = f\left(P_{01},;P_{02},;\ldots.P_{0n},;\theta\right)^{rs}$$

$$= f\left(P_{01,},\theta)(P_{02},\theta\right)\ldots.\left(P_{0n};\theta\right)^{rs}$$

Let $L\left(\hat{P}_{01}\right) = \max_{\theta \in p_0} L(\theta) = L\left(\hat{\theta}_0\right)$; MLE s of under null hypothesis for P_0

$L\left(\hat{P}_{11}\right) = \max_{\theta \in p_1} L(\theta) = L\left(\hat{\theta}_0\right)$; MLE s of under null hypothesis for P_1

$$\text{LRT function} = L\left(\mu,\theta / P_0 P_1\right) = \mu^n \left(\prod_i P_0\right)^{\mu-1} \theta^n \left(\prod_j P_1\right)^{\theta-1} \tag{1.5}$$

Maximizing the Eq. (1.5) by differentiating the likelihood (Tables 1.1 and 1.2).

1.55 Randomized Clinical Trial

The objective of a clinical trial is to evaluate the effect of an intervention. Evaluation implies that there must be some comparison, no intervention, placebo and best source for the available therapy. The important goal of clinical trial is to know the response between the groups and may not be due to the treatments under. The history of clinical trials dates back to approximately 600 B.C., when Vandenbroucke et al. (2001) conducted what is probably the earliest recorded clinical trial. He compared the health effects of the vegetarian diet with those of a royal Babylonian diet over a 10-day period. The trial had obvious deficiencies by contemporary medical standards (allocation bias, ascertainment bias and confounding by divine intervention), but the report had remained influential for more than two millennia. The nineteenth century saw many major advances in clinical trials. In 1836, the editor of the American Journal of Medical Sciences wrote an introduction to an article, that he considered "one of the most important medical works of the present century, marking the start of a new era of science" and stated that the article was "the first formal exposition of the results of the only true method of investigation in regard to the therapeutic value of remedial agents." The article that evoked such effusive praise was the French study on bloodletting in treatment of

Table 1.1 Experimental design of $p_1 - p_0 = 0.20$ values

	Optimal design					Minimax design			
		Reject drug if response rate				Reject drug if response rate			
P_0	P_1	$\leq r1/n1$	$\leq r1/n$	EN (P_0)	PET (P_0)	$\leq r1/n1$	$\leq r1/n$	EN (P_0)	PET (P_0)
0.05	0.25	0/9	2/24	14.50	0.63	0/13	2/20	16.4	0.51
		0/9	2/17	12.0	0.63	0/12	2/16	13.8	0.54
		0/9	3/30	16.8	0.63	0/15	3/25	20.40	0.46
0.10	0.30	1/12	5/35	19.8	0.65	1/16	4/25	20.40	0.51
		1/10	5/29	0.74	0.74	1/15	5/25	19.50	0.55
		2/18	6/35	0.71	0.71	2/22	6/33	26.20	0.62
0.20	0.40	3/17	10/37	0.55	0.55	3/19	10/36	28.3	0.46
		3/13	12/43	0.75	0.75	4/18	10/33	22.3	0.50
		4/19	15/54	0.67	0.67	5/24	13/45	31.2	0.66
03.0	0.50	7/22	17/46	0.67	0.67	7/28	15/39	35.0	0.36
		5/15	18/46	0.72	0.72	6/19	16/39	25.7	0.48
		8/24	24/63	0.73	0.73	7/24	21/53	36.6	0.56
0.40	0.60	7/18	22/46	0.56	0.56	11/28	20/41	33.8	0.55
		7/16	23/46	0.72	0.72	17/34	20/39	34.4	0.91
		11/25	32/66	0.73	0.73	12/29	27/54	38.1	0.64
0.50	0.70	11/21	26/45	0.67	0.67	11/23	23/39	31.0	0.50
		8/15	26/43	0.70	0.70	12/23	23/37	27.7	0.66
		13/24	36/61	0.73	0.73	14/27	32/53	36.1	0.65
0.60	0.80	6/11	26/38	0.47	0.47	18/27	24/35	28.5	0.82
		7/11	30/43	0.70	0.70	8/13	25/35	20.80	0.64
		12/19	37/53	0.69	0.69	15/26	32/45	35.9	0.48
0.70	0.90	6/9	22/28	0.54	0.54	11/16	20/25	20.10	0.55
		4/6	22/27	0.58	0.58	19/23	21/36	23.20	0.95
		11/15	29/36	0.70	0.70	13/18	26/32	22.7	0.67

Note: For each value of ($p_0 - p_1$) design are given for three sets of error probabilities (α, β). The first, second, and third rows correspond to error probability limits (0, 10, 0, 10), (0.05, 0.20), and (0.05, 0.10), respectively. For each design, EN (p_0) and PET (p_0) denote the expected sample size and the probability of early termination, when the true response probability is p_0

pneumonia by Louis et al. Credit for the modern randomized trial is usually given to Sir Austin Bradford Hill. The Medical Research Council trials on streptomycin for pulmonary tuberculosis are rightly regarded as a landmark that ushered in a new era of medicine. Since Hill's pioneering achievement, the methodology of the randomized controlled trial has been increasingly accepted and the number of randomized controlled trials reported has grown exponentially. The Cochrane library already listed more than 150,000 such trials and they have become the underlying basis for what is currently called "evidence-based medicine." Stratified randomization is random assignment within groups defined by participant characteristics, such as age or disease severity, intended to ensure good balance of these factors across intervention groups (Fig. 1.14).

Randomization trail are gold standard of study design because the potential for bias (Selection into treatment groups) is avoided.

1.55.1 Simple Randomization

The most commonly encountered situation in practice is a two treatment comparison with a predetermined overall sample size N with a predetermined sample size of '*n*' for Treatment 1 and size for Treatment 2 (+ = *N*). A total of "*N*" opaque envelopes, containing an identifier for Treatment 1 and containing an identifier for Treatment 2, may be shuffled. The order of the shuffled envelopes determines the allocation of participants to treatments. This process is relatively simple to organize, preserves the prede-

Table 1.2 Experimental design of $p_1 - p_0 = 0.15$ values

	Optimal design					Minimax design			
		Reject drug if response rate				Reject drug if response rate			
P_0	P_1	≤$r1/n1$	≤$r1/n$	EN (P0)	PET (P0)	≤$r1/n1$	≤$r1/n$	EN (P_0)	PET (P_0)
0.05	0.20	0/12	3/37	23.50	0.54	0/18	3/32	26.40	0.40
		0/10	3/29	17.60	0.60	0/13	3/27	19.8	0.51
		1/21	4/41	26.70	0.72	1/29	4/38	32.9	0.57
0.10	0.25	2/21	7/50	31.20	0.65	2/27	6/40	33.7	0.48
		2/18	7/43	24.7	0.73	2/22	7/40	28.8	0.62
		2/21	10/66	36.8	0.65	3/31	9/55	40.0	0.62
0.20	0.35	5/27	16/63	43.6	0.54	6/33	15/58	45.5	0.50
		5/22	19/72	35.4	0.73	6/31	15/53	40.4	0.57
		8/37	22/83	51.4	0.69	8/42	21/77	58.4	0.53
03.0	0.45	9/30	29/2	51.4	0.59	16/50	25/69	56.0	0.68
		9/27	30/81	41.7	0.73	16/46	25/65	49.6	0.81
		13/40	40/110	60.8	0.70	27/77	33/88	78.5	0.86
0.40	0.55	16/38	40/88	54.5	0.67	18/45	34/73	57.2	0.56
		11/26	40/84	44.9	0.67	28/59	34/70	60.1	0.90
		19/45	49/104	64.0	0.68	24/62	45/94	78.9	0.47
0.50	0.65	18/35	47/84	53.0	0.63	19/40	41/72	58.0	0.44
		15/28	48/83	43.7	0.71	39/66	40/68	66.1	0.95
		22/42	60/105	62.30	0.68	28/57	54/93	75.0	0.50
0.60	0.75	21/34	47/71	47.1	0.65	25/43	43/64	54.4	0.46
		17/27	46/67	39.4	0.69	18/30	43/62	43.8	0.57
		21/34	64/95	55.6	0.65	48/72	57/84	73.2	0.90
0.70	0.85	14/20	45/59	36.2	0.58	15/22	40/52	36.8	0.51
		14/19	46/59	30.3	0.72	16/23	39/49	34.4	0.56
		18/25	61/79	43.4	0.66	33/44	53/68	485	0.81
0.80	0.95	5/7	27/31	20.8	0.42	5/7	27/31	20.8	0.42
		7/9	26/29	17.7	0.56	7/9	26/29	17.7	0.56
		16/19	37/42	24.4	0.76	31/35	35/40	35.3	0.94

Note: For each value of $(p_0 - p_1)$ design are given for three sets of error probabilities (α, β). The first, second, and third rows correspond to error probability limits (0, 10, 0, 10), (0.05, 0.20), and (0.05, 0.10), respectively. For each design, EN (p_0) and PET (p_0) denote the expected sample size and the probability of early termination when the true response probability is p_0

termined design parameters, and can be readily extended to situations where multiple treatments are to be compared.

1.55.2 Block Randomization

Block randomization is commonly used in the two treatment situation where sample sizes for the two treatments are to be equal or approximately equal. The process involves recruiting participants in short blocks and ensuring that half of the participants within each block are allocated to treatment "A" and the other half to "B." Within each block, however the order of patients is random. Conceptually there are an infinite number of possible block sizes. Suppose we consider blocks of size four. There are six different ways that four patients can be split evenly between two treatments: (1) AABB, (2) ABAB, (3) ABBA, (4) BAAB, (5) BABA, (6) BBAA. The next step is to select randomly among these six different blocks for each group of four participants that are recruited. The random selection can be done using a list of random numbers generated using statistical software, e.g., SPSS, Excel, Minitab, STATA, and SAS (Fig. 1.15).

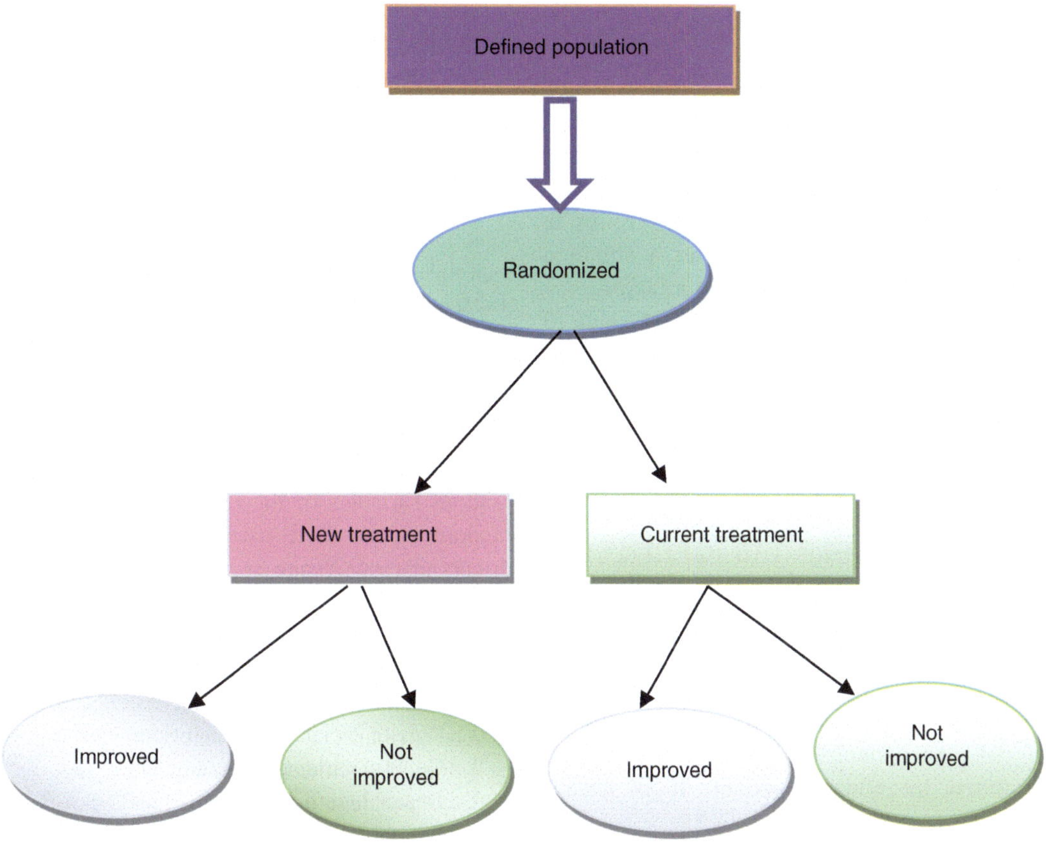

Fig. 1.14 Schematic diagram of Randomized control trail study design

Fig. 1.15 Block randomization

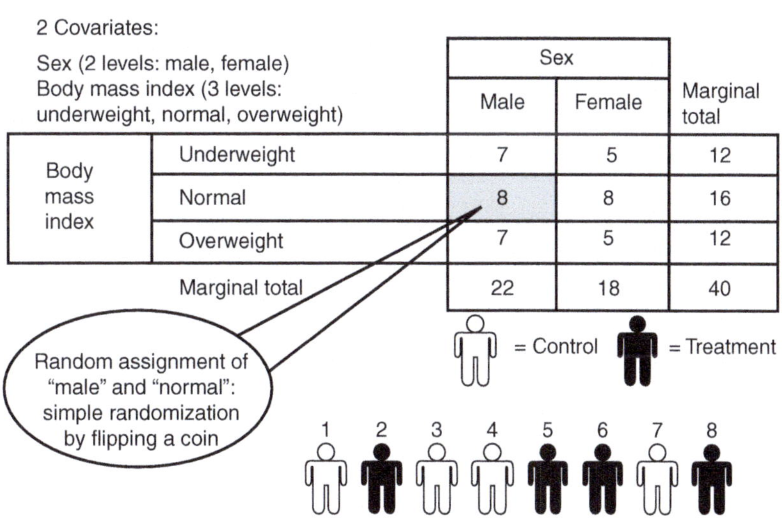

1.55.3 Minimization Method Stratification

Using this method, the first patient is truly randomly allocated; for each subsequent patient, the treatment allocation is identified, which minimizes the imbalance between groups at that time. For example, consider a situation where there are three stratification factors: sex (2 levels), age (3 levels), and disease stage (3 levels). Suppose there are 50 patients enrolled and the 51st patient is male, age 63, and stage III disease.

1.55.4 Stratified Randomization Method (Figs. 1.16 and 1.17)

1.55.5 Results of Randomization

Drug efficacy = efficacy can signify the reduction of risk, the administered drug prognosis was measured by efficacy variant. It is always expressed in percentage (Fig. 1.18).

$$\text{Efficacy}(\%) = \frac{\text{Rate in placebo} \\ -\text{Rate in treated}}{\text{Rate in placebo}} \times 100$$

$$\text{Efficacy}(\%) = 1 - \frac{\text{Rate in treated}}{\text{Rate in placebo}} \times 100$$

1.56 Model Formulation

This section discusses to determine the maximum response or potency (E-max) of the drug and therapeutic index was demonstrated based on the following model; $f(y) = (X_1, X_2, X_3 \ldots X_n)$ is the random variables of the interest, the following random factors were used to demonstrate the drug potency or E max

X_1: Rate and extent of drug absorption
X_2: Body size composition
X_3: Distribution in body fluids
X_4: Plasma protein bindings
X_5: Rate of metabolism excretion
X_6: Genetic variants or parameters
X_7: Desensitization
X_8: Path physiological condition, etc.

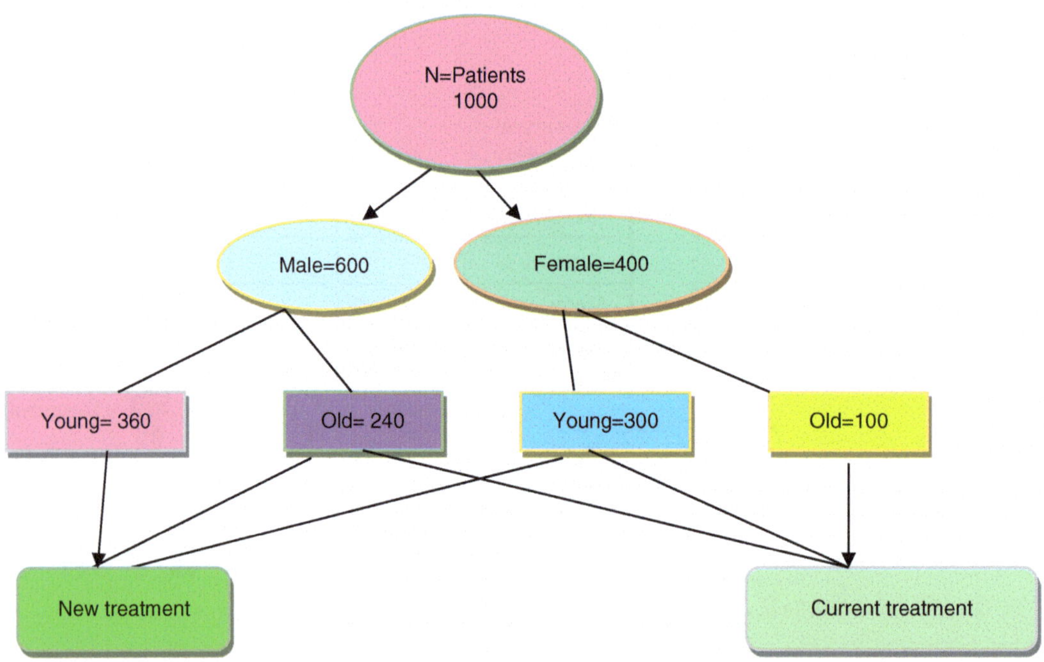

Fig. 1.16 Schematic diagram of stratification

Fig. 1.17 Schematic diagram of Planned crossover trail

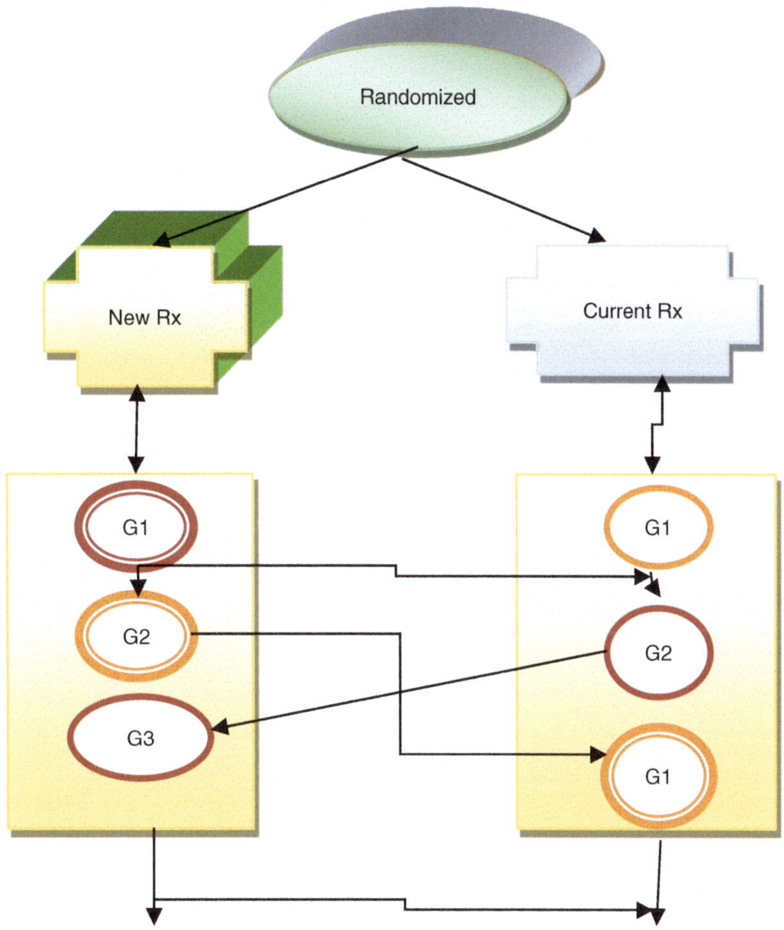

Fig. 1.18 Therapeutic and toxic effect of dose

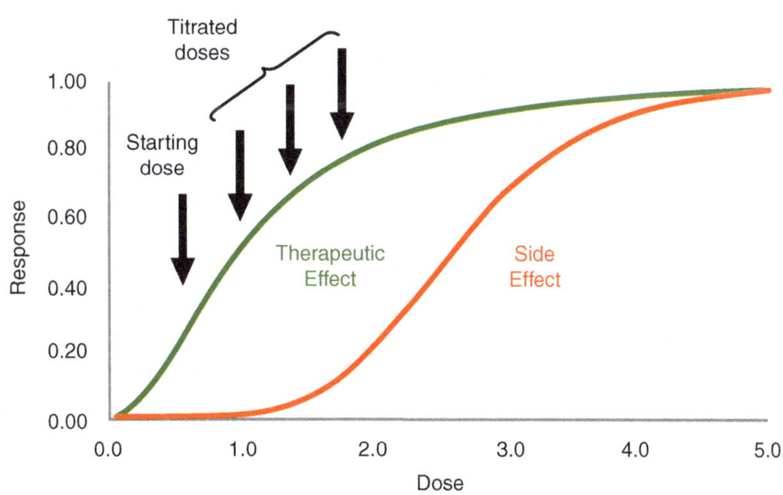

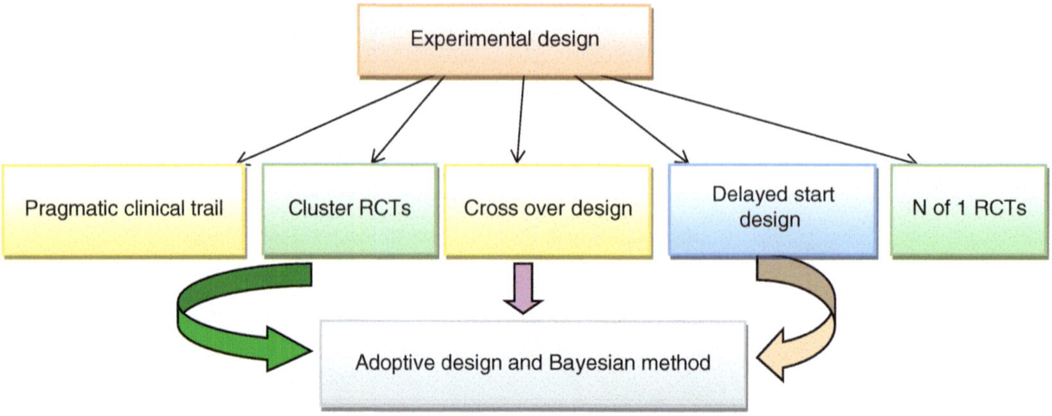

Fig. 1.19 Classification of advanced experimental design in clinical research

The logit exponential model distribution was used to know the accurate response and index of the *E*-max, the probability distribution was formulated by using the above concomitant variables.

$$P\left(x_{i=1\text{to}8}\right)=\frac{e^{\beta_0+\beta_1X_1+\beta_2X_2\ldots\beta_8X_8}}{e^{\beta_0+\beta_1X_1+\beta_2X_2\ldots\beta_8X_8}+1}$$

$$=P\left(e^{\beta_0+\beta_1X_1+\beta_2X_2\ldots\beta_8X_8}+1\right)=e^{\beta_0+\beta_1X_1+\beta_2X_2\ldots\beta_8X_8}$$

$$=P.\left(e^{(\beta_0+\beta_1X_1+\beta_2X_2\ldots\beta_8X_8)}+P\right)=e^{\beta_0+\beta_1X_1+\beta_2X_2\ldots\beta_8X_8}$$

$$=e^{\beta_0+\beta_1X_1+\beta_2X_2\ldots\beta_8X_8}-P.\left(e^{(\beta_0+\beta_1X_1+\beta_2X_2\ldots\beta_8X_8)}+P\right)$$

$$=P.\left(e^{(\beta_0+\beta_1X_1+\beta_2X_2\ldots\beta_8X_8)}(1-P)\right)$$

$$\text{logit}\left(\frac{P}{1-p}\right)=e^{(\beta_0+\beta_1X_1+\beta_2X_2\ldots\beta_8X_8)} \quad (1.6)$$

$$L(\beta,y)=\prod_{i=1}^{n}\frac{\left[e^{\beta_0+\beta_1X_1+\beta_2X_2\ldots\beta_8X_8}\right]^{y_i}}{(1+e^{\beta_0+\beta_1X_1+\beta_2X_2\ldots\beta_8X_8})} \quad (1.7)$$

From Eq. (1.7), the maxium likelihood estimation (MLE's) of β_1, β_2, …β_n were extrapolated from minimization and maximization techniques (Fig. 1.19).

1.57 Pragmatic Clinical Trials (PCTs)

Pragmatic clinical trials are nothing but randomized controlled trail Vandenbroucke et al. (2001). This design will help us to determine the various risk benefits and cost intervention, precluded by the routine clinical practices (e.g., carefully chosen the treatment coherent parameters and protect from the risk). The PCT would evaluate the effect of treatment in a real-world setting with positive results and also the Pragmatic clinical trials (PCT) is appropriate design provide research information to the researcher and facilitate scientific evidence and treatment effect in usual clinical practices (Whiteside et al. 2006).

Illustration

In Mumbai city, the health care specialist conducted experiment on prophylactic Oseltamivir to know the number needed to treat the patients who are affected by flu from household contact.

Subjects	Flu	No flu	Total	Risk
Oseltamivir drug	03	206	209	3/209 = 1.40%
Placebo	26	180	206	26/206 = 12.61%
Total	29	386	415	

Risk ratio = 1.41%/12.6% = 0.11; Relative risk reduction (RRR) = 1 − RR = 0.89; Absolute risk reduction (ARR) = 12.6− 1.4 = 11.20%; Number needed to treat (NTT) = 1/

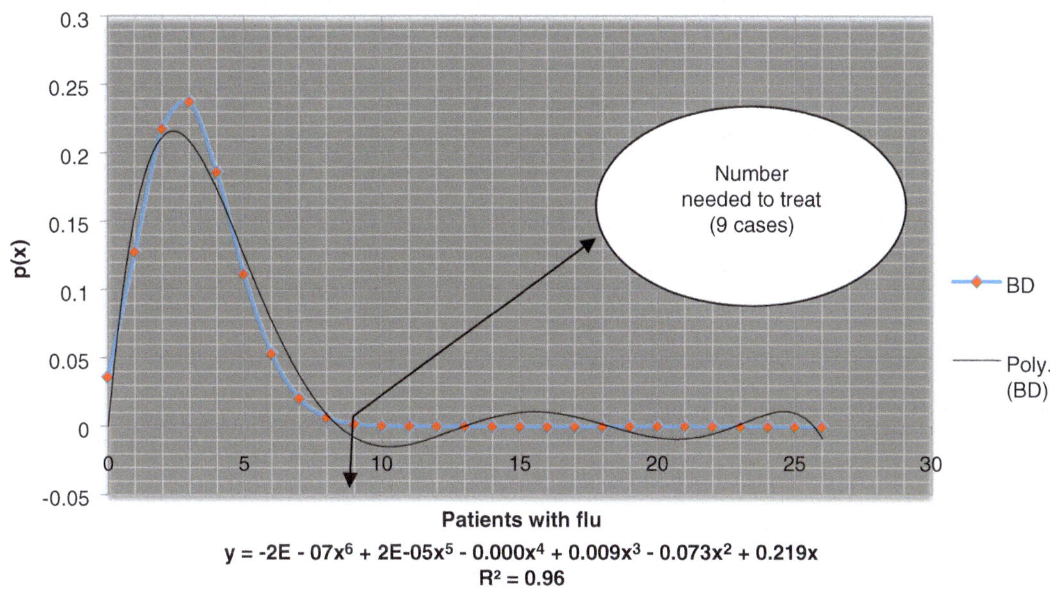

Fig. 1.20 Binomial distribution model experiment on prophylactic Oseltamivir drug

ARR = 1/11.20% = 9 cases will be needed for intend to treat for testing the subjects (Fig. 1.20).

Number needed (N) tends to finite number, the risk factors were modeled by using binomial probability distribution. The Binomial distribution can be defined in terms of the expansion of the binomial $(q + p)^N$, where $(q + p = 1)$; $p > 0$, $q > 0$ and N is a positive. The $(k + 1)$th term in the expansion of $(q + p)^N$ is

$$\binom{N}{k} p^k q^{N-k} = \frac{N!}{k!(N-k)!} p^k q^{N-k} \tag{1.8}$$

The BD with parameters N, p is defined as distribution of a random variable x for which

$$\Pr(x = k) = \binom{N}{k} p^k q^{N-k} \tag{1.9}$$

At two sample level, the probability generating function of x is $(q + p)^N$. If x_1,x_2 are independent random variables having BD parameters N_1,p and N_2,p, respectively, then the probability generating function $(x_1 + x_2)$ is $(q + pt)^{N}{}_1$, $(q + pt)^{N}{}_2$

$$\Pr[X_1 = k / X] = \frac{\binom{N}{k} p^k q^{N_1-k} \binom{N}{X-k} p^{X-k} q^{N_2-(X-k)}}{\binom{N1+N2}{X} p^X q^{N_2+N2-X}} \tag{1.10}$$

From Eq. (1.10) we get the following equation

$$= \frac{\binom{N1}{k}\binom{N2}{x-k}}{\binom{N1+N2}{X}} \tag{1.11}$$

The $n \to \infty$, probability will be nearer to zero, (p is very small), the binomial distribution (BD) tends to Poisson distribution, Eq. (1.8) describes Poisson distribution (PD); A random variable x is said to have Poisson distribution with parameters λ if the probability density function was modeled by the following equation

$$\Pr[x = X] = \frac{e^{-\lambda}\lambda^X}{X!}, \text{The mean and variance of PD is } \lambda\,(\lambda = np) \tag{1.12}$$

In Eq. (1.12) PD is the limiting of binomial distribution (BD); the distribution may also arise for events occurring randomly and independently in time factors; we have simulated the Poisson distribution by using the above illustration on prophylactic Oseltamivir to know the number of patients who affected by flu from house hold contact. Figure 1.18 shows nine cases 9 (34.61%) were intended to treat the patients on prophylactic Oseltamivir –75 mg (Tamiflu) drug adminstered longer duration (> 5 days) in severely ill patients who remain severely ill after 5 days of therapy for H1N1influenza cases (exposed population) when compared to without flu. The parameters were simulated based on the mean and variance of PD ($\lambda = 5.46$, $\lambda = 6.5$ and $\lambda = 13$). As per the model demonstration, the clinician intend to draw nine cases in stage I drug trail. If the experimentation is not found to be significantly correlated, it switches on to the stage II trail inclusion to draw 18 cases or subjects for testing the effectiveness of the Oseltamivir drug when compared to naïve or control group (Fig. 1.21).

The relationship between the PD and chi-square distribution can be implied from Eq. (1.12),

$$\Pr\left[x \le X\right] = \Pr\left[\chi^2_{(r-1)(c-1)} > 2\theta\right] \quad (1.13)$$

$\lambda \sim N(\chi^2_{(r-1)(c-1)}) \Rightarrow n \rightarrow \infty$; Probability is very large

$$Pr\left[x = X\right] = e^{-\lambda_k}\left(\sum_{i=1}^{n}\frac{\lambda_1^{X_1}}{X_1!} + \frac{\lambda_2^{X_2}}{X_2!} + \frac{\lambda_3^{X_3}}{X_3!} .. \frac{\lambda_k^{X_k}}{X_k!}\right) \quad (1.14)$$

$$\Pr\left[x = \chi^2\right] = N \sim e^{-\lambda_k}\left(\sum_{i=1}^{n}\frac{\left(O_{ij} - E_{ij}\right)^2}{E_{ij}}\right) \quad (1.15)$$

$$\Pr\left[x = \chi^2\right] = N \sim e^{-\lambda_k}\left(\sum_{i=1}^{n}\chi_1^{\ 2} + \chi_2^{\ 2} + \chi_2^{\ 2} .. \chi_n^{\ 2}\right)_{df\,(c-1)(r-1)} \quad (1.16)$$

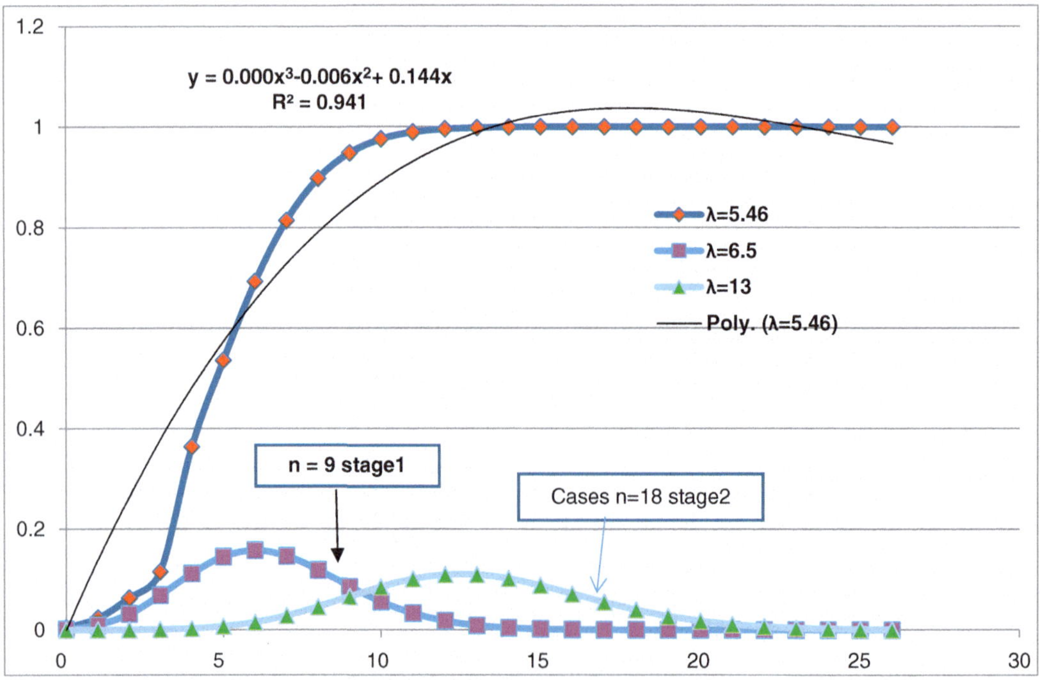

Fig. 1.21 Poisson distribution simulation intended to treat the patients on prophylactic Oseltamivir drug

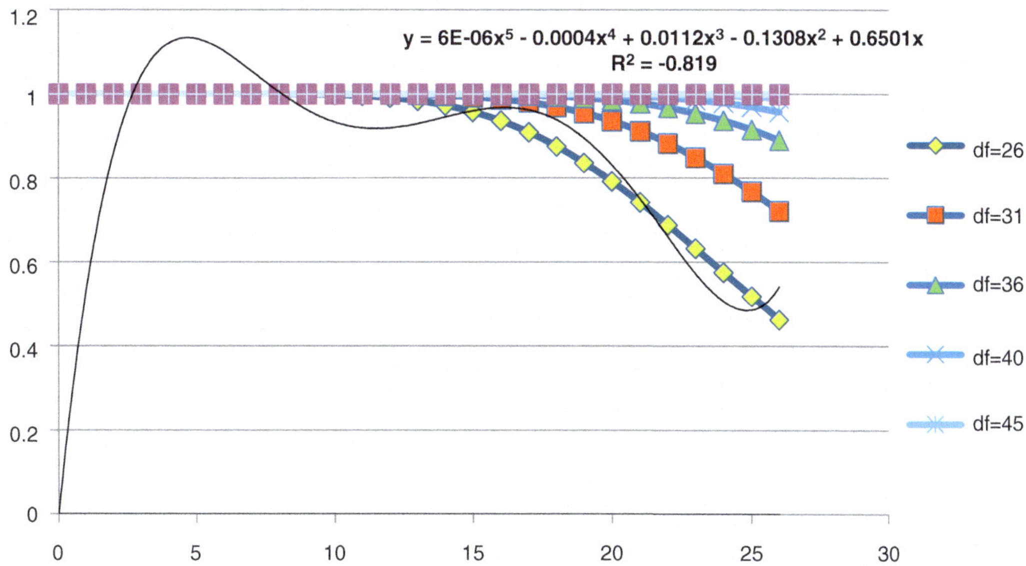

Fig. 1.22 Simulation of chi-square distribution (PD approximation) considering (Probability =1) with varied degrees of freedom $df = (c - 1) \times (r - 1)$

Differentiating w.r.t "X" the above Eq. (1.16) becomes

$$\Pr\left[x = \chi^2\right] = N \sim -e\sum_{i=1}^{n}\left(X_i\right)^{\lambda_{ki}}\left(\sum_{i=1}^{n}\chi_n^{\ 2}\right)'_{df(c-1)(r-1)} \tag{1.17}$$

Figure 1.18 clearly depicted the variation of Poisson distribution with varied parameters "λ."

As per the model results, the clinician intend to draw nine cases in stage I and eighteen cases in stage II drug trail experiment (if trail becomes failure). The fitted model was smoothened by using Thompson singleton iteration method; the polynomial trend was adjusted to know the goodness of fit and extraction of maximum likelihood (MLE's). The Thompson singleton iteration simulation techniques smoothened the numerical equation $Yt = 0.000x^3 - 0.006x^2 + 0.144x$; $R^2 = 0.941$ (t = treatment duration). According to the results obtained from the model, the **P**rophylactic Oseltamivir –75 mg drug was strongly associated ($p < 0.01$) for preventing flu when compared to untreated population (associated 94.10%) (Fig. 1.22).

$$\Pr\left[x = \chi^2\right] = N \sim -e\sum_{i=1}^{n}\left(X_i\right)^{\lambda_{ki}}\left(\sum_{i=1}^{n}\chi_n^{\ 2}\right)'_{df(c-1)(r-1)} \tag{1.18}$$

Squared deviation taken from the population mean "μ," the equation becomes

$$\Pr\left[x = \chi^2\right] = N \sim -e\sum_{i=1}^{n}\left(X_i - \mu\right)^{\lambda_{ki}} + e^{-\lambda i}\left(\sum_{i=1}^{n}\frac{\left(\chi_n - \mu\right)^2}{\sigma}\right) \tag{1.19}$$

Substitute $z = \frac{(\chi_n - \mu)^2}{\sigma}$

$$\Pr\left[x = \chi^2\right] = N \sim -e\sum_{i=1}^{n}(X_i - \mu)^{\lambda_{ki}} + e^{-\lambda i}\left(\sum_{i=1}^{n} z^2\right) \tag{1.20}$$

$$\Pr\left[x = \chi^2\right] = N \sim -e\sum_{i=1}^{n}(X_i - \mu)^{\lambda_{ki}} + e^{-\lambda i}\left(\frac{1}{\sqrt{2\pi\sigma}}\exp - \frac{1}{2\sigma^2}\left(\sum_{i=1}^{n} z^2\right)\right) \tag{1.21}$$

Equation (1.20) $\chi^2 \approx N(\mu, \sigma^2)$ is normally distributed with population mean μ and variance σ^2

$$\Pr\left[x = \chi^2\right] = N \sim -e\sum_{i=1}^{n}(X_i - \mu)^{\lambda_{ki}} + e^{-\lambda i}\left(\frac{1}{\sqrt{2\pi\sigma}}\exp - \frac{1}{2\sigma^2}\left(\sum_{i=1}^{n} z^2\right)\right)$$

In case of lognormal distribution, the equation will be precluded the log scale for each individual observations

$$\Pr\left[x = \chi^2\right] = N \sim -e\ln\left[\sum_{i=1}^{n}(X_i - \mu)\right]^{\lambda_{ki}} + e^{-\ln \lambda i}\left[f(x)\right] \tag{1.22}$$

where $f(x) = \frac{e\left[\ln(x-\theta)/m\right]^2 2\sigma^2}{(X-\theta)\sigma\sqrt{2\pi}} X > \theta; m\sigma > 0$

$\mu = \log m$, σ is the shape; θ is the location; m is the scale parameter (Figs. 1.23 and 1.24).

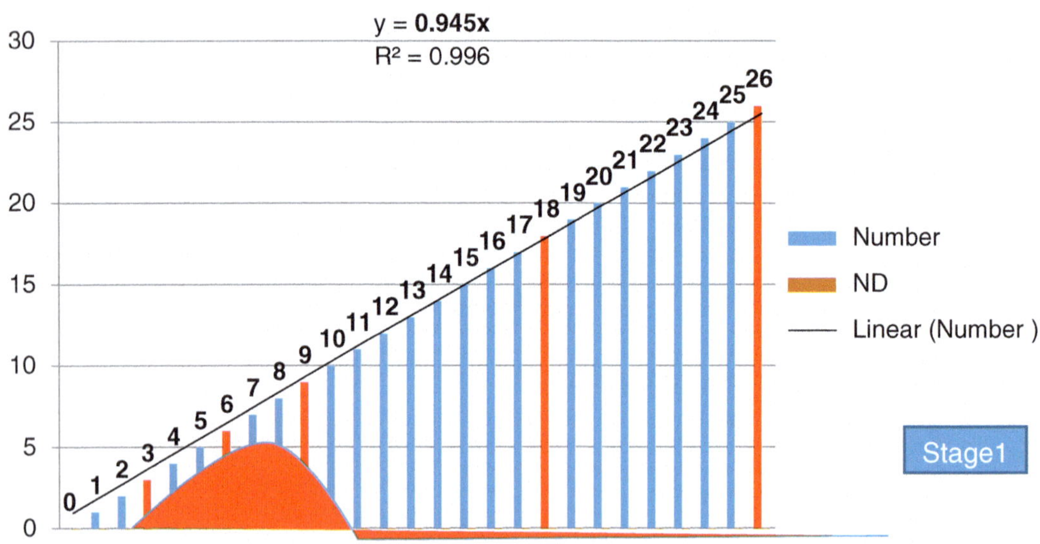

Fig. 1.23 Normal distribution simulation intended to treat the patients on prophylactic Oseltamivir drug

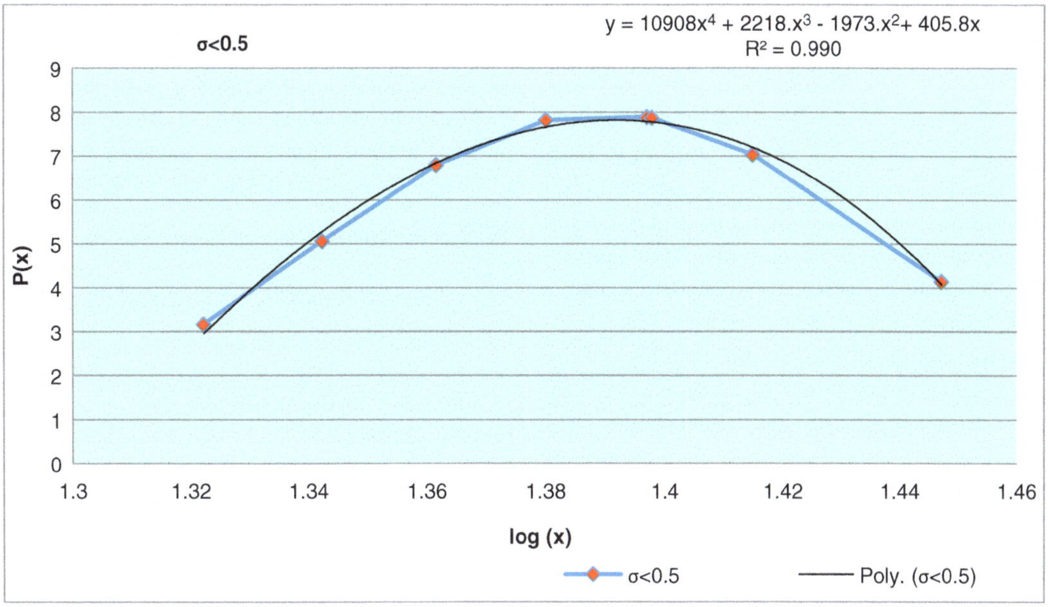

Fig. 1.24 Normal distribution simulation intended to treat the patients on prophylactic Oseltamivir

Table 1.3 Difference between explanation and pragmatic design

Explanatory	Criteria	Pragmatic
Narrow	Eligibility	Broad
Highly targeted	Recruitment	In clinic
Single,special centre	Settings	Usual care
Research Infrastructure	Organization	Clinical infrastructure
Strict protocol	Delivery	Flexible protocol
Incentives,censoring	Adherence	Usual encouragement
Specific to trail	Follow up	Available metrics
Surrogates Bio markers	Out comes	Relevant to patients
As treated	Analysis	Intention to treat

1.58 Limitation

A negative result in a PCT cannot provide whether the *Rx*/intervention is effective under optional conditions; an investigator may need to invest more time and resources to conduct PCT compared to explanatory trails. The PCTs are more pragmatic design to extrapolate various challenges as comapred to RCT because its potential heterogeneity of the treatment in large setup (Table 1.3).

1.59 Statistical Implications of Pragmatic Design

The pragmatic design has been demonstrated by logistic regression model; this prevailing statistical model will help us to know the effect of drug interventions with multiple clinical and historical data sets of patients. The analysis was designed by using one dependent variable and group of independent variables. Model setting was claimed based on the response of the drug. Since the response of administered drug was categorized into two interventions (1 coded as good response and 0 coded as poor response), the criteria of these two dichotomous variables were regressed with group of independent variables (age, sex, demographic profile, complications, drug reaction, duration of drug, clinical findings, etc.) (Wittes and Wallenstein 1987).

$$y = a + \beta_0 x_0 + \beta_1 x_1 + \beta_2 x_1 \ldots \beta_n x_n \quad (1.23)$$

$$y = \frac{1}{1 + e^{-\beta_0 x_0 + \beta_1 x_1 + \beta_2 x_1 \ldots \beta_n x_n}} \quad (1.24)$$

$$\text{Logit}\left[\frac{y}{1-y}\right] = \text{odd}\left(\frac{1}{1 + e^{-\beta_0 x_0 + \beta_1 x_1 + \beta_2 x_1 \ldots \beta_n x_n}}\right) \quad (1.25)$$

By putting "*Y*" in sigmoid function we will get the above results

1.60 Cluster RCTs Design

Custer RCTs studies in which patients are grouped (cluster) on the basis of geography of practice (caregivers, hospitals, community) and then Randomized as a group to either intervention or control arm. Community-based cluster RCTs are generally characterized by small number of cluster with a large number of patients in each cluster. They are reviewed as a pragmatic methodology to measure the effectiveness of intervention on large scale. More recently researcher have suggested that, the cluster RCTs can be used to determine the comparative effectiveness of two or more therapies on simultaneously where there exists a natural variation in practical approach. The longitudinal studies sometimes use cluster techniques to study the impact of intervention on the same group of patients over time (Fig. 1.25).

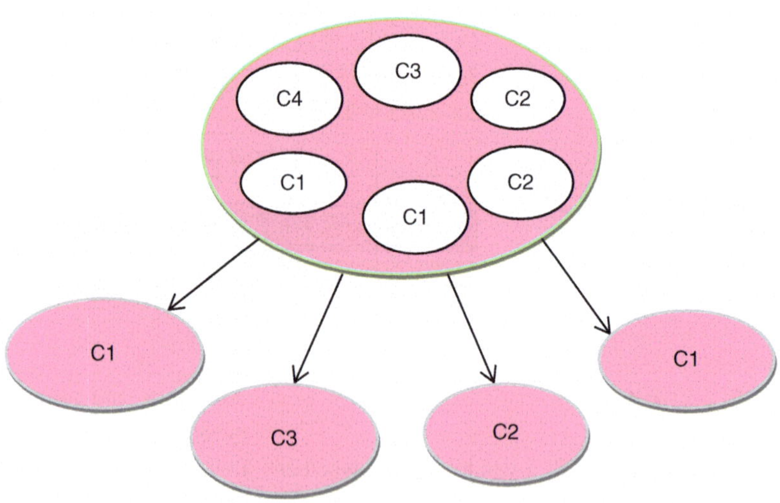

Fig. 1.25 Cluster RCTs design approach

1.60.1 Statistical Implications of Cluster Design

$$cc(\omega)=\frac{\sum_{r=induction}^{r=t} C_1(r_1)C_2(r_2)C_3(r)....C_n(r_3)}{\sqrt{\sum_{r=induction}^{r=t} y_1^2(r_1)\sum_{r=induction}^{r=t} y_2^2(r_1)\ldots\sum_{r=induction}^{r=t} y_n^2(r_1)}} \tag{1.26}$$

where $C_1,C_2..C_n$ is the cluster selected based on the geographical location

$r_1,r_2,r_3..r_n$ is the correlation co efficient will be obtained from data sets

$y_1,y_2,y_3..y_n$ is the dependent variables, i.e., drug response (0–200 scale)

1.61 Crossover Design

A crossover design is adopted based on the time or situation, design which can allow patients to act as their own control of intervention, enabling comparisons between and within groups (>one groups). Arbitrary 1–2 Patients receive a sequence of treatments (S_1,S_2) over successive time periods; crossing over is done at an alternative therapy as part of the sequence group. At the inception of the study intervention, each patient is assigned to a sequence (e.g., AB vs. BA) or (ABC, BCA, ACB, CBA) with successive treatments typically separated by a washout period (a specified period of nonuse prior to initiation of therapy or trail). Because all the participants received the same number of treatments, usually in different sequences, it is merely possible to determine how patient attributes or characteristics will influence drug response to treatment. There are several types of crossover designs (CD) with different numbers of periods and sequences, and all these designs have their own sets of considerations on subjective conditions (Fig. 1.26).

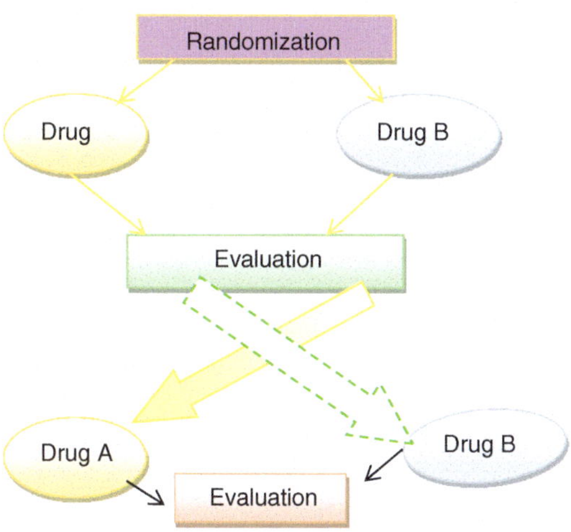

Fig. 1.26 Schematic diagram of crossover design

1.61.1 Statistical Implication

The analysis is being done on two-way or three-way analysis, if the experimentation could be conducted using RCBD, LSD, and lattice design. After obtaining data sets from the RCT trail, analysis will be carried out in R studio or SAS statistical software. An attempt to apply standard analysis methods on a subjective interest (Table 1.4).

1.61.2 Limitations

There are several shortfalls of crossover design in clinical experimentation; there is no guarantee that washout periods will completely control car-

Table 1.4 ANOVA for crossover design

Source of variation	*df*	SS	MSS	F_{Cal}	F_{table} @error *df*
Treatment	$(t-1)$	SSt	MSSt	MSSt/MSSe	$F_{Cal} \geqq F_{tab}$, reject H_o
Subjects	$(t-1)$	SSb	MSSb	MSSb/MSSe	$F_{Cal} \geqq F_{tab}$, reject H_o
Periods	$(t-1)$	SSp	MSSp	MSSp/MSSe	$F_{Cal} \geqq F_{tab}$, reject H_o
Error	$(t-1)(t-2)$	SSe	MSSe		
Total	(t_n-1)	SST			

ryover effects in the interest of researcher. Profusely, long washout periods might unavoidably increase the duration of the experiment. Ethical concerns (how long can a patient be refused treatment during a washout period) and incomplete knowledge (what washout period length is sufficient) may sometimes lead to inadequate washout periods drawn by the researcher. Within each unit, or patient, responses to therapy are likely to be correlated (e.g., a single patient's response to treatment A is correlated with that patient's response to treatment B; the responses are not independent). This causes complexities in both the design and the analysis work.

1.62 Delayed Start Design

Delay start design (DST) design will allow us to know the reducing stage of symptoms or modifying disease in particular time period, e.g., evaluation of people living with HIV (PLHIVs) who are receiving highly active antiretroviral therapy (HAART) treatment for stage or phase of reduction of virus in the body, also to know exponential distribution of CD_4 counts in defined time interval. A delayed-start study is being conducted in two phases. In Phase I, patients are randomized to receive either the active HAART treatment or a control treatment (Not receiving HAART). Phase I should be long enough in duration to allow the effects of the treatment on the disease symptoms to be fully captured based on patient record. At the end of Phase I, we evaluate if any significant differences between the two groups (if present) reflect differences in symptomatic effects, disease modifying effects, or both. In Phase II, the patients in the control group are switched to receive a "delayed-start" of the active treatment, so that every patient in the study receives the active treatment. The patients are then followed for a predetermined length of time. Any beneficial symptomatic effects should be equal in the two groups, and any remaining differences must be attributable to the disease-modifying effect of the treatment group (Fig. 1.27).

An Alzheimer disease is an age-related neurodegenerative disorder characterized by progressive reduction in cognitive function. The course of AD can involve progressive memory loss, behavioral deciles, gait and motor disturbance and the inability to perform activities of daily living, eventually leading to a complete dependence on caregivers, usually followed by nursing dependent palliative care. Medical ethics clearly depicted that, the course of treatment is comparable to delay and early start for the neurodegenerative disorder.

1.62.1 Indicators

Indicators can be used to assess disease progression as well as disease relapses (or other short-term outcomes).

The treatment period is sufficiently long for a therapeutic effect to be obtained with minimal attrition and the same number in both groups.

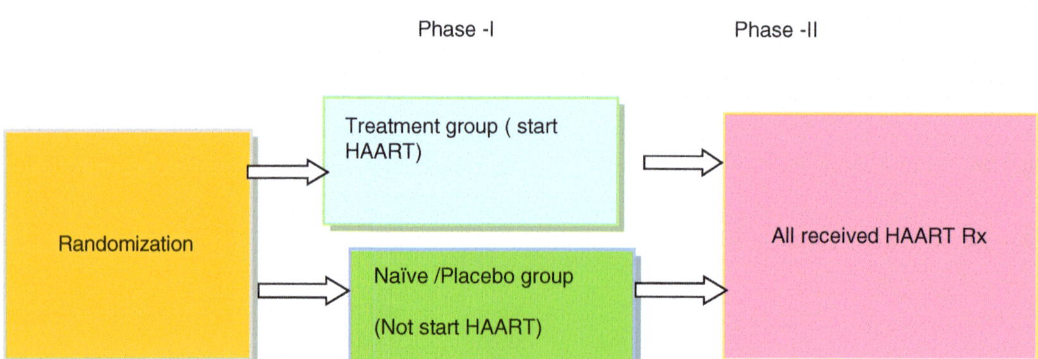

Fig. 1.27 Schematic diagram of delayed start design

Sufficient number of follow-up visits to measure the treatment effect to allow a precise estimator of the treatment effect slope.

1.62.2 Merits

Allow more patients to receive an active treatment and can distinguish effects on symptoms and effect on the disease evolution (progression and relapse)

1.62.3 Demerits

At the start of second phase, the patient is not comparable

No real binding for the second period (phase II) carry over effect possible

1.63 Randomized with Drawl Design

On broad perspective randomized withdrawal design subject to receiving a test treatment for a specified time is randomly assigned to perceiving treatment with test treatments or to placebo (i.e., withdrawal of active therapy). Subject for such trail could be derived from an organized open single arm study, from an existing clinical cohort (but usually with a protocol specified wash—in phase to establish initial therapy base line) to the active arm of controlled trail or from one or both arms of an active control trail. Any difference that emerges between the group receiving continued treatment and the group randomized to placebo would demonstrate the effect of the active treatment. The pre-randomized observation period on treatment can be of any length; this approach can therefore be used to study long-term persistence of effectiveness when long-term placebo treatment would not be acceptable. The post-withdrawal observation period could be for a fixed duration or could be early escape or time to event (e.g., relapse of depression) approaches. As with early escape design, careful attention should be paid to procedure for monitoring patients and assessing study endpoints to ensure that patients failing on an assigned treatment are identified rapidly (Fig. 1.28).

1.63.1 Merits

1. Used to assess *Rx* continuation in patients who are responding to the *Rx*.
2. Randomization of responders to continue *Rx* or switch to placebo.

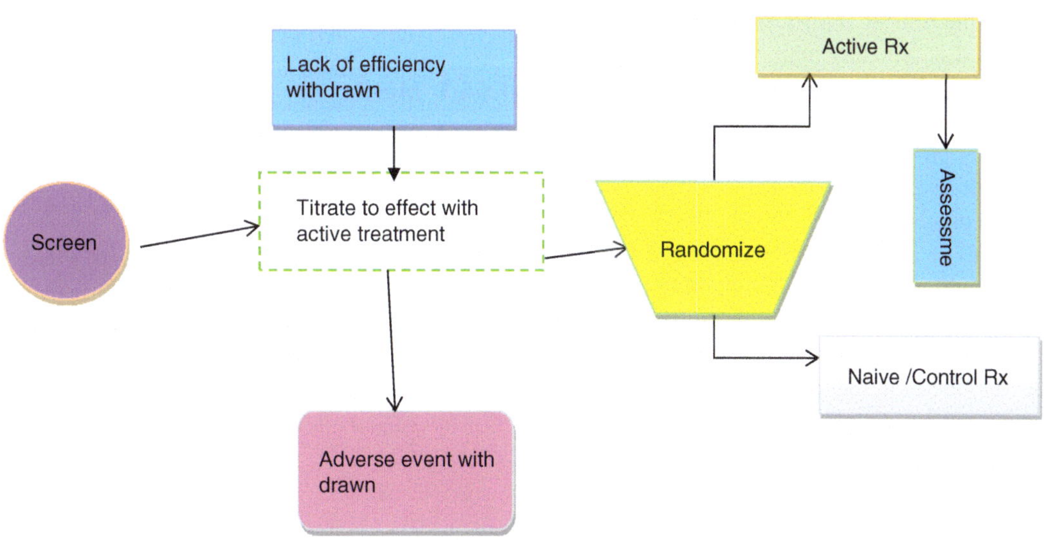

Fig. 1.28 Schematic diagram of Randomized with drawl design

3. The *Rx* effect is overestimated since only respondents are included.
4. All patients initially receiving the tested *Rx* respondents are randomized.
5. Reduce the time on placebo since only respondents randomized to placebo for use in chronic disease can assess if *Rx* needs to be continued or can be stopped.

1.63.2 Demerits

1. Not suitable for unpredictable disease (e.g., spontaneous remission or those with slow evolution), possible carryover effect for adverse effect.

1.64 Adaptive Design

An adoptive design is defined as a study that includes a prospectively planned opportunity for modification of one or more specified aspects of the study design and hypothesis based on the analysis of data (usually interim analysis) from subjects in the study. Further, an adaptive design accomplish for acculturating data sets to decide how to modify clinical aspects of the trail as it continues without determining the validity and integrity of the experimental study. In case of adoptive design we will find many ways in which the trail or statistical procedures may be modified is typically defined prospectively, but can also occur during the trail. An adoptive study designs will include pre-specified interim points or phases in the protocol where investigators can re-evaluate hypothesis or planned statistical procedures. At every planned phase, data set analysis is performed and updated information can be utilized efficiently and to make certain adaptation is being followed. Various categories of adaptation are utilized for conducting the trail, that can be classified into three major categories.

Prospective adaptation—These adaptations are pre-specified in the protocol before the trail begins. Some examples include adaptive randomization stopping a trail due to safety, futility, or efficacy at interim analysis or dropping inferior treatment groups.

Concurrent adaptation—These are the changes that are incorporated as the trail continues. Concurrent adaptation are not specified as priority, but are incorporated when need arises, such as modifying inclusion/exclusion criteria, evaluability criteria (defining what it means to be treated) dose, regimen or treatment duration or changing hypothesis or study endpoints (Fig. 1.29).

Retrospective adaptations—These adaptations are typically made to the statistical analysis plan. They can occur after data set collection, but prior to off blinding of treatment modalities.

Traditional	Adoptive
Accept or reject H_0 in a well-defined population (no modification with amendments)	Pre-specified modification are allowed based on interim analysis
Not more than two or three study arms	Many study arms
Standard Phase I-II phases with clearly separated phase II and III and allows for little learning	Allows early detection at early stage if warranted
Standard statistical methods	Different sets of risks and decision points than conventional statistical methods

1.64.1 Merits

1. More efficient data collections at any point of time, the design will produce massive data sets.
2. It is more applicable to short-term study duration inclusion with less number of patients.
3. To increasing probability of success in achieving the study objectives.
4. Improved understanding of investigational protocol and efforts at larger extent.

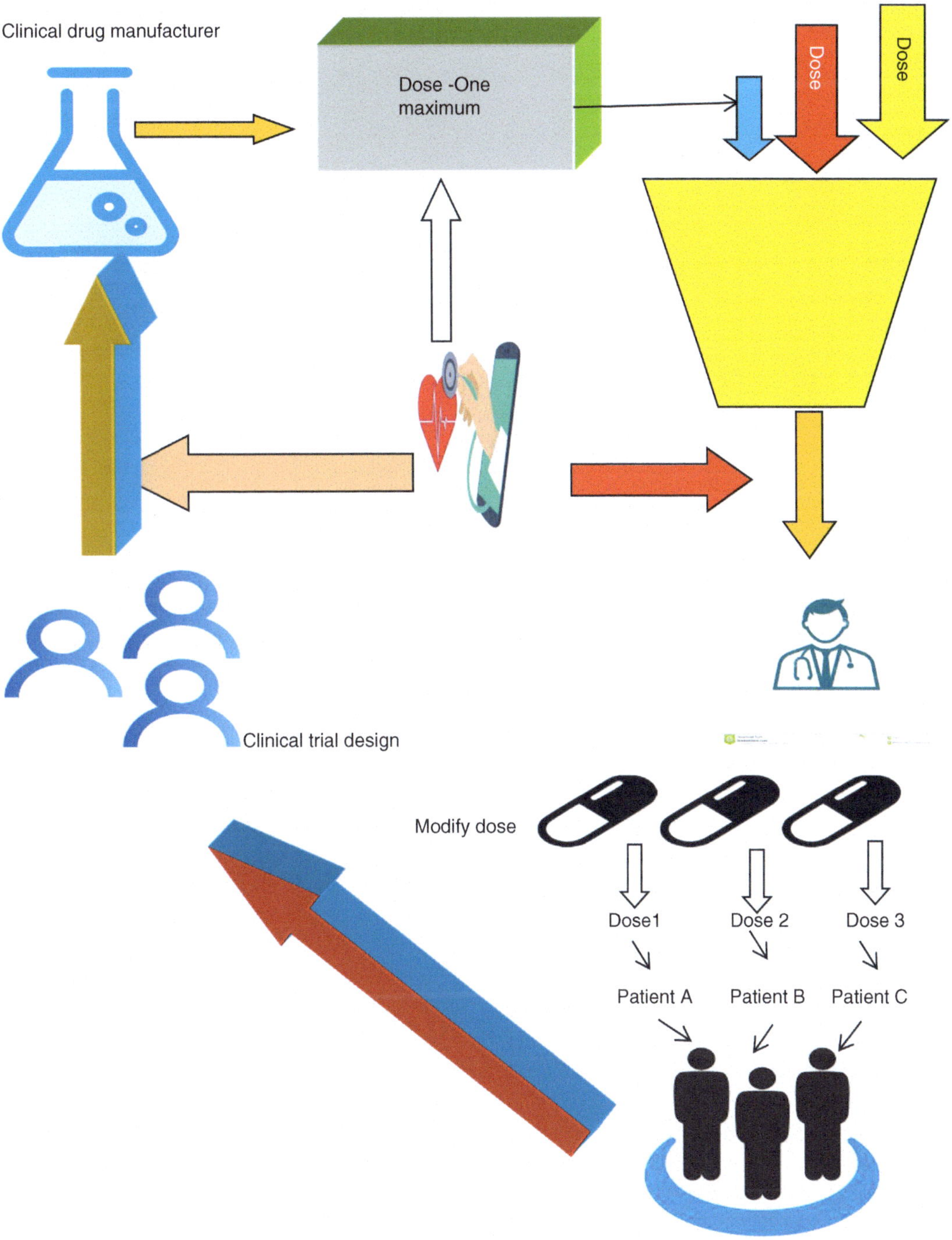

Fig. 1.29 Adoptive design flow diagram

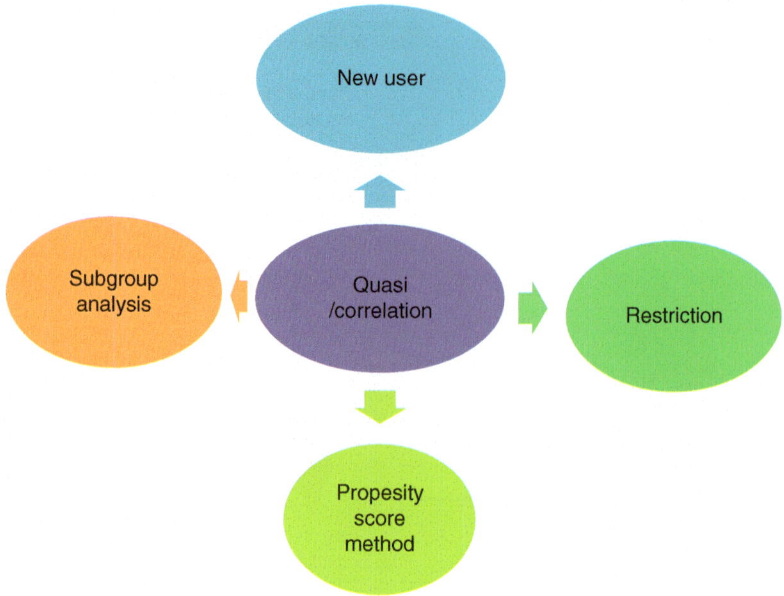

Fig. 1.30 Nonexperimental methods

1.65 Nonexperimental Methods

The essence of nonexperimental methods in clinical research lacks the manipulation of criterion variables of interest, random assignment of patients or participants to be done on certain conditions or order of their conditions with greater accuracy (Garraway et al.1980). In a sense, it is unfair to define this large and diverse set of approaches collectively by what they are not. Nevertheless by doing so reflects the fact that most researchers in clinical research consider the distinction between experimental and nonexperimental research to be an extremely important one. This distinction is just because of obtaining relevant results; although experimental research can provide strong evidence, those changes in an independent variable cause differences in a dependent variable, nonexperimental research generally cannot. As we will see, this inability does not mean that nonexperimental research is less important than experimental research or inferior to it in any general sense. The research questions frame about single variable rather than a statistical relationship between two variables (How accurate the patients responding drug). The cited research questions can be about a noncasual statistical relationship between variables (correlation between drug interaction and efficacy). The research questions can be about a casual relationship, but the independent variable cannot be manipulated or participants cannot be randomly assigned to conditions or order of conditions (the patients memory loss due to high dosage of drug); the research question can be broad and exploratory or it can be about what is likely to have particular experience. Further, the choice between the experimental and nonexperimental approaches is generally dictated by the nature of the research question. The nonexperimental methods may be classified as follows (Fig. 1.30).

1.66 New-User Design

A new-user design is a novel type of nonexperimental study that identifies all patients in defined population "*N*" at treatment inception. This type of design can eliminate certain biases by excluding prevalent users, only retaining those patients with a minimum period of nonuse and/or no use prior to the treatment. Given the critics in identifying new users especially in Pharmacoepidemilogical studies, the patients can be identified as new users if they have specified period of nonuse prior to inception of *Rx* (washout period). The chance of an initiator being true new users can be increased by requiring longer washout periods before the start of follow-up (Langlands et al. 1980). Choosing a comparison group can be a

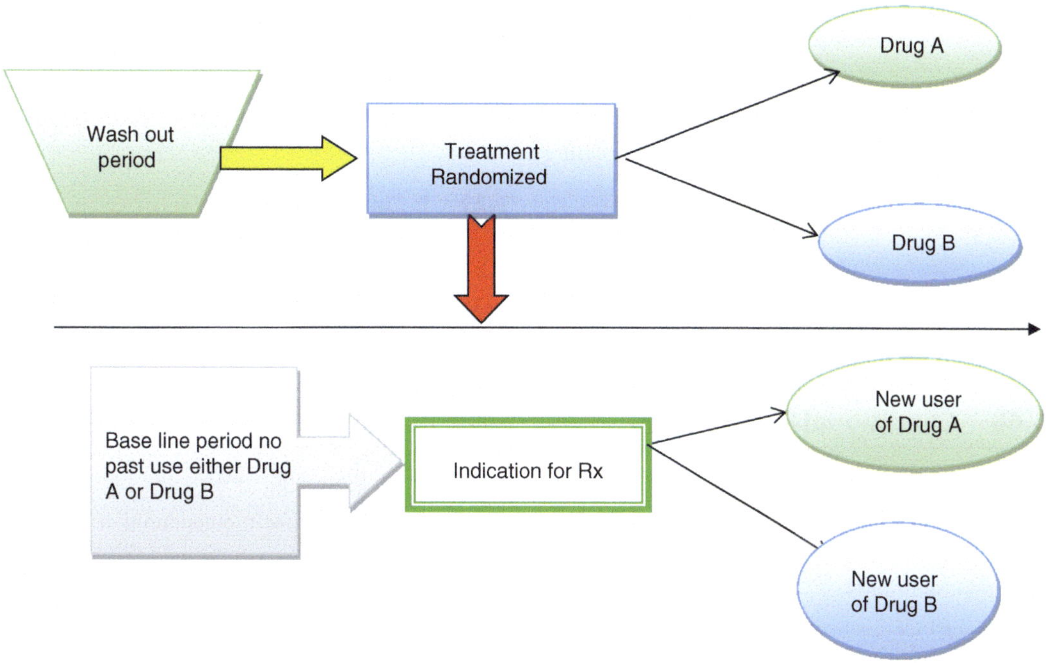

Fig. 1.31 New-user design flow diagram

complex and subjective issues, with the ideal comparison being with patients having uniform distributions of estimated risk factors (RF) for the study outcome. New-user design can be initiated as cohort study or as a nested case–control study (a case–control study performed within existing cohort with the comparison group ideally consisting of alternative treatment users or nonusers). However, the new-user design could be considered when the rate at which treatment-related outcomes varies with the time elapsed since inception of *Rx*. In such being the case, the period of early use of pharmacotherapy is significantly associated with a declining trend of risk outcome, i.e., the bias will be introduced if prevalent user groups included and the risk of outcome does in fact vary with time intervals. For example, clinically we consider past studies done in the way back 1990s; it was reported that there was an excess risk of venous thromboembolism in users of third-generation oral contraceptives as compared to users of earlier agents ($p < 0.001$). Since the risk of venous thromboembolism was found to be greater earlier in therapy, and the users of third generation oral contraceptives have started using more recently than the users of earlier therapies, the results conclude that excess risk identified and attributable to the significant difference was found in duration of therapy between comparison groups. If the user of earlier therapies were observed from the time of treatment inception, additional events might be eventually ascertained with certain conditions (Dupont 1988). The new-user designs can eliminate this type of under-ascertainment bias because compilation begins with the start of the current course of treatment for recruited patients (Fig. 1.31).

1.67 Glossary

1.67.1 Random Variable

A variable which is attached to the probability value, usually denoted by capital Roman letter such as $X, Y \ldots$, is a function that assigns a number to each outcome in the sample space. For example, the HIV patients who are taking HAART treatment where we sample one individual from the population

$X(\omega)$= The survival time for HIV infected patient ω

$Y(\omega)$= CD4 and RNA plasma viral load changes for HIV infected patient ω

$Z(\omega)$= Duration of HAART taking of HIV patients

The probability distribution of random variable "X" is just a list of all different possible values that "X" can take together with corresponding probabilities.

The mean expectation of X is $E(X)=\sum_{\omega\in©}X(\omega)p(\omega)=\sum_{x}xP(X=x)$, and the variance of X is

$$\operatorname{var}(X)=\sum_{\omega\in©}\{x(\omega)-E(X)\}2p(\omega)=\sum_{x}\{x-E(x)\}2P(X=x)$$
$$=E\{X-E(X)\}2=E(X^2)-\{E(X)\}2 \tag{1.27}$$

1.68 Conditional Expectation

Suppose we have two random variable X and Y considered for the same probability of the experiments, then we ascertained the expectations of "X" conditional on knowing that $Y=y,$ by $E\left(\frac{X}{Y}=y\right)$ and this is computed as $E(X/Y=y)=\sum_{\omega:Y(\omega)=y}X(\omega)P^{p(\omega)}P(Y=y)$. The conditional expectation of "X" given by "Y" was denoted by $E(X/Y)$ is itself a random variable which assign the value $E(X/Y=y)$ to every outcome ω for which $Y(\omega)=y$. Specifically we note that $E(X/Y)$ is a function of "Y."

Since $E(X/Y)$ is itself considered a random variable, we have an expectation $E\{E(X/Y\}$. By the definition of expectation this equals to $E\{E(X/Y\}=\sum_{\omega\in©}E\{E(X/Y)(\omega)p(\omega)\}$.

By rearranging this sum, first within the partition $\{\omega: Y(\omega)=y\}$, and then across the partitions for the different values of y, we get the following equations

$$E\{E(X/Y\}=\sum_{y}\left\{\frac{\sum_{\omega:Y(\omega)=y}X(\omega)p(\omega)}{P(Y=y)}\right\}P(Y=y)$$
$$=\sum_{\omega\in©}X(\omega)p(\omega)=E(X)$$

Thus we have proved the very important results that

$$E\{E(X/Y\}=E(X)$$

1.69 Conditional Variance

There is also a very important relationship involving the conditional variance. Just like expectation, the conditional variance of X given Y, denoted by var (X/Y), is a random variable, which assigned the value $\operatorname{var}(X/Y=y)$ to each outcome ω, where $Y(\omega)=y$ and

$$\operatorname{var}(X/Y=y)=E\left[\{X-E(X/Y=y)\}2/Y=y\right]$$
$$=\sum_{\omega:Y(\omega)=y}\{X(\omega)-EE(X/Y=y)\}2\frac{p(\omega)}{p(Y=y)}$$

Equivalently, $\operatorname{var}(X/(Y=y))=E[\{X\wedge 2/Y=y)-E((X)/(Y=y)\}2]$

It turns out that the variances of a random variables X equals

$$\operatorname{var}(X)=E\{\operatorname{var}(X/Y)\}+\operatorname{var}\{\operatorname{var}(X/Y\}$$

This followed because of

$$E\{\operatorname{var}(X/Y)\}=E\left[E(X\wedge 2/Y)-\{E(X/Y)\}2=E(X\wedge 2)-E\left[\{E(X/Y)\}\right]2\right] \tag{1.28}$$

And the equation becomes

$$=\operatorname{var}\{E(X/Y)\}=E\left[\{E(X/Y)2\}\right]-\left[E\left[\{E(X/Y)\}\right]\right]^2 \tag{1.29}$$

The clinician will be acquainted to adopt the hierarchical models for conducting "*N*" studies from a population, for each study """we sample n_i individuals at random from the *i*th study group and count the number of responses *Xi* variables. We shall also assume that the sample size $n_1, n_2, \ldots N_n$ are random variables from some distribution.

1.70 Conclusion

The practical aspects of present chapter has described the advanced study design; these study designs shows how research questions are articulated with hypothetical assumptions applied in the field of medical and clinical research. Methodological procedures on this above-said design will claim the significance of the research. These advanced techniques deal with practical implications of the research than how research is organized, planned, and conducted effectively and also provides theoretical and practical explanation of clinical or medical research on broad perspectives. The chapter is very useful for the researcher to obtain systematic results from the experimental areas and confirming the reliable research gap for future line of research work. Various study designs show different series of steps for well constructing of research in the interdisciplinary field as well as in-house research.

References

Ademex (2002) A prospective randomized controlled trial. J Am Soc Nephrol 13:1307–1320

Aggarwal R, Ranganathan P (2019) Study designs: part 2: descriptive studies. Perspect Clin Res 10:34–36

Anturane Reinfarction Trial Research Group (ARTRG) (1980) Sulfinpyrazone in the prevention of sudden death after myocardial infarction. N Engl J Med 392:250–256

Bello AK, Peters J, Wight J, de Zeeuw D, El Nahas M (2008) A population-based screening for microalbuminuria among relatives of CKD patients: the Kidney Evaluation and Awareness Program in Sheffield (KEAPS). Am J Kidney Dis 52:434–443

Biberstein M, Parker BA (1985) Enema-induced hyperphosphatemia. Am J Med 79:645–646

Byron J, Kenward MG (2003) Design and analysis of cross-over trials, 2nd edn. Chapman and Hall, London

Campbell MJ, Machin D (1999) Medical statistics: a common-sense approach, 3rd edn. Wiley, Chichester

Casagrande JT, Pike MC, Smith PG (1978) An improved approximate formula for calculating sample sizes for comparing two binomial distributions. Biometrics 34:483–486

Chambers G, Fairbarn M (1998) Clinical trial design; An introduction to good clinical trial design and the protection of human subjects. Appl Clin Trials 7(9):60–66

Chavalarias D, Ioannidis JP (2010) Science mapping analysis characterizes 235 biases in biomedical research. J Clin Epidemiol 63:1205–1215

Choi B, Noseworthy A (1992) Classification, direction, and prevention of bias in epidemiologic research. J Occup Med 34:265–271

Dalma A, Petralias A, Tsiampalis T, Nikolakopoulos S, Veloudaki A, Kastorini CM et al (2019) Effectiveness of a school food aid programme in improving household food insecurity; a cluster randomized trial. Eur J Public Health 30(1):171–178. https://doi.org/10.1093/eurpub/ckz091

Detsky A, Naglie I (1995) Subgroup analyses: primary and secondary. ACP Journal Club May/June:A12-A14 12. Cook D, Sacket D (1992) On the Clinically Important Difference. ACP Journal Club September/October:A16–A17

Dupont WD (1988) Power calculations for matched case-control studies. Biometrics 44:1157–1168

Dupont WD (2008) Statistical modeling for biomedical researchers, 2nd edn. Cambridge University Press, Cambridge

Dupont WD, Plummer WD (1990) Power and sample size calculations: a review and computer program. Control Clin Trials 11:116–128

Dupont WD, Plummer WD (1998) Power and sample size calculations for studies involving linear regression. Control Clin Trials 19:589–601

Durack DT et al (1981) Opportunistic infections and Kaposi's sarcoma in homosexual men. N Engl J Med 305(24):1465–1467

Ebrahim G, Sullivan K (1999) Mother and child health research methods, 1st edn. Book-Aid, London

Fleiss JL (1981) Statistical methods for rates and proportions, 2nd edn. Wiley, New York, pp 38–46

Freedman M, Osicka T (2006) Reader variability: what we can learn from computer-aided detection experiments. J Am Coll Radiol 3:446–455

Gabbe B, Finch C, Bennell K, Wajswelner H (2003) How valid is a self-reported 12 month sports injury history? Br J Sports Med 37:545–547

Garraway WM, Akhtar AJ, Presscott R et al (1980) Management of acute stroke in the elderly: preliminary results of a controlled trial. Br Med J 280:1040–1043

Gottlieb MS, Schroff R, Schanker HM et al (1981) Pneumocystis carinii pneumonia and mucosal candidiasis in previously healthy homosexual men: evidence of a new acquired cellular immunodeficiency. N Engl J Med 305(24):1425–1431

Grimes D, Schulz K (2002) Bias and causal association in observational research. Lancet 359:248–252

Hopewell S, Dutton S, Yu LM, Chan AW, Altman DG (2010) The quality of reports of randomised trials in 2000 and 2006: comparative study of articles indexed in PubMed. BMJ 340:723

Hulley S, Cummings S, Browner et al (2001) An epidemiologic approach, 2nd edn. Lippincott Williams & Wilkins Publishers, Philadelphia

Indian Council of Medical Research (ICMR) (1991) Multi-centric randomized controlled clinical trial of Kshaarasootra (Ayurvedic medicated thread) in the management of fistula-in-ano. Indian J Med Res 94:177–185

Jorgensen HS, Kammersgaard LP, Nakayama H et al (1999) Treatment and rehabilitation on a stroke unit improves 5-year survival. A community-based study. Stroke 30(5):930–933

Kaerlev L, Lynge L, Sabroe S, Oslen J (2004) Colon cancer controls versus population controls in case-control studies of occupational risk factors. BMC Cancer 4:15

Langlands AO, Presscott RJ, Hamilton T (1980) A clinical trial in the management of operable cancer of the breast. Br J Surg 67:170–174

Lazarus RP, John J, Shanmugasundaram E, Rajan AK, Thiagarajan S, Giri S et al (2018) The effect of probiotics and zinc supplementation on the immune response to oral rotavirus vaccine: a randomized, factorial design, placebo-controlled study among Indian infants. Vaccine 36:273–279

Lilienfeld AM, Lilienfeld DE (1980) Foundations of epidemiology. Oxford University Press, London

Mantel N, Haenszel W (1959) Statistical aspects of the analysis of data from retrospective studies of disease. J Natl Cancer Inst 22:719–748

Mapes DL, Lopes AA, Satayathum S, McCullough KP, Goodkin DA, Locatelli F, Fukuhara S, Young EW, Kurokawa K, Saito A, Bommer J, Wolfe RA, Held PJ, Port FK (2003) Health-related quality of life as a predictor of mortality and hospitalization: the Dialysis Outcomes and Practice Patterns Study (DOPPS). Kidney Int 64:339–349

Masur H, Michelis MA, Greene JB et al (1981) An outbreak of community-acquired Pneumocystis carinii pneumonia: initial manifestation of cellular immune dysfunction. N Engl J Med 305(24):1431–1438

Medical Research Council Working Party (MRCWP) (1977) Randomized controlled trial of treatment for mild hypertension: design and pilot trial. Br Med J 1:1437–1440

Moseley JB, O'Malley K, Petersen NJ et al (2002) A controlled trial of arthroscopic surgery for osteoarthritis of the knee. N Engl J Med 347(2):81–88

Paniagua R, Amato D, Vonesh E, Correa-Rotter R, Ramos A, Moran J, Mujais S (2008) Effects of increased peritoneal clearances on mortality rates in peritoneal dialysis: Tripepi G, Jager KJ, Dekker FW, Wanner C, Zoccali C: bias in clinical research. Kidney Int 73:148–153

Pearson ES, Hartley HO (1970) Biometrika tables for statisticians, vol I, 3rd edn. Cambridge University Press, Cambridge

Pocock S (1983) Clinical trials: a practical approach. Wiley, Chichester

Price DD, Finniss DG, Benedetti F (2008) A comprehensive review of the placebo effect: recent advances and current thought. Annu Rev Psychol 59:565–590

Quinn TJ, Dawson J, Walters MR, Lees KR (2009) Reliability of the modified Rankin Scale: a systematic review. Stroke 40:3393–3395

Ranganathan P, Aggarwal R (2018) Study designs: part 1—an overview and classification. Perspect Clin Res 9:184–186

Ranganathan P, Aggarwal R (2019) Study designs: part 3—analytical observational studies. Perspect Clin Res 10:91–94

Schlesselman JJ (1982) Case-control studies: design, conduct, analysis. Oxford University Press, New York, pp 144–152

Schoenfeld DA, Richter JR (1982) Nomograms for calculating the number of patients needed for a clinical trial with survival as an endpoint. Biometrics 38:163–170

Spilker B (1996) Fundamental principles, considerations, and techniques in the interpretation of clinical data. In: Guide to clinical trials. Lippincott-Raven T, Philadelphia, pp 505–558

Stel VS, Jager KJ, Zoccali C, Wanner C, Dekker FW (2007) The randomized clinical trial: an unbeatable standard in clinical research? Kidney Int 72:539–542

Tuccinardi D, Farr OM, Upadhyay J, Oussaada SM, Klapa MI, Candela M et al (2019) Mechanisms underlying the cardiometabolic protective effect of walnut consumption in obese subjects: a cross-over, randomized, double-blinded, controlled inpatient physiology study. Diabetes Obes Metab 21(9):2086–2095. https://doi.org/10.1111/dom.13773

Vandenbroucke JP (2001) In defense of case reports and case series. Ann Intern Med 134:330–334

Whiteside JL, Hijaz A, Imrey PB, Barber MD, Paraiso MF, Rackley RR, Vasavada SP, Walters MD, Daneshgari F (2006) Reliability and agreement of urodynamics interpretations in a female pelvic medicine center. Obstet Gynecol 108:315–323

Wittes J, Wallenstein S (1987) The power of the Mantel-Haenszel test. J Am Stat Assoc 82:1104–1109

2 Advanced Designs of Experiment Approach to Clinical and Medical Research

2.1 Introduction

Some set of rules and regulations that have been imposed for conducting the drug trial or experiment is called as an experimental design. A clinical researcher wishes to compare the response rate on newly manufactured drugs (approved by the FDA) of A and B. Primarily, the researchers will make an architectural plan or layout of the experimental design with an equal number of patients for each trial (Subramanian et al. 2005). The presumption of the estimation of efficacy of drugs for each dose has been measured based on the objective of the interest. If the administered drugs can yield a better response rate on the basis of different confounders, then the experimentation is said to be success. With valid reason despite simplicity and commonsense appeal of the clinical trial, the experimental procedure is just to be outlined by the researchers before induction; it has been a considerable part of the subjects; it is one of the good moves, which can presume that any significant differences will be found in the (prognosis) two drugs or it may be caused by the formulation and other chance factors, etc. (Wu et al. 2004). Certainly, it is not being a true factor even if the same formulation of the drugs A and B has been administered by the physician; the efficacy of the particular drugs will differ based on the drug formulation, food intake, physical exercise/activity, and mental status of the patients; meanwhile, other factors such as patient illness, residual effect of past illness, duration of illness, immunity, body condition, and many confounders will be affected by the negative response rate. Besides all the above factors, the nursing and palliative care support is greatly affected drug response rate. The factors affecting drug trial and pharmokinetic differences from other sources of variation was studied by (Subramanian et al. 2005) (the clinical researchers must be able to design the architectural plan for conducting experimentation before inception). The experimentation can allow him to estimate the drug efficacy and formulation from suitable statistical tools without any ambiguity (difference and environmental factors). The logic behind the above-cited decision is yet to be simple, e.g., two kinds of drug trials are conducted in different geographical locations with many confounders (temperature, humidity, relative humidity food habit, water, and other climatic factors). The relative confounding factors of the intervention would greatly affect the dose response of the administered drugs. In this section, an observed response rate of marginal differences is smaller than the expected value of realized response and also alienated with many confounders achieved to know the drug response; obviously, the response will be negatively associated with selected subjects or cases in case if both drug trials will be conducted under the identical condition at controlled environmental condition (age and sex-matched clinical trial); the response rate is

B. D. M., B. Narasimha Murthy, *Design of Experiments and Advanced Statistical Techniques in Clinical Research*, https://doi.org/10.1007/978-981-15-8210-3_2

larger than the expected values, and the research findings will be positively associated with selected subjects. Hence, the researchers need to forecast the effectiveness and efficacy of the drug differences, which can be determined by suitable experimental designs or statistical methods. The differences among dose–response rate are treated alike and it is called as experimental error. These errors are aroused from the experimental area and human intervention; it is a primary source for deciding experimentation, whether an observed difference is real or just it may be aggravated due to chance factors. Every clinical experimentation must be designed to measure the experimental errors at greatest accuracy. There are three basic principles adopted to prevent or curb the experimental errors, i.e., replication, randomization, and local control.

2.1.1 Replication

In the same way, there are at least two kinds of drugs with same formulation necessary to determine the observed and expected differences on the estimation of response rate (treated alike), since the experimental error can be measured only if there are at least two drug trials conducted at the same geographical location (or receiving the same treatment or subjects). Thus, the researcher should obtain a measure of experimental error through replication (repetition of treatment or subjects more than once); the replication is necessary for the control of experimental error. In general, more number of replications will be able to reduce the sample and population probable error (minimization of PE) (sampling and nonsampling error).

2.1.2 Randomization

The Randomization procedure ensures that each drug will have an equal chance of being assigned in any particular experimental unit or ward. Consequently in agriculture field experimentation, the randomization procedure can evolve for testing the subjects or treatment at larger area and also it has been replicated in any particular environmental condition in various experimental site. Fisher (1926) (renowned statistician) coined the term randomization procedure or scheme. He employed the randomization techniques in agricultural research experimentation to evaluate the treatment effects in various plots.

2.1.3 Control of Error

It is an ability to detect excising observed differences among treatment groups. However, an increasing number of subjects resulting to appear smaller standard errors in experimental area, (the size of the experimental error decreases) a good experimental site is able to incorporate all possible means of various errors (which are minimizing the experimental error) (SE). The following techniques are used for controlling experimental error.

(a) Blocking
(b) Proper plot techniques
(c) Data analysis or compilation

2.1.4 Blocking

The researcher assigning the treatment groups in experimental units that are as similar as possible together in the same groups (generally referred to as block) and there by assigning all possible homogeneous treatments into each block separately. An independent heterogeneous variation among blocks shall be measured at greater accuracy and higher precision (received from experimental error). In case of clinical experimentation, the substantial variation within experimental unit is expected to correlate significant reduction of experimental error; it is usually achieved from proper blocking techniques.

2.1.5 Proper Experimental Techniques

Almost in all types of clinical and drug trial experimentation, the selected parameters are absolutely essential to measure the drug potency and efficacy at singleton drug trial; overwhelmingly, all factors have been kept at constant and normal distribution assumption was applied for measuring the errors in selected experimental area or subjects beside with estimation of maximum likelihood (MLEs) of individual factors is very important for testing the null hypothesis. In this accord, the treatment group shall be maintained uniformly in all experimental sites or units or hospital wards.

2.1.6 Data Analysis

In case of compilation of resulted findings, blocking is a very essential tool to incorporate the standard error at greater extent, whereas blocking is alone at the time of assignment of treatment in experimental sites; it may not be able to achieve a good control of experimental error; and the proper choice of data analysis will help the researcher greatly for the estimation of standard error (SE) in selected sites. Many clinical and patient oriented research, covariance analysis is most commonly used technique for estimation of SE in homogeneous subblocks or units (e.g., yield response of paddy crop was measured in association with weed). In this propinquity, one or more covariate analysis will be employed to test the null hypothesis and also the characters are measured on the basis of scientific evidence (historical data) whose functional relationship with respect to the characters has measured by suitable statistical methods (data analysis) simultaneously on the primary objective of interest.

2.2 Design on Single Factor Clinical Experiments

The researcher may conduct a clinical trial in different level of settings; in case the trial is attempted to evaluate the potency of drug with respect to age, the trial is said to be a single factor. However, the single factor experimentation has derived only one factor to assess the potency of the drug over a period of time. The factor variation has been measured in terms of only one attribute while rest of the attributes are kept constant. The experimental unit or treatment solely consists of different levels on the single variable or factor. All other factors are applied uniformly to experimental units at desired level of significance, for example, the clinical trial consists of age for the validation of drug with the use of confounder variables like sex, history of the patients, illness, coinfection, etc. On the other hand, single factor experiment is a favorable tool (Shan et al. 2013, 2016) in clinical trial where several doses of drugs are tested under the identical condition/control condition, (the trial on several kind of drugs are tested with age factor). The randomized clinical trial on several confounders has been tested only on a single defined factor (sex, geographical area, etc.). There are two groups of experimental designs applicable for a single factor clinical experimentation. One group of the experimentation is the family of complete block design which is more suited for experimentation considering a small number of patients (it is characterized by blocks or units); each unit consists of at least one complete data set of treatments. The other group is the family of incomplete block design which is more suited for experimentation with a large number of patients (treatment or subjects) considered on the different geographical location and it is characterized by different blocks/units/wards.

2.3 Complete Randomized Design

A complete randomized design (CRD) is only appropriate for the experimentation conducted under homogeneous condition (pot culture, drug trial, and laboratory experiment). In other manner, the complete randomized design (CRD) is one of the basic designs suitable for small-scale experiment (treatment group <9). The treatment groups are assigned or allocated randomly so that each experimental unit has received the subjects on equal chance (receiving any one of the treatment: T_1, T_2, T_3, etc). For example, in drug trial experimentation, the researcher has categorized the patients or subjects based on the homogeneous groups with respect to age, gender, and location. The design is formulated by the researcher considering the above factors. The factors should not be overlapping; each factor is independent and identical in nature and also the errors are associated normally distributed with mean 'μ' and common variance 'σ^2' respectively. The randomization techniques have not been adopted for the allocation of treatment or subjects to the experimental area during the study period.

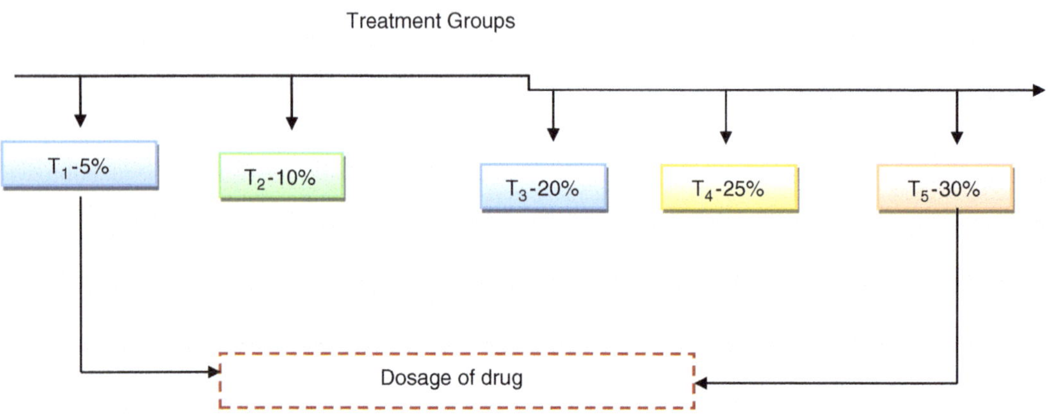

Layout of a design of CRD

2.3.1 Randomization

Treatment randomization with respect to unit

1-(T_1)	2-(T_2)	3-(T_1)	4-(T_2)
5-(T_3)	6-(T_3)	7-(T_3)	8-(T_4)
9-(T_5)	10-(T_2)	11-(T_4)	12-(T_1)
13-(T_2)	14-(T_5)	15-(T_2)	16-(T_2)
17-(T_4)	18-(T_4)	19-(T_5)	20-(T_3)

Method 1: Determine the total number of experimental plots (n) as the product of the number of treatments (t) and the number of replication (r), *i.e.*, $n = r * t = (4)(5) = 20$.

Method 2: Assign a plot number to each experimental plot in any convenient manner, for example, 1...20.

Method: Assign the treatment to the experimental plot (read above table) by pipette random number table or by drawing play card method.

2.3.2 Analytical Method

There are two sources of variation among the "n" observations obtained from a CRD trial. One is the treatment variation, and the other is experimental error. The following analytical methods are for compilation of data.

Assumption of the model

$$y_{ij} = \alpha_i + \beta_j + \epsilon_{ij}, \qquad (2.1)$$

where y_{ij} = Observed prognosis value of ith patient and j^{th} ward or hospital

α_i = Effect of trial drug on i^{th} patient

β_j = Effect of trial drug in j^{th} ward or hospital

ϵ_{ij} = Error associated with effect of trial drug on i^{th} patient j^{th} ward or hospital, $\epsilon_{ij \sim N(\mu,\sigma^2)}$

In case of interaction between the patients on trial drug and hospitals, the Eq. (2.1) becomes

$$y_{ijk} = \alpha_i + \beta_{ij} + \gamma_{jk} + \epsilon_{ijk} \qquad (2.2)$$

α_i = Effect of trial drug on i^{th} patient

β_j = Effect of trial drugs on i^{th} patient and j^{th} ward or hospital

γ_{jk} = Interaction effect between i^{th} patient j^{th} ward and k^{th} location

ϵ_{ij} = Error associated with effect ith patient j^{th} ward and k^{th} location, $\epsilon_{ijk \sim N(\mu,\sigma^2)}$

2.3.3 Analysis of Variance (ANOVA)

Total $df = (r)$ (t) − 1 = eg (4) (7) − 1 = 27

Treatment $df = (t - 1) = (7–1) = 6$

Error $df = t(r - 1) = 7(4–1) = 21$

The error df can also be obtained through subtraction from

Error df = Total df – Treatment df = 27–6 = 21

$$\text{Correction factor}(\text{CF}) = \frac{G^2}{(r)(t)}$$

$$\text{Total SS} = \sum_{I=1}^{n} Xi^2 - \text{CF}$$

$$\text{Treatment SS} = \frac{\sum_{i=1}^{n} Ti^2}{r}$$

$$\text{Error SS} = \text{Total SS} - \text{Treatment SS}$$

495063	df	Sum of square	Mean sum of square	Computed "F"
Treatment	$(t - 1)$	St^2	$\text{MST} = \frac{St^2}{(t-1)}$	$F = \frac{\text{MST}}{\text{MSE}} = \frac{S1^2}{S2^2}$
Experimental error	$t(r - 1)$	Se^2	$\text{MSE} = \frac{Se^2}{t(r-1)}$	
Total	$(r)(t) - 1$			

Illustration 1: The researcher wishes to determine the adherence of HIV drug (Stavudine + ZN + EFV) in the calendar years 2020. He has divided the data sets into three groups based on the age criteria G_1: <30 years, G_2: 31–40 years, and G_3: 41–50 years, respectively. The hypothesis he tested was at 1% level of significance (Any significant differences between the groups and adherence level)

Data summary					
Groups	N	Mean	Std. dev.	Std. error	
Group 1 (<30 years)	5	5.4	4.1593	1.8601	
Group 2 (31–40 years)	5	2.8	2.3875	1.0677	
Group 3 (41–50 years)	5	10.4	3.4351	1.5362	
ANOVA Summary					
Source	df	Sum of squares SS	Mean square MS	F-stat	P-value
Between groups	2	149.2	74.6	6.4311	0.0126
Within groups	12	139.1994	11.5999		
Total	14	288.3994			

$F_{\text{calculated}} >= F_{\text{Table}}$ value, the results found to be significant at 1% level of significance. Null hypothesis was rejected. As per the resulted findings, drug adherence level was found to be statistically significant irrespective of groups.

Analytical methods

Between Groups Degrees of Freedom: $df = k - 1$, where k is the number of groups.

Within Groups Degrees of Freedom: $df = (N - k)$, where N is the total number of subjects.

Total Degrees of Freedom: $df = (N - 1)$.

Sum of Squares Between Groups: $SS_B = S_{i=1k} n_i(x_i - x)^2$, where n_i is the number of subjects in the i-th group.

Sum of Squares Within Groups: $SS_W = S_{i=1}^{k}(n_i - 1)S_i^2$, where S_i is the standard deviation of the i-th group.

Total Sum of Squares: $SS_T = SS_B + SS_W$

Mean Square Between Groups: $MS_B = SS_B/(k - 1)$

Mean Square Within Groups: $MS_W = SS_W/(N - k)$

F-Statistic (or F-ratio): $F = MS_B/MS_W$

2.4 Randomized Complete Block Design

The randomized complete block design (RCBD) is most widely used architectural research plan in medical, agricultural, biological, and engineering sciences. It is a basic experimental design demonstrated in clinical research. RCBD design especially suited for randomized control trial (RCT) employed at different geographical locations, where the number of patients and treatment groups should not be large and the experimental area is known for demonstrating the predictable productive gradient. The primary distinguished features of RCBD is the formation of blocks; in each blocks, treatments were allocated randomly and blocks were comprising an equal size and shape, also each unit of experimental material consists of homogeneous treatment groups (number of patients) (Shan et al. 2017).

2.4.1 Blocking Techniques

The primary aim of blocking is to condense or reduce the experimental error by eliminating the contribution of known source of variation (e.g., environmental, permanent and temporary environment, drug interaction, age, gender, past residual effect of drug) among the experimental units. This was done by grouping the experimental units into homogeneous blocks; such being the case, variability within each block (grouping of patients with similar characteristics) is minimized and variability between the blocks has been maximized. Because only the variation within a block becomes part of the experimental error, blocking is most effective tool when the experimental unit (selected patients groups) has been estimated a predictable pattern of the variability. Further, the predictable pattern of patient's selection is a very important domain to correlate the clinical trials at larger manifesto. After identifying the specific source of variability, the estimation of gradient is one move and it should be used as the extrapolation of blocking. As per the research modalities, the sample size and type of drugs used in clinical trial is prime and researcher must be included to maximize the variability among experimental units or blocks. When the error gradient is unidirectional (i.e., there is only one gradient) that was used in long horizontal basis of the patients, recruitment will be necessary to carry out the research. Further, orient these blocks in similar condition, so that the length of the study is perpendicular to the known source of error gradient, respectively. When the drug prognosis factors occur in two directions with one gradient much stronger than the other, ignore the weaker gradient and follow the preceding guideline of unidirectional gradient. If error prognosis gradient occurs in two directions with both gradients equally strong and perpendicular to each other, choose one of these alternatives to formulate the study design and also use proper blocking techniques to concur the square as possible; use long narrow blocks with their length perpendicular to the direction of one gradient and use covariance techniques (Pocock et al. 1975).

2.4.2 Randomization and Layout

The randomization process of RCBD is applied separately and independently to each of the blocks. For example, a clinical experimentation with six treatment groups A,B,C,D,E, F and four replications to illustrate the following procedure.

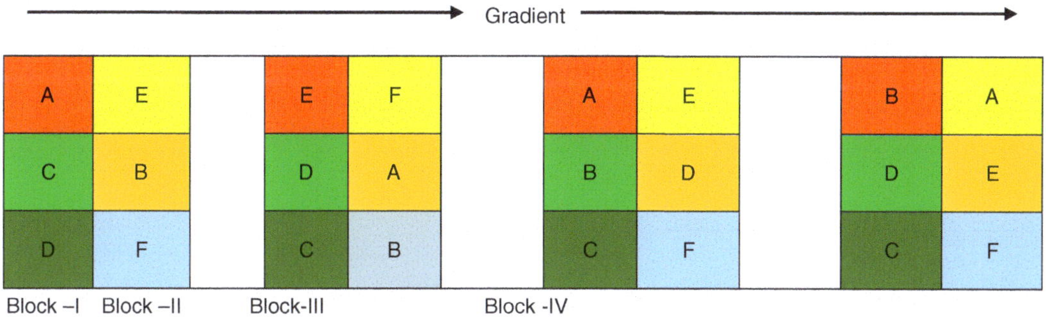

In randomized clinical trial, we can involve human subjects; we often use gender and age classes that are the blocking factors. We simply divide our subjects into age classes; however, this parameter does not consider gender variable. Therefore, we partition our subjects by gender and from there into homogeneous age classes. Thus, we did a block of subjects that is defined by the combination of factors like gender and age class. Often in medical studies or research, the blocking factors used the type of institution. This provides a very useful blocking factor, hopefully removing institutionally related factors such as size of the institution, types of populations served, and hospitals versus clinics that would influence the overall results of the experimentation (Fisher 1918, 1925c; Kerr and Churchill 2001).

2.4.3 Analytical Method

There are three basic sources of variability aroused from the randomized control block design (RCBD), viz. treatment, replication (or blocks), and experimental error. The clinical researcher's noted a slight change in analytical method, there is one more factor inclusion for testing the null hypothesis at desired level significance and greater precision, because of the addition of replication, which corresponds to the variability among blocks were studied simultaneously in RCBD.

2.4.4 Assumption of the Model

The RCBD can utilize the salient principles of additive and multiplicative linear models—one in which there is no interactions between the treatments and blocks. The error term signifies the randomized complete block model, which can reflect how the treatment effects will be varied from one block to another. In case of RCBD, both the treatments and blocks can be focus at random effects rather than fixed effects if the different levels were selected based on the objective interest at randomly from a population (treatments or blocks). The researcher has been considering this as an inherent procedure discussed in the latter part of the chapter. The RCBD mathematical model with interaction effect was modeled systematically and presented as follows:

$$y_{ijk} = \alpha_i + \tau_j + \beta_{ij} + \epsilon_{ijk}, \quad (2.3)$$

where

y_{ijk} = Observed value of ith patient and j^{th} ward k^{th} hospital

α_i = Effect of trial drug on i^{th} patient

τ_j = Treatment effect of jth block or ward

β_{ij} = Effect of tria drugs on i^{th} patient and jet hospital

ϵ_{ijk} = Error associated with effect of trial drug on i^{th} patient j^{th} ward k^{th} hospital, $\epsilon_{ij \sim N(\mu, \sigma 1^2)}$

2.4.5 Analysis of Variance (ANOVA)

Total $df = (r\,t) - 1$

Replication $df = (r - 1)$

Treatment $df = (t - 1)$

Error $df = (t - 1)\,(r - 1)$

The error df can also be obtained through subtraction as

Error df = Total df – Treatment df – Rep df

$$\text{Correction factor}(\text{CF}) = \frac{G^2}{(r)(t)}$$

$$\text{Total SS} = \sum_{i=1}^{t}\sum_{j=1}^{r} Xij^2 - \text{CF}$$

$$\text{Treatment SS} = \frac{\sum_{i=1}^{t} Ti^2}{r} - \text{CF}$$

$$\text{Replication SS} = \frac{\sum_{j=1}^{r} Ri^2}{t} - \text{CF}$$

$$\text{Error SS} = \text{Total SS} - \text{Treatment SS} - \text{Rep SS}$$

Source of variation	*df*	Sum of Square	Mean sum of square	Computed "*F*"
Treatment	$(t-1)$	St^2	$\text{MST} = \frac{St^2}{(t-1)}$	$\text{Ft} = \frac{\text{MST}}{\text{MSE}}$
Replication	$(r-1)$	Sr^2	$\text{MSR} = \frac{Sr^2}{(r-1)}$	$\text{Fr} = \frac{\text{MSR}}{\text{MSE}}$
Experimental error	$(t-1)(r-1)$	Se^2	$\text{MSE} = \frac{Se^2}{t(r-1)}$	
Total	$(rt)-1$			

$$\text{Co efficient of Variation}(\%) = \frac{\sqrt{\text{Error MS}}}{\text{Grand mean}} \times 100$$

The magnitudinal reduction on experimental error due to blocking by computing the relative efficiency (RE) parameter is as follows

$\text{RE} = \frac{(r-1)E_b + r(t-1)E_e}{(rt-1)E_e}$, where E_b is the replication mean square and E_e is the error mean square in the RCBD-ANOVA.

Illustration 2: The experiment was conducted in double-blind RCT to know the drug efficacy of novel regimen new drug (Interim analysis) G_1 to G_6 is different blocks (homogeneous) arranged in four treatment (various dosage) we test the H_0: All the Treatments' effects are zero; H_0: All the Blocks' effects are zero.

Data sets (mean efficacy)

	G_1	G_2	G_3	G_4	G_5	G_6
A	98	88	86	88	86	93
B	89	84	84	86	84	96
C	84	79	89	83	82	93
D	83	82	92	81	81	87

Treatment variation	36.94	Block variation	50.96
Within the variation	13.07	Total variation	24.42
Treatment statistics	2.82	Its *P*-value	0.054
Block statistics	3.89	Its *P*-value	0.030

Inference: The experimental result was not found to be statistically significant; there is a significant difference between the treatment group and age of the person at 1% level of significance. Accept the null hypothesis $F_{\text{Cal}} > F_{\text{table}}$ value. All the Blocks' effects are not zero.

2.5 Latin Square Design (LSD)

In biological essence or insight, a single piece of information is very important to test the null hypothesis without any loss of research information from the experimental material. The researcher should modify the design based on the relevancy, field condition, and precision of the experimentation. If the experimentation is conducted at larger area, we need to encompass or modify the design to control sampling and nonsampling errors. In most of the agricultural and medical science research, the modification of the design is a prime factor for testing the null hypothesis and objective of the interest (Fisher 1935; Federer and Meredith 1992), for example, we have more than one blocking factor for estimation of predictable errors. Latin square design (LSD) attempt to prove or disprove the null hypothesis at desired level of significance α. The Latin square design will allow you to remove the two source error variations simultaneously. So, when we consider agriculture experimental research, we are using the blocking techniques on the basis of row and column wise, i.e., each row is considered as level of the row factor, and each column considered as level of the column factor. However, we can remove the variation from our measured response in both directions. Note that the Latin square is an incomplete block design, which means that it does not include the observations for all possible combinations of *i, j,* and *k*. This is the reason we are using the notation $k = d(i, j)$. Once we know the row and column of the design, then the treatment is specified at desired level of significance and randomization will be done in accordance with randomization procedure. In other words, if we know *i* and *j*, then *k* is being specified by the Latin square design (Fisher 1996). In case of laboratory trial experiments, researcher considering replication over time, such that the observed differences were noticed among the experimental units, since the experimentation has been conducted at the same time and the experimental trial was constituted into two known sources of variability (drug formulation and time). In the presence of rows and columns, the blocking will be done in a Latin square design, while it is very useful for taking care of two independent source of variations, and also it can be relied upon too many restrictions for the formulation of design. The major restriction of designing on the Latin square design (LSD) is as follows:

1. It must be perfect square (The number of rows equal to the number of columns) 3 × 3, 4 × 4, and 5 × 5.
2. Every treatment will appear once in rows and once in columns, respectively.
3. The treatments were allocated randomly with some restrictions.
4. The population or treatment should not be overlapping at any point of time, and in the two ways error gradient will be estimated by using LSD.

This is so because the requirements appear in each row block and each column block can be satisfied only if the number of replications is equal to the number of treatments. As a result, when the number of treatment is very large the design becomes impractical because of the large number of replications is being required. On the other hand, when the number of treatment is small the degree of freedom is closely associated with the experimental error (Efron, 1976)

2.5.1 Randomization and Layout

The process of randomization and layout for an LS design is presented below considering an experiment with four treatments (A, B, C, D)

A	B	D	C
C	D	C	B
B	C	B	D
D	A	A	A

4x4 Latin square design

2.5.2 Analytical Method

There are four sources of variability in a Latin square design (LSD); rows, treatment, replication (or blocks), and experimental error. Mathematical model is presented below:

$$y_{ijk} = \alpha_i + \tau_j + c_{ij} + \gamma_{jk} + + \epsilon_{ijk}, \qquad (2.4)$$

where

y_{ijk} = An observed value of ith patient (rows) and j^{th} ward (replication) k^{th} hospital (treatment)

α_i = Effect of trial drug on i^{th} patient

τ_j = Treatment effect of jth block or ward

c_{ij} = Effect of trial drugs on i^{th} patient and j^{th} hospital

γ_{jk} = Interaction effect between j^{th} ward and k^{th} hospital

ϵ_{ijk} = Error associated with effect of trial drug on i^{th} patient j^{th} ward k^{th} hospital, $\epsilon_{ij\sim N(\mu,\sigma 1^2)}$

Analytical section for analysis of variance (ANOVA)

Total $df. = t^2 - 1$

Row $df. = (r - 1)$

Column $df = (c - 1)$

Treatment $df = (t - 1)$

Error $df. = (t - 1)(t - 2)$

The error df can also be obtained through subtraction as

Error df = Total df – Row df – Column df – Treatment df

$$\text{Correction factor}(\text{CF}) = \frac{G^2}{t^2}$$

$$\text{Total SS} = \sum_{i=1}^{n} Xi^2 - \text{CF}$$

$$\text{Row SS} = \frac{\sum_{j=1}^{r} Ri^2}{t} - \text{CF}$$

$$\text{Column SS} = \frac{\sum_{j=1}^{n} Ci^2}{t} - \text{CF}$$

$$\text{Treatment SS} = \frac{\sum_{i=1}^{t} Ti^2}{t} - \text{CF}$$

$$\text{Error SS} = \left(\begin{array}{l}\text{Total SS} - \text{Row SS} - \text{Column SS} - \\ \text{Treatment SS}\end{array}\right)$$

Source of variation	df	Sum of Square	Mean sum of square	*Fisher F*-computed value
Treatment	$(t - 1)$	St^2	$\text{MST} = \frac{St^2}{(t-1)}$	$Ft = \frac{\text{MST}}{\text{MSE}}$
Row	$(r - 1)$	Sr^2	$\text{MSR} = \frac{Sr^2}{(r-1)}$	$Fr = \frac{\text{MSR}}{\text{MSE}}$
Column	$(c - 1)$	Sc^2	$\text{MSR} = \frac{Sc^2}{(c-1)}$	$Fc = \frac{\text{MSC}}{\text{MSE}}$
Experimental error	$(t - 1)(r - 1)$	Se^2	$\text{MSE} = \frac{Se^2}{t(r-1)}$	
Total	$(rt) - 1$			

$$\text{Co efficient of Vvariation}(\%) = \frac{\sqrt{\text{Error MS}}}{\text{Grand mean}} \text{x}100,$$

magnitude of the reduction in the experimental predictable errors due to blocking by computing the relative efficiency (RE) parameter is as follows:

Relative efficiency (RE) of $\text{CRD} = \frac{E_r + E_{c+}(t-1)E_e}{(t+1)E_e}$, where E_r is the row mean square, E_C is the column mean square, and E_e is the error mean square.

Illustration 3: The drug trial was conducted 4 × 4 LSD, and the efficacy obtained from study sites. The resulted observations were presented in the following table matrix. We wish to calculate any significant difference between treatment, blocks

		Rows			Means
Blocks	A(88)	B(79)	C(84)	D(93)	86.0
	B(96)	C(85)	D(82)	A(94)	89.25
	C(81)	D(80)	A(89)	B(88)	84.5
	D(78)	A(83)	B(91)	C(86)	84.5
Means	85.75	81.75	86.50	90.25	86.06

ANOVA Summary

Source of variation	df	Sum of square	Mean sum of square	F-computed
Treatment	$(t-1)=3$	$St^2=96.19$	$\text{MST}=\frac{St^2}{(t-1)}=32.06$	$Ft=\frac{\text{MST}}{\text{MSE}}=1.23\text{ns}$
Row	$(r-1)=3$	$Sr^2=60.19$	$\text{MSR}=\frac{Sr^2}{(r-1)}=20.06$	$Fr=\frac{\text{MSR}}{\text{MSE}}=0.77\text{ns}$
Column	$(c-1)=3$	$Sc^2=145.69$	$\text{MSR}=\frac{Sc^2}{(c-1)}=48.56$	$Fc=\frac{\text{MSC}}{\text{MSE}}=1.86\text{ns}$
Experimental error	$(t-1)(r-1)=6$	$Se^2=156.88$	$\text{MSE}=\frac{Se^2}{t(r-1)}=26.15$	
Total	$(rt)-1=15$	$ST^2=458.94$		

Note: The trial was found to be significant $Ft > F$ table value, accept the H_o

2.6 Crossover Design (COD)

This design is most widely used in agricultural field experimentation and drug equivalence trial at a larger extent. A crossover design is a repeated measurements that has been taken from the data sets, the design is such that each experimental unit (patient) can receive different treatment groups during the different time period (winter, summer, and rainy season). In case of COD, the patients were crossed over from one treatment to another treatment groups during the course of drug trial. This is in contrast to a parallel design in which patients are randomized to a particular treatment and remain on that same treatment throughout the duration of the trial. One more cited example driven by animal science, the experimentation was demonstrated to know the response rate of the milk yield considering feed supplementation (effective feed ratio). The feed has been fed to the animals in half and full season with defined time interval 't'; the response of the milk yield data sets was collected half yearly and annually for extrapolation of response variable (milk yield) contrasting the preceding values of milk yield. The reason behind to consider a crossover design at large scale, an each every individual observations is very important to approximate the response variables and also the planning of experiment on clinical trial and agricultural field experiments (varietal trial), considering COD can yield good results at the time of data compilation and testing of hypothesis (DeLury 1946). It is more efficient comparison of treatments groups when compare to parallel design simultaneously. eg The designing of COD will able to include less number of patients required for constructing the crossover design efficiently in order to meet the requirement of novelty of subject interest at desired level of statistical power (β) or precision of the experiment ($1-\alpha$). Intuitively, this design seems to be reasonable and researcher able to conduct the experiments in half season period because each patient can be served as real group. The patient will be received both treatment type A and B (naive and control). However, the crossover design is more popular in medical, agricultural, manufacturing, education policy intervention, and many other disciplines of science. Since the response variable comparison has made of the subjects of the interest. The concept of design cross over design is serving as their own control to extrapolate the predictable errors appealing to the researcher (biomedical investigators). The crossover design is not to be preferred on a routine basis because of the problem of inherent coercive effect. Many medical and clinical research has been noticed that, the disease may have triggered *chronic and stable*, the *treatments should not be prevailing to control diseases progression, the researcher should extrapolate the causation factors at defined time intervals 't'; since the incumbent results shows a total cure,* but apparently can alleviate the disease condition. If the treatment "A" cures the patient during the first period, then treatment B will not have the opportunity to demonstrate its effectiveness when the patient crosses over to treatment /B in the second period or subsequent period, respectively. Therefore, this type of design will work only for those conditions that are chronic illness (e.g., asthma where there is no cure and the treatment can attempt to improve the quality of life (QOL) of patients) (Duncan 1955; Dunnett 1955).

Design	Period 1	Period 2
Sequence AB	A	B
Sequence AB	B	A
Sum	A + B	B + A

A: New Rx and B: Old regimen

Design	Period 1	Period 2	Period 3
Sequence ABB	A	B	B
Sequence BAA	B	A	A
Sum	A + B	B + A	B + A

A: New Rx and B: Old regimen

Examples of three-period, three-treatment crossover designs are

Design	Period 1	Period 2	Period 3
Sequence ABC	A	B	C
Sequence BCA	B	C	A
Sequence CAB	C	A	B
Sum	A + B + C	B + C + A	C + A + B

A: New Rx and B: Old regimen C: Ayurveda base

The compilation of crossover design is very simple for any patient in the sequence AB with respect to period (period 1 versus 2) difference that has expectation $\mu_{AB} = \mu_A - \mu_B + 2P - \lambda$. Similarly, we wish to know the BA sequence, the period 1 versus 2 differences has expectation $\mu_{BA} = \mu_B - \mu_A + 2P - \lambda$. Therefore, we construct these differences for every patient and compare the two sequences with respect to these differences using a two sample *t* test or Wilcoxon Rank Sum Test. Thus, we obtain the relevant resulted part.

Illustration

The data sets obtained from Department of Pediatrics, BMCRI, consists of 13 children enrolled in a double-blind RCT trial to investigate the effects of two bronchodilators, formoterol, and salbutamol, in the treatment of asthma. The outcome variable shows peak expiratory flow rate (liters per minute) and is measured in 8 h after treatment intervention. There is a 1-day washout period between treatment periods.

FS	SF	SF	FS	SF	FS	FS	SF	FS	FS	SF	SF	FS	SF
270	370	310	260	380	300	390	290	210	350	260	90	365	361
310	385	400	310	410	370	410	320	250	380	340	220	330	320

The estimated treatment $\overline{x}$ difference is 46.6 L/min in favor of formoterol ($p = 0.0012$) and the CI-95% for the treatment $\overline{x}$ difference is 22.9, 70.3. The Wilcoxon Rank Sum Test also indicates statistical significance between the treatment groups ($p = 0.0276$).

2.6.1 Data Collection and Documentation

1. Treatment—assigned and received
2. Outcomes—including beneficial and adverse effects
3. Prognostic profile at entry
4. Randomization procedure
5. Method used to generate the random allocation sequence
6. Method used to implement the random allocation
7. Personnel who generated the allocation sequence, enrolled participants, and assigned participants to groups

2.6.2 Masking or Blinding

Masking or blinding is used to increase the objectivity of the persons dealing with the randomized study (to prevent prejudice).

Subjects who can be masked/blinded are as follows:

8. Study participants
9. Caregivers/treaters
10. Data collectors/assessors of outcome—Data analysts
11. Investigators level of masking/blinding
12. Non-blinded (open)
13. Single–Double–Triple

A placebo (from the Latin for "I will please") is a medical treatment (operation, therapy, chemical solution, pill, etc.), which is administered as if it were a therapy, but has no therapeutic value other than the placebo effect. A nocebo (from the Latin for "I will harm") is treatment like a placebo but which has a harmful result.

Compliance is the willingness of the participants to carry out the procedures according to the established protocols (adherence).

Drop-outs are the participants, who do not adhere to the experimental regimen during follow-up. Drop-ins are the participants, who do not adhere to the control regimen during follow-up.

2.7 Ethical Issues

(a) Is randomization ethical?
(b) Can a truly informed consent be obtained from the patients?
(c) Institutional ethical clearance obtained from your organization.
(d) When can a placebo be used?
(e) Under what condition should a randomized clinical trial be stopped earlier than originally planned?

2.8 Sampling Techniques Associated with Bayesian Analysis

A common theme in medical research is a two-stage sampling, that is, sampling of responses within experimental units (e.g., patients) and sampling of experimental units within populations. For example, in prospective longitudinal studies, the patients are repeatedly sampled and assessed in terms of a variety of endpoints such as mental and physical levels of functioning or in terms of the response of one or more biological systems to one or more forms of treatment. These patients are in turn sampled from a population, often stratified on the basis of treatment delivery, for example, in a clinic, in a hospital, or during space missions. Like all biological and behavioral characteristics, the outcome measures exhibit individual differences. Investigators should be interested in not only the mean response pattern but also the distribution of these response patterns (e.g., time trends) in the population of patients. One can then address the number or proportion of patients who are functioning more or less positively at a specific rate. One can then describe the treatment–outcome relationship not as a fixed law but as a family of laws, the parameters of which describe the individual biobehavioral tendencies of the subjects in the population. This view of biological and behavioral research may lead to Bayesian methods of data analysis. The relevant distributions exist objectively and can be investigated empirically by Bayesian emulator approach (Draper et al. 1993, 1994) (Figs. 2.1 and 2.2).

Many researchers are fitted predictive modeling for assessment of risk of stroke patients by using traditional frequentist statistical approach such as estimation of MLEs based on the assumed hypothesis (normality). In the vague of frequentist analysis, entire data sets are repeatable process and various parameters, which are fixed in nature. Furthermore, confidence intervals are used to draw the significant inference, but in real life the clinician/policymakers do not have fully developed prior beliefs about clinical, biological, behavioral, and drug interaction information, and also estimated parameters (traditional way) providing spurious decisions about the population without estimation of credibility intervals. However, in case of Bayesian approach, the decision is based on subjective basis and using prior beliefs to define a prior probability distribution on the probabilistic values of unknown parameters. Although the parameters of interest are

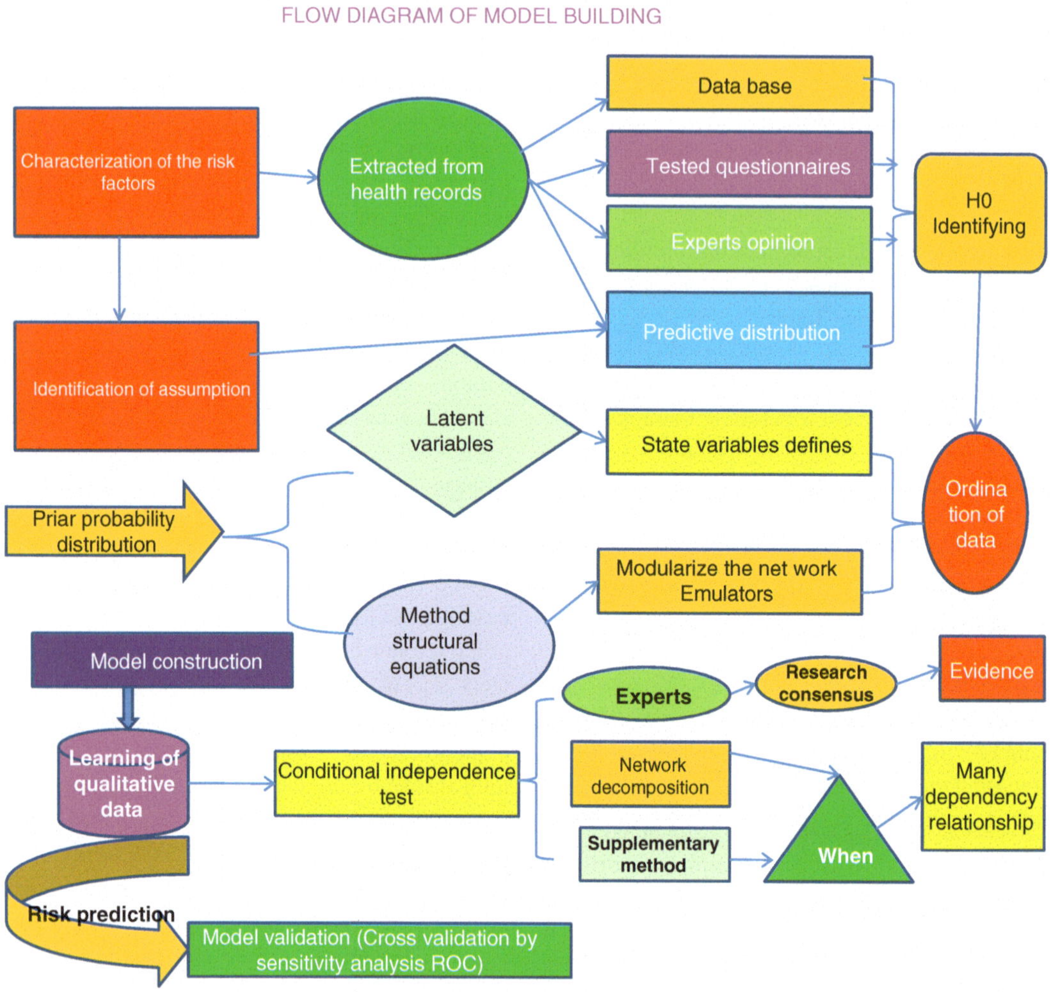

Fig. 2.1 Flow diagram of Bayesian model fitting

interpreted differently by adopting practical approach, from a frequentist viewpoint, the parameters are fixed but unknown quantities and also random variables. Hence, Bayesian approach is affordable to derive the convenience of basic probability computations in accordance with credibility intervals and getting rid of nuisance distribution state (Baker et al. 2001; Craig et al. 2001; Currin et al. 1991; Chu et al. 2005; Dragic et al. 1998). Most importantly, Bayesian network model makes conditional inferences on the data observed (but does not consider hypothetical life data sets that were not observed). A Bayesian approach is very natural when constructing predictive emulators with the chosen statistical model treated as a prior distribution on the simulator outputs and prediction, with associated uncertainty quantification via posterior predictive distribution parametric state. The "nascent" line of this research pressing to build predictive modeling of health care data for the automatic detection of risk, genetic, and environmental interactions, recently health delivery practices for specific population such as patient suffering from chronic disability, for example, stroke, terminal illness, life-threatened disease such as HIV. The elderly people are shifting towards the constant health monitoring 24 h/day or 24 × 7 per day at defined state. Health monitoring may be determined not only in hospital envi-

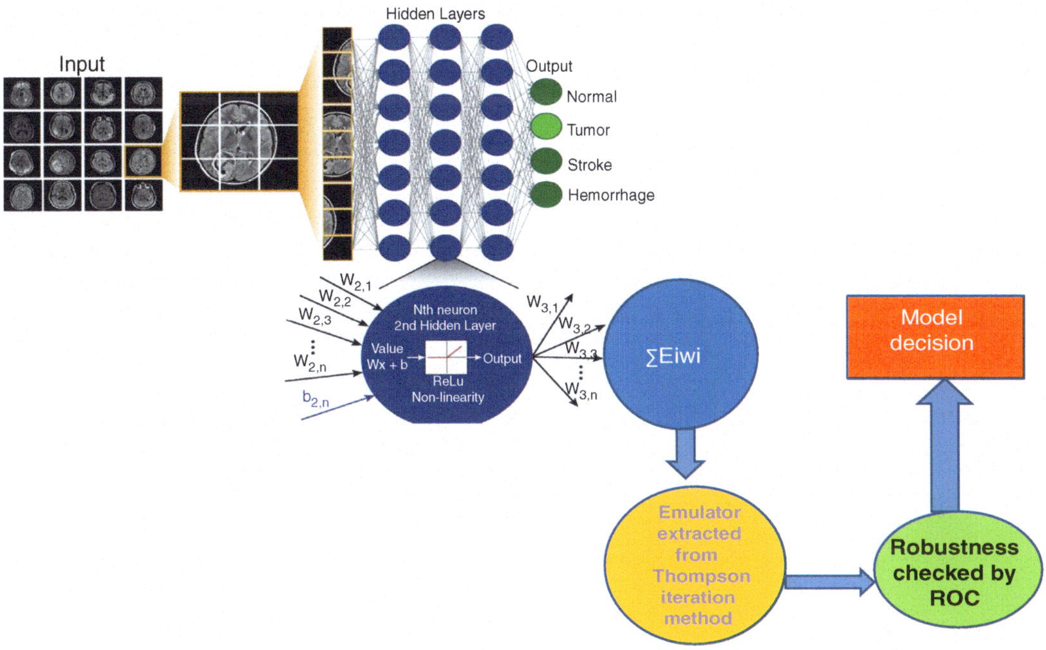

Fig. 2.2 Extraction of trainer data from Bayesian model

ronment but also at home, through establishment of modern patient tale-monitoring system. The above cited reason to obtain better possibilities for managing chronic care, controlling health delivery cost, increased quality life domain, and distinct possibility of predicting and thus avoiding serious complications. Therefore, the execution of a risk analysis is necessary to assure health information system safety and quality services (QOS), estimation of DALYs to estimates the credibility risk as well as life span index. In this context, traditional statistical approach is not able to predict the Bayesian probabilities and MLEs of long entries of continuous state variable function. In view of the existing analytical research gap, the present study aims to fit new probabilistic model by Bayesian emulator approach.

2.9 Probabilistic Diagnostic Gaussian Model for Risk Analysis

Self-learning probabilistic diagnostic which can be implemented in medicine are reported by many authors (Wei et al. 1988). This general approach towards creating self-learning risk assessment can also be used in other disciplines (e.g., detect spam, credit and debit financial risk flow, and biological science). In general, a risk assessment of real-time medical massive data sets consists of pertinent database, the comprehension skills, decision support by practical approach, etc. This is the reason why these plausible interventions of the risk element probabilistic diagnostic model are discussed and simulated at greater accuracy and reduced error. Probabilistic diagnostic methods fitted based on the Gaussian simulator Bayesian method is discussed below. Let us assume that there are "*N*" events mutually exclusive, independent, and identical in nature; β_n is normally distributed with "μ" and variance "σ^2" variance $\beta_n \sim N(\mu, \sigma^2)$ which are excluded from each other and are mutually independent

$$P(\beta_n) = N(\mu, \sigma^2) = 1 \tag{2.5}$$

The event β_n denoted as occurrence of assumed that P ($A_n > 0$, if ($n = 1, 2, 3. . n$). Further, we assume that there are "*M*" independent events

$A_m = m = 1, 2...Mi$ which do not exclude each $\left\{\sum_{i=1}^{m} A_m = m\right\}$ where the probability of this conjunction is determined as

$$p(A) = \prod_{I=1}^{N} P(A_m) = 1. \quad (2.6)$$

Events "β_n" and "A" are mutually exclusive and dependent because nth unknown parameters come into being by defined symptoms of evaluation A_m, $m = 1, 2, , M$. The unknown Bayesian parameters are normally distributed with conjunction of dependent events.

$$p('\beta_n \hat{} A) = P(\beta_n).P(A / \beta_n) \quad (2.7)$$

$$= P(A_i).P(\beta_n / A_i) \sim N(\mu, \sigma^2)$$

$$\mu = 0, \sigma^2 = 1$$

$$\therefore = \mathrm{P}(A_i)P(\beta_n / A_i) \sim N(0,1),$$

where the conditional probability

$P(\beta\ \_\ n/Ai)$ is obtained from the formula (solved by using Eqs. 8.2 and 8.3)

$$P(\beta_n / Ai) = P(A_i)P(\beta_n / A_i) / P(A_i) i = 1,2,..n$$

As it was assumed that event A_m is not independent, so it can be written as

$P(Ai / \beta_n) = \prod_{i=1}^{n} P(A_i / \beta_n)$. Assuming normalcy, the equation becomes

$$P(Ai / \beta_n) = p(Ai)P(Ai / \beta_n) / \sum_{i=1}^{n} p(Ai) +$$

$$P(Ai / \beta_n) \sim N(\mu^2, \sigma).$$

The probability of nth risk assessment can be determined from the Bayesian matrix conditions that the conjunction of Ai symptoms comes into being if the following probability is known. Asper the cited model, the emulators on each probability values eagerly tend to Gaussian approach (Table 2.1).

The expected value of probability or credibility has been calculated as

$$P(E_i) = \sum_{i=1}^{n} P(\beta_{n11}) \times P(A_{11}) \times \sum_{i=1}^{n} P(\beta_n \cdot) \times$$

$$P(A_{1.}) / \sum_{i=1}^{n} \sum_{i1}^{n} P(\beta_n) \times P(A_n).$$

Therefore, the true credibility of genetic linkage was calculated by

$$\chi_{(n-p)df}{}^2 = \sum_{i=1}^{n} \frac{\left(O_{ij} - E_{ij}\right)^2}{E_{ij}} \sim N(\mu^2, \sigma).$$

Further, we continued to test risk credibility by seeing whether the observed data's summary statistics is inside the Gaussian approach around the parameters tested by the estimation of likelihood unknown parameters $\hat{\theta}$ (Fig. 2.3).

The whole series of risk outcomes $\hat{\theta}(x \in \theta)$ can be finite series of real Bayesian probability values; the extension random variable is mutually exclusive and independent with MLEs $(\hat{\theta})$. Therefore, intuitive variation was estimated at $\hat{\theta} = [X_0, X_1]$.

$$\hat{\theta} = P[X_0 \le \theta \le X_1],$$

$$\hat{\theta} = \left(X - \frac{\delta X}{2} \le \theta \le X + \frac{\delta X}{2}\right) = F(X)\delta X; \int f(x)\delta x$$

$\hat{\theta} = \left(X - \frac{\delta X}{2} \le \theta \le X + \frac{\delta X}{2}\right) f(x)$ are the probability Gaussian density functions. An experiment approaches the Bayesian trial with "k" independent outcomes with MLEs $\hat{\theta} = \mathrm{I} = 1,2,..K \sum \theta_i 1 = 1$. Probability distribution of "N" outcomes of the same experiment getting n_i occurrences of outcomes "i" $\sum n_i = N$.

$$M\left(\frac{N}{\theta}\right) = \frac{N!}{\pi n_i!} \prod_{i=1}^{K} \theta_i^{n_i} \quad (2.8)$$

From Eq. (2.8) Bayes probability outcome is generated (without overlapping loop).

Let us assume that $\hat{\theta} = (\hat{\theta}_1, \hat{\theta}_2, \hat{\theta}_3, \hat{\theta}_4 .....\hat{\theta}_k)$ with constant values $\alpha_1, \alpha_2, \alpha_3.... \alpha_k$ which gives different probability distribution over $\hat{\theta}_i$ (MLEs) the density function of Bayesian risk probability "DALY" is formulated in the following manner

$$f(\theta / x) = \prod_{i=1}^{n} \theta_i^{\alpha_i - 1} \delta\left(\sum_{i=1}^{n} \theta_i - 1\right) \quad ((2.9))$$

Table 2.1 Bayesian matrix table for risk assessment (diagnosis test table)

Ai / β_n	$P(A_1)$	$P(A_2)$	$P(A_3)$	$P(A_4)$	$P(A_5)$	$P(A_n)$	Row total
$P(\beta_1)$	$P(\beta_1)xP(A_1)$	$P(\beta_1)xP(A_2)$	$P(\beta_1)xP(A_3)$	$P(\beta_1)xP(A_4)$	$P(\beta_1)xP(A_5)$	$P(\beta_1)xP(A_n)$	$\sum_{i=1}^{n} P(\beta_n.)xP(A_{1.})$
$P(\beta_2)$	$P(\beta_2)x\ P(A_1)$	$P(\beta_2)xP(A_2)$	$P(\beta_2)xP(A_3)$	$P(\beta_2)xP(A_4)$	$P(\beta_2)xP(A_5)$	$P(\beta_2)xP(A_n)$	$\sum_{i=1}^{n} P(\beta_n)xP(A_1)$
$P(\beta_3)$	$P(\beta_3)\ xP(A_1)$	$P(\beta_3)xP(A_2)$	$P(\beta_3)xP(A_3)$	$P(\beta_3)xP(A_4)$	$P(\beta_3)xP(A_5)$	$P(\beta_3)xP(A_n)$	$\sum_{i=1}^{n} P(\beta_n)xP(A_1)$
$P(\beta_4)$	$P(\beta_4)x\ P(A_1)$	$P(\beta_4)xP(A_2)$	$P(\beta_4)xP(A_3)$	$P(\beta_4)xP(A_4)$	$P(\beta_4)xP(A_5)$	$P(\beta_4)xP(A_n)$	$\sum_{i=1}^{n} P(\beta_n)xP(A_1)$
$P(\beta_5)$	$P(\beta_5)\ xP(A_1)$	$P(\beta_5)xP(A_2)$	$P(\beta_5)xP(A_3)$	$P(\beta_5)xP(A_4)$	$P(\beta_5)xP(A_5)$	$P(\beta_5)xP(A_n)$	$\sum_{i=1}^{n} P(\beta_n)xP(A_1)$
$P(\beta_n)$	$P(\beta_n)\ xP(A_1)$	$P(\beta_n)xP(A_2)$	$P(\beta_n)xP(A_2)$	$P(\beta_n)xP(A_2)$	$P(\beta_n)xP(A_2)$	$P(\beta_n)xP(A_2)$	$\sum_{i=1}^{n} P(\beta_n)xP(A_1)$
Column total	$\sum_{i=1}^{n} P(\beta_{n11})xP(A_{11})$	$\sum_{i=1}^{n} P(\beta_{n2})xP(A_{21})$	$\sum_{i=1}^{n} P(\beta_{n3})xP(A_1)$	$\sum_{i=1}^{n} P(\beta_n)xP(A_1)$	$\sum_{i=1}^{n} P(\beta_n)xP(A_1)$	$\sum_{i=1}^{n} P(\beta_n)xP(A_1)$	$\sum_{i=1}^{n}\sum_{i1}^{n} P(\beta_n)xP(A_n)$

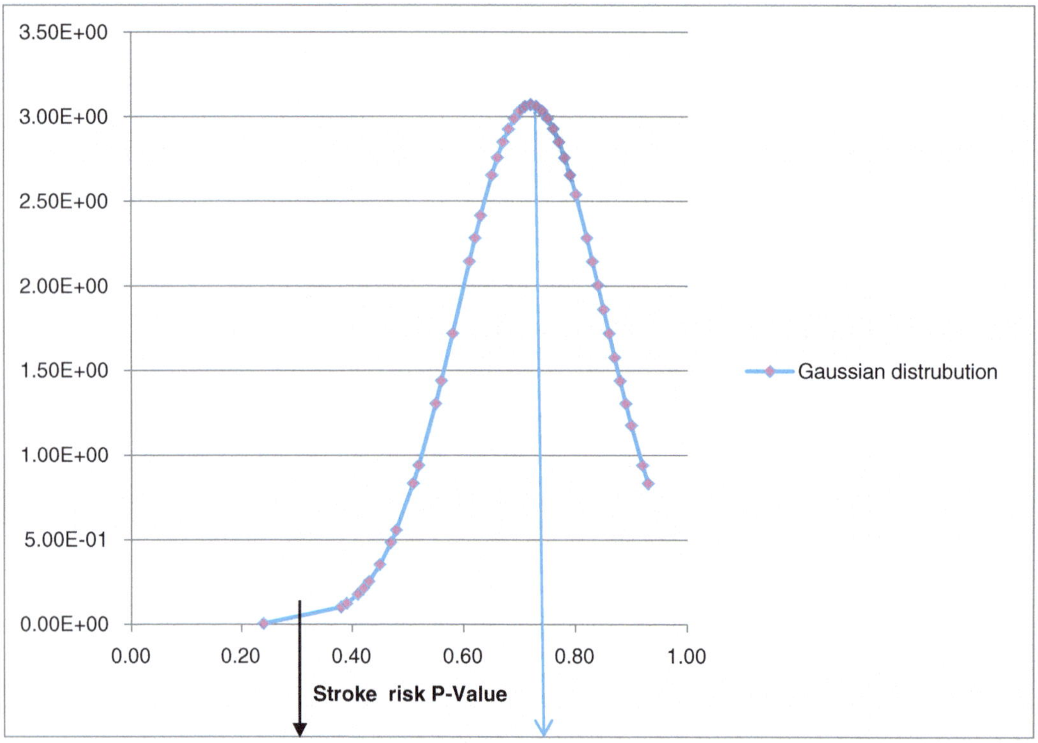

θ (MLE's) = 0.72

Fig. 2.3 Gaussian distribution probabilistic curve of stroke risk

2.10 Practical Component of DALY (Stroke)

Disability-adjusted life year is a measure of overall burden of disease it adds the years of life lost due to early death and years spent living with disability or ill health together. One important component of "DALY" can be thought of as one lost year of healthy life. The sum of the "DALY" across the population or the burden of diseases can be thought of as a measurement of the gap between current health status and an ideal health situation where the entire population lives to an advanced age, free of disease and disability. The following diagram depicted major diseases of "DALY" (Fig. 2.4).

DALYs = YLD + YLL

(Years lived with disability = Years of life lost)

Years of life lost: Number of deaths at each age multiplied by the expected remaining years of life according to a global standard life expectancy.

Years lost to disability: Number of indirect cases due to injury and illness is multiplied by the average duration of diseases and a weightage factor reflecting the severity of diseases on scale from 0 and 1 (0 perfect health and 1 dead from diseases). The estimated net health effect, the "QALIBRA" (Quality of life for benefit risk assessment).

$$\mathrm{DALYY}_{a,s} = \left[P_{\mathrm{eff}(a,s)} * \left(P_{rec} * YLD_{rec} * w + P_{\mathrm{die}} * (YLD_{\mathrm{die}} * w + LE_{a,s} - CA - YLD_{\mathrm{die}} \right) + \left(1 - P_{\mathrm{die}} - P_{rec} \right) * (LE_{a,s} - CA * w \right],$$

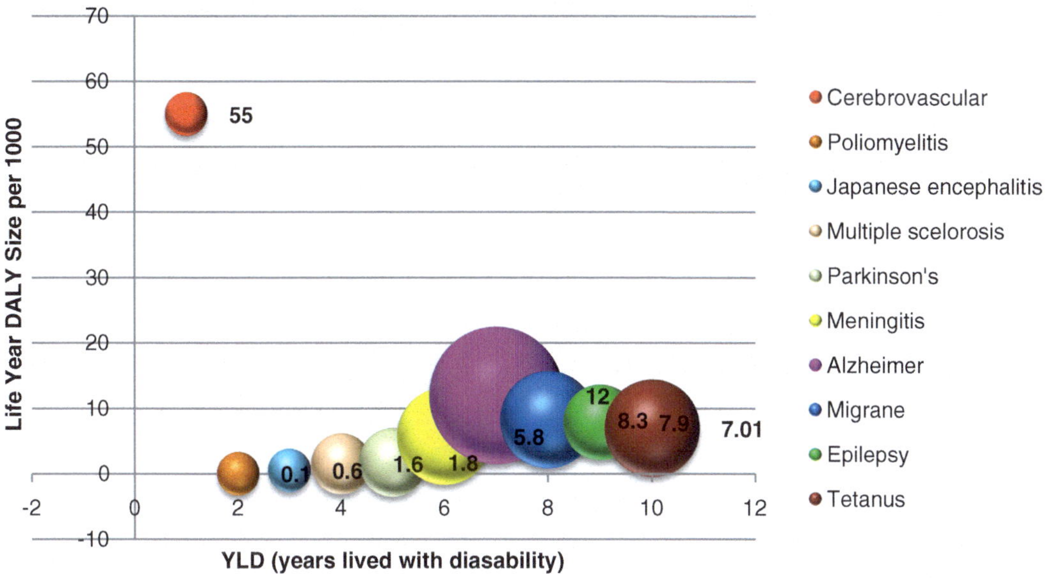

Fig. 2.4 Distribution of disability with years lived

where $DALYY_{a,s}$ = Disability-adjusted life years at age group "a" and sex "s".

$P_{eff(a,s)}$ = Probability of onset of the diseases at age and sex per year.

P_{rec} = Probability of recovery from the diseases.

P_{die} = Probability that the diseases cause death.

YLD_{die} = Mean duration of disease for those who die.

YLD_{rec} = Mean duration of disease for those who recover.

CA = Current age of individuals in year of disease onset.

$LE_{a,s}$ = Normal life expectancy (*i.e.*, expected year death) with "*w*" disability weight for disease.

DALY is only quantitative indicator of burden of disease that reflects the total year lost (premature mortality) or some degree of disability (morbidity) during a period of time.

Maximum likelihood estimation of DALYs = {Age at onset $* e^{-r\theta}$}, θ is parameter constant (MLEs) or number of years to be discounted, *i.e.*, (45–35). The DALY age at 35 $=19.95 * e^{-0.03\times 10} = 14.50$. Hence, the total DALY lost = YLD + YLL = 6.95 + 14.50 = 21.75.

For practical approach, we apply with a 3% discount rate, the YLL becomes

$$\text{YLL} = \frac{N^*\left(1-e^{-0.032}\right)}{0.03},$$ where N is number of deaths = standard life expectancy at age of death and r = discount rate.

$$\text{YLD} = \frac{I^*\text{DW}^*\left(1-\text{e}^{-0.032}\right)}{0.03},$$ where I = number of incident cases, DW = disability weights, L = duration of disability, and r = discount rate (Fig. 2.5, Tables 2.2, 2.3 and 2.4).

The results showed risk analysis of DALYs, it was optimized by real data and would be served as an advanced method, specifically when simulating data from Bayesian emulators; the ability of the model are indicated in the (Table 8.1). Note that a disability-adjusted life years combine years of potential life lost due to premature death is predicted in accordance with Bayesian risk analysis approach of DALYs. The results were correlated life lost due to premature death event, it has been happened unfavored between the age group 20 and above, the MLE's is less associated with DALY. Although the patients are profusely suffer-

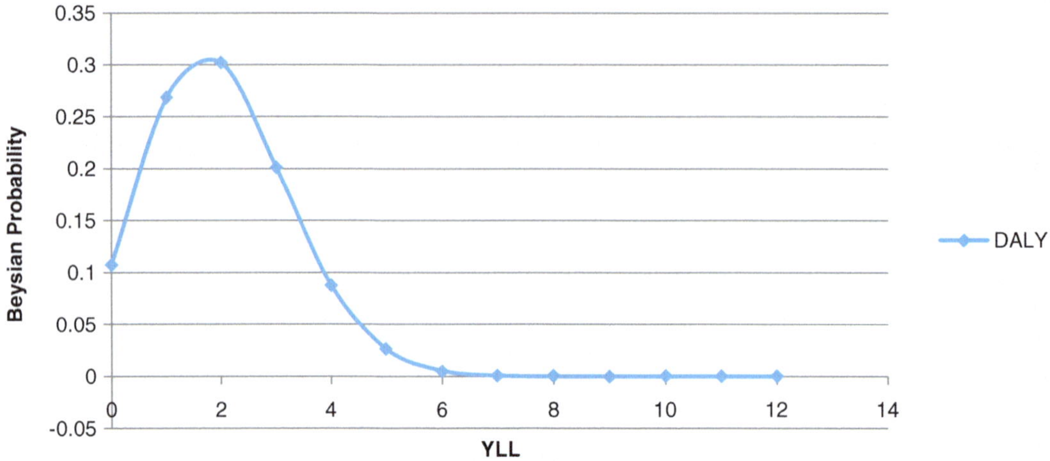

Fig. 2.5 Overview of potential life lost due to stroke (Population based)

Table 2.2 Disability-adjusted life years combine years of potential life lost due to premature death with years of productive life lost due to disability (age standardized)

Life lost due to premature death (PYLL)	Bayesian *P*-value	MLE Bayesian *P*-value $(\hat{\theta})$
20 and above	0.13	0.88
1588*n*	0.27	0.97
1097*n*	0.76	5.85
5.8	0.82	8.11
Below 5	0.86	9.02

Model statistically significant (AUC = 0.86–0.92, $P < 0.01$)

Table 2.3 Distribution of Disability weighting classes

Disability weighting classes	Bayesian ANN *P*-value
Limited ability to perform at least one activity in one of the following areas: recreation, education, procreation, or occupation	0.033
Limited ability to perform most activities in one of the following areas: recreation, education, procreation, or occupation	0.45
Limited ability to perform activities in two or more of the following areas: recreation, education, procreation, or occupation	0.56
Limited ability to perform most activities in all of the following areas: recreation, education, procreation, or occupation	0.66
Needs assistance with instrumental activities of DALY living such as meal preparation, shopping, or housework	0.84
Needs assistance with activities of DALY living such as eating, personal hygiene, or toilet use	0.93

Table 2.4 Bayesian emulator estimation of DALYs and final result

	Bayesian emulator estimation (age standardized)			
Age class	YLLs	YLDss	DALYs	AUC
30–35	253	30.16	283.16	0.73
36–40	325	35.22	360.22	0.77
41–45	368	36.22	404.22	0.76
46–50	385	40.96	425.96	0.78
51–55	392	43.25	435.25	0.76
56–60	452	44.44	496.44	0.80
61–65	563	45.66	608.66	0.82
66–70	665	47.25	712.25	0.84
71–75	675	48.55	723.55	0.88
>76	886	49.50	935.5	0.92

ing from the illness due to comorbid conditions. Moreover, risk bearing of potential life lost due to premature death event accrued 5–9 and 10–14 years after the event happened (stroke), were emulators statistically signifies the incidence of the happening of the event (Diagnosis test AUC = 0.92), original data extracted from Disability weighting classes (Table 8.4), data sets was simulated based on the Bayesian approach; Monte Carlo simulation techniques method.

Model uncertainty and risk assessment is essential for disease management and informed decision-making has been drawn at population level. In this study, we apply a continued test to risk credibility by seeing whether the observed data summary statistics is inside of the Gaussian approach around the parametric value. The "MLEs" were calibrated a risk of stroke approaches with Bayesian trial with "k" independentoutcomeswithMLEs $\hat{\theta} = I = 1,2,..K \sum \theta_i 1 = 1$. In the covet of data scarcity in modeling of stroke, follow-up data lead to using bootstrapping as a way to estimate the uncertainty of relations in Gaussian distribution approach. The idea of the model is as follows: parameters estimation can be used as a nonparametric estimate of a statistics of interest, for which we can take the probabilistic risk of an event (stroke) as we can see in Fig. 2.1. The intuition behind the normalcy curve is that if we assume a generative probabilistic model, the actual data sets are traversed in real value. However, each of the estimation has some latency which is attached to it, so as better approximation to the real probability can be obtained from the "Gaussian emulators." The diagnosis and evaluation of the model and their performance will use standard matrices from classified matrices (Table 8.1). Classification and evaluation of Bayesian emulators is often based on measuring true positive (TP) cases that are correctly classified as positive; false positive (FP), incorrectly classified as positive; and analogously for true/false negative (TN;FN). The true positive rate (TPR) is then defined as TP/(TP + FN) and the false positive rate (FPR) as FP/(FP + TN), plotting a curve of TP-FPR of different cut-off points results in an "ROC" curve which is often summarized in a single number by computing the AUC.

Table 2.5 Distribution of comorbidities

Comorbidities	DALY score	MLEs $(\hat{\theta})$	Bayesian ANNs emulator *P*-value
Ataxia and dysarthria	80.20	10.21	0.66
Attention deficit hyperactivity disorder	56.34	4.28	0.52
Left and right hemiparesis	74.32	3.63	0.28
Psychosis	24.90	0.98	0.11
Valproate-induced tremor	48.70	0.43	0.16

2.11 Discussion

The increasing burden of stroke health transition is pushing the scientific community towards the development of computational tools to support decision-making when defining health risk, such as estimation of MLEs of DALY (disability-adjusted life year) at population level by taking into account the progression of stroke incidence and health care needs. To this end, decision analysis is an early paramount tool to assess the better outcomes, and increasingly using, simulation of MLEs to derive Bayesian simulators (Table 2.5) about decision-making correlate with health outcomes in target population. The most reliable practical approach of this model outcome is represented by the Gaussian emulator method $G{\sim}N(\mu, \varepsilon)$. The model was fitted with time course of comorbidities with a probabilistic finite continuous state–time representation of different state function or events. According to the model, an entire stroke data set is simulated by Gaussian approach, the value of emulators were determined based on "Monte Carlo simulation techniques." Although the emulators describe the state function of DALY (Bayesian emulator) with respect to different health indicators of stroke disability health score. Similarly, the temporal evaluation of the patients is then obtained by sampling, at each continuous state treatment follow-up period, state of Bayesian risk p value will be generated on his/her state in the previous time in accordance with a transition probability matrix. Annually 15 million people worldwide suffer a stroke; of these five million die and another five million are left permanently disabled, placing a burden on family and community. Stroke is uncommon in people under 40 years; when does it occur, the main cause is high blood pressure. Stroke also occurs in about 15% of adults between age group 45–55 years associated with type I diabetes complications. The major risk factors are similar to those for coronary heart disease with high blood pressure and tobacco usage is the most significant modifiable risks. Atrial fibrillation, heart failure, and heart attack are other important risk factors. As per the literature, the incidence of stroke is declining in many developed countries, largely as a result of better control of high blood pressure, and reduced levels of smoking. However, the absolute number of strokes continues to increase because of the aging population. Between 1990 and 2016, there was a significant increase in prevalent cases, total deaths, and DALYSs due to smoking, sedentary life style, elevated BMI 35–42 in younger adults aged 35–46 years. Deaths and DALY rates increased in Indian context but a significant increase in absolute number of stroke deaths among younger adults was found to detect new incidence of stroke. Minimum DALY scores were attained in the age group 30–35 years (283.16 years,area under curve AUC 0.73, Bayesian probability is $P = 0.78$; followed 36–40 years (360.22, AUC; 0.77; 41–45 years 404.22; AUC 0.76; significantly increased DALY's trend was observed in the age group 56–76 years age class intervals, the mean DALY's was 935.50; AUC 0.92 (Table 8.4). The greater burden was due to ischemic stroke. While the trends in declined death and DALY's rates in developing countries like India are encouraging, this is a more aggressive approach towards primary prevention and increased access to adequate health care services for stroke is required to substantially narrow these disparities. The total health loss due to stroke as measured by DALY's risk analysis was similar for men and women for stroke both types in 2012–2016, with hemorrhagic higher than ischemic stroke, earning its inherent weakness in mind, DALY is still a very useful measure because it is the first comprehensive attempt made to summarize the world's burden of injury, disease, and premature death. It has initiated a debate and new research to find even better complex indicators for global comparisons. The DALY measures are useful to describe the burden across the world and to make projections for the future. At present, many countries are exploring the possibilities of using DALY's as a measure of trends in disease burden and as tool for cost-effectiveness studies and priority setting. Summing up the results, the present study concludes that Bayesian predictive risk analysis model gives a good consistent result, replicated as an automated tool to predicting the DALY risk emulators of stroke. This can be particularly useful in developing countries for implementation of policy intervention. Furthermore, with a larger health record database the results will be more consistent and accurate.

2.12 Summary

In practical point of view many researchers have fitted innumerable predictive models for the assessment of stroke risk by using traditional frequentisitc statistical approach; the edifice of fitted traditional frequentisitc models produce less consistent and inexact results because the results were simulated based on the assumed hypothesis. Frequentist analysis, entire data sets are repeatable process; the parameters are fixed in nature, and credibility of the parameters is undefined. Correspondingly, in case of Bayesian artificial neural network "ANN" emulator approach, the decision of the population has been drawn on the subjective basis with prior beliefs (prior probability). In this impression, the traditional statistical approach is incompetent to predict the unknown parameters of MLEs of long standing entries of continuous state variables "x". In this uneven penuriousness research gap, the present study aims to derive the new probabilistic model (Bayesian "ANN" emulator approach and disability adjustment life year score—DALY's) from the continuous state variables $x_1, x_2, x_3..x_n$. we assumed "N" events mutually exclusive, independent, and identical (IIDs) in nature; β_n is normally distributed with "μ" and variance "σ^2" variance $\beta_n \sim N(\mu, \sigma^2)$. The Bayesian risk probability was obtained with maximization of $f(\theta / x) = \prod_{i=1}^{n} \theta_i^{\alpha_i - 1} \delta\left(\sum_{i=1}^{n} \theta_i - 1\right)$; MLE's and DALY's probability values were obtained from the Bayesian simulation techniques (Thompson-iteration method). As per the resulted findings of the model, the life lost due to premature death event has waft between the age group ≥20 years and above; the MLEs more associated with DALYs as wells as a large number of patients suffering from the illness due to comorbid conditions. The risk bearing of potential life is lost due to premature death (5–9 years and 10–14 years after the stroke incidence). The artificial neural network "ANN" emulators statistically signify ($p < 0.01$) the higher incidence of stroke in developing countries. The entire summing of the results concludes that the Bayesian predictive risk analysis ANN model is the best simulation model to produce consistent result for estimation of DALYs at greater accuracy and lesser time intervals ($R^2 = 0.96$). Particularly, the present fitted models can be very useful in developing countries for implementation of policy interventions and reduction of high dimensional data sets with continuous state variables. In addition to that, the consistency and accuracy of the model can be enhanced with a larger health record database.

2.13 Factorial Design

Factorial design (FD) is one in which two or more variables or factors are employed to conduct the research in such a way that all the possible treatment combinations of selected subjects, each subjects are used (Mcburney et al.) for the practical point of view. The factorial design (FD) is a unique design in which selected parameters of two or more independent variables are certainly manipulated in all possible combinations so that the independent variables as well as interactive effects dealt upon the dependent variable may be studied. On the basis of the above-cited definition, the factorial design (FD) is more suited for clinical, drug trial, and biological experimentation. The FD is one in which two or more independent variables were assigned in all possible combinations, and thus the FD will provide practical insight information to the researcher at greater accuracy. The design will inculcate the interest of the researcher to know the effect of independent variables as well as combination of interactive effects of two or more independent variables simultaneously. In a broad sense, the factors were defined by the scientist in many ways; the term factors is broadly described and inclusion with all independent variables that are manipulated by the researcher in the experimentation or trial (manipulated through selection of the subjects and randomization techniques). In the advent of research pedagogy, sometimes it is possible to manipulate the independent variables directly, for example, in case of the clinical trial, the researcher may preclude to know the effect of different drugs or novel regime on the prognostic factors or recovery from the diseases; all the parameters of estimates were likely to be estimated at greater accuracy and more precision. In contrast to illustration, the researcher may select three dosages 2, 4, and 6 mg of norflox novel regime, and administered subjects are classified based on the different age criteria. Further, he wishes to evaluate the efficacy and prognosis effect by considering the age of the patient, previous history and adherence level, and also another important variable; the rate of recovery from the diseases was also considered. One more interesting practical experience was noted that the second independent variable (age) cannot be directly manipulated by the researcher; the manipulation of the variable of age will be achieved through the selection of the sample (at the time of inception of drug). The researcher willing to classify the subjects in different age groups is based on the objective of the interest.

2.13.1 Main Effect

This is the simplest effect of a factor on a dependent variable, the effect on each factors alone average across the level of other factors (Mourney et al. 2005) main effect in a factorial experiment, the effect of one independent variable averaged overall levels of another independent variables.

2.13.2 Interaction

An interaction means when the effect of one independent variable is dependent on the levels of another independent variable. An interaction is the variation among the difference between means of different levels of one factor over different levels of other factor. For example, a cholesterol reduction of obese cases driven by the two diets and exercise regime. It was found that, the exercise and diet alone was found to be effective (diet alone was effective for reducing cholesterol levels) (main effect of exercise and main effect of diet), also for those patients or cases who did not t practiced exercise, the two diet has worked equally well (the main effect of diet) those who follow diet "A" and exercised got the benefits of both intervention. Since it was found that the cases that followed diet "B" and exercised got the benefit of both plus a bonus, an interaction effect. The bio-statistician classified interaction effects broadly into three subtypes (Cook and Nachtsheim 1980).

1. Antagonistic interaction: The main effect is found to be insignificant and interaction is significant. In this situation, the two independent variables tend to reverse each other effect.
2. Synergistic interaction: When higher level of one independent variable enhances the effect of another independent variable it is called synergetic effect (e.g., age versus body mass index).
3. Celling effect interaction: When the higher level of one independent variable reduces the differential effect of another variable, i.e., one variable has a smaller effect when paired with higher level of a second variable (high dosage of fertilizer can yield fewer effect on response).

Asper the literature, three basic types of regular experimental designs, which are distinct relationships and applications on the research pedagogy (Fig. 2.6).

In factorial clinical trial, we learnt the outcomes of individual and interaction effect of selected factors. Design will permit us for assessment of potential impact among the treatments. There are two or more factors with multiple levels that are crossed, e.g., three dose levels of drug A and two levels of drug B can be crossed to yield a total six treatment combinations.

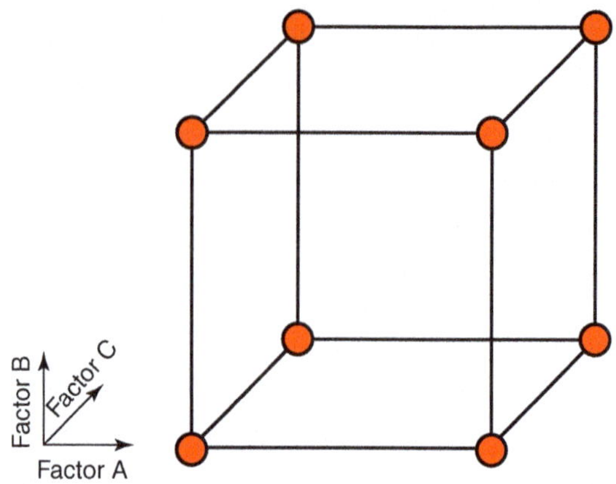

Fig. 2.6 Full factorial design

Low dose of A with low dose of B drug
Low dose of A with low high of B drug
Mid dose of A with high dose of B drug
Mid dose of A with low dose of B drug
High dose of A with low dose of B drug
High dose of A with high dose of B drug

In clinical trial setup, factorial design (FD) 2 × 2 factorial with two levels of factor A crossed with two levels of factor B to produce four treatment combinations. A special case of the 2 × 2 factorial design FD with a placebo and an active formulation of factor A crossed with a placebo and an active formulation of factor B. This yields the four treatment regimens.

Rx	Treatment	Placebo	
Active		A	B
	A	AA	AB
	B	BA	BB

Placebo A + Placebo B; Placebo A + Active B; Active A + Placebo B; Active A + Active B

FD provide the only way to determine the interaction between RxA and B. This is because the design formulation has treatment groups with all possible combination of Rx. The researcher wishes to know the interaction that may be dependent on the scale of measurement. Factorial designs provide the only way to study interactions between treatment A and treatment B. This is because the design has treatment groups with all possible combinations of treatments (Fig. 2.7).

Fig. 2.7 Interaction effects of A and B drug

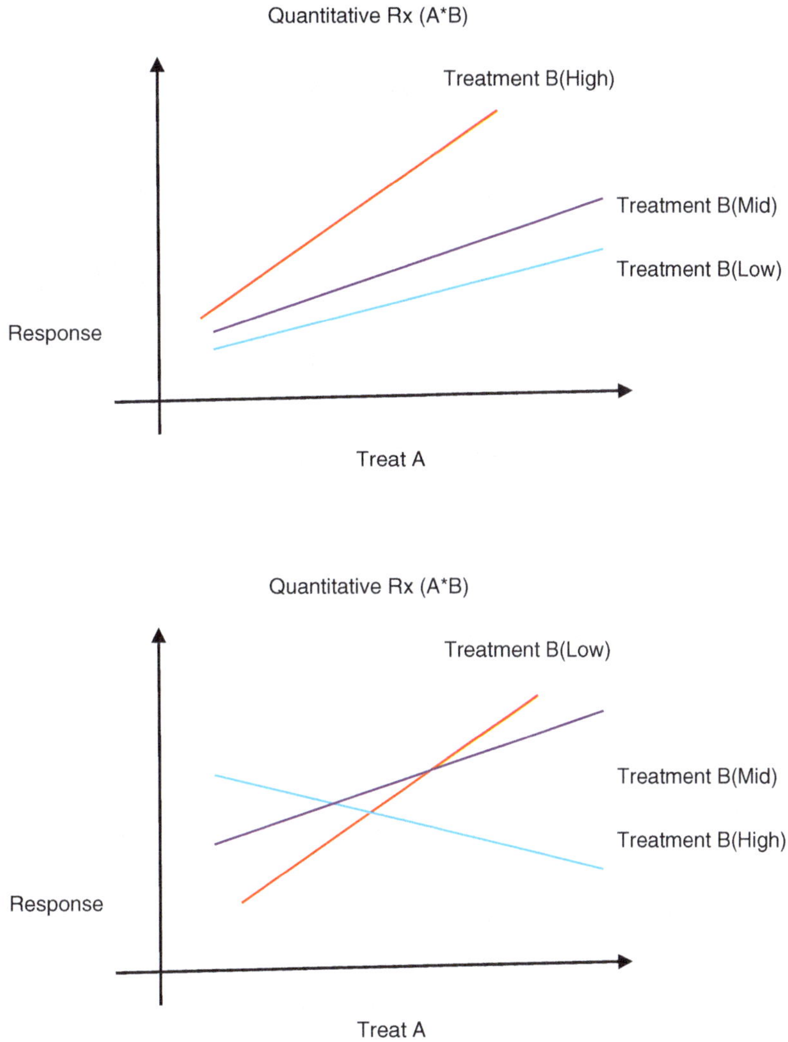

Note: Between the treatment groups are more heterogeneous and within the treatment comparison is more homogeneous in nature

A special case of PFD is occasionally used in clinical research in 2 × 2 factorial design (FD) with three treatments consisting of drug A, B, and D_A with D_B

Placebo A + Active B

Active A + Placebo B

Active A + Active B

Placebo A + Placebo B group is not included in the design hence the incompleteness. The combination of therapy can be marketable and profitable. In general situation, we have noticed in the PLHIVs lifelong therapy. The combination of ZN + STV + EFV increases the life longevity of patients and also increases the CD_4 counts in a particular period of time. Therefore; one pill or immunotherapy can increase the survivability of the patients and good response yielded from the administered drugs (monotherapy or combination). Suppose that the response is continuous, we want to compare the mean response μ_A, μ_B and interaction effect μ_{AB} which represents the population means for A immunotherapy, the B monotherapy and AB combination of therapy, respectively. The null hypothesis becomes

$$H_0 = \mu_A \le \mu_{AB}, H_0 = \mu_B \ge \mu_{AB}; H_1 = \mu_A < \mu_{AB}; \mu_B < \mu_{AB}$$

"Mini" test statistics is an appropriate method to test the null hypothesis for the above intervention and examine the Gaussianity (normality) and construct the two sample test statistics "*t*".

$$t_{\mathrm{A}} = \frac{\left(\bar{Y}_{\mathrm{AB}} - \bar{Y}_{\mathrm{A}}\right)}{S\sqrt{\frac{1}{n_{\mathrm{AB}}} + \frac{1}{n_{\mathrm{A}}}}}$$

$$t_{\mathrm{B}} = \frac{\left(\bar{Y}_{\mathrm{AB}} - \bar{Y}_{\mathrm{B}}\right)}{S\sqrt{\frac{1}{n_{\mathrm{AB}}} + \frac{1}{n_{\mathrm{B}}}}}$$

$$\bar{Y}_{\mathrm{A}} = \frac{1}{n_{\mathrm{A}}}\sum_{i=1}^{A} Y_{\mathrm{A}};\bar{Y}_{\mathrm{B}} = \frac{1}{n_{\mathrm{B}}}\sum_{i=1}^{B} Y_{\mathrm{B}};\bar{Y}_{\mathrm{AB}} = \frac{1}{n_{\mathrm{AB}}}\sum_{i=1}^{\mathrm{AB}} Y_{\mathrm{B}}Y_{\mathrm{A}}$$

$$s^2 = \frac{1}{n_{\mathrm{A}} + n_{\mathrm{B}} + n_{\mathrm{AB}} - 3}\left[\sum_{i=1}^{\mathrm{A}}\left(Y_{\mathrm{A}} - \bar{Y}_{\mathrm{A}}\right)^2 + \sum_{i=1}^{\mathrm{B}}\left(Y_{\mathrm{B}} - \bar{Y}_{\mathrm{B}}\right)^2 + \sum_{i=1}^{\mathrm{AB}}\left(Y_{\mathrm{AB}} - \bar{Y}_{\mathrm{AB}}\right)^2\right]$$

Minimum $(t_{\mathrm{A}} - t_{\mathrm{B}}) > tn_{\mathrm{A}} + tn_{\mathrm{B}} + tn_{\mathrm{AB}} - 3, (1 - \alpha)$, reject H_0.

2.14 Bioequivalence Trial

The drug trial experimentation we wish to see the potency and efficacy of drug. The objective of bioequivalence trial is to estimate whether test (*T*) and reference (*R*) formulation of a pharmaceutical product are equivalent with respect to blood concentration × time profile of the subjects. The researcher is interested in focusing on two situations: (1) Company A demonstrates the safety and efficacy of a drug formulation, but wishes to market a more convenient formulation (i.e., an injection versus time release capsule). This situation is less common in clinical trial; (2) Company B wishes to market a drug formulation similar to approved formulation of company A with an expired patent. Company B has to approve that they can deliver the same amount of active drug into the bloodstream which the approved formula does. Pharmaceutical scientists use crossover design for such trials in order to mitigate each trial participant to yield a profile for both formulations. The blood concentration x time profile is multivariate response and is a surrogate measure of therapeutic response. The pharmaceutical company does not need to demonstrate the safety and efficacy of the drug because that already has been established (Fig. 2.8).

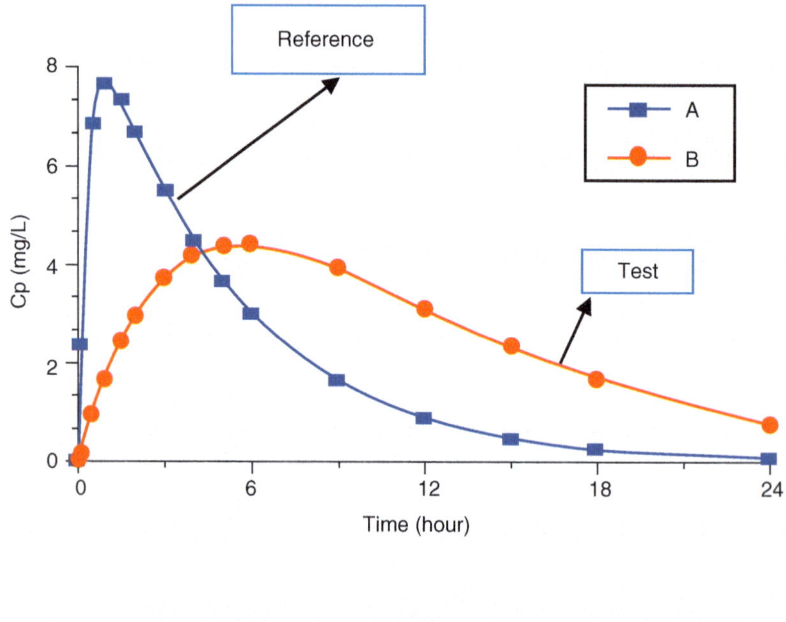

Fig. 2.8 Bioequivalence trial for 150 mg of bupropion capsule

2.15 Full Factorial Design

The first design shown in (Fig. 2.6) is a full factorial design; we call it full because the whole cube, including all its corners has been investigated. In addition to this, some replicated center point experiments are made. The factors have two levels of investigation; so far, the factors need 2^k design runs. This type of design is normally used for screening of various combinations with a linear or an interaction model. Especially, this type of design is more suited for the evaluation of progeny breeding trial experimentation in agriculture and animal science breeding trial at larger scale (Cox et al. 1989; Conover et al. 1981). All the treatment effects are estimated from every corner with greatest accuracy and more number of treatment subjects. The randomization procedure was allowed for the estimation of predictable errors. FD are the basis for certain principles besides with blocking at individual or group level and also which can examine the several factors simultaneously. We will start by looking at just two factors and then generalize the several factors, imputing with multiple factors in the same design automatically, it will generate replications for each of the selected factors or parameters.

2.16 Fractional Factorial Designs (FFD)

A fractional design does not consider all possible corners and reduces the number of design runs by choosing only a fraction of the $2k$ runs of the full factorial design (Fig. 2.9) shown as an example, where only four of the possible eight points are investigated. FFD are normally used for screening and robustness tests (Erikson et al.). FFD is very useful, when we cannot afford even one fall replicate of the FD. In a typical situation our, total number of runs is $N = 2^{k-p}$ which is the fraction of total number of treatments $k = 3$, $p = 1$; $N = 2^2 = 4$, so in this case either one of these blocks above is one half fraction of a 2^3 design. ABC produce 1/2 fraction of the 2^3 factorial design,

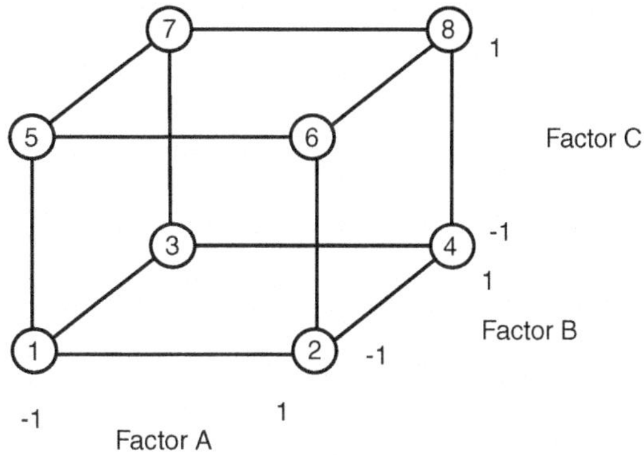

Fig. 2.9 Fractional factorial design (FFD)

Table 2.6 Treatment combination in FFD

Treatment	A	B	C	AB	AC	BC	ABC	I
(1)	–	–	–	+	+	+	–	+
ab	+	+	–	+	–	–	–	+
ac	+	–	+	–	+	–	–	+
bc	–	+	+	–	–	+	–	+

now we take just the fraction of FD where ABC = −1 and we place it within its following table (Table 2.6).

The goal is to create design that allow us to screen a large number of factors but without having a very large experiment. In this context, we are screening a large number of factors we are operating under the assumptions that only a few are very important. Here we wish to consider $k = 5$ and $p = 1$, again, so that we have a one half fraction of a 2^5 design. Extended to have five factors, A, B, C, D, and E, each at two levels. The runs that were obtained is as follows. Since we are picking up only on one generator, we should choose the highest order interaction as possible. So our likelihood of interaction effect I = ABCDE, the five-way interactions were obtained from the FFD.

Fractional Factorial Design

Factors:	5	Base design:	5, 16	Resolution:	*V*
Runs:	16	Replicates:	1	Fraction:	1/2
Blocks:	1	Center pts (total):	0		

Design Generators: E = ABCD

Alias Structure

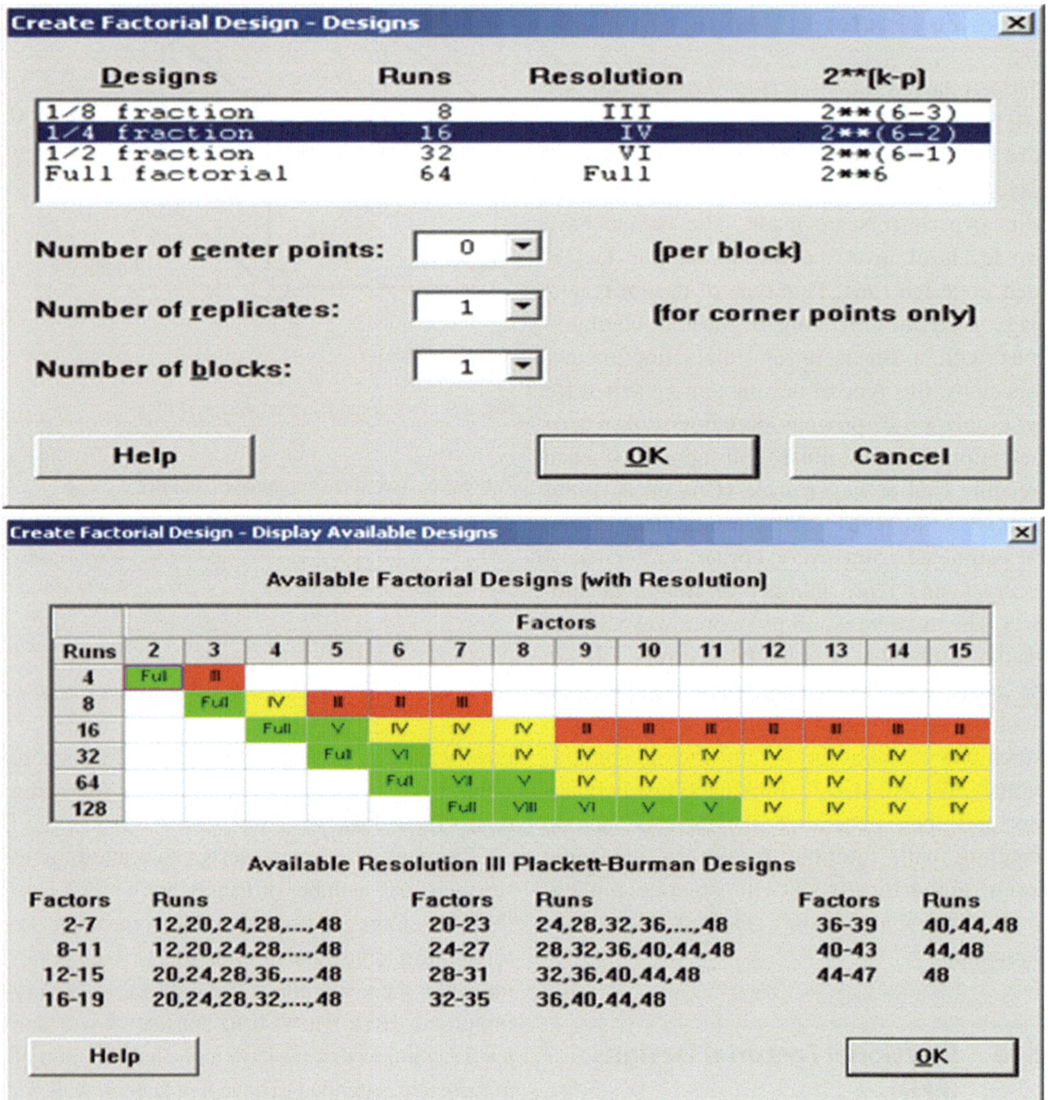

Fig. 2.10 Resolution IV design generated from Minitab software

I + ABCDE,A + BCDE,B + ACDE,C + ABD E,D + ABCE,E + ABCD,AB + CDE

AC + BDE,AD + BCE,AE + BCD,BC + AD E,BD + ACE,BE + ACD,CD + ABE

CE + ABD,DE + ABC, E = ABCD gives us the basis for the resolution of the design.

From the resulted alias structure we obtained a main and effective two-way and three-way interaction and overwhelmingly two-way interaction are very clear of each other but are aliased with three-way interaction effects (Fig. 2.10).

2.17 Composite Designs

The last design type for a rectangular experimental area is the composite design; it combines the investigations done by a factorial design, the corner, and replicated center points, with the use of axial experiments. Right hand cube shows axial experiment are placed on the six squares. Factors normally have three or five levels of investigations, and due to this quadratic models are used (Erikson et al.). Box–Wilson central composite design, commonly called as central composite

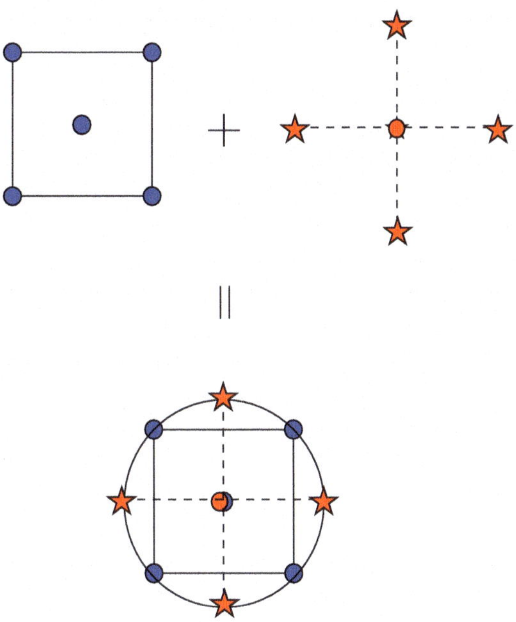

Fig. 2.11 Show center, factorial, and axial points of the CCD

design inclusion with imbedded factorial or FFD design with center points, i.e., augmented with a group of star ostrich or points that allow us to estimation of full-blown curvature. If the distance from the center of the design space to factorial point is ±1 unit for each factor, the distance from the center of the design space to a start point is $|\alpha| > 1$. The precise random value of α depends on certain properties desired for the design and on the number of factors involved. A number of center point's runs the design in association with certain properties required for the design (Concato et al. 2000; Cox and Reid 2000) (Fig. 2.11).

The value of α is chosen to maintain rotatability, practical insight of the CD, and the value of α depends on the number of experimental runs in the factorial portion of the central composite design. The α values were obtained from the following eqn.:

$$\alpha = [\text{Number of factorial runs}]^{1/4}$$

If the factorial is full factor, then the above equation becomes

$$\alpha = \left[2^k\right]^{1/4}.$$

Table 2.7 Demonstration of α rotatability values

Number of factors	Factorial portion	Scaled value for **α relative to ± 1**
2	2^2	$2^{2/4} = 1.44$
3	2^3	$2^{3/4} = 1.68$
4	2^4	$2^{4/4} = 2.00$
5	2^{5-1}	$2^{5/4} = 2.00$
5	2^5	$2^{5/4} = 2.37$
6	2^{6-1}	$2^{5/4} = 2.37$
6	2^6	$2^{6/4} = 2.82$

However, the factorial portion can be a fractional factorial design of fifth resolution (v). In practical essence, the α rotatability will be very much required for the formulation of the design. Various scaled values were derived by using Minitab fundamental software (Table 2.7).

The values of alpha also depend on whether or not the design is orthogonally blocked by the hypothesis and whether or not the design is divided into blocks such that the block effects do not affect the estimates of the coefficient in the second-order model.

2.18 Factorial Design 2 × 2 ($2^2 = 2 \times 2$)

In case of 2 × 2 factorial designs, the experiment has two independent variables, each of which has two values or levels. This is known as factorial design. 2 × 2 is simplest factorial design (FD), whereby participants are randomly allocated to one of four combination of two subjects (A&B), these combinations are a alone b alone both a&b, Neither A nor B, C is control. This type of design allows the researcher to compare the experimental interest with the placebo or unexposed population (control population) to compare the experimental intervention with each other and investigator can also derive the possible combination of interactions between them. If there is no interaction between the subjects, the factorial design will have greater statistical power then a traditional multiple arm trial. This implies that two interventions can be studied in the same trial without increasing the required number of participants (Akey et al. 2007).

Illustration: The drug trial experts conducted the experiment to know the effect of drug on omega-3 supplementation with Marvistatin 5 and 8 mg considering placebo, the outline of 2 × 2 factorial design is as follows (Table 2.8):

2.18.1 Effect of Interaction A&B, AB

Let experiment preclude (*I*), (*a*), (*b*), and (*ab*) combination of four runs, *n* represents the total of all observations.

Main effect of A = 1/2*n* {*a* + *ab* − b − (1)}

Main effect of B = 1/2*n* {b + ab − a − (1)}

Effect of AB = 1/2*n* {*ab* + (*I*) − *a* − *b*} brackets are called contrasting effect

Contrast A = {*a* + *a b* − b − (1)}

From illustration, an effect of A, B, and AB is determined by the following:

$$\bar{y}_{a+} - \bar{y}_{a-} = 40 + 52/220 + 30/2 = 21$$
$$\bar{y}_{b+} - \bar{y}_{b-} = 30 + 52/2 - 20 + 40/2 = 11$$
$$52 + 20/2 - 30 + 40/2 = -1$$

2.19 Factorial Design 2 × 2 × 2 (2^3)

In any clinical research, the oncologist wishes to evaluate the tumor size after the intervention of chemotherapy to know the efficacy of the drug at desired level at 99% (α = 0.01 level of significance) level of significance; he considered the treatment aspects of chemotherapy in association with different length of period (<90 days and >90 days follow-up period) considering gender-matched frequency (male and female population) administered by different dosage of chemo drugs. The layout of design is formulated as follows (Tables 2.9, 2.10 and 2.11).

2.20 3^2 Factorial Design (2 Factor at 3 Level)

A multicentric diabetes drug trial which was conducted in three selected regions comprises of male and female subjects at 24 months duration;

Table 2.8 Intervention of Marvistatin on different dosage

Intervention	A_1 Marvistatin 5 mg +	A_2 Marvistatin 8 mg −	Total
Omega 3 Supplementation (B_1) +	30 (b_1×a_1) ++	52 (b_1×a_2) + −	82
Placebo (B_2) −	20 (b_2×a_1) − +	40 (b_2×a_2) − −	60
Total	50	92	142
2 × 2 = 4			

Trial run	A	B	AB	Combination
1	+1	−1	−1	(1)
2	+1	+1	+1	(*a*)
3	−1	−1	+1	(*b*)
4	−1	+1	−1	(*ab*)

Table 2.9 Interaction effect of factor A, B, and C in male and female

	Factor A				
	FA_1 (< 90 days assessment)		FA_2 (> 90 days assessment)		
	Factor B				
Factor C (Tumor size)	FB_1 (male)	FB_1 (female)	FB_2 (male)	FB_2(female)	Average total (%)
C_1 (0–100 cc)	88%	78%	85%	79%	82.51%
C_2 (100–200cc)	92%	86%	84%	81%	85.75%
Average total (%)	90%	82%	84.5%	80%	84.12%

Table 2.10 Number of runs iterated

Runs	A	B	C	Label
1	–	–	–	(1)
2	+	–	–	(*a*)
3	–	+	–	(*b*)
4	+	+	–	(*ab*)
5	–	–	+	(*c*)
6	+	–	+	(*ac*)
7	–	+	+	(*bc*)
8	+	+	+	(*abc*)

the design will be formulated in the following ways (Tables 2.12 and 2.13).

2.21 Merits of Factorial Design

Many merits are enlisted; the factorial design is easy to permit the researcher for the assessment of the presence of interaction between two or more factors, and if no interaction is present it

Table 2.11 Analysis of variance (table ANOVA)

Source of variation	*df*	SS	MSS	F_{cal}	$F_{cal} > F_{table}$ @ error *df*
Factor A	$(a - 1)$	SS^2a	MSa	Fa = MSa/MSe	*Ho* accept
Factor B	$(b - 1)$	SS^2b	MSb	Fb = MSb/MSe	*Ho* accept
Factor C	$(c - 1)$	SS^2c	MSc	Fc = MSc/MSe	*Ho* accept
AB	$(a - 1)(b - 1)$	SS^2ab	MSab	Fab = MSab/MSe	*Ho* accept
AC	$(a - 1)(c - 1)$	SS^2ac	MSac	Fac = MSac/MSe	*Ho* accept
BC	$(b - 1)(c - 1)$	SS^2bc	MSbc	Fbc = MSbc/MSe	*Ho* accept
ABC	$(a - 1)(b - 1)(c - 1)$	SS^2abc	MSabc	Fabc = MSabc/MSe	*Ho* accept
Error	*n-abc*	SS^2Error	MSe		
Total	$(abc - 1)$				

Table 2.12 Hierarchical table interaction with A and B factors

	Levels (regions)			Total
	Northern Mean temp (35 °C)	Southern Mean temp (31 °C)	Eastern Mean temp (28 °C)	
Gender	$A_{1(+)}$	$A_{2(-)}$	$A_{3(+)}$	
Male (500 mg) B_{1+}	$A_1B_{1\,(++)}$	$B_1A_{2(+\,-)}$	$B_1A_{3\,(++)}$	$A_1B_1 + B_1A_2 + B_1A_3$
Female (500 mg) B_{2-}	B_2A_1 (– +)	B_2A_2 (– –)	A_3B_2 (– +)	$B_2A_1 + B_2A_2 + A_3B_2$
Total	$A_1B_1 + B_2A_1$	$B_1A_2 + B_2A_2$	$B_1A_3 + A_3B_2$	*N*

Runs	B_{1+}	B_{2-}
$B_1 \times A_1$	–1	–1
$B_1 \times A_2$	–1	0
$B_1 \times A_3$	–1	+1
$B_2 \times A_1$	0	–1
$B_2 \times A_2$	0	0
$A_3 \times B_2$	0	–1
$A_1B_1 \times B_2A_1$	+1	–1
$B_1A_2 \times B_2A_2$	+1	0
$B_1A_3 \times A_3B_2$	+1	–1

Table 2.13 Matrix of combination of various factors at each level

	Factors			
Levels	2	3	4	5
2	4	8	16	32
3	9	27	81	243
4	16	64	256	1024
5	25	125	625	3125
6	36	216	1296	7776
7	49	343	2401	16,807
8	64	512	4096	32,768

can simply reject the null hypothesis. The design is more efficient than two separate studies, one for each of the two factors. As such interaction is present when the differences between the levels for one factor are different for the different levels of the other factor. That is, when differences are different. In this following two-factor example, participants received one of four drugs and also participated in one of four exercise programs. Hence, each factor has four levels and there are 16 treatment combinations altogether. Three participants were assigned to each of the 16 treatment combinations, so that a total of n = 48 participants were involved.

An activity intensity score was recorded for each participant (Fig. 2.12).

Note:-If the null hypothesis of no interaction is rejected, then a test for overall drug effect or overall exercise effect has no meaning. Under these circumstances, these tests should not be done; however, it is likely to be insightful to examine the patterns of interaction between the two factors.

Activity response score

Drug	Type of exercise				Total
	A	B	C	D	
1	4 3 7	2 2 1	9 7 3	3 4 3	
Total	14	5	19	10	48
2	2 4 6 12	5 3 7 15	5 2 3 10	5 4 7 16	
					53
3	3 6 3 14	4 8 5 17	7 5 4 16	9 5 6 20	
					67
4	2 2 3 7	9 4 5 18	4 6 5 15	9 5 8 22	
					62
Total	47	55	60	68	230

ANOVA results

Source of variation	df	SS	MS	F Critical
Exercise (E)	3	19.42	6.47	1.95
Drug (D)	3	18.42	6.14	1.85
$E * D$	9	70.08	7.79	2.35
Treatments	15	107.92	7.19	
Within	32	106.00	3.31	
Total	47	213.92		

$$F(\text{interaction}) = 7.79 / 3.31 = 2.35 F 0.95(9,32) = 2.19$$

$$F(\text{exercise}) = 6.47/3.31 = 1.95 F 0.95(3,32) = 2.90$$

$$F(\text{drugs}) = 6.14/3.31 = 1.85 F 0.95(3,32) = 2.90$$

2.22 Practical Approach of Fractional Factorial Design (FFD)

As the number of factors to be tested increases, the complete set of factorial treatment may become too large to be tested simultaneously in a single clinical experiment. Say for example in clinical research HAART drug trial (multicentric study) for PLHIVs, cancer drug trial, evidence-based medicine, etc. This type of study has been generated numerous and countless number of treatment groups and attributes; each attribute is very essential for the researcher to know the effectiveness of drug or potency. In this proximity, a large number of treatment groups and experimental areas would be needed for practical

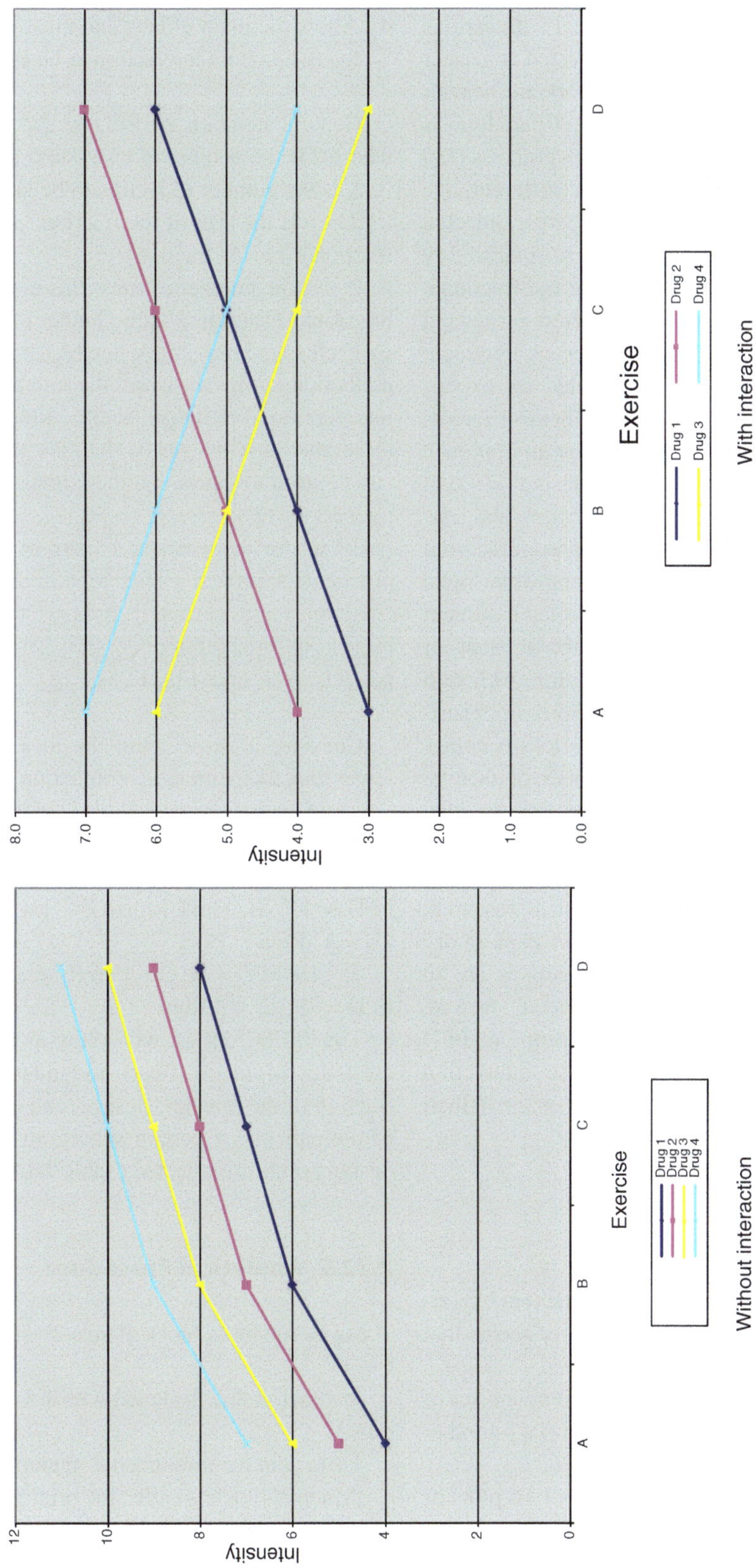

Fig. 2.12 Interaction with and without effect of various factors

wpoint of view; the exposure indeed with various multiplicative factors have to be tested at greater accuracy. Eventually, certain factors are heavier than the others. A logical treatment paradigm is very essential for testing the null hypothesis (H_0) (e.g., potency of the drug with different age group, gender-matched potency with selected sites, correlation with risk factors, comorbidity and quality of life domain). Since the fractional factorial design allows the parameters for testing only fraction of the total number of treatment groups. A design is uniquely suited for experiment involving a large number or heavier factors that could be tested systematically; an approach is nothing but fractional factorial design (FFD). It provides a systematic way for selecting and testing only a fraction of the complete set of factorial treatment combinations. In exchangeable logic, loss of information of some preselected treatment group has precluded effect in the interest of objectives of the research intervention. Although this information loss may be serious in experiment with one/two factors, such a loss becomes more tolerable with a large number of factors. Since the number of interaction efforts may increase rapidly with a number of factors involved which allows flexibility in the choice of particular effect to be scarified. In clinical research, "FFD" is most commonly used in exploratory clinical trial where the main objectives are to determine the interaction between factors. The above cited trial is the most appropriate FFD are those that scarifies only those interaction effects that involve more than two factors (Bhatt et al. 2008).

2.22.1 Features

1. Apply clinical or drug trial 2^n factors experiment where "n" is the number of factor that ranges from 5 to 7.
2. Involves only one half of the complete set of factorial treatment combination (i.e., number of treatment 1/2 of 2^n, 2^{n-1}).
3. Have a block size (ward units) of 16 plots or less.
4. Allow the main effects and most, if not all of the two factors interaction to be estimated.

General notation of FFD is $2R^{k-p} \neq$ runs, where 2 is the number of levels for each factors.

K is the number of factors to be investigated.

$2 - p$ is the size of the fraction ($p = 1 \Rightarrow 1/2$ fraction $p \Rightarrow 1/4$ fraction).

2^{k-p} is the number of runs, R is the resolution; Standard (2^3 design $2 \times 2 \times 2 = 8$).

Run	A	B	C
1	−1	−1	−1
2	+1	−1	−1
3	−1	+1	−1
4	+1	+1	−1
5	−1	−1	+1
6	+1	−1	+1
7	−1	+1	+1
8	+1	+1	+1

Note: −1 means set factor to low level in this run, +1: means set factor to high level in this run

Consider a $2k$ set with the idea of running fewer than $2k$ treatment combination

2^3 design run 4 times, 2^{3-1} (1/2 of 2^3), 2^5 design in 8 (2^{5-2} 1/4 of 2^5)

2^7 full factor = 7F, 2L = 128 Runs, 2^{7-1} 1/2 FFD = 7F, 2L = 64 Runs, 2^{7-2} 1/4 FFD = 7F, 2L = 32 Runs

2^{7-3} 1/8 FFD = 7F, 2L = 16 Runs and 2^{7-4} 1/16 FFD = 7F, 2L = 8 Runs

The "FFD" design will allow us to get good estimates of main effects and interaction at a fraction of the potency, dosage, and body weight of the patients. A certain subsets of $2k$ possible design points are selected (Table 2.14).

2.22.2 Analytical Procedure

2^k can be run in $2q$ block of size 2^{k-q} for $q = 1,\ldots, k - 1$.

2^{k-q} factorial is designed with k factors in 2^{k-q} runs I.

1 Block of a confounded 2^k factorial

Principal block is called the principal fraction; other blocks are called alternate fractions.

Table 2.14 Overview of runs with respect to contrast

Runs	A	B	C	D	E	F	G	γ
1	−1	−1	−1	1	1	1	−1	1.18
2	1	−1	−1	−1	−1	1	1	22.30
3	−1	1	−1	−1	1	−1	1	23.10
4	1	1	−1	1	−1	−1	−1	1.73
5	−1	−1	1	1	−1	−1	1	27.00
6	1	−1	1	−1	1	−1	−1	1.72
7	−1	1	1	−1	−1	1	−1	0.56
8	1	1	1	1	1	1	1	39.00
Contrast	12.91	12.19	19.97	21.23	13.41	9.49	106.21	14.57

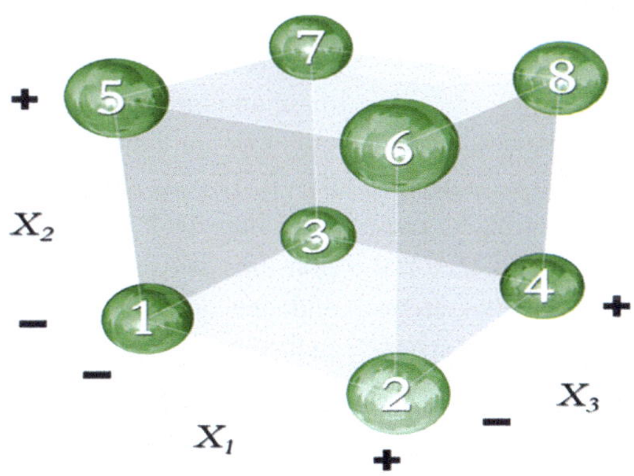

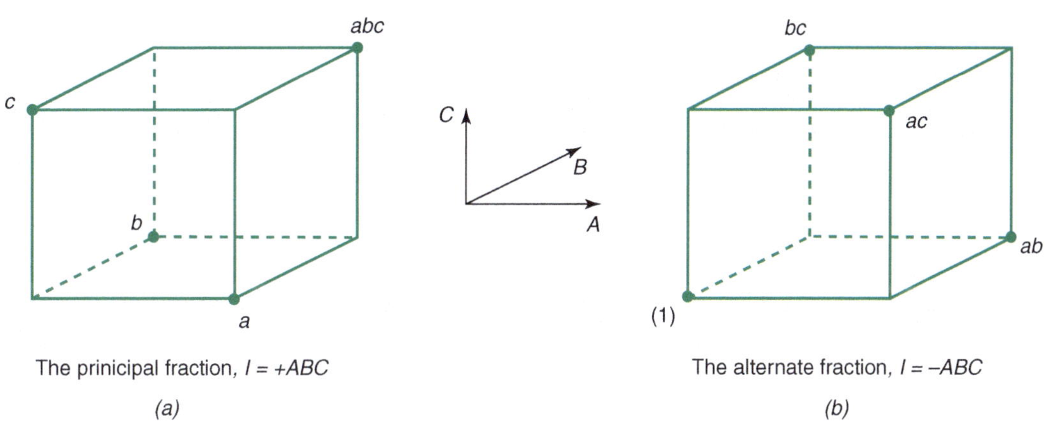

Fig. 2.13 Graphical view of RSD with associated principal of fraction and alternate fraction (*I*)

Augment table of two series with column of "+", labeled "*I*".

Defining contrasts are effects to be confounded together.

Generators are used to create the blocks by +/− structure.

Generalize the interactions of generators and also extrapolate the constant sign in particular blocks.

Defining the relations: I = A, I = −B * I = −AB.

Determining the selection of subset of 4 runs from a 2^3 = 8-run design. The driven methodology has generated many possible "fractional" designs in large-scale experiment.

The one-half fractions of the 2^3 design. (a) The principal fraction, I = +ABC. (b) The alternate fraction, I = −ABC. Figure 2.13 describes that

Table 2.15 FFD on a full 2^3 factorial design experiment

Treatment combination	A	B	C	D	E
ad	+1	−1	−1	+1	−1
e	−1	−1	−1	−1	+1
abde	+1	+1	−1	+1	+1
b	−1	+1	−1	−1	−1
ac	+1	−1	+1	−1	−1
cde	−1	−1	+1	+1	+1
abce	+1	+1	+1	−1	+1
bcd	−1	+1	+1	+1	−1

Note: Fractional factorial design allows us to get good estimates of main effects and interaction at a fraction of time and greater precision. A certain subsets of $2k$ possible design points are selected for the experiment

the random factors of $X_1, X_2..Xn$ have assigned in the corner of the cube in association with principal and alternate fraction; the iteration of runs were shown in the table matrix. The factorial design (FD) will estimate the parameters systematically without any loss of information in accordance with factorial analysis of variance nested type (nested ANOVA with and without interaction) (Table 2.15).

2.23 Response Surface Design (RSM)

In biological and medical research, the response surface design is very useful to evaluate the relationship between the response and the different input variables say for example, in case of life-threatened diseases like cancer or malignancy and HIV, the physician has been administered a new drug to improve the Quality of Life (QOL) domain since the researcher wishes to know the efficacy and dose response in defined time or follow-up period. Again he can optimize the response or understand the underlying mechanism of various input variables in association with multiple coaxial variables among massive data sets. However, the RSD are simple polynomial designs, which include many terms of interaction and curvature. The coefficients are usually established by regression analysis by computer program and insignificant variants are discarded at early inception of the treatment intervention. The response surface design (RSD) has been classified into I, II, and III order interactions, based on the different degree of polynomials. In historical perspective, way back in 1966 the response surface designed was coined by Prof. R A Fisher published numerous articles and also has reviewed the response surface methodology by using medical life data sets. Similar in a study done by Benson et al. (2000) derived the RSD by multiplicative and polynomial structure modeling techniques, the RSD is unique design and more suited for medical and agricultural research. In a similar extended study done by Prof. R A Fisher (1926) opined that the RSD is very compressive and allows us to get estimation of main and interaction effects simultaneously without any ambiguity. Box et al. (1978) describe the RSD way back in 1978; his assumptions regarding for RSD, the design explores the relationships between several explanatory variables and one or more response variables included for reduction of experimental runs in convenient manner without loss of any information from research settings (no ambiguity between the selection of treatment runs). The above research intervention for selection of runs from the treatment groups is apparently correlated by various scientists at global level (Box 1957; Hunter et al. 1966). Main purpose of the research study to review the practicability of RSD in chemical and related problems of biology. Further recent research work done by (Oehlert et al. 2019; Myers et al. 1995) published research findings on RSD from a biometrical point of view for validation of design effects and smoothening of explanatory variables on selected variables. The Response surface design (RSD) uses various applications for formulation statistical modelling, graphical presentation, and advanced mathematical techniques to develop and improve the data points driven by the resulted findings or optimize a entire process of massive types of research data sets.

2.23.1 Analytical Procedure RSM

1. RSD able to resolve around the certain salient assumptions that the response is a function of a set of independent variables $X_1, X_2, X_3 \ldots X_K$

and function can be approximated in variant of polynomial model.

$$Y = f(X_i), Y = f(X_1, X_2, X_3 \dots X_k) \quad (2.10)$$

Here, response variable is "Y" that depends on the "kth" independent variable.

2. Factors directly estimates the effect and interaction of the model as describe in (Fig. 2.12).
3. And if the factors are unknown, then first you have to calculate the parameters by using screening method.
4. To estimate the interaction effects by using first-order polynomial model, the equation of polynomial is as follows:

$$Y = \beta_0 + \beta_1 x_1 + \beta_2 x_2 + \beta_3 x_{12} + \beta_4 x_{22} + + \beta_5 x_1 x_2 + \varepsilon \quad (2.11)$$

5. If curvature is found, use RSM and second-order polynomial model and it will be very easy to approximate the response variable.
6. To make the graph and find stationary points, the maximum response and saddle points were estimated by using the values of $X_1, X_2, X_3 \dots X_k$.

2.23.2 Types of Model

First-order model: Often in RSD, the relationship between response variable and independent variable is not given; after screening, we use first-order model to find curvature situation and to find either there is a curvature or not existing in the data sets.

Second-order model**:** If we have to find curvature after making figure from the result of first-order model, then we use second-order model to find our optimum point.

Response Surface Model modelled with two factors: assumed X_1 (age) and X_2 (drug dosage) and measured response Y (regardless of number of levels) considered as two factors, extrapolate the model by three phase, namely screening, steepest and optimization techniques or methods.

$$\text{Screening}\, y = \beta_0 + \beta_1 x_1 + \beta_2 x_2 + \beta_3 x_{12} + \beta_4 x_{22} + \beta_5 x_1 x_2 + \varepsilon \quad (2.12)$$

Variable = constant + main effects + curvature + interaction + error

$$\text{Steepest}\, y = \beta_0 + \beta_1 x_1 + \beta_2 x_2 + \varepsilon \quad (2.13)$$

Optimization

$$Y = \beta_0 + \beta_1 X_1 + \beta_2 X_2 + \beta_{12} X_1 X_2 + \beta_{11} X_1^2 + \beta_{22} X_1^2 + \varepsilon$$

The same variables were considered to know the effect of response on three factors at two levels.

Three factors at two level

$$Y = \beta_0 + \beta_1 x_1 + \beta_2 x_2 + \beta_3 x_3 + \beta_{11} x_{12} + \beta_{22} x_{22} + \beta_{33} x_{32} + + \beta_{12} x_1 x_2 + \beta_{13} x_1 x_3 + \beta_{23} x_2 x_3 + \varepsilon \quad (2.14)$$

Response (Y) = Constant + main effects + curvature + interactions + error

Second-order model

$$y = \beta_0 + \sum_{i=1}^{k} \beta_i x_i + \sum_{i=}^{k} \beta_{ij} x^2{}_i + \sum_{i=1}^{k} \sum_{j=1}^{k} \beta_{ij} x_i x_j + e \quad (2.15)$$

$$\hat{y} = \hat{\beta}_0 + x^1 b + x^1 B x$$

$$x = \begin{bmatrix} x \\ x \\ \cdot \\ \cdot \\ x \end{bmatrix} b = \begin{bmatrix} \beta \\ \beta \\ \beta \end{bmatrix} B = \begin{bmatrix} \beta_{11} & \beta_1^2 & \beta_0^2 \\ . & \beta_2 & \beta_{11}^2 \\ . & .. & \beta^2{}_K \end{bmatrix}$$

$$\frac{\hat{\partial} Y}{\partial X} = b + 2BX$$

$$X_s = -\frac{1}{2} B^1 b$$

$$y = \hat{\beta}_0 + \frac{1}{2} X^1{}_s b \quad (2.16)$$

The stationary points represent a point of maximum response, a point of minimum response or saddle point. The design of second order may be classified as follows:

(1) Center composite design (2) Box–Behnken design (3) Face-centered design (4) Equi-radial design, and (5) Small composite and hybrid design.

Before deciding whether to build a response surface model, it is important to assess the adequacy of a linear model, the linear model represents constant and sum of coefficient of *Xi* variables, the equation becomes

$$Y = \beta_0 + \sum_{i=1}^{N} \beta_i X_i + \sum_{i=1}^{N}\sum_{j=1}^{N} \beta_{ij} X_i X_j \quad (2.17)$$

The lack of fit method is a unique method of estimation in RSD, and it will be considered for any model, $Y = f(\beta,Xi) + \varepsilon$, where $f(\beta,Xi)$ is an arbitrary function of the factors and the statistical parameters. The error term "ε" in the model is comprised of two parts, viz. modeling error (lack of fit, LOF), experimental error (pure error, PE), which can be calculated from replicate points. The lack of fit will help us to determine if the modeling error significantly differs from the pure error. In the method of comparison of LOF and PE by using fisher "*F*" ratios (determined from sum of squares and methods of ANOVA techniques).

2.23.3 Determining *F*-Ratio for the Lack of Fit

The "*F*" ratio statistics test is the ratio between the estimates of error due to lack of fit (LOF) and the estimate of error due to pure error (PE). The estimates are obtained from the two components which make up the total sum of squares for error (SSE)

$$\text{Sum of squares for error SSE} = (\text{SSPE} + \text{SSLOF}),$$

where SSE = Total sum of squares for error or residual sum of squares

SSPE = Sum of squares due to pure error

SSLOF = Sum of squares due to lack of fit

Determining pure error, suppose we have "*n*" repeated points at some *Xj*th matrix, then the sum of square probable error was

$$\text{SSPE} = \sum_{i=1}^{N} (y_i - \bar{y})^2, \quad (2.18)$$

where y_i's are the *n* different measured value at *Xj*. Then the estimate of pure error (PE) is

MSPE = SSPE/(n − 2). If there are "*m*" points available ($m \gg n$), with grand mean, the sum of squares due to lack of fit is driven by the following equation:

$$\text{SSLOF} = \text{SSE} - \text{SSPE}, \text{MSLOF} = \text{SSLOF}/(m-n) \quad (2.19)$$

F_{obs} = MSLOF/MSPE with $m - n$ and $n - 2$ degree of freedom, respectively.

Hypothesis testing: If $F_{obs} > F_{cal}$ (*df* LOF, *df* PE, α) (from Eq. 2.19), then there is a lack of fit. Several points are repeated, the general approach is to determine the SSPE for each set of replicates and then "pool" these sum of squares will be forming overall SSPE weighted values by the employed sufficient degree of freedom (*df*) for each set. Then, the estimate of probable error (PE) is obtained by dividing the SSPE by the appropriate number of degree of freedom and continuing as above derivation.

2.24 RSM Methods

A sequential nature of RSD we often to estimate the predictable error at greater accuracy and less profound time, when we use at a point on the response surface, i.e., response surface is remote (for away) from the optimum point and also we move rapidly from the current point to the optimum point with same sequence, resulted values shows significant digits (Box et al. 1988; Berry 1989). In this context, we have employed RSD design at greatest view for estimation of predictable error by using desired level of significance. However, we want the optimum point where the sources are minimum but output is maximum then we move rapidly towards points of conjunction. Two methods of RSD were used to obtain optimum response, and we move towards our optimum point with the following methods. (The objective is to lead the experimenter rapidly and efficiently along a path of improvement towards the general vicinity of the optimum.)

2.24.1 Methods of Steepest Ascent

This is the procedure for moving sequentially in the direction of the maximum increase in the response getting optimum response. The objective of the experimenters to move rapidly to the general vicinity (nearest point) of the optimum, we wish to use a simple economically efficient experimental procedure where we remote from the optimum point, usually assume that first-order model is an adequate approximation to the true surface in a small region of the Xs.

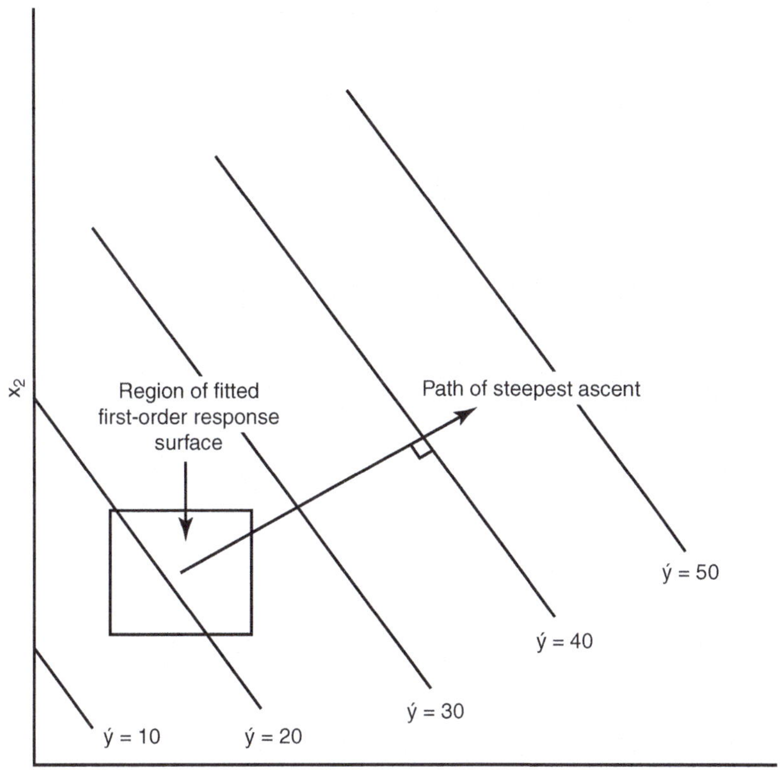

$$\overline{y} = \beta_0 + \sum_{i=1}^{k} \overline{\beta_i} x_i$$

$$\overline{y} = \beta_0 + \sum_{i=1}^{k} \overline{\beta_i} x_i \tag{2.20}$$

The actual step size was determined by the experimenter based on the process of technical and scientific knowledge or other practical considerations (Table 2.16).

$$\hat{y} = 40.44 + 0.775x_1 + 0.325x_2$$

Steepest descent

If minimization is desired, then we call these techniques as the method of steepest descent.

3^2 Factorial experiments Geometric Presentation is as follows

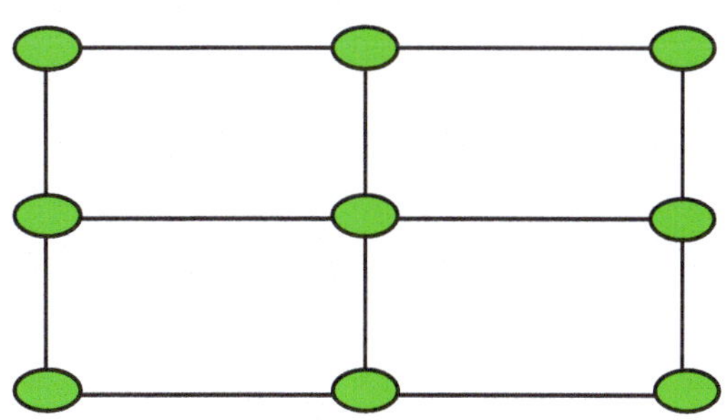

Table 2.16 Overview of runs with respect to factor 1 and 2

Std	Runs	Blocks	Factor 1 A:Time (Min)	Factor2 B:Temp (0 °C)	Response Yield (%)
1	7	{1}	1	1	39.34
2	6	{1}	1	1	40.91
3	5	{1}	1	1	40.22
4	2	{1}	1	1	41.51
5	9	{1}	0	0	40.32
6	4	{1}	0	0	40.58
7	1	{1}	0	0	40.71
8	3	{1}	0	0	40.20
9	8	{1}	0	0	40.63

Mathematical Model

$$y = \beta_0 + \beta_1 x_1 + \beta_2 x_2 + \beta_3 x_{12} + \beta_4 x_{22} + \beta_5 x_1 x_2 + \beta_6 x_{12} x_2 + \beta_7 x_1 x_{22} + \beta_8 x_{12} x_{22} + \varepsilon \quad (2.21)$$

3^3factorial experiment

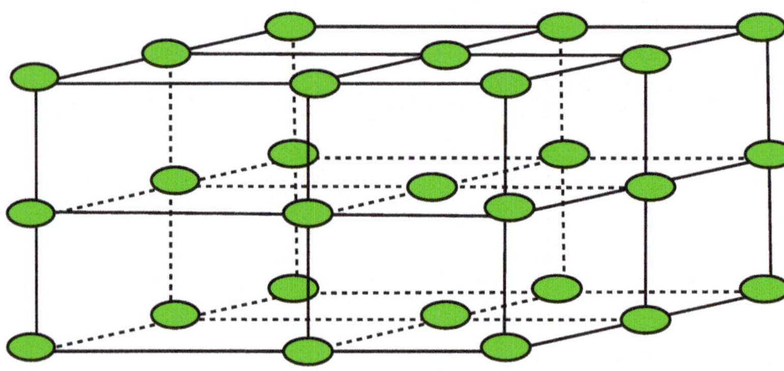

Geometric Presentation

Mathematical Model

$$\begin{aligned} y = {} & \beta_0 + \beta_1 x_1 + \beta_2 x_2 + \beta_3 x_3 + \beta_4 x_1 x_2 + \beta_5 x_1 x_3 + \beta_6 x_2 x_3 + \beta_7 x_{12} + \beta_8 x_{22} + \beta_9 x_{32} + \beta_{10} x_{12} x_2 \\ & + \beta_{11} x_{12} x_3 + \beta_{12} x_1 x_{22} + \beta_{13} x_{22} x_3 + \beta_{14} x_1 x_{32} + \beta_{15} x_2 x_{32} + \beta_{16} x_{12} x_{22} + \beta_{17} x_{12} x_{32} + \beta_{18} x_{22} x_{32} + \beta_{19} x_1 x_2 x_3 \\ & + \beta_{20} x_{12} x_2 x_3 + \beta_{21} x_1 x_{22} x_3 + \beta_{22} x_1 x_2 x_{32} + \beta_{23} x_{12} x_{22} x_3 + \beta_{24} x_{12} x_2 x_{32} + \beta_{25} x_1 x_{22} x_{32} + \beta_{26} x_{12} x_{22} x_{32} + \varepsilon \end{aligned} \quad (2.22)$$

The following designs are widely used for fitting a quadratic model.

Central composite design (uniform precision of effect estimates): The Box–Behnken design almost maintains uniform precision of effect estimates, but usually fewer runs are required for estimation of parameter than for CCD. The choice between these models is usually decided by the availability of these designs for a given number of runs and number of factors were considered. Importantly, note that there are other suitable designs usually available in statistical software that support DOE. Let we assume that the optimum we are looking for is a maximum. The steepest ascent direction is the clear path which gives or extrapolates the maximum increase in response as estimated from the coefficients of the mathematical modeling association with a full factorial (FD) or fractional factorial experiment (FFD) (i.e., the first-order term of a Taylor's series of expansion) (Fig. 2.14).

2.25 Plackett–Burman Design

The Plackett and Burman (1946) showed analytical intervention about the factorial interaction, how full fractional design (FFD) can be fractionalized in a different manner than traditional 2^k fractional factorial design (FFD), in order to screen the maximum number of main effects in the least number of experimental run, whereas "FFD" used for studying (K = N − 1) the variables of "N" runs, where "N" is a multiple of "U". It is a type of screening design that helps us to find which factors are favorable for the experiment. We noted that, this design screen out unimportant factors (noise), which means that you researcher avoid for collecting large amounts of data on relatively important factors. Commonly used PB design exists total run (N = 8,12,16,20,24,28, and 36) since the total number of runs for the 2^{k-P} design are powers of 2; the PB design has total number of runs that generally fall between those for the 2^{k-P} fractional factorial (FFD) (note that a few PB design exists where n is power of 2). The PB designs are considered resolution of third type because they are orthogonal for main effect estimates, but each main effect is partially aliased with numerous ways of interactions (two-way interaction). For each interactions, we estimate predictable errors. If they are estimable the coefficient estimates may be highly correlated because two-way interaction effects are non-orthogonal and as noted partially aliased with main effects. illustration: The messy aliasing structure suppose we

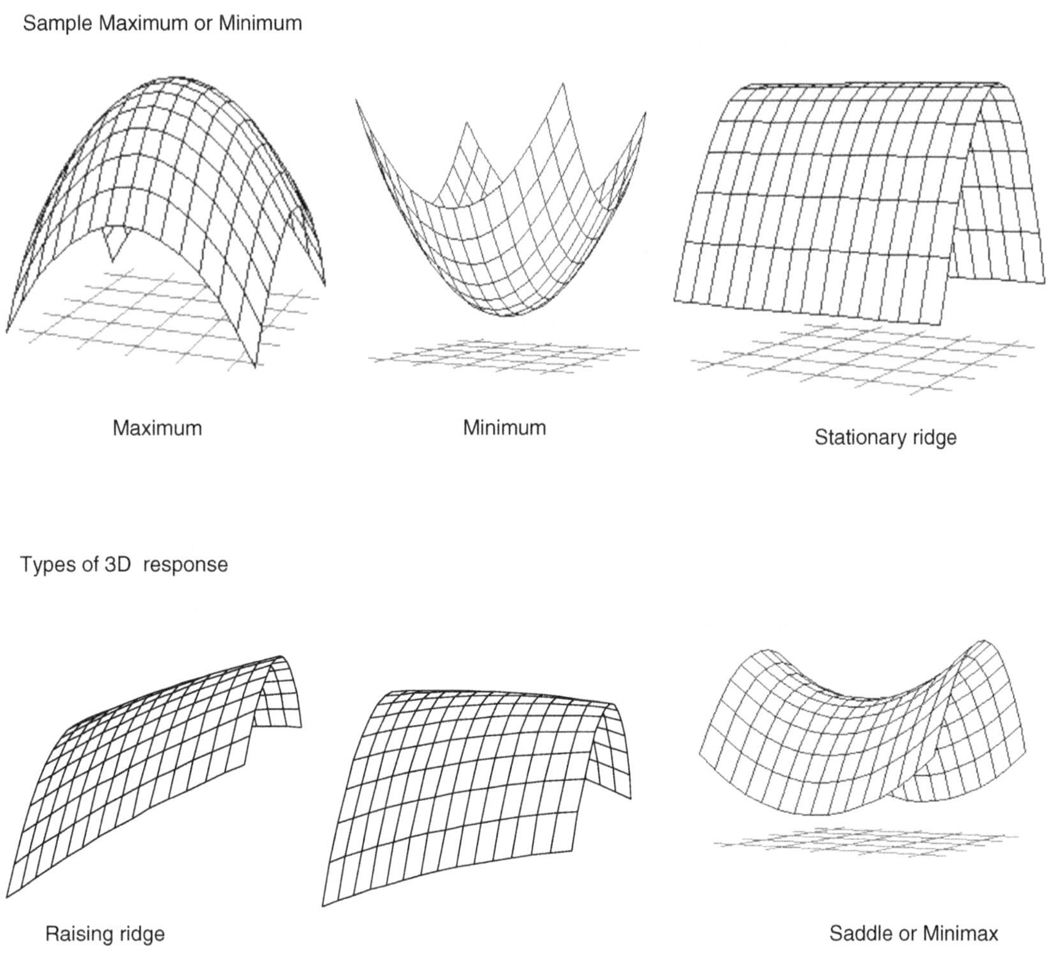

Fig. 2.14 RSM constructed by various methods

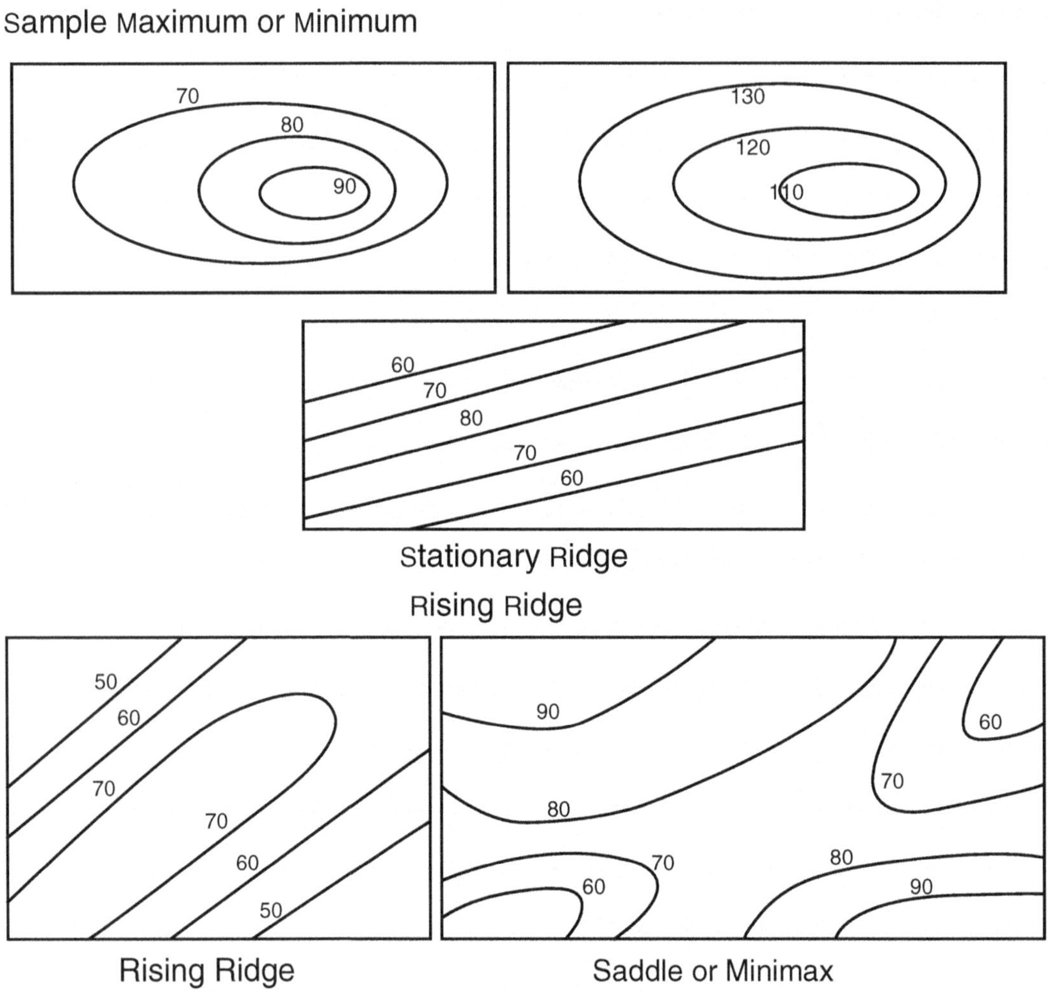

Fig. 2.14 (continued)

study five factors A through E using a 12 runs of PB design the table below gives the aliasing structure for all 11 columns notice interaction AB appears in different aliens chains (Box and Draper 1987).

2.25.1 Properties and Assumptions of PB Design

Fractional factorial design (FFD) for studying $k = (N - 1)$ variables in "N" runs, where "N" is a multiple of four. Only main effects are of interest to extrapolate the efficacy. In case of standard orthogonal arrays, we are not defining the relationship of aliens chains since interactions are not independent and identically equal to main effects and also all framed information is used to estimate the parameters not to leave triangle degrees of freedom to estimate the error term from the ANOVA techniques.

2.25.2 When to Use PB Design

Screening of patients on drug response is possible to neglect higher order interactions two-level multifactor experiments. More than four factors, since for 2–4 variables a full factorial can be performed. Economically we detect the large main effects. Particularly, it is very useful for the following number of runs (N = 12, 20, 24, 28, and 36).

Factors: we selected the sharpness of vision, distance from target to eye, target shape, illumination level.

Target size, target density was also considered for screening of cases. The subject of cases were screened at higher order due to cause and effect relation. Screening was done at two levels, each factor is considered while higher order interactions are negligible and required to economically identify the most important factors during the time of study intervention.

View of aliens chains

Effects	Aliens chain
A	*−bc + bd − be − cd − ce − de*
B	*−ac + ad − ae − cd + ce − de*
C	*−ab − ad − ae − bd + be − de*
D	*+ab − ac − ae − bc − be − ce*
E	*+ab − ac − ad + bc − bd − cd*
1	*−ab − ac − ad + ae − bc − bd − be + cd − ce − de*
2	*−ab − ac − ad + ae − bc + bd + cd + cd − ce + de*
3	*+ab + ac − ad − ae − bc + bd − be − cd + ce + de*
4	*−ab − ac − ad − ae + bc + bd − be − cd − ce − de*
5	*−ab − ac + ad − ae − bc − bd −be + cd + ce − de*
6	*−ab + ac + ad − ae − bc − bd + be − cd − ce + de*

PB-8 run matrix

Runs	*a*	*b*	*c*	*d*	*e*	*f*	*g*
1	+	–	–	+	–	+	+
2	+	+	–	–	+	–	+
3	+	+	+	–	–	+	–
4	–	+	+	+	–	–	+
5	+	–	+	+	+	–	–
6	–	+	–	+	+	+	–
7	–	–	+	–	+	+	+
8	–	–	–	–	–	–	–

Above-cited illustrative example conclusively state that PB is likely that all of these factors contribute to estimation of response variable, but that some are much more important than others. Within design of experiment methods, the Plackett–Burman design is a good choice for figuring out which factors are most important and signify the better way in research paradigm. After the Plackett–Burman experiment was done, researcher could use a different experiment to answer questions like "does the effect of response variable depend on how to control the extraneous error and prediction of various interaction effects on selected sites?" (Box et al. 1978)

Illustration: Trick to determine the effect of drug response

Effects	A	B	AB	Response of the drug
(i)	−1	−1	+1	85
b	−1	+1	−1	90
a	+1	−1	−1	92
ab	+1	+1	+1	86

$$\text{Effect of A} = 1/2\{-85-90+92+86\} = -3$$

$$\text{Effect of B} = 1/2\{-85+90-92+86\} = -11$$

$$\text{Effect of AB} = \{1/2(86-90) - 1/2(92-85\}$$
$$= -2-(3.5) = 5.5$$

Note:-As "k" increases, the runs specified for a $2k$ or $3k$ full factorial quickly become very large and outgrow the resources of most experimenters. The solution is used to solve the above-cited problem, viz. (1) researcher should assume that certain high-order interactions are negligible by using only a fraction of the runs specified by the full factorial design (2) chosen fractional factorial designs for two-level experiments at desirable properties like balanced (In this assumption, all runs have the same number of observations.).

Illustration: the researcher conducted the experimentation at *in vitro* condition to know the plasma concentration level of newly administered drug significance, he has included the 31 geographical areas with the following factors CD_4: X_1, gender X_2, BMI: X_4, RBS X_5, PPBS: X_6,WBC: X_7; he wishes to determine the experimental reliability in PB design (Table 2.17).

Estimated parameters of age: X_1, gender X_2, BMI: X_4, RBS X_5, PPBS: X_6,WBC: X_7

	Effect	Coefficient	*t*-test	*P*-value
CD4 count: X_1	–	25.52	339.96	0.000
Gender X_2	0.492	0.27	3.27	0.047
BMI: X_3	6.311	3.15	41.95	0.000
X_4, PPBS	−4.85	−2.4	−32.28	0.000
X_5: WBC	−5.27	−2.65	−35.03	0.000
X_6: SGOT	0.82	0.410	5.45	0.012
X_8:SGPT	1.01	0.507	6.75	0.000
X_6:Blood urea	1.84	0.921	12.24	0.000
X_7: TC	0.75	0.372	5.01	0.015

Table 2.17 Estimated Aspergillus production by PBD

Source of variation	*df*	Seq SS	Adj SS	Adj MS	Fisher F	*P*-value
Regression	14	2609.91	2609.91	186.42	63.27	<0.000
Linear	4	712.62	358.82	89.70	30.45	<0.000
Square	4	1801.61	1801.61	450.40	152.86	<0.000
Interaction	6	95.68	95.68	15.94	5.41	<0.000
RE	16	47.14	47.14	2.94	–	
Lack of fit	10	32.48	32.48	3.24	1.33	0.38
Probable error	6	14.66	14.66	2.49	–	
Total	30	2657.05	–	–		

Runs	Observed (IU/mL) Plasma concentration at initial stage	Predicted (IU/mL)
1	23.35	23.75
2	27.32	27.30
3	27.11	27.29
4	16.28	16.40
5	29.19	29.24
6	29.73	29.55
7	24.24	24.06
8	18.32	18.30
9	22.32	22.33
10	29.0	29.18
11	34.75	34.94
12	25.20	25.02

2.26 Box–Behnken Design

Box–Behnken designs are equivalent to Plackett–Burman designs for the case of $3(k - p)$. The BBD is an independent quadratic design that does not contain an embedded factorial or fractional factorial design. In this design, the treatment combinations are at the mid points of edges of the process space and at the center. These designs are rotatable and require three levels of each factor. The design has limited capability for orthogonal blocking when compared to central composite design (CCD) (Fig. 2.15).

Table 2.18 describes that the contrast of the structure of four common quadratic designs might be used when investigating three factors. The embedded table combines CCC and CCI designs because they are structurally identical. For including three factors, the BBD design offers some advantages in requiring a fewer number of runs. Inclusion of four or more factors and the merits have disappeared.

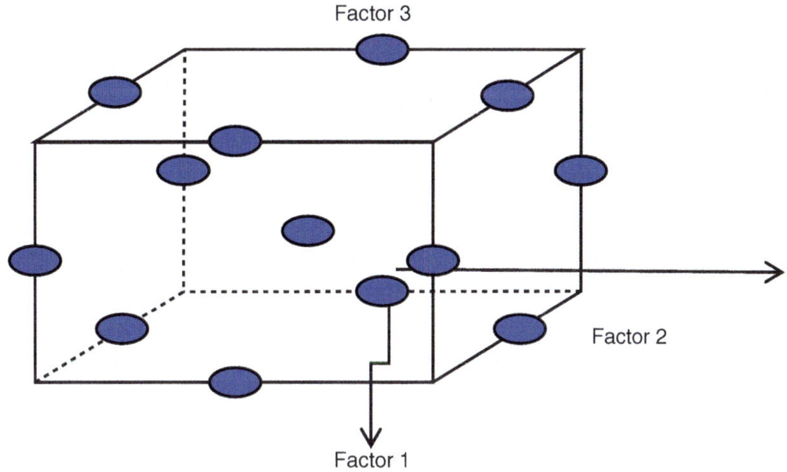

Fig. 2.15 Box–Behnken design outline structure with different factors

Table 2.18 Structural comparison of CCC, CCF, and BBD

	Central composite circumscribed			Central composite circumscribed/ inscribed				Box–Behnken design			
Rep	X_1	X_2	X_3	Rep	X_1	X_2	X_3	Rep	X_1	X_2	X_3
1	−1	−1	−1	1	−1	−1	−1	1	−1	−1	0
1	+1	−1	−1	1	+1	−1	−1	1	+1	−1	0
1	−1	+1	−1	1	−1	+1	−1	1	−1	+1	0
1	+1	+1	−1	1	+1	+1	−1	1	+1	+1	0
1	−1	−1	+1	1	−1	−1	+1	1	−1	0	−1
1	+1	−1	+1	1	+1	−1	+1	1	+1	0	−1
1	−1	+1	+1	1	−1	+1	+1	1	−1	0	+1
1	+1	+1	+1	1	+1	+1	+1	1	+1	0	+1
1	−1.65	+1	0	1	−1	0	+1	1	+1	−1	−1
1	1.65	0	0	1	+1	0	0	1	0	+1	−1
1	0	−1.65	0	1	0	−1	0	1	0	−1	+1
1	0	−1.65	0	1	0	+1	0	1	0	−1	+1
1	0	0	−1.65	1	0	0	0	1	0	+1	+1
1	0	0	−1.65	1	0	0	−1	3	0	0	0
6	0	0	0	6	0	0	+1				
Total	20 runs			20 runs				15 runs			

2.26.1 Properties and Assumptions

The salient properties of BB designs have ascertained in so many ways; the researcher focuses on certain regularity assumptions before evaluating the BB design. The experimental setup area would be conducted at three-level multifactor experiments which allow to combine two-level factorial designs with incomplete block designs. The complexity of interaction effects would be estimated by BB design, the design bring back the economic feasibility to estimates different variants of the experimentation. Finally, the treatment combinations are at the mid points of edges of the process space and at the center and design must be rotatable in nature (varimax and equimax) (Table 2.19).

2.26.2 Conditions to Apply Box–Behnken Designs

With three-level multifactor experiments (e.g., multicentric drug trail), the novelty of this design has been required to economically detect large main effects, especially when it is expensive to perform all the necessary runs and also it determines the linear and quadratic effects of each variable. (Notable point for applying the BB design, the researcher or experimenter should avoid combined factor extremes.) This property will prevent a potential loss of data sets in particular cases. For example, experiment to study the yield of a chemical process; we have considered the response and factors; the response was considered chemical process; yield is the factor or parameter while other parameters like temperature, pH, pressure, viscosity, mixer speed, screening experiment, etc. extrapolate the variants (Box 1954; Box and Hunter 1957) (Fig. 2.16, Table 2.20).

The BBD permit us estimate the parameters on the quadratic model, building of sequential designs, detection of the lack of fit of the model, and use of blocks in varied parameters. Rayanne et al. (2019) demonstrated fat-based nanostructured lipid carriers for nail drug delivery of ketoconazole: development and optimization using Box–Behnken design. Similar application of BBD reported by Swami et al. (2013) demonstrated the proximate/fatty acid composition and the antioxidant activity of breads using a Box–Behnken design composed of 15 experiments and three factors. The study findings revealed that the breads had significantly altered baking times and the wheat flour, it was partially substituted by chia seeds, carrot leaves, etc. The total antioxidant capacity of results were significant correlated ($p < 0.001$) to those obtained from control bread (495.33 μmol TEAC g^{-1} for DPPH assays and 413.85 μmol TEAC g^{-1} for FRAP assays), the results showed the increased levels of 97 and 102% for DPPH and FRAP assays, respectively. The addition of chia seeds and car-

Table 2.19 Number of runs required by Central Composite and Box–Behnken designs

Number of factors	Box–Behnken	Central composite
2	–	13 (5 center points)
3	15	20 (6 center point runs)
4	27	30 (6 center point runs)
5	46	33 (fractional factorial) or 52 (full factorial)
6	54	54 (fractional factorial) or 91 (full factorial)

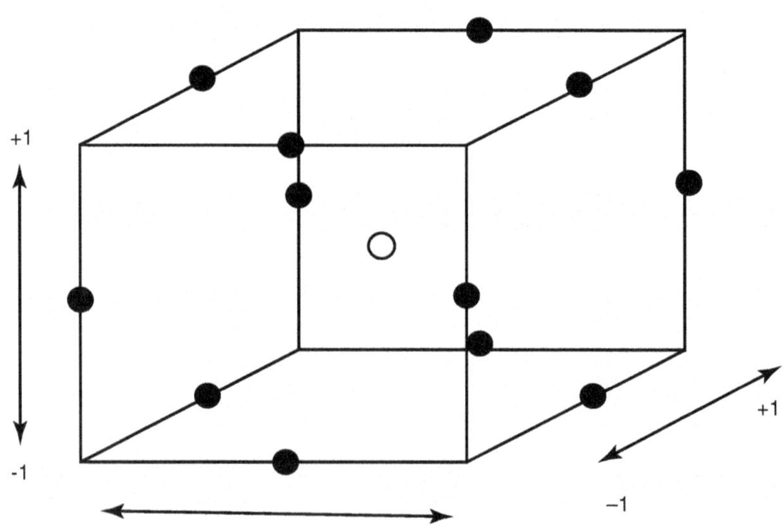

Fig. 2.16 Box–Behnken design for three factors

Table 2.20 Three-factor runs of Box–Behnken design for three factors

Runs	X_1	X_2	X_3
1	−1	−1	0
2	−1	0	0
3	1	−1	0
4	1	1	0
5	−1	0	−1
6	−1	0	1
7	1	0	−1
8	1	0	1
9	0	−1	−1
10	0	−1	1
11	0	1	−1
12	0	1	1
13	0	0	0
14	0	0	0
15	0	0	0

rot leaves led to maximal alpha-linolenic acid and simultaneously drew up to 216.69% and maximum PUFA:SFA ratio increase of 18.88% in relation to control bread (with alpha-linolenic acid amount of 34.03 mg g^{-1} total lipid and a 2.86 ratio value), as well as a maximum omega-3:omega-6 ratio reduction (70.01%) was noticed during the study period (15.59 ratio value for control bread).

Jun et al. (2003) demonstrated BBD by optimization techniques to evaluate the fungal contamination of grains during the post-harvest period aggravated with health hazards. The experiment was intervened to escalate the remedial measures for optimization of contaminated fungal grains, a UV light system is being used to inactivate the fungal spores of Aspergillus niger in corn meal. Three factors in the UV light process are kept as varying parameters: treatment time (number of pulses), distance from the UV strobe, and input voltage for UV lamp.

Factor	Name	Units	Low level	High level
A	Time	s	20	100
B	Distance	cm	3	13
C	Voltage	v	2000	3800

The following data metrics shows corresponding effect of the different UV light settings of fungal spores

Standard order	Run order	Time A(s)	B: Distance (cm)	C:Voltage	Response
1	12	20	3	2900	0.449
2	10	100	3	2900	3.255
3	5	20	13	2900	0.321
4	2	100	13	2900	2.954
5	7	20	8	2000	0.176
6	6	100	8	2000	1.352
7	14	20	8	3800	0.507
8	8	100	8	3800	4.954
9	9	60	3	2000	0.724
10	4	60	13	2000	0.477
11	13	60	3	3800	2.109
12	3	60	13	3800	1.954
13	15	60	8	2900	1.301
14	1	60	8	2900	1.301
15	11	60	8	2900	1.301

ANOVA Summary of BBD

Source of variation	*df*	SS (Partial)	MSS (partial)	*F*-ratio	*P*-value
Model	9	245,497	27,277	92.3389	0.0000
A:Time	1	15,296	15,296	517.79	0.000
B:Distance	1	0.086	0.0863	2.922	0.1484
C:Voltage	1	5.7715	5.7715	195.37	0.000
AB	1	0.0075	0.0075	0.2533	0.6362
AC	1	2.6749	2.6749	90.548	0.0002
BC	1	0.0021	0.0021	0.0716	0.7997
AA	1	0.7067	0.7067	23.924	0.0045
BB	1	0.0001	0.0001	0.0049	0.947
CC	1	0.0003	0.0003	0.0096	0.9259
Residual	5	0.1477	0.0295		
Lack of fit	3	0.1477	0.0492		
Pure error	2	0	0		
Total	14	24.6975			

The optimal settings $A = 100$, $B = 3$ cm, and $C = 3800$ voltage the expected number of logarithmic reduction is found to be 4.90 and it was found to be statistically significant ($p < 0.01$) and more reliable gain of optimal factors.

2.26.3 Summary BB Design

The satisfactory distribution of information is obtained from BBD across the experimental region (rotatability); the fitted values are as close at real value as possible to overcome the observed values (minimize residuals or error of prediction) and showed good lack of fit detection. Internal estimate of error is possible by BB design. The constant variance has been extracted at any point of time, and the transformations of data sets are very easy and precluded at greater accuracy. It is very suitable for blocking without loss of any information. Sequentially, the construction or building of any model (linear and nonlinear) has been made at higher order designs from the use of simpler designs; a minimum number of treatment combinations is possible to know the effect of final response of the variable. Practically, BBD will facilitate good graphical representation through simple data patterns or data sets. It showed an excellent behavioral expression on the estimation of predictable errors (PE) in the even and odd experimental setup (Input variables) (Bose and Nair 1939).

2.27 D-Optimal Design

Many of the clinical trials are complex in nature and irregular because due to some accidental causes, besides these above-cited families of design are not applicable to conduct the research at large-scale population level (mixed factors). We have made use of other families of alternative design that are useful in certain critical situations. In this present section, we describe the D-optimal design and its application. In previous design, we describe the experimental is regular without any juxtapose on overlapping between the observations, these present design uniquely differ from other design due to its proximity of the results i.e. an experimental region is irregular as such being the case D-optimal design is very useful to congruent the information and compilation, the number of designs runs has to be reduced by D optimal, special regression model must be fitted through linearity of the observations, the process and mixture factors are used for formulation of the design (Cummings et al. 2012).

$$y \approx p(y/t,x,\theta)$$
$$y/t = obseved/controlled$$
$$x = controlled$$
$$\theta = unknownparameter$$
$$utility = u(t,x,\theta), reliability(\theta,x,t)$$

The following table matrices showed the minimum number of runs of fractional factorial design (FFD), full factorial (FD) and D-optimal design.

Factors	Full FD	FFD	D-optimal
5	32	16	16
6	64	32	28
7	128	64	35
8	256	64	43
9	512	128	52

$$Y_t = \frac{1}{1+\text{expo}^{(-\theta_1-\theta_2X)}} \text{Nonlinear model}$$

θ_1 and θ_2 have half of the observations on each of the two doses, and we also get the incremental changes of dose variations obtained from the following equation:

$$Y_t = \int \frac{1}{1+\text{expo}^{(-\theta_1-\theta_2X)}}$$

2.27.1 Regression Models for D-Optimal

In a study by Cummings et al. (2012), the D-optimal designs will give an opportunity to alter or modify the underlying model in various methodological ways. The following equation showed that it is possible to delete the selected items or terms if the experimenter knows that they are unimportant for the response explored during the study period or intervention. This will allow in reducing the number of runs alternatively without any loss of information and overlapping of experimentation or population structure.

$$y = \beta_0 + \beta_1x_1 + \beta_2x_2 + \beta_{12}x_1x_2 + \beta_{11}x_{12} + \beta_{22}x_1^2 + \varepsilon, \quad (2.23)$$

e.g., the bold letter deleted term

In case, we consider the second-order possible model, the modification of the cited addition will show precursor changes bearing a single higher order term. The classical designs have approached by the analytical researcher for the improvement of accuracy and precision of the experiment. Since it is only possible to change or alter the whole model setup, e.g., from an interaction to a quadratic model (higher order). In the contrast to this above gap, the D-optimal designs are most suited for reducing the number of factors and runs. We can allow the addition of independent model inclusion. Practically, we have run the D-optimal design for reduction of sampling error. In another manner of definition, it is full of computer program because it is a computer-aided design which contains the best subset of all possible experiments in a single platform which depending upon a selected criterion and a given number of design runs at greater accuracy, the best design is created by a selection process run program run by computer-aided softwares, etc.

2.27.2 Important Criteria for D-Optimal Design

The D-optimal design having several criteria and pitfalls, the following section, we discuss the different criteria for a D-optimal design from mathematical equations. All of them belong to the group of information-based criteria because they try to maximize the information matrix (*X'X*). The D-Optimality is the most common criterion which seeks to maximize |*X'X*| the determinant of the information matrix (*X'X*) of the design. This means that the optimal design matrix *X** contains the "*n*" experiments which maximizes the determinant of (*X'X*) or in other words, the "*n*" runs "span the largest volume possible in the experimental region". Equation of D optimal design shows the selection of *X** out of all possible design matrices chosen from "*N*". This connection between the design matrix and the "determinant also explains the use of the D in the term D-optimal designs" (Cook et al. 2001).

2.28 Allowable Drug Resistance Design (ADRD)

Allowable drug resistance design is unique method and valuable tool for medical and clinical research , the formulation of model construction is very easy, any kind of drug trail, the safety and efficacy of drug is very important to achieve better results from the experimentation on practical approach. In realistic problem, the new drug is an inbuilt mechanism to change biologically as well as behaviorally. Many scientists opined that the clinical trial is always focused on biological and clinical aspects; firstly, we have assumed the hypothesis "the drug resistance of respondent ≥ effect of drug (efficacy)" on respondents or subjects (Cook et al. 1989). From this hypothesis it is essential that both sides are evaluated for same conditions, e.g., the stress on soil should be compared with bearing capacity of soil.

2.28.1 The Limits of Resistance or Loading

Practically, we noticed that, many clinical trials, the loading factor (drug resistance) could be reached its limits; the success is the next process of arbitrary results, *i.e.,* the resistance condition becomes success modes; such a condition is referred to as limit state and it can be defined as "a condition beyond which a clinical and biological component has positively expressed to fulfill the function for which it is designed clinically." The limits state has been broadly classified into four categories (1) Strength on limit state (Strength of drug), (2) serviceability (Tolerability), (3) survivability limit states (Mortality reduction), (4) Special limits-damage, death of respondents, some accidental cause cases will withdraw the trial in mid time.

Serviceability Limit States: The drug failure, lost to follow-up (LFU), decline the trial, migration and no stability of the patients, etc.

The "ADRD" approach must ensure that the probability of a limit state being reached in the design or serviceability limit within the acceptable hypothesis; the design will provide an adequate margin of drug safety irrespective of trial or experiment; this state of method was applied by structural engineer for formulation of planning on the building of modeling techniques (Cook and DeMets 2008). Further, the ADRD should take into account the estimation of probability occurrence bearing an event of success in the entire formulation of design of experiment or research process. The research is in full-blown state of limit encompassed with many attributes and each variable can be tested by suitable statistical methods Barbáno et al. (2008). If the state of limits is accurate (cent percent) at early stage of formulation of drug trials, an experimentation can achieve good results (success of trial).

Note: To determine the acceptable margin of safety, opinion should be sought from the practical experience and expert opinion (qualified group of clinicians before conducting experiment).

Allowable Stress Design (ASD), FOS = Resistance, R/Effect of load, $Q = \text{fy}/0.5\text{fy} = 2$

Since, the specifications set limit on the stresses, it becomes allowable stress design (ASD), and it is mostly reasonable criteria where the relative stresses are uniformly distributed over the drug trial process.

Mathematical formulation of ASD

$$\frac{\Phi R_n}{\gamma} \geq \sum Q_i \tag{2.24}$$

$$\frac{0.85*(0.52)}{1.0} x100 \geq \sum Q_i \tag{2.25}$$

Rn = Resistance or Strength of the drug being designed, Φ = the resistance factor or strength reduction factor, Q = overload or load factors (additional formulation) with factor of safety (FS)-γ. From the above illustrations the left hand side equation becomes 44.22% ASD≧ additional formulation of (Q_i). That means a total of 44.42% has led overloading for the formulation of new drug in accordance with regularity guidelines (Fig. 2.17).

$$\text{Drug safety}(\%) = \text{Drug strength} / \text{Resistance} \times 100$$

2.29 Taguchi Design for Orthogonal Array

This modest technique was propounded by Prof. Taguchi, the intervention involving estimation of multiple factors on orthogonal effects; it was first proposed by Prof. RA Fisher (1925a, b) and the method is popularly known as the factorial design of experiments (FDE). A full factorial (FD) will overwhelmingly identify all possible combinations in a given set of factors. Since, most of the clinical experimentation will usually involve a significant number of factors or attributes, which can reduce the number of experimental parameters at practical level or essence, only a fewer number or small set of observations were selected from the population (all the possibilities are being selected). The method of selecting a limited number of experiments can produce the most cited information to the researcher; this newer method is known as partial fractional experiment (PFE). Since, this method is well known to see in agricultural breeding trial or in-house experiment, there are no general regularity guidelines for its own application or the analysis of the resulted findings. The data sets were obtained by experiment in performing the clinical experimentation. Box et al. (1988), Bhatt et al.(2016) formulated a special set of general (modified) design for conducting the research on full-blown basis considering full factorial design (FFD) that bears with too many applications or algorithms (Fig. 2.18. Table 2.21).

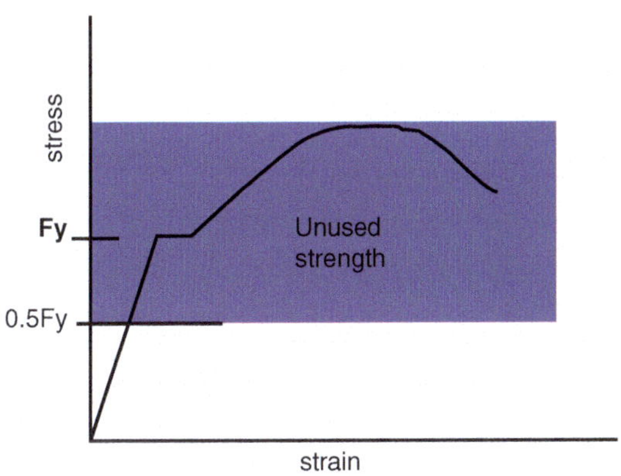

Fig. 2.17 ADRD design overview

2.29.1 Properties of Orthogonal Array

An orthogonal data set or array bearing the following cited properties reduces the number of experiments to be conducted.

1. The vertical column matrix data set under each independent variable of the table showed special combinations of the level of settings. All the level settings should appear an equal number of times.
2. All the levels on their values of independent variables are being used for conducting the experiments.
3. The sequence of level of each value was considered for conducting the experiments; it shall not be altered or changed.

Fig. 2.18 Inner 2^3 and outer 2^2 arrays show robust design with "*I*" the inner array and "*E*" the outer array

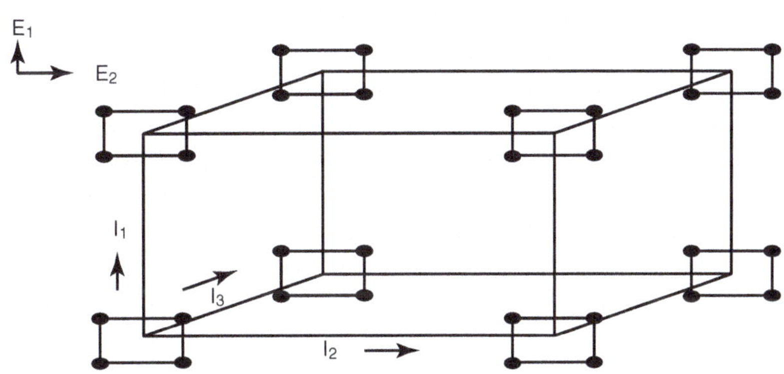

Table 2.21 Layout of the Taguchi design

	$L_{9},3^{4}$ (orthogonal arrays)				
Trial number	V_1	V_2	V_3	V_4	Performance of parametric values
1	1	1	1	1	P_1
2	1	2	2	2	P_2
3	1	3	3	3	P_3
4	2	1	2	3	P_4
5	2	2	3	1	P_5
6	2	3	1	2	P_6
7	3	1	3	2	P_7
8	3	2	1	3	P_8
9	3	3	2	1	P_9

The design of experiment (DOE) using the orthogonal arrays is most cited parameter for almost all subjects or cases, respectively; an orthogonal array is more efficient when compared to many other types of statistical design of DOE. The minimum number of experiments that are required to perform the "Taguchi method" can be determined by Taguchi method based on the different degrees of freedom of practical approach.

$$N_T = 1 + \sum_{i=1}^{NV} (L_i - 1) \tag{2.26}$$

2.29.2 Assumptions

In this section, we describe salient assumptions employed for the Taguchi method. The Taguchi design implies additive assumptions that each individual factor or main effects of the independent variables on the performance parameters are separable. Under this salient assumption, the effect of each factors cross-checked interns of their linearity, quadratic, or of higher order Chow et al. (2011). In addition to the above assumptions, we diagnose the model robustness (the model assumes that there exists no cross-product effects (interactions) among the individual factors). The effect of an independent variable bearing number one on the performance parameter does not depend on the different or various levels on the varied type of settings at any independent variables and vice versa. If at any time of action, this assumption has been violated from the objective of interest or modalities of research. Therefore, the additive main effect or model effectiveness does not hold good at the level of higher order interactions.

2.29.3 Experimental Designing

1. Selection of independent variables (define independent variables).
2. Selection of number of level settings for each independent variables.
3. Selection of orthogonal arrays.
4. Assigning the independent variable in each column.
5. Conducting the experiment.
6. Compiling the data and finding the robustness of the experiment.

2.29.4 Experimental Loss or Trial Loss

An experimental loss or trial loss is caused due to various factors (accidental, biotic intervention, and natural calamities); it is more valid and highly accountable for the validation of research program. The insight experimental loss will significantly reduce the fidelity of the entire research and also it is negatively affected on the precision of the experiment. In clinical research or drug trial, the loss occurs due to drug performance variation proportional to the square of the deviation of the performance characteristics from its normal variation, i.e., the equation used to determine the loss of performance is as follows:

$$L(y) = k(y - m)^2 \quad (2.27)$$

Loss at a particular period

$$L(x) = K * (k - t)^2, \quad (2.28)$$

where k = loss coefficient, x = measure coefficient, and t = target value

Average loss of $L = k(S^2 + (\text{pm} - t)^2$

S = SD, pm = process mean, the total reduction = Average loss * number of trial conducted

2.29.5 Rules of Trial

1. The researcher must ensure the system of designing which can involve creativity and innovations.
2. Parameter design: A detailed design phase is described as early as possible; the parameters are to be chosen at the right time with good precision so as to minimize the effects of the various subjects; sometimes we called this as robustness of the model.
3. Tolerance of the drug: The main resources should focus on reducing the variation (in the critical few dimension) (Tables 2.22 and 2.23).

Table 2.22 Taguchi orthogonal array selection overview matrix

No. of parameters	No. of levels 2	3	4	5
2	L_4	L_9	L_{16}	L_{25}
3	L_4	L_9	L_{16}	L_{25}
4	L_8	L_9	L_{16}	L_{25}
5	L_8	L_{18}	L_{16}	L_{25}
6	L_8	L_{18}	L_{32}	L_{25}
7	L_8	L_{18}	L_{32}	L_{50}
8	L_8	L_{18}	L_{32}	L_{50}
9	L_{12}	L_{18}	L_{32}	L_{50}
10	L_{12}	L_{27}		L_{50}
11	L_{12}	L_{27}		L_{50}
12	L_{16}	L_{27}		
13	L_{16}	L_{36}		
14	L_{16}	L_{36}		
15	L_{16}	L_{36}		
16	L_{32}	L_{36}		
17	L_{32}	L_{36}		
18	L_{32}	L_{36}		
19	L_{32}	L_{36}		
20	L_{32}	L_{36}		
21	L_{32}	L_{36}		
22	L_{32}	L_{36}		
23	L_{32}	L_{36}		
24	L_{32}			
25	L_{32}			
26	L_{32}			
27	L_{32}			
28	L_{32}			
29	L_{32}			
30	L_{32}			

Table 2.23 Choice of design based on the *S*/*N* ratio

Choose	*S*/*N* ratio	Goal
Smaller the better one	$S/N = -10\log\left[\frac{1}{n}\sum_{i=1}^{n} y_i^2\right]$	Minimize the response
Nominal the better one	$S/N = 100 Log \frac{\mu^2}{\sigma^2}$	Target the response and want to base the *S*/*N* ratio means and SD
Larger the better one	$S/N = -Log\left[\frac{1}{n}\sum_{i=1}^{n}\frac{1}{y_i^2}\right]$	Maximize the response

2.30 Conclusion

Clinical research is an organized way of science for conducting drug and vaccine trials on human and animal intervention, intended to provide adequate information on the use of novel new regimens or vaccines to evaluate therapeutic agents with regard to usefulness, safety, and adverse effects. In a broad sense, all clinical researches will be conducted scientifically and also the researcher willing to know various effects of therapeutic, drug dosage, risk, efficacy, and health benefits of a new drug. These processes will be carried out by many steps and analytical procedures (design, state, and drug delivery space), prior to release of any kind of drug in the market shall undergo various steps for its validation and evaluations based on the advanced design of experiment (DOE); these designs will assist the researcher, drug developers, clinicians, and researchers effectively to know the congruence risk of drug from inception till FDA approval or release. In this practical point of view, this chapter deals with different types of advanced design of experiments which are demonstrated with real data sets for the benefit of researchers, clinicians, and drug manufacturers.

References

Akey JM et al (2007) On the design and analysis of gene expression studies in human populations. Nat Genet 39:807–808

Barbáno Y et al (2008) Predictability of designs which adjust for imbalances in prognostic factors. J Statist Plann Inference 138:756–767

Benson K et al (2000) A comparison of observational studies and randomized, controlled trials. N Engl J Med 342:1876–1886

Berry DA (1989) Comments on "Investigating therapies of potentially great benefit: ECMO". Stat Sci 4:306–310

Bhatt L, Mehta C (2016) Adaptive designs for clinical trials. N Engl J Med 375:65–74

Bose RC, Nair KR (1939) Partially balanced incomplete block designs. Sankhya 4:337–372

Box G (1957) Evolutionary Operation: A Method for Increasing Industrial Productivity", Journal of the Royal Statistical Society (Applied Statistics) 6:81–101

Box GEP (1954) Some theorems on quadratic forms applied in the study of analysis of variance problems, I. Effect of inequality of variance in the one-way classification. Ann Math Stat 25:290–302

Box GEP, Draper NR (1987) Empirical model-building with response surfaces. Wiley, New York

Box GEP, Hunter JS (1957) Multi-factor experimental designs for exploring response surfaces. Ann Math Stat 28:195–241

Box GEP, Hunter WG, Hunter JS (1978) Statistics for experimenters. Wiley, New York

Box GEP, Bisgaard S, Fung CA (1988) An explanation and critique of Taguchi's contributions to quality engineering. Qual Reliab Eng Int 4:123–131

Brown MB (1975) Exploring interaction effects in the ANOVA. Appl Stat 24:288–298

Carroll MB, Dykstra O (1958) Application of fractional factorials in a food research laboratory. In: Chew V (ed) Experimental designs in industry. Wiley, New York, pp 224–234

Chow SC, Chang M (2011) Adaptive design methods in clinical trials (Chapman & Hall/CRC Biostatistics Series), 2nd edn. Chapman and Hall/CRC, Boca Raton

Cochran WG, Cox GM (1957) Experimental designs. Wiley, New York

Cochran WG, Autrey KM, Cannon CY (1941) A double changeover design for dairy cattle feeding experiments. J Dairy Sci 24:937–951

Concato J et al (2000) Randomized, controlled trials, observational studies, and the hierarchy of research design. N Engl J Med 342:1887–1892

Connor WS (1958) Experiences with incomplete block designs. In: Chew V (ed) Experimental designs in industry. Wiley, New York, pp 193–206

Conover WJ et al (1981) A comparative study of tests for homogeneity of variances, with applications to the outer continental shelf bidding data. Technometrics 23:351–361

Cook TD, DeMets DL (2008) Introduction to statistical methods for clinical trials. Chapman & Hall/CRC, Boca Raton

Cook RD, Nachtsheim CJ (1980) A comparison of algorithms for constructing exact D-optimal designs. Technometrics 22:315–324

Cook RD, Nachtsheim CJ (1989) Computer-aided blocking of factorial and response-surface designs. Technometrics 31:339–346

Cook TD et al (2001) Experimental and quasi experimental designs for generalized causal inference. Houghton Mifflin, Boston

Cox DR, Reid N (2000) The theory of the design of experiments. Chapman & Hall/CRC, London

Cummings J et al (2012) Advances in designs for Alzheimer's disease clinical trials. Am J Neurodegener Dis 1:205–216

DeLury DB (1946) The analysis of covariance. Biometrics 4:153–170

Draper NR et al (1993) Mixture designs for four components in orthogonal blocks. Technometrics 35: 268–276

Draper NR et al (1994) Isolation of degrees of freedom for Box-Behnken designs. Technometrics 36:283–291

Duncan DB (1955) Multiple range and multiple F tests. Biometrics 11:1–42

Dunnett CW (1955) A multiple comparisons procedure for comparing several treatments with a control. J Am Stat Assoc 50:1096–1121

Efron B (1976) Forcing a sequential experiment to be balanced. Biometrika 58:403–417

Federer WT, Meredith MP (1992) Covariance analysis for splitplot and split-block designs. Am Stat 46: 155–162

Fisher RA (1918) The correlation between relatives on the supposition of Mendelian inheritance. Trans R Soc Edinburgh 52:399–433

Fisher RA (1925a) Applications of "student's" distribution. Metron 5:90–104

Fisher RA (1925b) Statistical methods for research workers. Oliver & Boyd, Ltd, London

Fisher RA (1925c) Statistical methods for research workers, 1st edn. Oliver and Boyd, Edinburgh

Fisher RA (1935) The design of experiments. Oliver & Boyd, Ltd, London

Fisher LD (1996) Comments on Bayesian and frequentist analysis and interpretation of clinical trials. Control Clin Trials 17:423–434

Hunter WG, Kittrell JR (1966) "Evolutionary Operation: A Review", Technometrics, 8:389–397

Kerr MK, Churchill GA (2001) Experimental design for gene expression microarrays. Biostatistics 2:183–201

Myers RA, Barrowman NJ (1995) Time series bias in the estimation of density-dependent mortality in stock-recruitment models. Canadian Journal of Fisheries and Aquatic Sciences 52(1):40–43. https://doi.org/10.1139/f95-022

Oehlert A M et al (2019) Multi-proxy constraints on the significance of covariant d13c values in carbonate and organic carbon during the early. Mississippian Sedimentology 66:241–261. https://doi.org/10.1111/sed.12502

Pocock S et al (1975) Sequential treatment assignment with balancing for prognostic factors in the controlled clinical trial. Biometrics 31:103–115

Rayanne R et al (2019) Fat-based nanostructured lipid carriers for nail drug delivery of ketoconazole: development and optimization using Box-Behnken design. Pharmaceutics 11(6):284. https://doi.org/10.3390/pharmaceutics11060284

Shan C et al (2013) Randomized two-stage phase II clinical trial designs based on Barnard's exact test. J Biopharm Stat 23:1081–1090

Shan G et al (2016) Optimal adaptive two-stage designs for early phase II clinical trials. Stat Med 35: 1257–1266

Shan G et al (2017) Efficient confidence limits for adaptive one-arm two-stage clinical trials with binary endpoints. BMC Med Res Methodol 17:22

Subramanian A et al (2005) Gene set enrichment analysis: a knowledge-based approach for interpreting genome-wide expression profiles. Proc Natl Acad Sci U S A 102:15545–15550

Swami A et al (2013) Application of Box-Behnken design to the study of fatty acids and antioxidant activity from enriched white breadJ. Braz Chem Soc 24(9):883–888. https://doi.org/10.5935/0103-5053.20130193

Wu Z et al (2004) A model-based background adjustment for oligonucleotide expression arrays. J Am Stat Assoc 99:909–917

3 Random Forest and Concept of Decision Tree Model

3.1 Random Forest Model

A random forest model is an advanced technique resembled with bootstrapping algorithms inclusion on various decision tree, say for example we have thousands of observations set in the complete population besides with ten different parameters or attributes, an extrapolation of individual decisions or results are very critical, so far the random forest will possibly build the multiple CART models with different sampled observations in associated with base or initial variables, etc. (Hajjem et al. 2014). For some instances, we will take a random sample of hundred observations and five randomly chosen initial variables to build a CART model; it will repeat the entire process at ten times and then obtain final prediction values on each observation (function of each predictions). This final prediction can simply be called as mean of each prediction; flow chart of random forest was shown in (Fig. 3.1).

Practically, much literature cited that the random forest is ensemble method, which makes to build various independent classifiers which can contribute towards the suitable classification as a whole (at population level). The important objective of interest on random forest (RF) is to achieve an independent opinion of each classifier which has been looked at the data points by using different features, so researchers can draw their own opinion about the research attributes. Although, the random selection of various features does not guarantee for obtaining conclusive results, always they will be in different set of functional features, as you do it enough times you expect them to be different. The random forest and random tree significantly will be differing in association with scientific and analytical ethos. Random forest is a well-known classifier nowadays. In its simplest form, it can be thought of using bagging and random subsets of meta-classifier (on the basis of tree classifications) (Harrell et al. 1996; Harville 1996). The researchers wish to improve the inherent performance of a tree classifier by summing, averaging, or voting between several weak tree classifiers. Since they have not been able to build multiple trees on the same data points, they will get the same results of analytical findings. Scientifically, we introduce two types of randomness; each tree is solely built and slightly different with various manifold of rows sampled with repetitions from the original bagging and columns on each trees (in some cases each branch decision) built by using small randomly selected subsets of columns. However, random tree usually refers to randomly built trees which have nothing to do with machine learning (ML) (Hajjem et al. 2014; James et al. 2014). Therefore, the popular machine learning framework uses the term to refer to a decision tree built on random subsets of columns.

B. D. M., B. Narasimha Murthy, *Design of Experiments and Advanced Statistical Techniques in Clinical Research*, https://doi.org/10.1007/978-981-15-8210-3_3

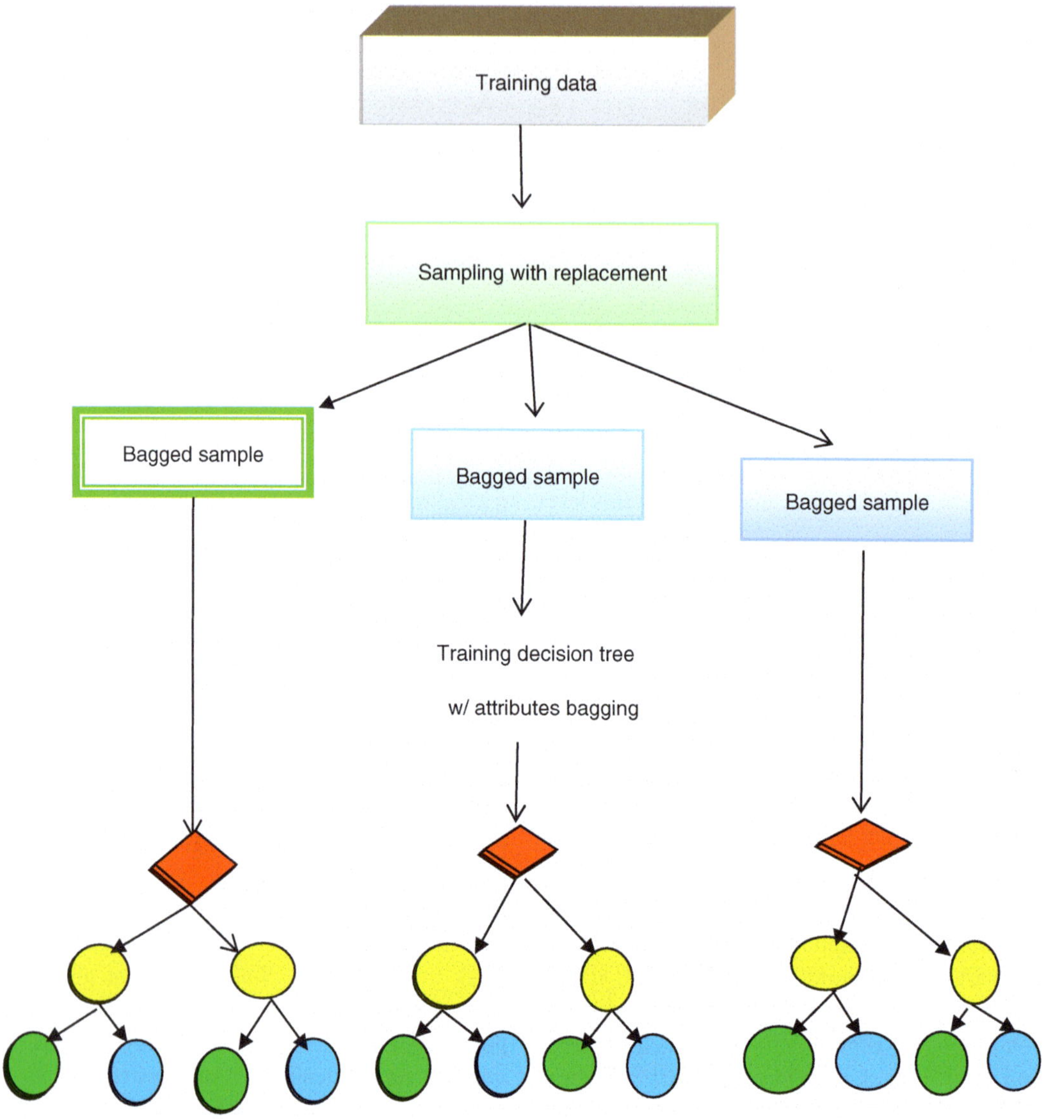

Fig. 3.1 Flow diagram of random forest

3.2 Tree Representation

In statistical perspective, the term tree is acyclic form of graphs (undirected) which comprises with a number of parent and child nodes. It was demonstrated that (Spjotvoll 1977; Strobl et al. 2009) the nodes have been simulated from the data structure and basic algorithms. On the other hand, a tree representation is a convenient way for representing different hierarchical attributes. In some sort of architectural plan or design, the tree will be considered as a major indicator to depict the full-blown information at multiple points (Fig. 3.2). It is clearly demonstrated that the tree is a sequential structure; it is connected to the deep network space; it can be represented as $T_1, T_2, T_{3,} \ldots T_n \left(\sum_{i=1}^{n} T_i \right)$ in association with known effect of random variables, e.g., the body mass index (BMI) effect on the intervention of type A drug. In the sequential structure, various dichotomous algorithms have been generated from the

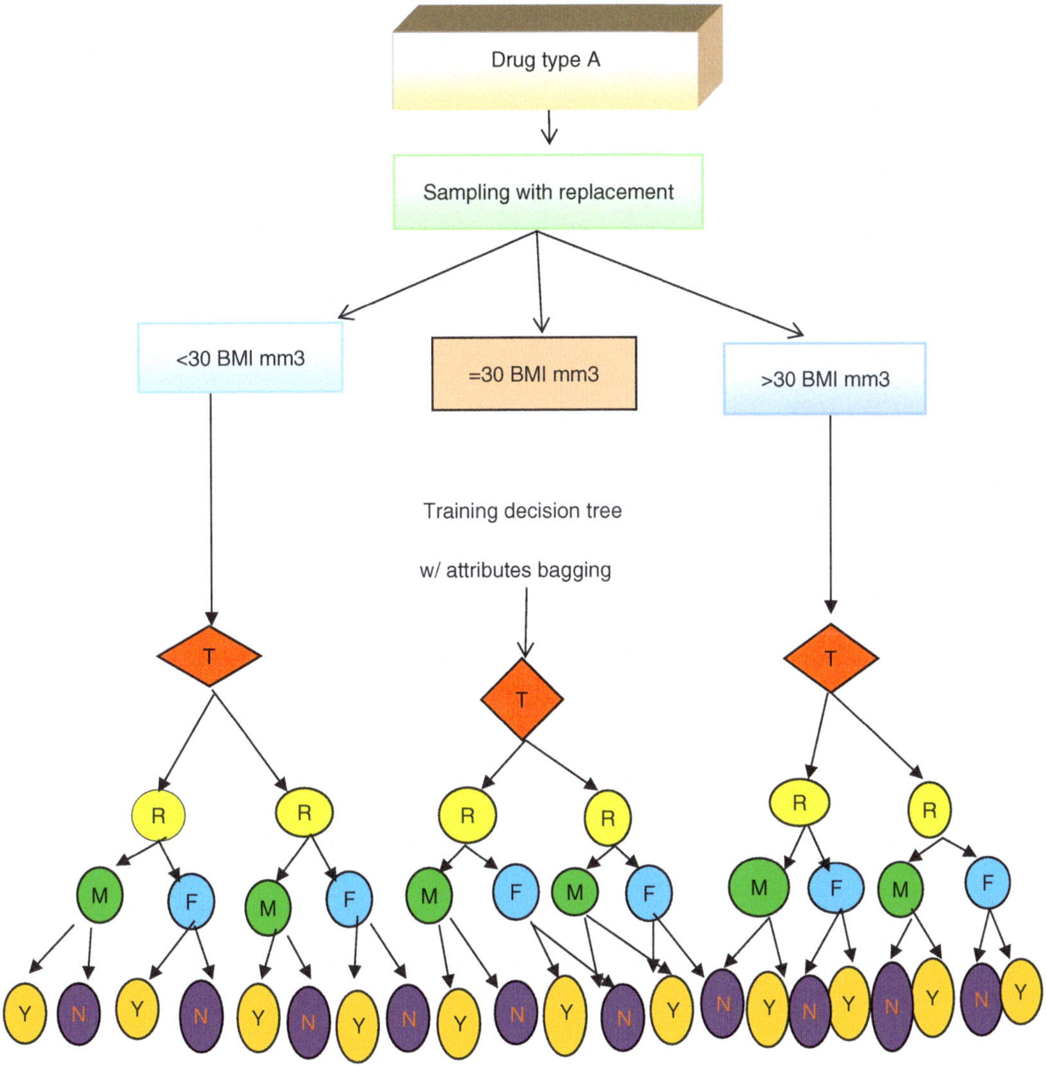

Fig. 3.2 Flow diagram of entropy random forest algorithms for drug trial. *R* Response, *M* Male, *F* Female, *Y* Yes, *N* No, *BMI* Body mass index

tree; in case of multicentric drug trial experimentation conducted at population level, researchers wish to extrapolate intervention on subjects with respect to response of the novel regimen. The novel regimen response will solely depend on various attributed data sets or characteristics, viz. gender, age, geographical location, type of food, morbid and comorbid condition, nursing care, peer supports, etc. Each variable of the response will preclude two dichotomous events. The response variable yes is coded as 1 and no coded as 0. The family of tree is usually considered as a preamble to build random forest by using different attributes or characteristics. In case of advanced computer science, it would be serving as a tool for formulating the computer languages (C^{++}, Java, python, and R script, etc.) and tree representation can facilitate full-blown decision about the computer programming language written by the various binary numbers or some pneumonic codes. An additional structures were consider to correlate by using various classification (classifier) and regression trees (CART models). The node is smoothly individuated as the root of the tree and subtrees which are attached to the node order between them. This is equivalent to deep specifying information with its own plan embedded with distinguishable subtrees dangling from a node with a left and right order, respectively, a new tree was obtained by appending a root on various sequences of a tree which already exists (tree representation, brief information theory, learning decision trees, bagging, random forests, etc.)

3.3 Decision Tree

The decision tree is one of the most widely used innovative methods for taking decision of random variants, in some consonance deductive and inductive inference drawn about the sampled observations from random variables (X_1, X_2, X_3,…, Xn) by using acyclic graphs. The sum of the random variables $\sum_{i=1}^{n} X_i$ will generate the decision tree representation, brief hypothesis, bagging and learning processes, etc. In previous section, we described the correlation on the effect of BMI on novel regimen in association with different attributes presented (Fig. 3.2). In this example, each parameter is represented with various acyclic form of graphs in association with dichotomous variables (binary number coded as 1 and 0). The following features or inclusions were considered for making decision about the theory of hypothesis: (1) methods of approximating random variables, (2) discrete-valued functions (including Boolean data), (3) learned functions—represented as decision trees (or if-then-else rules), (4) expressive hypotheses deep learning space inclusion disjunction, and finally we have to assess (5) the robustness of the random tree with noisy data which is demonstrated by Thompson iteration and Runge–Kutta method. Further, decision trees (DTs) are a supervised learning technique that predicts values of responses by learning decision rules derived from the random variables or attributes. Researchers can use both a regression and a classification context for testing null hypothesis underlying with assumed statement of the research problem. For this reason, they are sometimes also referred to as classification and regression trees (CART).

Note: The regression tree analysis is when the predicted outcome can be considered a real number (e.g., the price of a house or a patient's length of stay in a hospital).

3.4 Building of Decision Tree

Different chain of reasoning was used to build or fit decision tree; first, domain is construction of tree starting from top of the tree (construction begins with binary numbers 0 and 1), simultaneously the tree grows by splitting binary numbers or attributes one by one. Tree presentation is embedded with many primary and secondary nodes (acyclic graphs called as parent and child nodes) using parent and child nodes, we determined which attribute splitted homogenously, look at node impurity. After intervention of diagnosis of impurity we assign to leaf nodes, the majority vote in the leaf node was comprised of Boolean form of data. When we get to the bottom, prune the tree to prevent overfitting of the model. Classification instance by sorting them down the tree from the root to some leaf node, the node ≈ test of some random variables or attributes, Branch ≈ designed one of the possible values for the attributed data, as a matter of fact tree represented disjunction of conjunctions of various constraints on the attributed values of instances, i.e., $(\ldots \wedge \ldots \wedge) \vee (\ldots \wedge \ldots \wedge) \vee \ldots.$ equivalent to a set of if-then rules, each branch represents one if-then rule. If-part: conjunctions of attribute tests on the nodes; then-part: classification of the branch represented by the following example:

Each internal node: test one attribute Xi, each branch from a node: selects one value for Xi

Each leaf node: predict Y (or $P(Y|X \in \text{leaf})$)

This decision tree is equivalent to:

if (Outlook = Sunny) ∧ (Humidity = Normal), then Yes.

if (Outlook = Overcast), then Yes.

if (Outlook = Rain) ∧ (Wind = Weak), then Yes.

From Fig. 3.3 each internal node was tested on one attribute Xi; each branch from a node selects one value for Xi.

Each leaf node predicted Y or P ($Y|X \in \text{leaf}$)).

This decision tree is equivalent to the following syntax:

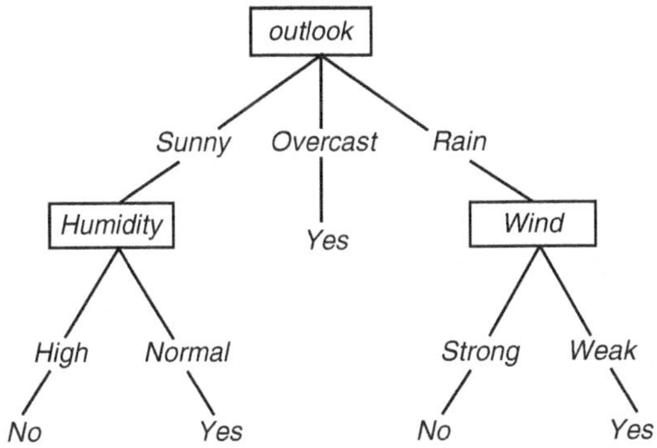

Fig. 3.3 Shows algorithms decision tree for humidity and wind

if (Outlook = Sunny) ∧ (Humidity = Normal), then Yes.

if (Outlook = Overcast), then Yes.

if (Outlook = Rain) ∧ (Wind = Weak), then Yes.

Illustration: A total of 1000 HIV-infected women pregnancy status was simulated by using random forest decision tree model; the following steps were used to simulation of results:

Positive HIV-infected women pregnancy status from CMIS data base

[833+, 167−] .83+ .17−

Fetal_presentation = 1: [822+, 116−] .88+ .12−

Previous _HIV test = 0: [767+, 81−] .90+ .10−

Primiparous = 0: [399+, 13−] .97+ .03−

Fetal _distress = 0: [334+, 47−] .88+ .12−

Birth _weight < 3349: [201+, 10.60−] .95+ .05

Birth _weight >= 3349: [133+, 36.4−] .78+ .25

Fetal _distress = 1: [34+, 21−] .62+ .38−

Previous _HIV test = 1: [55+, 35−] .61+ .39−

Fetal _presentation = 2: [3+, 29−] .11+ .89−

Fetal _presentation = 3: [8+, 22−] .27+ .73−

3.5 Rationality of the Decision Tree

The rationality of the decision tree will be varied from individuals. As we noticed in many literature survey, the rationality of decision tree profusely depends on the various attributes selected by the researcher during the time of research intervention. If the attributes have positive phrase with our statement of the problems, they yield positive response. In this rationality, the decision tree provides fallacious conclusive results for taking the right conclusion at the right time (Scarborough 1998). Therefore, as per the effective interpretation of research hypothesis by using decision tree, we have to ascertain the problems or attributes on various random variables (characteristics) in each instances. Further, we describe our salient objective of interest by various attributed data sets or variable since naturally the target function bears with discrete-valued observation, the hypothesis of our objective of interest is tested by CART disjunctive paradigm inclusion with noisy data sets. Therefore, the robustness of the fitted model shall be tested by using some set of mathematical approximation or derivation (errors in training data are obtained from Thompson iteration method); finally, the target values were estimated at greater accuracy, highest precision, and lower time intervals with precise cost function (e.g., different classification problem on drug trial, medical diagnosis, credit risk analysis in banking sector, and several tasks derived from building real computer language: C++, Java, python).

3.6 Top-Down Induction Decision Trees

Rao (1965) derived the quantification of induction on decision trees; he defined "it is a basic algorithm for learning decision trees (DTs)." Practically, a training set was built on CART; each algorithm was propagating decision trees (DTs); it performs search in the space of decision trees (Borst 1989; Michael 1992; Farmer et al. 1992). CART is the logical way for construction of decision tree would be done at top down with greedy algorithms (coded 1 and 0) (the fundamental question is which attribute should be tested next and which question gives us more information). After logic way, the construction of algorithms was selected based on the characteristics of CART. Further, we have to select the best attributes based on the subjective and objective approach or else experienced with data sets. Further, a descendant node is then created for each possible value or selected parameters on this attributes, for example, a CART induction was propagated or partitioned in accordance with trainer values. Since the process has been repeated

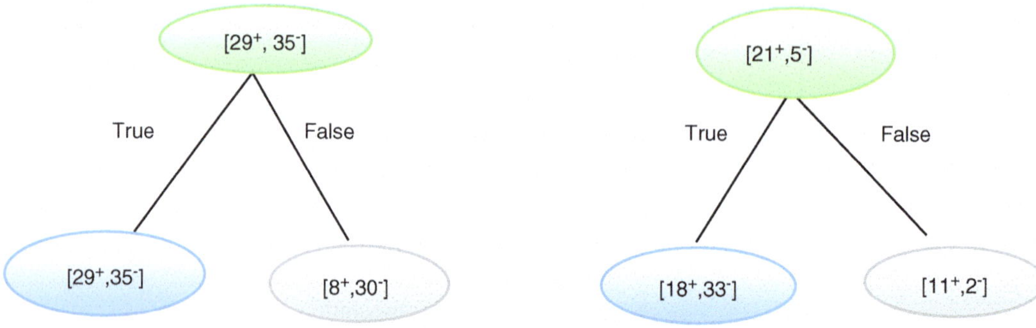

Fig. 3.4 Attribute classified based on deduction factors

in each successor node until all the examples are classified correctly or there are no attributes left out (Fig. 3.4).

A random forest is nothing but meta-estimator that fitted a number of decision tree classifiers on various subsamples of the data sets and uses averaging to improve the predictive accuracy and control overfitting of the model. The subsample is always the same as the original input sample size, but the samples are drawn with replacement if bootstrap is true (default). However, the statistical property bears with all pertaining information gained from trainer CART model; it can measure how well a given attribute separates the training. Examples usually the information gain use the notion of entropy, commonly used in information theory the formula for information gain is "IG" = expected reduction of entropy (Pilz 1991).

Entropy will measure the impurity of a collection of examples. It depends from the distribution of the random variable "p". Where

S is a collection of training examples,

$p+$ the proportion of positive examples in "S",

p^- the proportion of negative examples in "S".

An entropy will measure the impurity of a collection of examples. It mainly depends on the distribution of the various random variable "p".

"S" is a collection of training examples.

$p+$ the proportion of positive examples in "S".

p^- the proportion of negative examples in "S".

Entropy (S) = $\sum -p+ \log_2 p+ - p - \log_2$

Entropy ([14+, 0−]) = $-14/14 \log_2 (14/14) - 0 \log_2 (0) = 0$

Entropy ([9+, 5−]) = $-9/14 \log_2 (9/14) - 5/14 \log_2 (5/14) = 0.94$

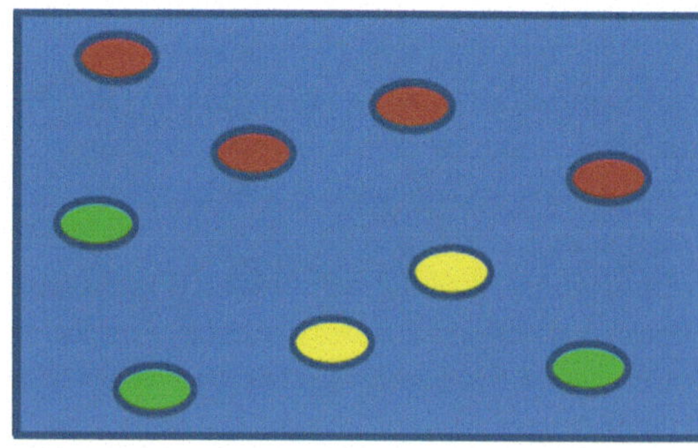

Fig. 3.5 Calculating information-based sampled observations

Entropy ([7+, 7−]) = $-7/14 \log_2 (7/14) - 7/14 \log_2 (7/14)$

$= 1/2 + 1/2 = 1$ [$\log_2 1/2 = -1$]

The entropy is the favorable convenience of the use of a logarithmic function in the definition of the entropies; it is practically useful because many important parameters for generating large multiplication of CART main node and subnodes; these nodes that are very useful for determination of valid entropy values at single point of CART is intuitive because we use to measure magnitudes by linear comparison with units of measurements; it is mathematically more suitable because many limiting operations in terms of the logarithm are simpler than in terms of the number of possibilities. In turn, the choice of a logarithmic base amounts to a choice of a unit for measuring information. If the base 2 is used, the resulting unit is called "bit" a contraction of binary unit (Fig. 3.5).

The information derived by choosing a ball from the bin is determined as follows:

I(red ball) = $-\log_2(4/9) = 1.1699$ bits
I(yellow ball) = $-\log_2(2/9) = 2.1699$ bits
I(green ball) = $-\log_2(3/9) = 1.58496$ bits

3.7 Entropy

The entropy of a variable is an amount of information including various attributes. This amount has been determined not simply, but it was just defined by the number of different values, and scientifically it is aroused from the subjective nature of the individuals. Since the variable can take on the basis of expression or different attributes measured from scale parameters, for example, we have experienced in the electronic mailbox, the information mentioned in the email is mainly quantified not just by the number of words in the email or the different possible words in the language of the email (Mallet 1986; Mentre et al. 1997). Informally, the amount of information presented in the mailbox is directly proportional to the amount of surprise its reading causes. For example, if an email is simply dealt with a repeat of an earlier email, then it is not informative at all. On the other hand, say if the email reveals the outcome of an event then it is highly informative. Information variable is tied to the amount of surprise that value of the variable causes when we revealed. This variable was modeled by using entropy techniques (Shannon's entropy), this was discussed above cited model, the model will quantify the amount of information in a variable which has been cited in different attributes, thus, fitted model has been providing the fundamental mechanisms or phenomena on the basis of salient theory of entropy scatteredness around the notation or information used by the analyst (Mentre et al. 1997). Bit is the basic unit of information, which represents two possible states (1) if you have "n" bits, then that information represents $2n$ possible states. For example, a byte is 8 bits; therefore, the number of states it represents is 28 = 256. This magnifies that a byte can store any number between 0 and 255. If you are given the total number of states, then you just take the log of that number to get the amount of information measured in the bits (log 2256 = 8). Analytically, the log of the number of total microscopic states corresponding to the particular macrostate of thermodynamics is the best example for the above interventions. This is an additional information to the researcher, tuning with order of magnitudinal and relative differences, estimated for completion of entire task with prior specification of microstate and besides with given knowledge of the macrostate, etc. In the above-cited example, there are three outcomes that have been aroused from the possible events; when you choose the ball, it can be red, yellow, or green (n = 3). So the following events to be generated simultaneously.

$$\text{Entropy} = -(4/9)\log(4/9) \pm (2/9)\log(2/9) \pm (3/9)\log(3/9) = 1.5305.$$

Therefore, observer expected to get 1.53 information each time you choose a ball from the bin equation for determining the range of Entropy: $0 \leq \text{Entropy} \leq \log(n)$, where "$n$" is number of outcomes. Entropy "0" (minimum entropy) occurs when one of the probabilities is "1" and rest are "0"s; Entropy log (n) (maximum entropy) occurs when all the probabilities have equal values of $1/n$ (Fig. 3.6).

$$E = \sum_{i=1}^{n} -p \log p_i \tag{3.1}$$

Drug trial was conducted in the year 1993 at Austria, the study reported that the response in target symptoms was found to be 40 children who attending nursery and special school for handicapped in Garz, Austria, seen over 55 consultations. Total 18 children responded well, rest of 11 cases showed improvement in some but not all target symptoms, 7 cases did not respond to the treatment, and results or outcomes of 4 cases were not assessed properly (Lindstrom and Bates 1988, 1990). The children with organic brain damage, autism, and definitive syndromes generally responded well, whereas those with lack of support and social deprivation generally failed to respond. Majority of the cases were found to significantly show good response and the rate was drawn up to 70%. Improvement in hyperactive and aggressive behavior, which enabled the children to benefit more from their education. Physical symptoms and problems such as stammering and enuresis also improved. The researcher wishes to calculate the expected entropy for the above-cited trial by using entropy techniques (Fig. 3.7).

Response in target symptoms (40,18),E(40,11), E(11,7),E(11,4)

$$E(p)=\sum_{i=1}^{n} -40\log 40-18\log 18$$

$E(P) = -64.08 - 22.59 = 0.86.$

$$E(p)=\sum_{i=1}^{n} -40\log 40-11\log 11$$

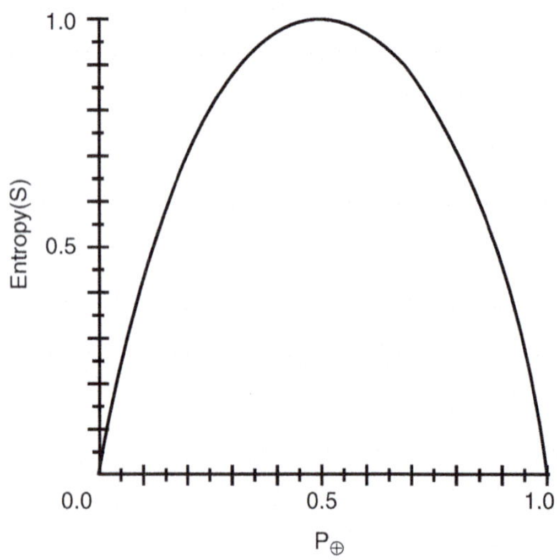

Fig. 3.6 Entropy distribution ($0 \le e \le 1$)

Not responded = 0.75

$$E(p)=\sum_{i=1}^{n} -11\log 11-7\log 7$$

Did not respond = 0.17%

$$E(p)=\sum_{i=1}^{n} -11\log 11-4\log 4$$

Could not be assessed = 0.03%

$$Giniindex(IG)=1-\sum_{i=1}^{c} p_j^{\,2}$$

3.8 Impurity

An impurity has been classified into two categories, namely left and right impurity.

$$Leftimpurity=1-(40/40+18)^2-(40/40+11)^2$$

$$Rightimpurity=1-(11/11+7)^2-(11/11+4)^2$$

Attributes Labels

X_1	X_2	Y	Count
T	T	+	2
T	F	+	2
F	T	–	5
F	F	+	1

$$\mathrm{IG}(X_1,Y)=H(Y)-H(Y|X_1) \quad (3.2)$$

Fig. 3.7 Algorithms of target symptoms of children attending nursery and special school for handicapped in Garz

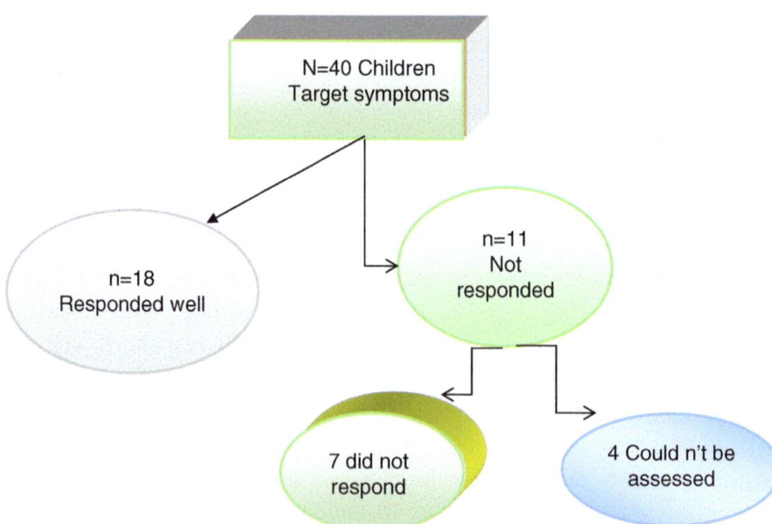

$$H(Y) = -(5/10)\log(5/10) - 5/10\log(5/10) = 1$$

$$H(Y|X_1) = P(X_1 = T)H(Y|X_1 = T) + P(X_1 = F)H(Y|X_1 = F)$$

$$= 4/10(1\log 1 + 0\log 0) + 6/10(5/6\log 5/6 + 1/6\log 1/6)$$

$$= 0.39$$

Information gain $(X_1,Y) = 1 - 0.39 = 0.61$

Entropy measures the amount of information in a random variable

$$H(X) = -p + \log_2 p \pm p - \log_2 p - X = \{+,-\}$$

for binary classification [two-valued random variable]

$$H(X) = -\underset{i=1}{\overset{c}{}} pi\log_2 pi = \underset{i=1}{\overset{c}{}} pi\log_2 1/pi \quad X = \{i,\ldots,c\} \tag{3.3}$$

for classification in "*c*" classes, for example, rolling a die with 8, equally probable, sides.

$$H(X) = -8 1/8\log_2 1/8 = -\log_2 1/8 = \log_2 8 = 3$$

The entropy can specify on the number of average length (in bits) of the message needed to transmit the outcome of a random variable. This depends on the probability distribution. An optimal length code assigns $\log_2$ "p_i"; bits to messages with probability *p*. Most probable messages get shorter codes.

For example, eight-sided [unbalanced] die

1	2	3	4	5	6	7	8
4/16	4/16	2/16	2/16	1/16	1/16	1/16	1/16
2 bits	2 bits	3 bits	3 bits	4bits	4bits	4bits	4bits

$$E = (1/4\log 24) * (2 + (1/8\log 28) * 2 + (1/16\log 216) * 4 = 1 + 3/4 + 1 = 2.75$$

Information gain is the expected reduction in entropy method which was caused by partitioning the examples of various attributes. As well as that higher the information gains lead to recieve more effective parameter from various attributes for classifying training data sets. An expected reduction entropy is known by "*A*".

$$\text{Gain}(S,A) = \text{Entropy}(S) - \text{Entropy}(Sv)\text{values}(A)$$

Values (*A*) possible values for *A*

Sv subset of "*S*" for which "*A*" has value "*v*"

$$H(X) = -\Sigma p_i \log_2 p_i \quad X = \{i,\ldots,c\} \quad i = 1 \quad \text{for classification in 'c' classes} \tag{3.4}$$

Example: Rolling a die with 8, equally probable has estimated by the followings

$$H(X) = -\Sigma 1/8\log_2 1/8 = -\log_2 1/8 = \log_2 8 = 3$$

Entropy specifies the number of average length (in bits) of the message needed to transmit the outcome of a random variable. This depends on the probability distribution. Optimal length code assigned was estimated by - $\sum p_i \log_2 p_i$ bits to messages with probability "*p*". Most probable messages will get shorter codes (Fig. 3.8).

The Gini impurity decreases each random forest tree node. Random forest feature selection relies on the bootstrap aggregation (bagging) and therefore does not preclude the training sets, validation sets, test sets, etc.

3.9 Shannon's Entropy

According to Shannon et al. (1949), a general communication system consists of five parts:

1. A source *S*, which generates the message to be received at the destination.
2. A transmitter "*T*" which turns the message generated at the source into a signal to be transmitted. In the cases in which the information is encoded, encoding is also implemented by this system.
3. A channel CH is the medium used to transmit the signal from the transmitter to the receiver.
4. A receiver *R*, which reconstructs the message from the signal.
5. A destination *D*, which receives the message.

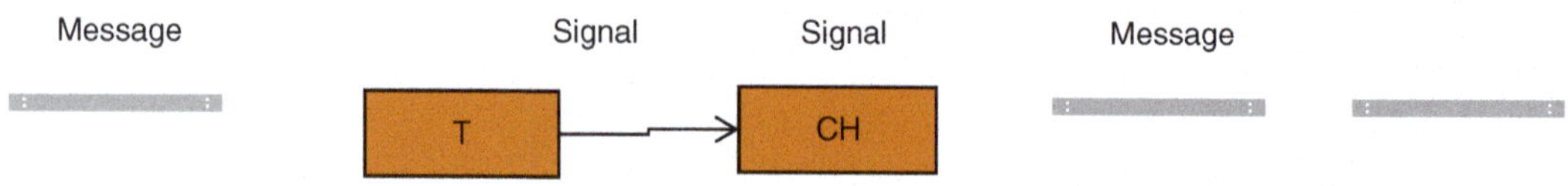

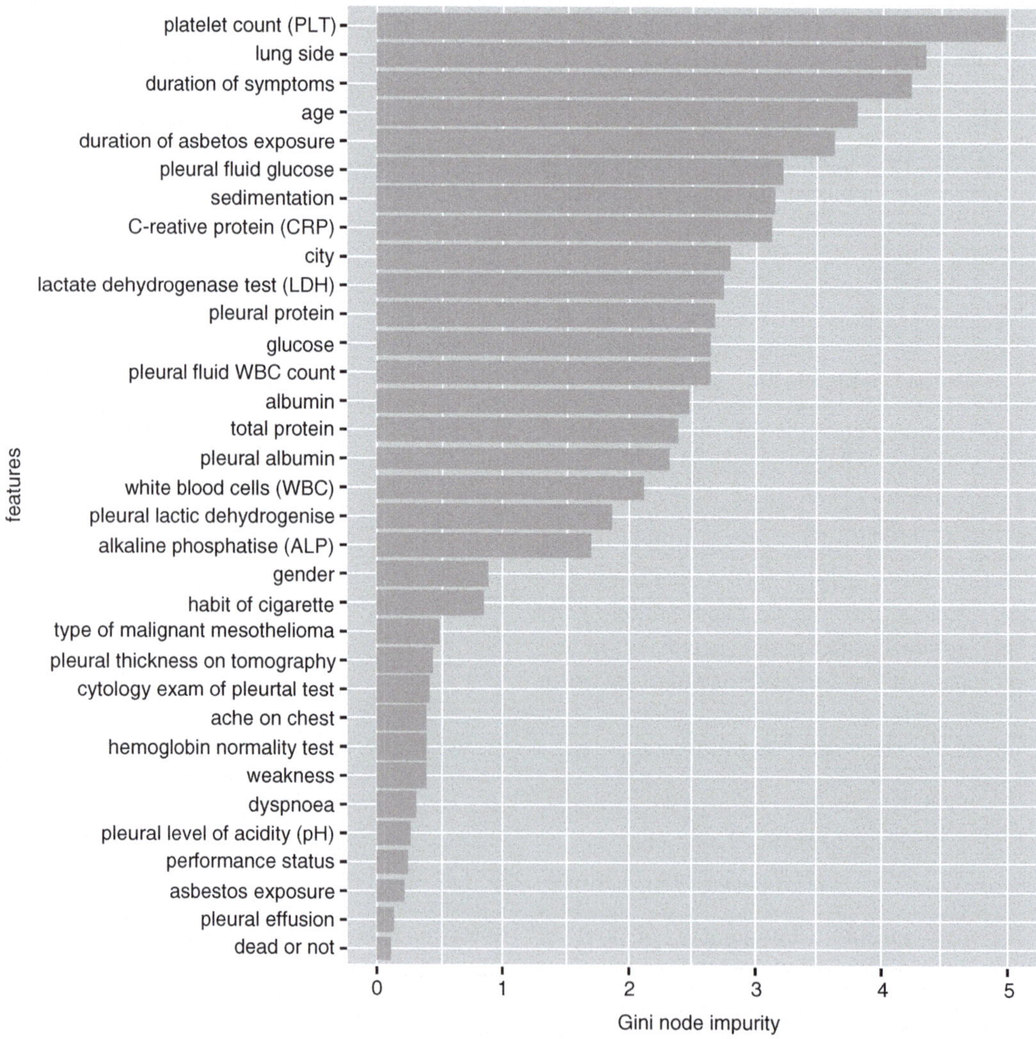

Fig. 3.8 Gini node impurity determined based on the random forest

Information reduction on the uncertainty has estimated by the following Eq. (3.5) (amount of surprise in the outcome):

$$I(E) = \log_2 \frac{1}{p(x)} = -\log_2 p(x) \quad (3.5)$$

If the probability of event is very small and happening of other event would be very large, the following model is formulated for calculation of information (I).

$$I = -\log_2 1/2 = 1$$

Observing the outcome of a coin flip is head. Observing the outcome of a dice is 6.

$$I = -\log_2 1/6 = 2.58$$

The expected amount of information when observing the output of a random variable "*X*" is as follows:

$$H(X) = E(I(X)) = \sum_i p(x_i) I(x_i) = -\sum_i p(x_i) \log_2 p(x_i)$$

If "*X*" can have eight outcomes and all are equally likely, the *H*(*x*) becomes

$$H(X) == -\sum_i 1/8 \log_2 1/8 = 3$$

Finally, the entropy was roughly estimated.

$$H(x) \le \log_2 k$$

However, equality holds when all outcomes are equally likely Probability distribution is the derivatives of H(x), which are uniformily distributed at the lower level of entropy, the conditional entropy has been formulated in the Eq. (3.6)

Conditional entropy

$$H(x) = -\Sigma\, p(x_i) \log 2\, p(x_i)$$

$$H(X/Y) = -\Sigma(P(y_j) H(x/y = yi)$$

$$= -\sum_j p(y_j) \sum_i p(x_i / y_j) \log 2\, p(x_i / y_j) \quad (3.6)$$

From Eq. (3.6) we calculate information gain of experiments IG(*X*,*Y*) = *H*(*X*) − *H*(*X*|*Y*) (information before split) − (information after split) (Table 3.1).

Table 3.1 Showed attributable difference between bagging and boosting of trainer data

Bagging	Boosting
No clear winner; usually depends on the entire data sets. Bagging is computationally more efficient when compared to boosting (note that bagging can train the "M" models in parallel, boosting can not) Both reduce variance (and overfitting) by combining different models The resulting model has higher stability when compared to the individual ones Bagging usually cannot reduce the bias, boosting can (note that in boosting, the training error steadily decreases) Bagging usually performs better than boosting if we do not have a high bias and only want to reduce variance (i.e., if we are overfitting)	Boosting is an ensemble technique where new models are added to correct the errors made by existing models. Models are added sequentially until no further improvements can be made. A popular example is the AdaBoost algorithm that weights data points that are hard to predict Gradient boosting is an approach where new models are created that predict the residuals or errors of prior models and then added together to make the final prediction. It is called gradient boosting because it uses a gradient descent algorithm to minimize the loss when adding new models This approach supports both regression and classification predictive modeling problems In boosting, the trees are built sequentially such that each subsequent tree aims to reduce the errors of the previous tree. Each tree learns from its predecessors and updates the residual errors. Hence, the tree that grows next in the sequence will learn from an updated version of the residuals
In contrast to bagging techniques like random forest, trees are grown to their maximum extent	Boosting makes use of trees with fewer splits Such small trees, which are not very deep, are highly interpretable. Parameters like the number of trees or iterations, the rate at which the gradient boosting learns, and the depth of the tree could be optimally selected through validation techniques like *k*-fold cross-validation Having a large number of trees might lead to overfitting. So, it is necessary to carefully choose the stopping criteria for boosting

3.10 *K*-Means Clustering

Initially, two centroids are assigned randomly; the Euclidian distance has been used to find out which centroid is closest to the data points that are assigned to the corresponding centroid. The cluster analysis tool was coined by Edwin Diday in 1985. One of the major clustering insight approaches was estimated based on the sum of squares criterion and on the various dichotomous algorithms that is today we are using well-known methods to know the patterns of *K*-means clustering analysis (Kazunaga et al. 2016; Jennrich and Schluchter 1986). The objectives of this intervention are to know the similarity of the observations in a Euclidian space; the estimation of the distance between two clusters has been determined analytically. Since various types of clustering are classified based on their characteristics and similarity or homogeneity, the following diagram represents the various classification of clusters (Fig. 3.9).

3.10.1 Agglomerative

Bottom-up approach begins with each element as separate clusters and merge them in successively larger cluster. The agglomerative approach has been classified based on the similarity of the characteristics and attributes; each data point would be clarified at preliminary stage of investigations and classification based on the successive appearance of the variables and similarity or homogeneity. For example, estimation of effect newly manufactured drug considering various attributes (age, sex, geographical residence, food types, diets, physical exercise, etc.); we have focused the single centroid point to determine the distance of the data points (Gladitz and Pilz 1982; Fedorov et al. 1993; Friedman et al. 2000) (Fig. 3.10).

Basic agglomerative hierarchical clustering algorithm

(1) Compute the proximity matrix, if necessary; (2) repeat; (3) Merge the closest two clusters; (4) Update the proximity matrix to reflect the proximity between the new cluster and the original clusters; (5) until only one cluster remains. The key operation of basic agglomerative clustering is the computation of the proximity between the two clusters.

Minimum proximity of the parameters were defined by the cluster variation of entire data sets, which is relatively measured by the normal distribution (SND) assumptions. The validation on each cluster was measured by the shortest distance between two points x and y, that are fully dependent on selected clusters of $X_1, X_2..X_n$ and $Y_1, Y_2..Y_n$ respectively. It was modeled in Eq. (3.7)

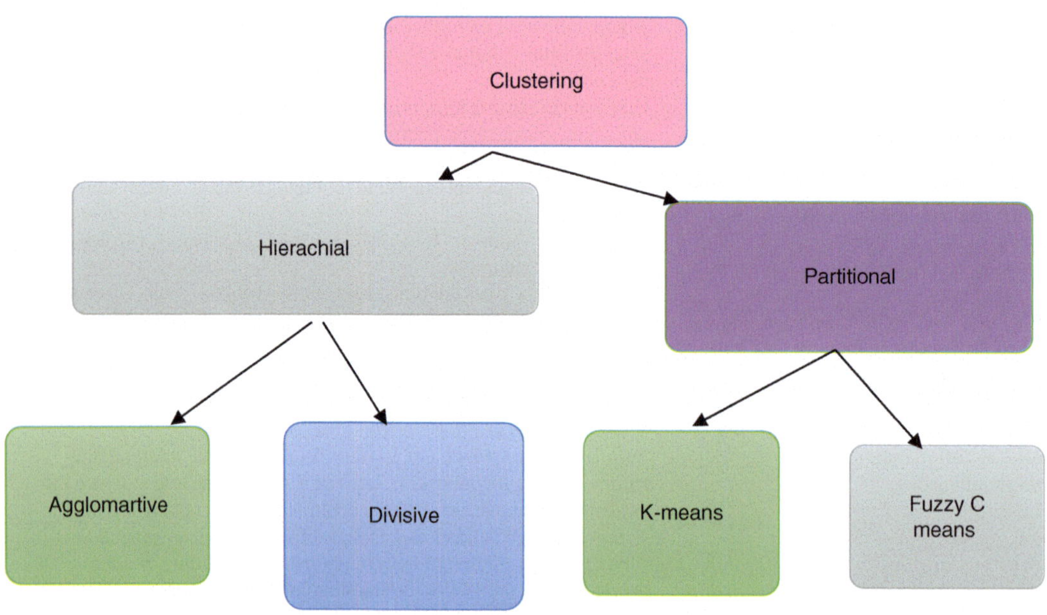

Fig. 3.9 Distribution of clustering types

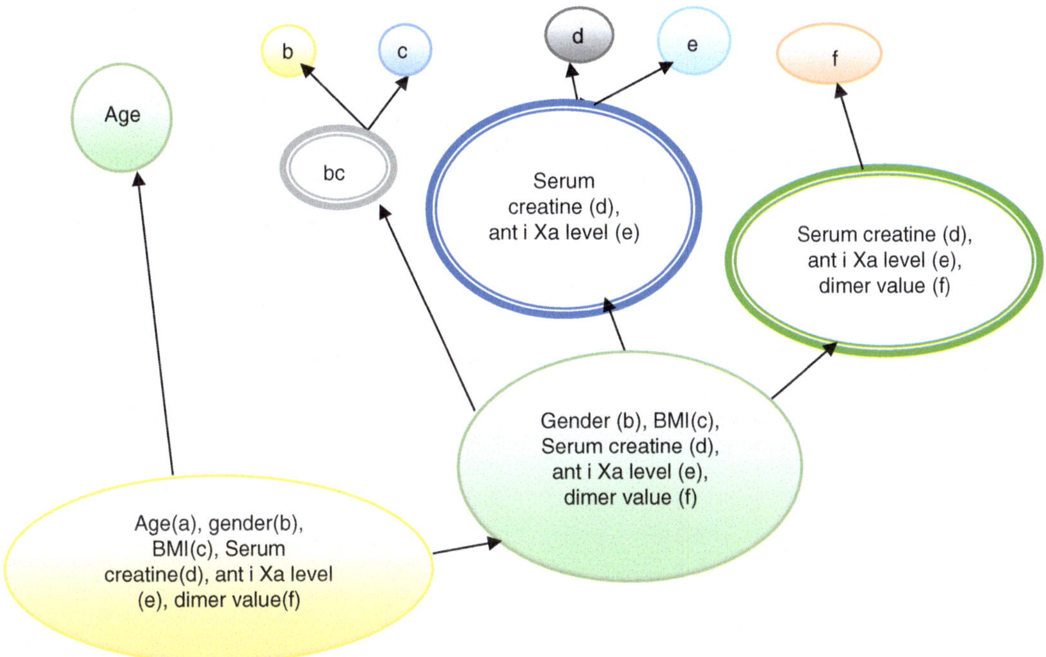

Fig. 3.10 Agglomerative classification

$$d(A,B) = \min_{X\epsilon A Y\epsilon B} d(A-B) \quad (3.7)$$

Max (Complete Link) Proximity defines cluster proximity as the furthest distance between two points, x and y, that are in different clusters, X and Y showed in Eq. (3.8)

$$d(A,B) = \max_{X\epsilon A Y\epsilon B} d(A-B) \quad (3.8)$$

As per the analytical approach, we define cluster proximity as the average distance between two points, x and y, that are in different clusters, A and B

$$d(A,B) = \left[\sum_{X\epsilon A Y\epsilon B} d(x-y) / n_A n_B \right] \quad (3.9)$$

Note: Single link is being called as chain-like and is good at handling nonelliptical shapes, but is sensitive to the outliers. A complete link is less susceptible to noise and outliers, but can break large clusters and favors globular shapes. A group average is an intermediate approach between the single and complete link approaches obtained from the Eq. (3.9)

3.10.2 Divisive Clustering

The division of objects into clusters such that each object or variable is exactly one cluster, not several. Also known as top-down approach, this algorithm does not require to pre-specify the number of clusters. The top-down clustering will require a suitable method for splitting a cluster that contains the whole axiom data points or sets and proceeds by splitting of clusters recursively until individual data points have been split into singleton cluster (Friedman 2001; Fedorov et al. 2002) (Fig. 3.11).

A distinction among different types of clustering is whether the set of clusters is nested or unnested. Partitioned clustering is a simple division of the set of data objects into nonoverlapping subsets (clusters), such that each data object is exactly in one subset. However, grouping of data objects within a group is similar in nature (or near) to one another and dissimilar (or far) from the objects in other groups; the salient objectives of clustering are to minimize intra-cluster distances and maximize inter-cluster distances (Figs. 3.12 and 3.13, Tables 3.2, 3.3 and 3.4).

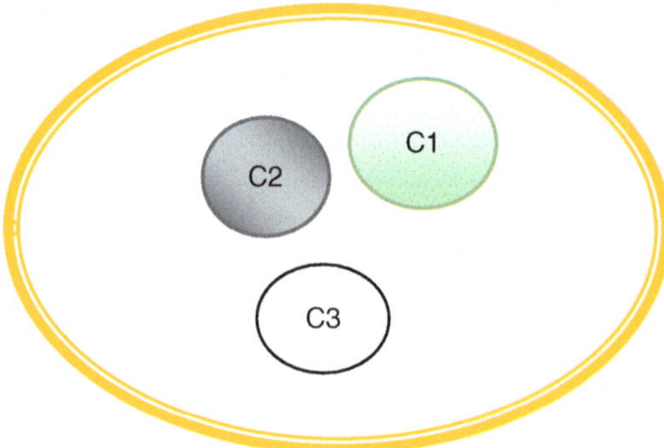

Fig. 3.11 Partitioned clustering sampling techniques

3.11 Applications

Radiographic image processing—cluster images based on their visual content.

Web mining/electronic health record—cluster groups users assessed the relevancy of results based on their access patterns on Web Pages and cluster Web Pages.

Bioinformatics—cluster similar proteins together (similarity with respect to chemical structure and/or functionality, etc.)

Fig. 3.12 Overview of partitioned clustering minimization

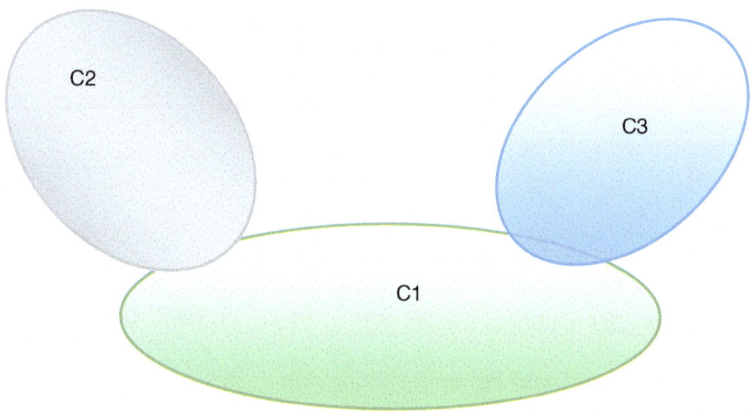

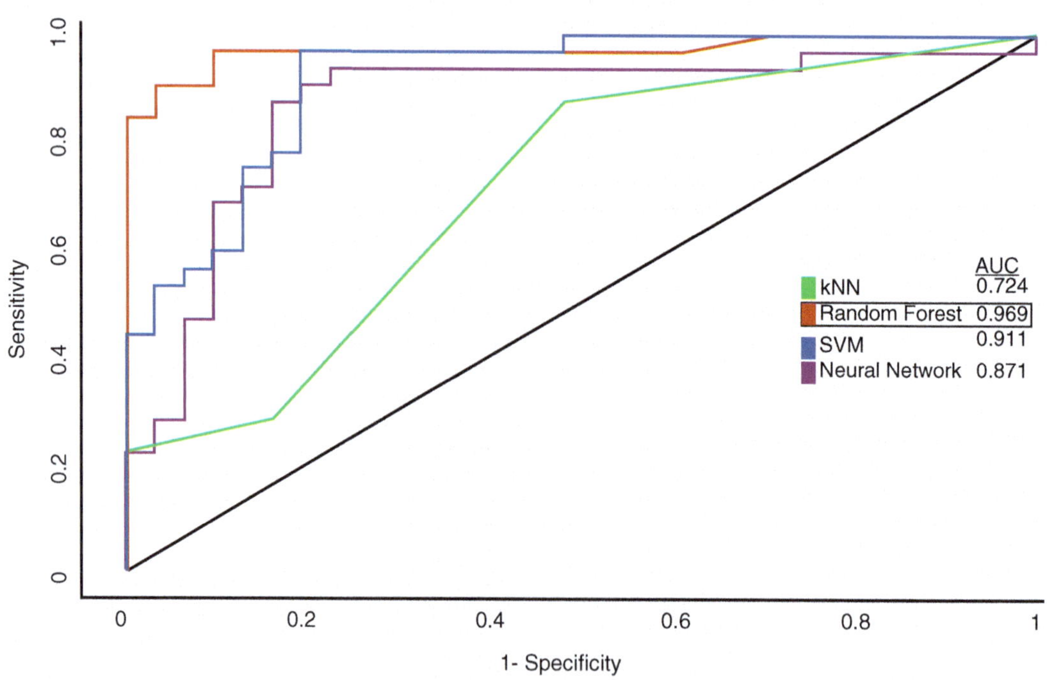

Fig. 3.13 Diagnostic analysis of random forest by using ROC techniques

Table 3.2 Various models used to calibrate the accuracy of the trainer results

Sl	Classification techniques	Accuracy	Correctly classified	Incorrectly classified
1	SVM	77.73	597	171
2	RF (random forest)	75.39	579	189
3	NB	73.48	129	61
4	Decision tree	73.18	562	206
5	KNN	63.04	145	85

Table 3.3 Relevancy of various steps for extrapolation of results

Sl	Steps	Sensitivity (%)	Specificity (%)	Overall predicted accuracy	Precision
1	Learning	0.938	0.969	0.953	0.968
2	External validation	0.938	0.938	0.938	0.938

Table 3.4 Performance metrics logistic regression and random forest

Sl	Performance metrics	Logistic regression	Random forest	Weighted average
1	Accuracy	0.931	0.983	0.990
2	Precision	0.953	0.967	0.975
3	Sensitivity (%)	0.843	0.972	0.984
4	Specificity (%)	0.978	0.977	0.924
5	*F*-measures	0.895	0.946	0.979

3.12 Fuzzy C-Means

Fuzzy *C*-means (FCM) is a unique method for classification of clustering in different approach, in broad sense which can be defined as the division of objects into different clusters, such that each sample data or object belongs to multiple cluster. On the other hand, it can allow one piece of data to belong to two or more clusters. This method was developed by Dunn in 1973 and improved by Friedman et al. (2002). The fuzzy means is analytically modeled by the following Eq. (3.10):

$$J_m = \sum_{i=1}^{N}\sum_{j=1}^{C} u^m{}_{ij} \| X_i - C_j \|^2, \quad (3.10)$$

where "m" is any real number greater than 1, "u_{ij}" is the degree of membership of "x_i" in the cluster j, x_i is the ith of D-dimensional measured data, c_j is the D-dimension center of the cluster, and ||*|| is any normative expressing the similarity between any measured data and the center. The fuzzy partitioning is carried out through an iterative optimization of the objective function showed in Eqs. (3.10) and (3.11), with the update of membership u_{ij} and the cluster centers c_j by

$$u_{ij} = \frac{1}{\sum_{k=1}^{c}\left(\frac{\| X_i - c_j \|}{\| x_i - c_k \|}\right)^{\frac{2}{m-1}}} \quad (3.11)$$

$$c_j = \frac{\sum_{i-1}^{N} u_{ij}^{m} \cdot x_i}{\sum_{i-1}^{N} u_{ij}^{m}}$$

Biologically, we have measured fuzzy means in terms of a monodimensional application of the FCM; we consider 25 patients data on the random sugar blood serum that was collected from the bedside record critically ill patients of diabetes and data points are divided into three clusters to initialize the base algorithms and to compute the "U" metrics. Figure 3.10 showed the family values of each datum at each cluster (interactive perception). The color of the data points is that of the nearest cluster according to the membership function (Francis et al. 2005; Demidenko et al. 2004) (Figs. 3.14 and 3.15).

Simulation technique was shown in Fig. 3.10; we used a fuzziness coefficient $m = 2$ and also we imposed to terminate the algorithms, when $\max_{ij}$ $\{|u_{ij}^{(k+1)} - u_{ij}^{(k)}|\} < 0.3$. Figures 3.14 and 3.16

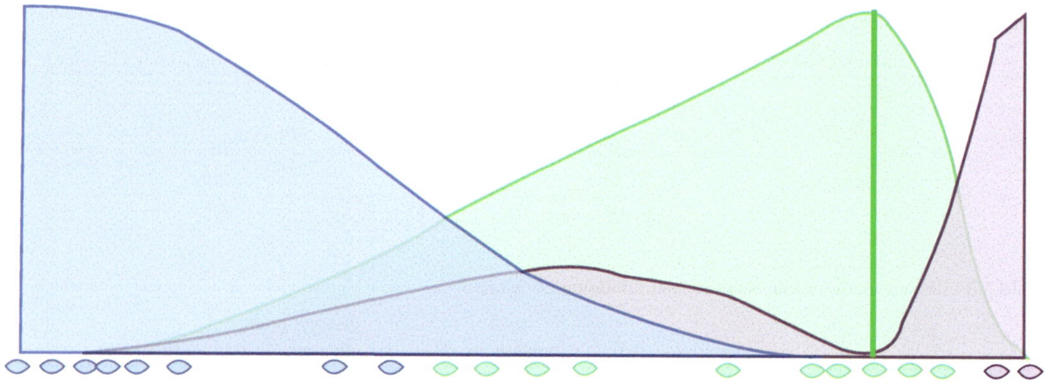

Fig. 3.14 Fuzzy means in terms of a monodimensional application

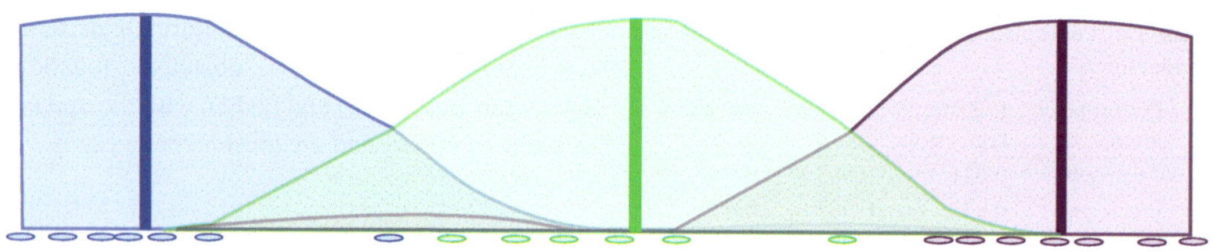

Fig. 3.15 Fuzzy means estimation $m = 2$

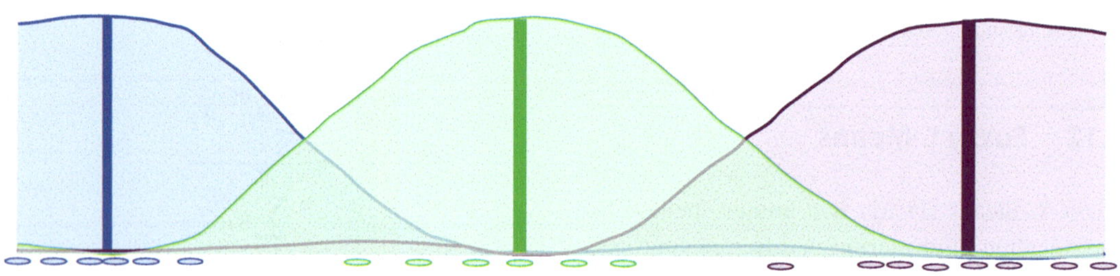

Fig. 3.16 Grouping of fuzzy means based on the distance $m = 2$

show the initial condition where the fuzzy distribution coherently depends on the particular position of the clusters.

3.13 *K*-Means Clusters

The "*K*"-means clustering algorithm is an object to categorize the different attributes based on the basic principles of clustering (data sets into k partitions, where $k < 1$). It is similar to the expectation algorithms used for mixture of Gaussian family $N\sim(\mu, \sigma^2)$ that they are attempted to find the center of natural clusters in the given attributed data points. Although it was assumed that the objective attributes were propagated from a vector space (Figs. 3.17, 3.18, 3.19 and 3.20).

Steps used for the determination of "K"-means clustering approach.

Given k, the k-means algorithm is implemented by the following four steps:

1. Partition objects into k non-empty subsets.
2. Compute seed points as the centroid of the clusters of the current partition (centroid is the center, the mean point of the cluster).
3. Assign each object to the cluster with the nearest seed points.
4. Go back to step 2, stop when no more new assignment.

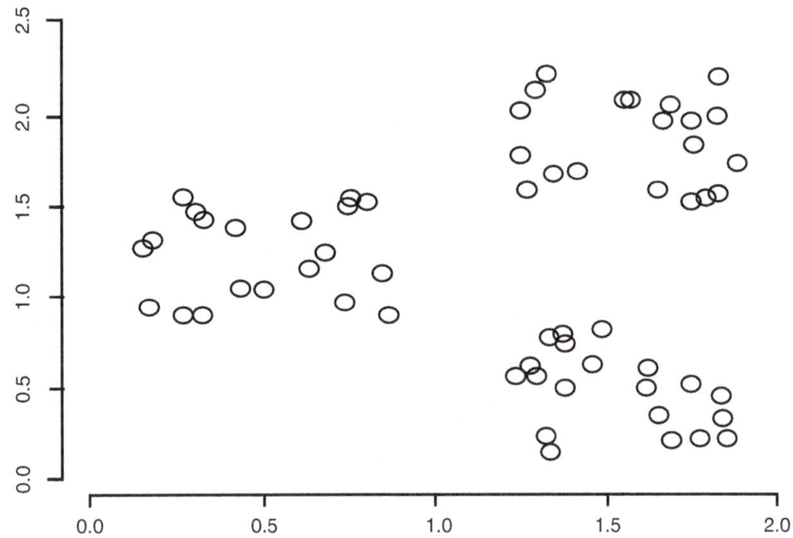

Fig. 3.17 Data for structure of cluster

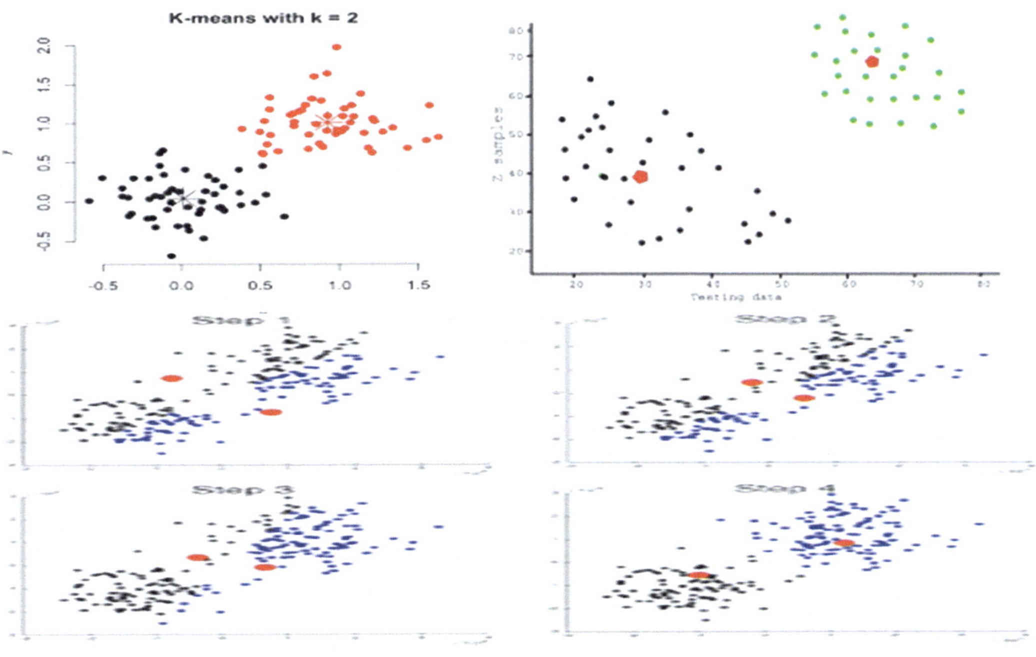

Fig. 3.18 Extrapolation method for the determination of "*K*"-means clustering approach

3.14 Application of *K*-Means Clustering in Medical Science

The cardiac imaging is an indispensable trivial gadget for determining the evaluation of coronary stenosis studied by Dilts (2013), Chevan and Sutherland (1991), Budescu (1993), and Breiman (2001); they demonstrated that cardiac images are used to detect and to know the correlation of coronary artery disease (CAD). A cardiac imaging is a method of choice, and the most important reason for choosing this method is the relatively noninvasive techniques. Even in "X" ray

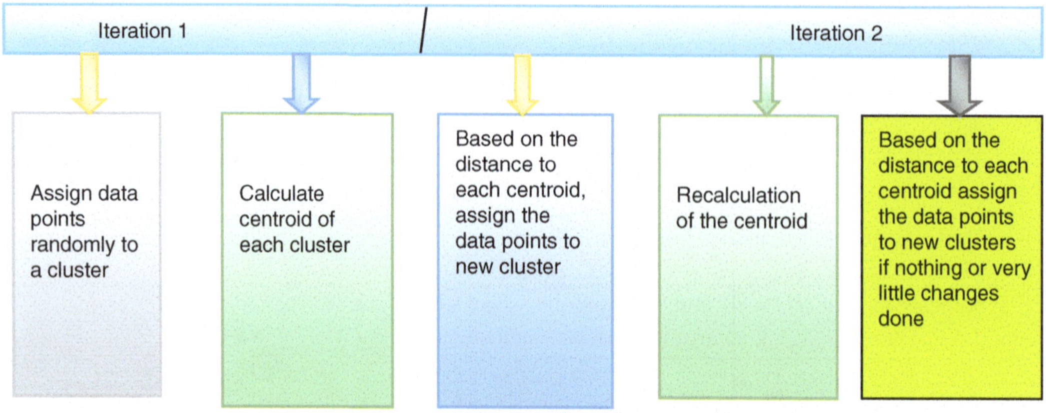

Fig. 3.19 Different classifications and optimization techniques used for *K*-means clustering in machine learning

angiography, the most invasive cardiac imaging condition will be choosing over excising a possible coronary lesion during cardiac surgery. Employing an intravascular approach instead of surgery for nonimaging measurement methods still requires cardiac imaging to set the arterial lesion. The *K*-means will extrapolate various subgroup analyses for the detection of standard error (SE) and means of the similar sampled data sets (Friedman 2001). Cardiac image analysis was done based on *k*-means clustering through segmentation; it is an operation that is used for portioning the image according to similarity and discontinuity or for determining the edge method to analyze the information with the help of multiple portion. It is an essential part that is used in medical image recognition tool (analysis). Different techniques were used to extrapolate the relation between the effectiveness of image rendering and smoothening of images. The following formidable methods are used for image processing, viz. (1) thresholding method, (2) region-based method, (3) edge-based method, and (4) clustering method.

3.14.1 Steps

1. The number of clusters must be known to "*k*".
2. The number of cluster centers should be obtained from each other.
3. Consider each data point and assign it to the number of clusters which is closest.
4. Recalculate the center by finding the mean of the data points.
5. Repeat third and fourth step until shifting centers among the cluster could observe.

3.15 Stenosis Intervention

Kakihara et al. (2008) describes the stenosis is a narrowing of the inner surface of the artery or valve, usually caused by atherosclerosis. According to human anatomy, there are two important cases of stenosis discussion; first is aortic stenosis and the second one is carotid stenosis, where the doctors are normally assuming the type of stenosis for further evaluation. First, aortic stenosis is a kind of disease which causes narrowing in the aortic valve, and it causes problem during the blood flow from heart to the body. Second, carotid artery disease stenosis is a kind of disease which causes the narrowing of the carotid arteries, and this kind of narrowing usually is caused by the providers of fatty material and cholesterol deposits on inner surface and it is called plaque. And it is important to know that carotid artery occlusion refers to complete blockage of the artery. An imaging modality needs to be fast to measure the cardiac function because the measurement of flow and influx requires a combination of high temporal resolutions and high spatial time (Fedorov and Leonov 2004). X-ray angiography is used in different medical imaging technique; the patterns of noiseless images are

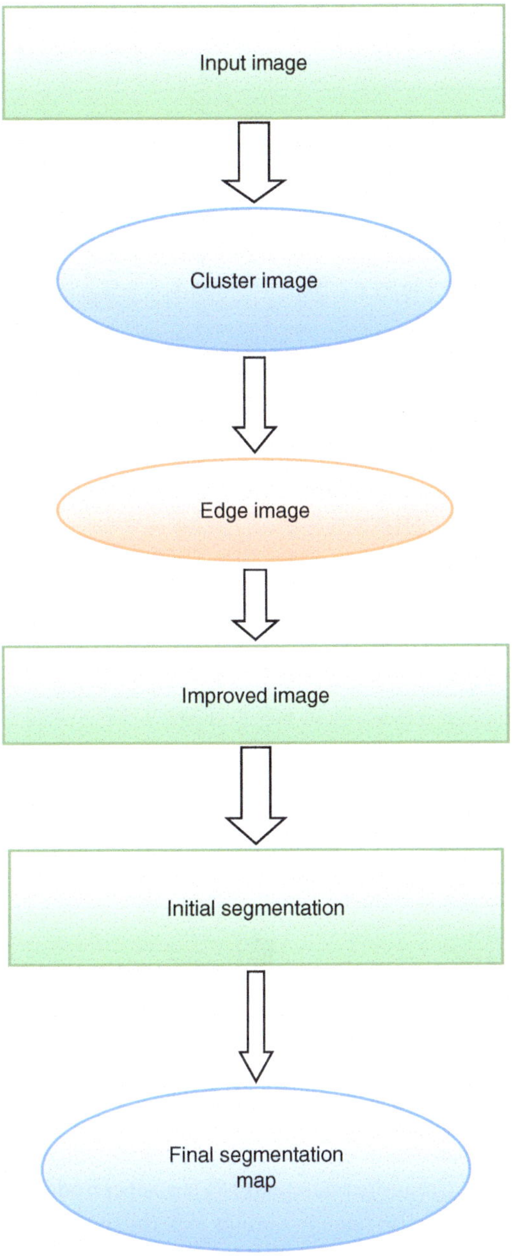

Fig. 3.20 Flow diagram of image processing by using *k*-means clustering method

obtained from fuzzification of *K*-means clustering and above-cited methods are used to visualize the blood-filled areas of the body, and it should be noted that these areas include various arteries or veins, where all are located throughout the body and also the chambers of the heart. The angiography is derived from the Greek words "to record" and "vessel." In most cases, the individual procedures needed to yield a modern angiogram for other purposes within developing a first model (Gladitz and Pilz 1982). Clearly heart catheterization in fuzzification model of machine learning would not be complex, during cardiac catheterization procedure doctor's inserted a tube directly into the arteries pervasive the heart and a substance is directly put into the blood which contrasts with the tissue of the heart (Schapire et al. 2012). Blood flow in the vessels encompassing the heart can then be easily seen. During the catheterization process, the catheter is injected into the body at a distant site and usually the wire and the femoral artery are threaded up the arterial system to the heart where the dye is present. This catheterization procedure is still used today and makes getting an angiography much safer as no sharp object needs to be introduced near the heart nor does it need to remain inside any vessels. Applying segmentation on the threshold pixels to be evaluated in the process of calculation of the percentage of that vessel blockage. Using *K*-means clustering method for the separation of vessel regions from the non-vessel regions for the calculation of the percentage of that vessel blockage.

3.16 Image Segmentation

Image segmentation is one of the first steps in image analysis and pattern recognition in the field of image processing, and it is important and is a necessary part of image analysis system, which is one of the most difficult tasks in image processing that determines the quality of the final result of analysis (Johnson 1977). It should be noted that image segmentation method is the process which divides an image into different regions where each region is homogeneous. For more understanding, we have categorized image segmentation methods as follows. A method of histogram thresholding and in this kind of segmentation we assumes that the images are compounded of regions with different gray ranges, and detaches it into a number of peaks, each corresponding to one region. The second type is edge-based approach where these kinds of seg-

Table 3.5 Evaluation of stenosis for Left Anterior Descending Artery in six samples

Sample	Doctor opinion method	Manual method	Threshold method	*K*-means method
1	55	51	31	50
2	70	58	67	59
3	55	56	70	56
4	75	73	76	78
5	61	53	55	67
6	70	68	33	60
Mean ± SE	36.93 ± 8.56	63.12 ± 3.33	56.99 ± 2.38	18.81 ± 0.12

mentation normally use edge detection operators such as sobel, prewitt, and laplacian and resulting regions may not be connected so edges need to be joined. The third one is region-based approach which is based on likeness of regional image data and some of the most common and widely used approaches in this category include thresholding, region growing, clustering, merging, and splitting. The fourth one is hybrid in which we consider both edges and regions on image (Table 3.5).

3.17 Distance Measures

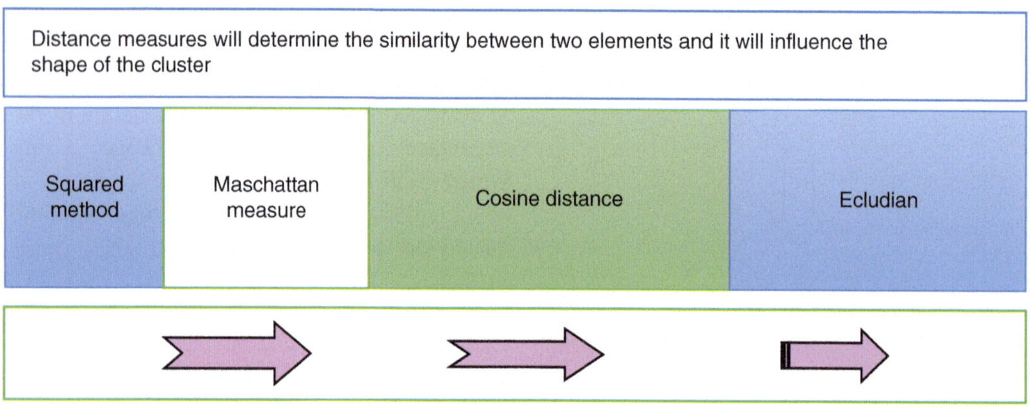

3.17.1 Squared Method

The Euclidian squared distance metric uses the same equation as the Euclidian distance metric but does not take the square root derived from Eq. (3.12).

$$d = \sum_{i=1}^{n} (q_i - p_i)^2 \tag{3.12}$$

The measurements were estimated and are often recorded at a relevant distance under different sets of experimental condition. Further, we can compile the data sets, whether the response on different factors differ significantly driven by the collected data sets (Karpievitch et al. 2009). For example, a clinical researcher wishes to know the efficacy of a new drug or an advertising campaign may be determined by comparing the measurements before the treatment (*Rx*) when compared to after intervention. In other situation, the two or more treatments (*Rx*) have been administered to the same or similar experimental units, and the response rate would be compared to know or assess the efficacy of the treatment (*Rx*). One rational approach has to compare the two treatments in the presence or absence of a single treatment, if the researcher has been assigned the treatment (*Rx*) to the same or identical units; the paired response on different sample data is analyzed by using the following equation:

$dj = (qi1 - pi2)$ $i = 1,2,\ldots n$; dj represents independent observations from an $N\sim(\mu, \sigma^2)$

$$t_{\alpha=0.05} = \frac{\bar{d} - \mu}{sd / \sqrt{n}} \quad (3.13)$$

$$S_d^{\,2} = \frac{1}{n-1}\left(d_i - \bar{d}\right)^2 \quad (3.14)$$

$S_d^{\,2} = \frac{1}{n-1}\left(d_i - \bar{d}\right)^2$ has a t distribution with $(n - 1)$ *df* consequently an "α" level test of H_0 : eve (zero means differences for distance); $H_0 : \mu \neq 0$

We may conduct by comparing $|t|$ with $t_{n-1}\alpha/2$ the upper 100(α/2)th percentile of a t-distribution with $(n - 1)$ *df*. A $100(1 - \alpha)\%$ confidence interval for the mean distance difference $\Delta = E(qi1 - pi2)$ is provided by the statement of normality assumptions.

$$\bar{d} - \frac{t_{n-1}\alpha}{2\frac{Sd}{\sqrt{n}}} \leq \Delta \leq \bar{d} + t_{n-1}\alpha / 2\frac{Sd}{\sqrt{n}} \quad (3.15)$$

A natural generalization of the squared distance has derived in the multivariate analog from the Eq. (3.16)

$$T^2 = \left(\bar{d} - \mu_0\right)'\left(\frac{1}{n}S\right)^{-1}\left(\bar{d} - \mu_0\right)$$

$$T^2 = N\left(\bar{\bar{d}} - \mu_0\right)'(S)^{-1}\left(\bar{d} - \mu_0\right) \quad (3.16)$$

Analytically, we consider $X_1, X_2, X_3, \ldots, Xn$ be the random sampled observation normally distributed $N_p(d, \sum))$ population. Then, $\bar{x}$ and "s" were determined by using standard mean and SD formula

$$\alpha = P\left[T^2 > \frac{(n-1)p}{(n-p)}F_{p,n-p}(\alpha)\right] \quad (3.17)$$

3.17.2 Manhattan Distance

It is the simplest equation determined from the sum of horizontal and vertical components triggered by the real data sets or the distance between two points was measured along the axes at right angle. The measured distance was calculated by using Eq. (3.18).

$$d = \sum_{i=1}^{n}\left|q_x - p_x\right| + \left|q_y - p_y\right| \quad (3.18)$$

3.17.3 Cosine Distance

The cosine distance always measures the distance between two similar vectors of data points. The formula for cosine distance is as follows:

$$d = \frac{\sum_{i=0}^{n=1}\left(q_i - p_x\right)}{\sum_{i=0}^{n=1}\left(q_i\right)^2 * \sum_{i=0}^{n=1}\left(p_i\right)^2} \quad (3.19)$$

$$\alpha = P\left[N\left(\bar{\bar{d}} - \delta\right)'(S)^{-1}\left(\bar{\bar{d}} - \delta\right) > \frac{(n-1)p}{(n-p)}F_{p,n-p}(\alpha)\right] \quad (3.20)$$

$$T^2 = (\text{Multivariate random variable})'\left(\frac{\text{Wishert random matrix}}{df}\right)^{-1}$$

$$(\text{Multivariate normal random vector})$$

$$= N_p(\mu, \Sigma))'\left[\frac{1}{n-1}\Sigma_{p,p-1}(\Sigma)\right]' N_p\sqrt{n}\left(\bar{x} - \delta\right) \quad (3.21)$$

This above equation is analogous to the following formula:

$$t_{n-1}^{\;2} = (\text{normal random variable})\left(\frac{\text{scaled random vari}}{df}\right)^{-1}(\text{normal}\,rv)$$

3.18 Convergence of *K*-Means

Reality, the convergence of *K*-means will provide the sufficient information to the researcher; the convergence is a very important parameter to minimize the cost and retrieval time for determining *k*-means cluster, the method of *k*-cluster means fascinating with awful methods inculcate the ambience of monotonic move of the random variables (Dragalin et al. 2006). However, the random variable has monotonically increased with cost and time at defined *k*-means, each gain of *K*-means cluster showed trivial changes for producing the estimated values when compared to other methods, we considered the selected variables with full-blown Gaussianity and our novelty of interest; the *K*-means consistently can generate the estimated values without any overlapping. In this advent, we minimize the distance of "*k*"-means cluster in the following eqn:

$$C\min = \sum_{i=1}^{n}(d_i - a)^2 \text{ drew up with minimum cost} \tag{3.22}$$

$$= \sum_{i=1}^{n} -(d_i - 0) = 0$$

$\sum_{i=1}^{n} d_i = \sum_{i=1}^{n} a$ right hand side we substituted the m_k (number of members in each cluster *k*)

$$mka = \sum_{i=1}^{n} d_i$$

$$a = \frac{1}{mk} \times \sum_{i=1}^{n} d_i \tag{3.23}$$

Obtained observations are sample based, we minimize the errors of closest clusters by the following eqn.:

$$a = \frac{1}{mk-1} \times \sum_{i=1}^{n} d_i \text{typically converges quickly} \tag{3.24}$$

Differentiating Eq. (3.24), we get the near closest points of each cluster point

$$\frac{\partial a}{\partial d} = \frac{1}{mk-1} \sum_{i=1}^{n} d_i^2 \, \partial a \tag{3.25}$$

The Eq. (3.25) has been minimized with respect to *a*; we will get full-blown information for the determination of convergence of the *K*-means (Figs. 3.21 and 3.22).

$$\frac{\partial a}{\partial d} = \frac{1}{mk-1} \sum_{i=1}^{n} d_i^2 \, \partial a_n \tag{3.26}$$

$$a_n = \frac{(n+1)!}{(n+2)!} a_n = \left[1 + \frac{1}{n}\right]^n$$

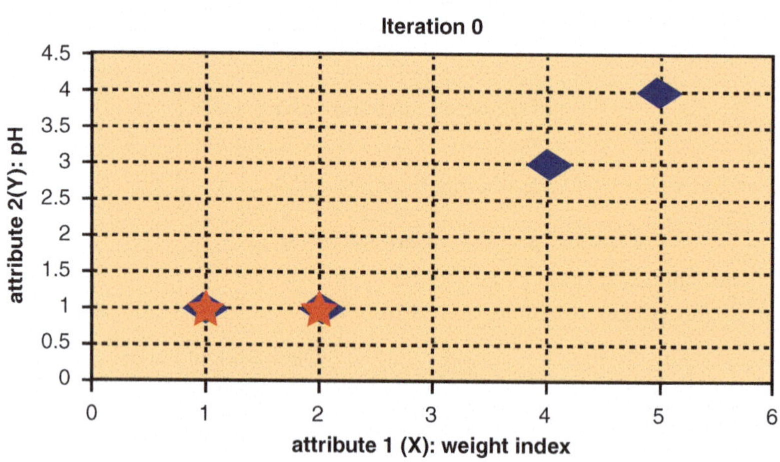

Fig. 3.21 Convergence of *K*-means attributes 1 with weight index "*a*" in pulmonary tuberculosis cases

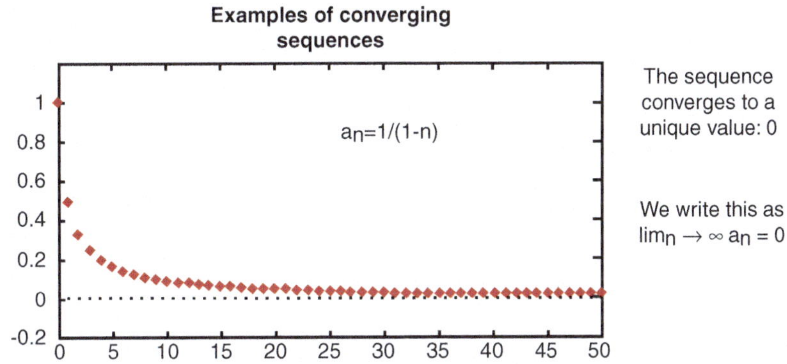

Fig. 3.22 Converging sequences with multiple data points

$$a_n = \frac{\sin(n)}{n}, \lim_{n\to\infty} a_n = L$$

3.19 Conclusion

The increasing availability of electronic health records offers a new resource to clinical, medical, and public health research. The researcher needs to focus on novel advanced statistical methods for compilation of electronic health records for many medical intervention, e.g., early diagnosis of disease, evidence-based medicine, robotic surgery, and formulation of newer clinical trials that have desirable biomedical tools that fulfill the statistical properties and feasibility of research at greatest accuracy and robustness. The conceptual framework of newer medical research will need to focus on the development of algorithms and predicative models from machine learning (ML) to test the research of hypothetical statement with real algorithms for something of voluminous health records (genetic algorithms for early identification of rare gene). In this broad perspective of analytical research gap, this chapter briefly describes various advanced techniques of machine learning to extrapolate research findings for effective testing of our objectives and how we can apply these methods in real life of medical research. An overall summary of this chapter concludes that the random forest methods will be able to classify the data sets in simple ways and provide valid results from the massive data sets and also apply small categorical data sets with varied setup.

References

Borst RA (1989) Artificial Neural Networks: The Next Modeling/Calibration Technology forthe Assessment Community?, Property Tax Journal (International Association of Assessing Officers) 10(1):69–94.

Breiman L (2001) Random forests. Mach Learn 45:5–32

Budescu DV (1993) Dominance analysis: a new approach to the problem of relative importance of predictors in multiple regression. Psychol Bull 114:542–551

Chevan A, Sutherland M (1991) Hierarchical partitioning. Am Stat 45:90–96

Demidenko E, Kiefer J, Wolfowitz J (2004) Mixed models, Wiley. Consistency of the MLE in the presence of infinitely many incidental parameters. AMS 27:887–906

Dilts P (2013) Modelling phonetic reduction in a corpus of spoken English using Random Forests and Mixed-Effects Regression. University of Alberta; Canada. Unpublished doctoral dissertation

Dragalin V, Fedorov V (2006) Design of multi-centre trials with binary response. Stat Med 25:2701–2719

Farmer RM, Medearis AL, Hirata GI, Platt LD (1992) The use of a neural network for the ultrasonographic estimation offetal weight in the macrosomic fetus, Am J Obstet Gynecol 166:1467–72

Fedorov V, Leonov S (2004) Parameter estimation for models with unknown parameters in variance. Commun Stat 33(11):2627–2657

Fedorov V, Hackl P, Mueller W (1993) Estimation and experimental design for second kind regression models. Inform Biometr Epidemiol Med Biol 24:134–151

Fedorov V, Gagnon R, Leonov S (2002) Design of experiments with unknown parameters in variance. Appl Stoch Model Bus Ind 18:207–218

Francis DJ, Fletcher JM, Catts HW, Tomblin JB (2005) Dimensions affecting the assessment of reading comprehension. In: Paris SG, Stahl SA (eds) Children's reading comprehension and assessment. Erlbaum, Mahwah, pp 369–394

Friedman JH (2001) Greedy function approximation: a gradient boosting machine. Ann Stat 29:1189–1232

Friedman JH et al. (2002) Addidive logestic regression; A statistical view of boosting. Annals of Statistocs 28:337–407

Friedman J, Hastie T, Tibshirani R (2000) Special invited paper. Additive logistic regression: a statistical view of boosting. Ann Stat 28:337–374

Gladitz J, Pilz J (1982) Construction of optimal designs in random coefficient regression models. Statistics 13:371–385

Hajjem A, Bellavance F, Larocque D (2014) Mixed effects random forest for clustered data. J Stat Comput Simul 84:1313–1328

Harrell FE, Lee KL, Mark DB (1996) Multivariable prognostic models: issues in developing models, evaluating assumptions and adequacy, and measuring and reducing errors. Stat Med 15:361–387

Harville D (1996) ML approaches to variance component estimation and related problems. J Am Stat Assoc 72:320–340

James G, Witten D, Hastie T, Tibshirani R (2014) An introduction to statistical learning: with applications in R. Springer Publishing Company, Incorporated

Jennrich R, Schluchter M (1986) Unbalanced repeated measures models with structured covariance matrices. Biometrics 42:805–820

Johnson L (1977) Stochastic parameter regression: an annotated bibliography. Int Stat Rev 45:257–272; (1980) 48, 95–102

Kakihara, Shinmyozu K, Kato K, Wada H et al. (2008) Conversion of plasma memerane topology during epithelial tube connection requires Arf-like 3small GTP Pase in drosophila. Mech Dev 125(3):325–3336

Karpievitch YV, Hill EG, Leclerc AP, Dabney AR, Almeida JS (2009) An introspective comparison of random forest-based classifiers for the analysis of cluster-correlated data by way of RF++. PLoS One 4(9):e7087

Kazunaga M et al (2016) The Random Forests statistical technique: an examination of its value for the study of reading. Sci Stud Read 20(1):20–33

Lindstrom M, Bates D (1988) N-R and EM algorithms for linear mixed-effects models…. J Am Stat Assoc 83:1014–1022

Lindstrom MJ, Bates DM (1990) Nonlinear mixed effects models for repeated measures data. Biometrics 46:673–687

Mallet A (1986) A MLE method for random coefficient regression models. Biometrika 73:645–656

Mentre F, Mallet A, Baccar D (1997) Optimal design in random-effects regression models. Biometrika 84:429–442

Michael L (1992) Astion and Peter Wilding, Application of Neural Networks to theInterpretation of Laboratory Data in Cancer Diagnosis, Clinical Chemistry 38(1)

Pilz J (1991) Bayesian estimation and experimental design in linear regression models. Wiley, New York

Rao CR (1965) The theory of least squares when parameters are stochastic. Biometrika 52:447–458

Scarborough HS (1998) Predicting the future achievement of second graders with reading disabilities: contributions of phonemic awareness, verbal memory, rapid naming, and IQ. Ann Dyslexia 48(1):115–136

Schapire RE, Freund Y (2012) Boosting: foundations and algorithms. MIT Press, Cambridge

Shannon et al. (1949) communication theory of secrecy system. The bell system technical journal 28(4): 656–715

Spjotvoll E (1977) Random coefficients regression models. A review. Statistics 8:69–93

Strobl C, Malley J, Tutz G (2009) An introduction to recursive partitioning: rationale, application, and characteristics of classification and regression trees, bagging, and random forests. Psychol Methods 14:323–348

Applications of Machine Learning in Medical Research

4

4.1 Introduction

Machine learning is a newer tool intricate with many methodological intervention; it is delighted to demonstrate various binary or layered algorithms to learn salient function of input data sets, i.e., the maps are input variables to the target and output accurate identification of geographical area (results) which has been generated from the training data series, e.g., we consider $Y = f(X)$, where "Y" is the input variable and function $f(x)$ is the output, the specific model of machine learning is written in statistical form, the learning is significantly associated with parametric predictive models, there is no matter how much data you throw the building of parametric model to test the hypothesis, it will not change its mind about how many parameters will be needed. Many remarkable merits have been enlisted from the machine learning (ML), viz. (1) feature selection is very less important, (2) requires fewer assumptions that can be driven superior performance, (3) it may require more training data sets, (4) risk of overfitting; it is often more difficult to explain the medical series data sets. Andrew et al. describes the machine learning (ML); it is a computer programming formulated by some pneumonic codes (programs that people write), in machine learning (ML) too many algorithms (programs) or principles are very yet to be simple in physical science and more complex in biological, medical, and agricultural sciences to draw the effective interpretation of multiple data sets or variables (e.g., evidence-based medicine for an increase of survival age who suffering from HIV, cancer, and Parkinson diseases in geriatric population). At a glance, the final decision about the population, the researcher clearly understood the hypothesis and complexity (structure) of the entire data sets. Much way we can automatically learn that structure (Bagirov et al. 2003; Demidenko 2004). From the above equation $Y = f(x)$ where "x" discrimination/Prediction (Regression):$f(x)$ continuous classification: $f(x)$ discrete Estimation: $f(x) = P(Y = c|x)$ for some class c.

4.2 Historical Background of Machine Learning

The first case of neural networks was developed way back in 1943 by the neurophysiologist Warren Mc Culloch and Mathematician Walter Pitts; they have published research paper on neurons and how it will work with massive data sets (Donchin et al. 2000). Further, the researcher decided to formulate a statistical models on the electrical circuits and therefore the neural network has been herald in the new era. In the way back 1950s, Alan Turing created the world famous Turing test, this test was fairly simple and it was computed by various physical traits and

B. D. M., B. Narasimha Murthy, *Design of Experiments and Advanced Statistical Techniques in Clinical Research*, https://doi.org/10.1007/978-981-15-8210-3_4

convince a human brain. In the year 1952, he demonstrated the first computer program which learns as it ran, designated as a game which played checkers, created by Arthur Samuel. Frank Rosenblatt designed the first artificial neural networks (ANNs) in 1958 called preceptors; the main goal of this network is to know the various patterns and shapes recognition at sampled level (Demir and Yener 2005). Another intervention at an early instance of a artificial neural network (ANN) is modeled in the year 1959. Bernard Widow and Marcian Hoff created two models at Stanford University, the first was called Adeline and it would detect binary patterns of the various system, an example in a stream of bits; it has predicted what the next one would be. The next generation was called Madeline and it could eliminate echo on phone lines, so this is useful for the real-world practical application of machine learning (ML) problem solving. In the year 1982, John Hopfield suggested that, the machine learning (ML) used for creating a network, which had bidirectional lines, similar intervention he demonstrated that, how neurons actually work in physical and medical science research at long term. Further, in the year 1982 Japan had announced ANN model and it was focusing on one more advanced neural networks, which incentivized American funding into the area and thus created more research in the area of physical and interdisciplinary sciences. Since the neural networks used back propagation method for validation of time series data, this tool is a very important footstep to inculcate the ecosystem of modeling research (came in the year 1986); another researcher intervention was done by Widrow and Hoff 1962 Stanford researcher decided to derived artificial neural network (ANN) algorithms. The ANN tool is allowble methods to derive multiple layers for producing trainers estimated values, the ANN construction is very easy with highest accuracy and reprodusability characters. Twenty-first century, many business and medical research line have realized that machine learning. They arbitrary assume that the ANN and machine learning (ML) will increase calculation potential. This is why they are researching more heavily in it, in order to stay ahead of the practical insight of machine learning at global level. In the mid-twentieth century, a large number of research groups have focused on the machine learning and its practical approach, for example, a Google Brain (2012) demonstrated a deep neural network invented by Jeff Dean of Google, which is focused on the various patterns for detection of textual and nontextual data sets (images and videos). It is possible to use Google's resources, which made it incomparable to much smaller neural networks operation (ANNs). Later, it is used to detect objects in Youtube online videos. Further, the AlexNet (2012) won the image net competition by a large margin in 2012, which led to the use of GPUs and Convolution neural networks in machine learning. They have also created ReLU, which is an activation function that greatly improves efficiency of CNNs. One more research intervention was demonstrated by Deep Face (2014). Deep space neural network (DNN) model is already created to access face book, which they claimed and can recognize people with the same precision as a human can; DeepMind (2014). Various company has bought by Google and can play basic video games to the same levels as humans. In 2016, it managed to beat a professional at the game-Go, which is considered to be one of the world's most difficult board games, Open artificial intelligence (2015). This is a nonprofit organization created by Elon Musk and others to create safe artificial intelligence (AIs) that can benefit humanity.

4.3 Machine Learning Model

Machine learning does an algorithm to learn a process or function that maps input variables to target the output from training data sets; mathematically, we defined $Y_i = I_f(X_i)$, where "$(X_i = x_1, x_2, x_n)$" group of independent vitiates and $(Y_i = y_1, y_2, y_n)$ is the group of dependent variants and "f" is nothing but function, the machine learning model abstains from different learning process to develop various algorithms of physical and biological traits; in the state of definition of machine learning (ML), it is the science of architecture that can facilitate the statistical, biological, and physical decision about the objects or biological indictors. The matter was concern how much would biological data sets throw for modeling of objects or data sets; it will not change its mind about how many parameters it needs to be inculcated (Dragalin and Fedorov 2006). The machine learning (ML) requires a fewer number of salient assumptions and can result in the superior performance of driven algorithms which was generated from the parametric, patrimonial, and complex mathematical models, it may require more training data sets in association with various less risk coverage (overfitting and cost-effective) (Fig. 4.1). The rationality of machine learning (ML) has been described as follows (Table 4.1):

1. The field has matured both in terms of identity and in terms of methods and tools.
2. There is an abundance of data available.
3. Ensure the abundance of computation to run methods or models.

Table 4.1 Glossary of machine learning and statistics

Machine learning (ML)	Statistics
Network and graphs approach	Model approach
Learning (Supervised and unsupervised)	Fitted or formulated some statistical models to describe random variables
Generalization of data sets	Test set performance
Supervised and unsupervised	Regression/classification
Data-driven models empirically optimized agnostic approach and exploratory data analysis insight	Empirically optimized by model fitting and unknown parameters were obtained based on the scale parameters
Came into existence and flourished in 1990s as computer power evolved Assumes nothing about the data necessary to handle big or voluminous data	Been around the centuries, understand how the data collected, statistical properties and population distribution was learnt Must determine appropriate parameters to provide predictive power

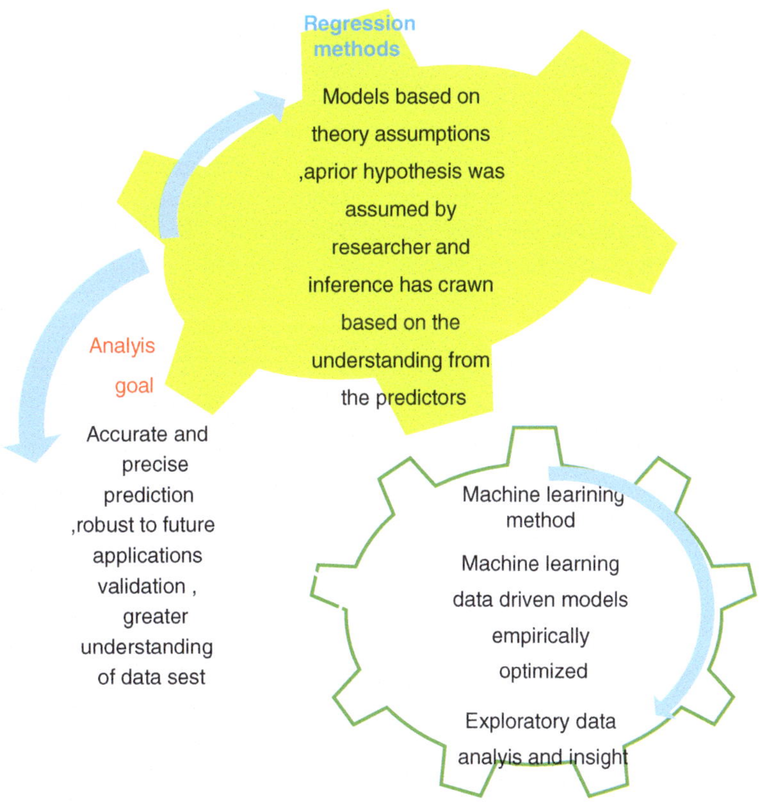

Fig. 4.1 Machine learning (ML) practical insight

4. Ensure machine learning produce impressive results.
5. Ensure the resources ingredients + tools + desire = population acceptance.

4.4 Models of Machine Learning

The linear model has been considered as main stem of statistics for the past 30 years and remains one of our most important tools. Given a vector of inputs $X^{T} = (X_1, X_2, \ldots\ldots X_p)$, we predicted the output of "*Y*" from the following eqn:

$$\hat{Y}_j = \alpha_i \widehat{+\beta_0} + \sum_{i=1}^{n} X_j \widehat{\beta_j} + u \qquad (4.1)$$

Equation (4.1) describes the term $\hat{\beta}_j$ which is the intercept, also known as the bias in machine learning and often it is convenient to include the constants in machine learning (ML)

$$\hat{Y}_j = X^{T} \widehat{\beta_j}' \qquad (4.2)$$

4.5 Measurement Error (*u*)

Reality, various analytical reasons were demonstrated to our question why "*Y*" and is measured incorrectly. Example we are measuring the crop yield in agricultural experiment, the error was precluded from the sloppy harvesting or inaccurate weights, assigned for the estimation of machine learning (ML) or it may be due to weighing of grains etc. example the study envisage to accomplish the consumption of alcohol individuals to tailored for assessment of family income at various levels, the measurement error was extracted from the person individuated parameter that was collected from tested questionnaires (Beumier and Acheroy 2001) (Fig. 4.2).

4.6 Stochastic Error (*u*)

The error occurred may have aroused due to inherent irreproducibility of biological and social phenomena (Bowyer et al. 2006; Bacciu et al. 2014). Even if there is measurement errors are continuously repeated in experimental area example experiment using exactly the same amount of fertilizer it would results to produce different yields; these differences is unpredictable and which is controlled by stochastic methods (differences). The stochastic method will be reduced by the tighter experimental control, for example, by holding constant soil conditions, amount of water and fertilizer, etc. But complete control is not possible, for example, the seeds cannot be duplicated. Stochastic error is greatly influenced on "*Y*" attributes with many omitted random variables of our interest, each with indi-

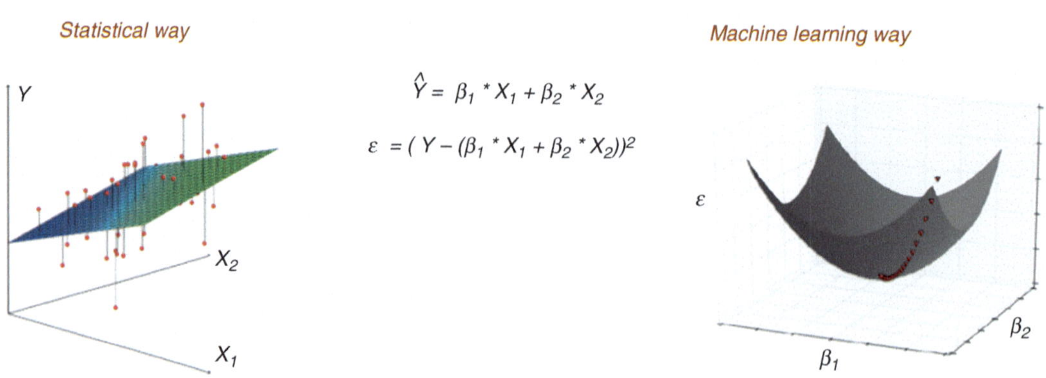

Fig. 4.2 Practical insight of machine learning (ML) way and statistics way for model fitting by using Gauss–Markov method; the nature of error has been aroused from the measurements taken from the data points and stochastic condition of random variables (rv). The error term includes the sum of two components, namely measurement and stochastic error, respectively

vidually yield short of small effects. Since the researcher cannot neutralize the extraneous influences by holding their constant factors, as per the practical findings, the best alternative measures would be taken to minimize the errors (explicitly) associated with fitting of regression model Y on X.

From Eqs. (4.1) and (4.2) we shall show to derive the random estimators $\hat{\alpha}_i$and $\hat{\beta}_j$

$$E\left(\widehat{\alpha_i}\right) = \alpha \tag{4.3}$$

$$\mathrm{Var}\left(\widehat{\alpha_\mathrm{i}}\right) = \frac{\alpha^2}{n} \tag{4.4}$$

$$E\left(\widehat{\beta_j}\right) = \beta \tag{4.5}$$

$$\mathrm{Var}\left(\widehat{\beta_j}\right) = \frac{\sigma^2}{\Sigma x_i^{\ 2}}, \tag{4.6}$$

where α^2 is the variance of the error ϵ_{ij} (the variance of Y). Because of its greater importance, we shall concentrate on the slope estimator $\hat{\beta}_j$ rather than $\hat{\alpha}_i$.

The Eq. (4.1) may be written as

$$\widehat{\beta_j} = \Sigma\left(\frac{x_i}{k}\right)k, \tag{4.7}$$

where $k = \sum x_i^2$

Thus,

$$\widehat{\beta_j} = \Sigma w_i Y_i = w_1 Y_1 + w_2 Y_2 + \ldots w_n Y_n, \tag{4.8}$$

where $w_1, w_2, w_3 \ldots. w_n$ the weights are assigned for simulation of machine learning supervised training (mean square errors), where $w_n = \frac{x_i}{k_i}$ since each x_i is a fixed constants, so for each $w_n$we establish the important and own conclusion about the population or objective of our interest.

4.7 Gauss–Markov Theorem (GMT)

The ordinary least square analysis or estimation (OLS) is the best linear unbiased estimation (BLUE), under the following salient assumptions we can prove the Gauss–Markov theorem (GMT) by using the above Eq. (4.8). Importantly, we consider analytical intervention to prove the Gauss–Markov theorem at population level (Bacciu et al. 2014).

1. Linear in parameters—All parameters were linearly related to $Y = \alpha + \beta 1X1 + u$.
2. Random sampling of "n" observations (X_i, Y_i); $i = 1, 2, ..n$.
3. Sampling variations would be self-explanatory of X_i and not all the same estimated values $X_i \neq (X_i = x_1, x_2. . x_n)$.
4. The zero conditional mean—The error "u" is an expected value of zero $E\left(\frac{u}{x}\right) = 0$.
5. Homoscedasticity—The errors have showed the same variance for given values of the explanatory variables $\mathrm{Var}\left(\frac{u}{x}\right) = \sigma^2$.

Note: Homoscedasticity, similar or identical distribution, normally distributed $X_{ij}{\sim}N(\mu, \sigma^2)$, are independent and uncorrelated.

From the Eq. (4.8) we estimated that $\hat{\beta}_j = C_{kxn}Y => \hat{\beta}_j$ is also linear estimators of "Y".

Let $C = (X'X)^{-1}X' + D_{kxn}$ and $\rho(D) = k$.

Then, estimated

$$\widehat{\beta_j} = \left[\left(X'X\right)^{-1} X' + D\right]\left[X\beta + u\right]$$

$$= \beta + \left[X^1 X^{-1} X' u\right] + DX\beta + Du\right]$$

$$E\left(\widehat{\beta_j}\right) = \beta + DX\beta = \left[l_k + DX\right]\beta. \tag{4.9}$$

GMT theorem is very important for estimation of likelihoods of unknown parameters because it follows in estimating the even form of weak set of assumptions and hence it will not require assumptions of shape parameters of the distribution precludes the error term. In the vague of interpretation of likelihood 'GMT' theorem is more favorable and gives consistent estimated values from machine learning, we consider $\hat{\beta}_j$, the least squares estimator of β, Eq. (4.9) we obtained from the linear estimator techniques because they are very easy to compile and understanding the concept of estimators (Banos et al. 2014; Baldi et al. 2015). We restrict ourselves even further, as shown in Fig. 4.2. within this set of linear estimators we consider only the limited class of weights assigned for prediction, and parameter is unbiased. The

Gauss–Markov theorem has an interesting corollary for estimation of unknown parameters considering massive data. As a special case of regression model, we can ask what happens if we explain Y, but $\hat{\beta}_j = 0$ so that no independent variable "x" will come into play.

Note: All equations are derived for the estimation of likelihood by using machine learning; the embedded equation will emphasize that the GMT is very much restricted applying only to estimator that is both linear and unbiased. It follows that there may be biased or nonlinear estimator that is better (smaller variance) than the least squares estimator (LSE).

Estimation of Confidence intervals and testing of hypothesis about 'β'. By using variance and mean, we have determined the Z-values; the condition of normality of estimator 'β' is now in order. Standardize 'β' we will obtained "Z"

$$Z = \frac{\hat{\beta} - \beta}{\sqrt{\sigma^2 / \Sigma X_i^2}}, \tag{4.10}$$

where "Z" is normally distributed $Z \sim N(0, 1)$, i.e., "Z" is normally distributed with mean and variance. Since the variance of "Y" is generally unknown, it was estimated from the following Eq. (4.11):

$$S^2 = \frac{1}{n}\sum_{i=1}^{n}\left(Y_i - \hat{Y}_i\right)^2, \tag{4.11}$$

where $\hat{Y}_i$ is the fitted value of "Y" on the estimated regression line that is

$$\hat{Y} = \hat{\alpha} + \beta X_i. \tag{4.12}$$

We have tested the hypothesis on sampled observations from t-test

$$t_{\alpha=0.05} = \frac{\widehat{\beta} - \beta}{\sqrt{S^2 / \Sigma X_i^2}} \sim (n-2)df. \tag{4.13}$$

Let $t_{\alpha=0.05}$ denotes the "t" value that leaves half of the distribution in the upper tail that is

$$\Pr\left(-t_{\alpha=.025} < t \text{ value} < t_{\alpha=.025}\right). \tag{4.14}$$

Substituting the above equation, we obtained the following eqn:

$$\Pr\left(-t_{\alpha=.025} < \frac{\widehat{\beta} - \beta}{\sqrt{S^2 / \Sigma X_i^2}} < t_{\alpha=.025}\right) = .95. \tag{4.15}$$

The inequalities within the bracket may be expressed as

$$\Pr(\beta - t_{\alpha=.025}\frac{S}{\sqrt{\Sigma Xi^2}} < \beta < \left(\beta + t_{\alpha=.025}\frac{S}{\sqrt{\Sigma Xi^2}}\right) = .95$$

which yields, the 95% confidence intervals for slope 'β'

$$\beta = \beta \pm t_{\alpha=.025}\frac{S}{\Sigma X_i^2} \sim (n-2)df \tag{4.16}$$

4.8 Maximum Likelihood Estimation (MLEs) of Gauss–Markov Theorem (GMT)

The Gauss–Markova theorem (GMT) derived by overall justification of least square analysis, and the selected parameters shall not require any salient assumptions of Gaussianity (estimation of normality of the error) (Aeberhard et al. 1992; Ahmed et al. 2015). In this section, the normality assumptions are required only for small sample estimation, and this is due to some quite general principles that were adopted for estimation of likelihoods; that small sample estimation will require limited observations and it should be normally distributed with parental population to validate the t-distribution status. We have made the strong assumptions for testing "t". In this paradigm, we derived the maximum likelihood estimation (MLE) of the various parameters of intercepts and slope of the curve (coefficients) on the distinct variables. The MLE techniques have been involved with various possible speculated population for the estimation of error rate. Question is how likelihood estimation to be accept in each of the sample give rise to the estimation of sampling errors and also the observed values are geometrically progressed, the cited problem, we will be able to resolve the research gap by using GMT theorem for testing the null hypothesis at sampled level (by moving the regression line and its surrounding distribution through all possible positions in each space of random variable). As per the moving regression line from intercept to another state of the random variable, the results were fascinatingly simulated by the likelihood function on each point of the variable of our interest. Let us consider $L(Y_1, Y_2 \ldots Y_n)$ is the likelihood or probability density function of sampled observations, which can be expressed as a function of the all possible population values of α, β, and σ^2. First, we consider the probability density (PD) of the first value of "Y" which was derived from the following eqn:

$$L\left(Y_1,Y_2\ldots Y_n\right)=\frac{1}{\sqrt{2\pi\sigma^2}}\text{expo}^{-\left(\frac{1}{2\sigma^2}\right)\left[Y_i-\alpha+\beta Xi\right]^2} \tag{4.17}$$

$$L\left(Y_1,Y_2\ldots Y_n\right)=\prod_{i=1}^{n}\left[\frac{1}{\sqrt{2\pi\sigma^2}}\ \text{expo}^{-\left(\frac{1}{2\sigma^2}\right)\left[Y_i-\alpha+\beta Xi\right]^2}\right]. \tag{4.18}$$

Recall that the observed Ys are given. We speculated on the various values of α, β, and σ^2 to emphasize the above Eqs. (4.17) and (4.18)

$$L\left(\alpha,\beta,\sigma^2\right)=\frac{1}{\left(2\pi\sigma^2\right)^{n/2}}\text{expo}^{-\left(\frac{1}{2\sigma^2}\right)\left[Y_i-\alpha+\beta Xi\right]^2}. \tag{4.19}$$

The values of α, β will become "L", largest values, α and β appears as the exponent of the Eq. (4.19); moreover, we maximizing the function with negative exponent involving for minimizing the largest magnitude of the exponent, we designating the Eq. (4.19) for estimation of MLEs, our estimation $\hat{\alpha}$ and $\hat{\beta}$ the problem is to select values for the minimizing the function of family of errors

$$minimize\sum\left\{Y_i-\hat{\alpha}-\hat{\beta}X_i\right\}^2. \tag{4.20}$$

Equation (4.19) differentiate w.r.t. x we will get accurate value.

4.9 Gauss-Markov-Weighted Least Squares Analysis

In any type of research pedagogy, the greater error occurs due to sampling and nonsampling methods; thus, observations will give a very less precise indications (precision is very less) for the estimation of true errors. Therefore, it is very reasonable for researchers to pay less attention; in this practical insight, the weighted least squares (WLS) analysis provides an efficient and meaningful information to the researchers for solving the real problem of machine learning program and also this method influence on propagating more precise values in machine learning process. Specifically, instead of minimizing the family of error in the above fitted model Eq. (4.20)

$$\sum_{i=1}^{n}\frac{1}{\sigma^2_{\ i}}\left\{Y_i-\hat{\alpha}-\hat{\beta}X_i\right\}^2. \tag{4.21}$$

This criterion will be justified for the estimation of MLEs assuming $\epsilon_{ij}{\sim}N(\mu,\sigma^2)$ for any hypothesis α and β, the likelihood function of our set of sampled observations $(Y_1, Y_2, Y_3\ldots\ldots Y_N)$ is

$$L(Y_1,Y_2\ldots Y_n)=\frac{1}{(2\pi)^{n/2}\prod_{i=1}^{n}\sigma^2}\text{expo}^{-\left(\frac{1}{2\sigma^2}\right)[Y_i-\alpha+\beta Xi]^2}+ui. \quad (4.22)$$

Likelihood function is maximized when negative exponent is minimized.

Suppose the researcher estimating the standard deviation of the distribution σ_i increases proportionally with X_i specifically

$$\sigma_i = k\,X_i \quad (4.23)$$

Or $\frac{\sigma_i}{X_i}=k$

From Eq. (4.21) the weighted least square analysis (WLAS) illustrated to minimized by the following Eq. (4.24)

$$\sum_{i=1}^{n}\frac{1}{k^2{}_i x^2{}_i}\left(Y_i-\hat{\alpha}-\hat{\beta}X_i\right)^2. \quad (4.24)$$

The data reduction term generated from the fitted Eq. (4.25) we modified the equation from $\frac{e_i}{X_i}$ and from its SD constant k, thus the equation becomes

$$\frac{Y_i}{X_i}=\alpha\frac{1}{X_i}+\beta_0+\beta_1+\ldots\beta_n+\frac{e_i}{X_i} \quad (4.25)$$

$$\sum_{i=1}^{n}\left(\frac{Y_i}{X_i}-\hat{\alpha}\frac{1}{X}-\hat{\beta}\right)^2=\sum_{i=1}^{n}\left(\frac{Y_i-\hat{\alpha}-\hat{\beta}X_i}{X_i}\right)^2 \quad (4.26)$$

$$\sum_{i=1}^{n}\frac{1}{X_i^2}\left(Y_i-\hat{\alpha}-\hat{\beta}X_i\right)^2 \quad (4.27)$$

Finally, the Eq. (4.27) will become WLA Sand modeled in the form of Eq. (4.24).

$$\sum_{i=1}^{n}\frac{1}{k^2{}_i x^2{}_i}\left(Y_i-\hat{\alpha}-\hat{\beta}X_i\right)^2. \quad (4.28)$$

The ordinary linear equation (OLS) will tend to be solved in multivariate form with "n" sampled observations of X and Y, we assumed to be generate from the following steps:

$$Y_{11}=\alpha_1+\beta_{11}X_{11}+\beta_{12}X_{12}\ldots\ldots+u_{11}$$
$$Y_{21}=\alpha_2+\beta_{21}X_{21}+\beta_{22}X_{22}\ldots\ldots+u_{21}$$
$$Y_{31}=\alpha_3+\beta_{31}X_{31}+\beta_{32}X_{32}\ldots\ldots+u_{31}$$
$$\cdots\cdots\cdots$$
$$\cdots\cdots\cdots$$
$$\cdots\cdots\cdots$$
$$Y_{n1}=\alpha_n+\beta_{n1}X_{n1}+\beta_{n2}X_{n2}\ldots\ldots+u_{n1}$$

$$\begin{bmatrix}Y_{11}\\Y_{12}\\Y_{13}\\\vdots\\Y_{n11}\end{bmatrix}=\begin{bmatrix}\alpha_{11}\\\alpha_{12}\\\alpha_{13}\\\vdots\\\alpha_{n11}\end{bmatrix}+\begin{bmatrix}\beta_{11}&\beta_{12}&\beta_{13}\\\beta_{21}&\beta_{22}&\beta_{23}\\\beta_{31}&\beta_{32}&\beta_{33}\end{bmatrix}\times\begin{bmatrix}X_{11}&X_{12}&X_{13}\\X_{21}&X_{22}&X_{23}\\X_{31}&X_{32}&X_{33}\end{bmatrix}+\begin{bmatrix}u_{11}\\u_{12}\\u_{13}\\\vdots\\u_{n11}\end{bmatrix}\ (4.28) \quad (4.29)$$

Response = Intercepts + Coefficient + Random variables +errors

From Eq. (4.28) we modeled the matrix from the following equation:

$$Y=\alpha'\beta(X)+ui. \quad (4.30)$$

$\beta=\beta'$ Without loss of generality if we take the partial derivatives with respect to each variable of interest $\beta_{21}=\beta_{12}'$

$$\frac{\partial}{\partial\beta}=\beta'\alpha\beta=2\alpha\beta \quad (4.31)$$

$$\beta'=(X'X)^{-1}X'Y$$

β' is a multivariate normal with the following equation:

$$E(\hat{\beta})=\beta\text{ and }\operatorname{cov}(\hat{\beta})=\sigma^2(X'X)^{-1}=\sigma^2V \quad (4.32)$$

Similarly, the above equation extended to test the different distribution with n $(n-k)$ df,

$$\chi^2=\left(c\hat{\beta}-c\beta\right)'\left(\sigma^2cvc'\right)^{-1}\left(c\hat{\beta}-c\beta\right) \quad (4.33)$$

$$\chi^2\sim(c-1)(r-1)df$$

$$\text{Fisher } F' = \frac{1}{r}\left(c\hat{\beta} - c\beta\right)'\left(\sigma^2 cvc\right)'\left(c\hat{\beta} - c\beta\right) \quad (4.34)$$

$F \sim (r, n - k)df$, where 'k' is the number of regression coeffcients and 'r' is the number being simultaneously tested.

From Eq. (4.30) we assumed that ui's are independent errors associated with mean zero and variance σ^2.

$$E(ui) = 0. \quad (4.35)$$

And the covariance matrix of ui's are independent errors so that $ui \sim N(0, \sigma^2)$

$$\mathrm{cov}(ui) = e(uu') = \sigma^2 I. \quad (4.36)$$

From eqn. (4.36) ui is normally distributed. The maximum likelihood function (MLEs) of the above parameters is as follows:

$$L(\beta, \sigma^2) = \frac{1}{(2\pi\sigma^2)^{n/2}} \text{expo} - \frac{1}{2\sigma^2}(y - x\beta)'(y - x\beta). \quad (4.37)$$

We can minimize the expression of the eqn. with respect to coefficient

$$\begin{aligned}&(y - x\beta)'(y - x\beta)\\&= yy' - 2y'x\beta + \beta'x'x\beta\\&= 0 - 2y'x\beta + \beta'x'x\beta\end{aligned}$$

Setting this equation equal to zero yields the maximum likelihood MLE's least squares estimator (LSE)

$$\hat{\beta} = (X'X)^{-1} X'Y \quad (4.38)$$

$$\hat{\beta} = \left(X^{-1}X'X^{-1}\right)^{-1}(X'Y) = X^{-1'}Y \quad (4.39)$$

MLEs of σ^2 derived from the following eqn:

$$\hat{\sigma}^2 = \frac{1}{n}(y - \hat{y})'(y - \hat{y})$$

$$\hat{s}^2 = \frac{1}{n-k}(y - \hat{y})'(y - \hat{y}) \quad (4.40)$$

4.10 Neural Network Modeling in HIV/AIDS

Artificial neural networks (ANNs) are prime forecasting methods that are modeled on simple mathematical models of the brain neurons. Neural network models were allow to know the complex nonlinear relationships between the response variable and its predictors. The ANN network will be thought of individual layers of neurons, which is organized in the manner of multiple nodes (circuit). The predictors (or inputs) are always presented in the bottom layer and the forecasted variables (or outputs) are presented in the top layer of the network. There may be intermediate layers containing hidden neurons. Simplest networks contain no hidden layers and are equivalent to linear regression model (Weiss and Provost 2003; Wang et al. 2010). Figure 4.3 showed the chief neural network architecture for linear regression method with four predictors. The coefficients attached with predictors are called weights (W). Model forecasted figures were obtained by a linear combination of the input data sets. Overwhelmingly, the assigned weights would be selected based on the acquition of input data sets from the network frame by using a learning algorithm that minimizes a cost function such as mean squared trainer data error (MSTE). In this cited simple example, we can use linear regression model for the estimation of likelihood values of predictors (Fig. 4.3)

Statistical modeling of neural network is a linear preceptor of $\sum_{i=1}^{n} X_i W_i = W.X$. The output or binary signal has been transferred to the brain where action and no action takes place. Neurons will provide "n" number of signals to the brain; the brain will act as an agent for action and no action, and the action coded as 1 and "np" action coded as 0 supplemented with success and failure of binary events. The outputs were modeled by weighted Bernoulli that is extended in the form of $\sum_{i=1}^{n} X_i W_i p_i (1 - p_i) = Wpq.X$, density function of binomial distribution modeled $P(x = X) = nc_x w\text{-}p^x q^{n-x}$, where $x = 0, 1, 2, .. n$ (Fig. 4.4).

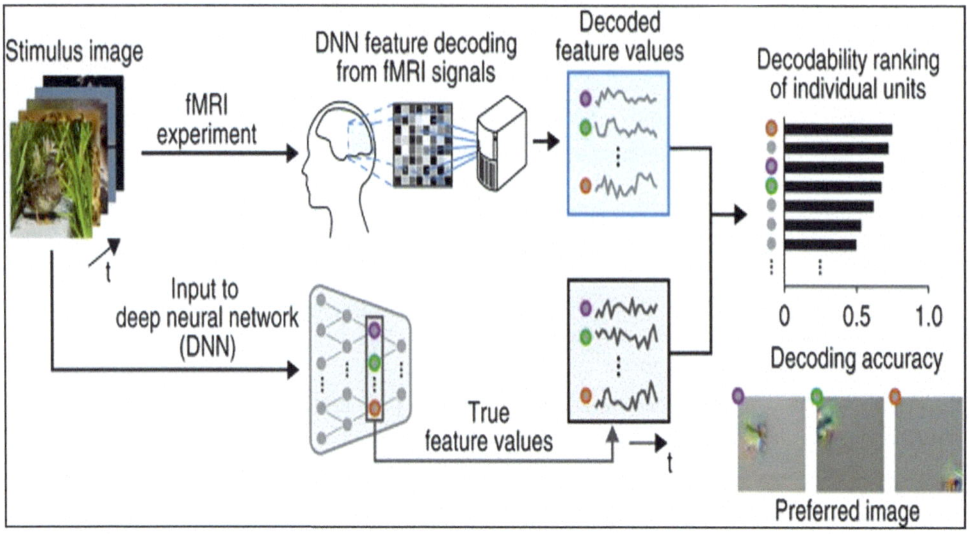

Fig. 4.3 Shows human brain works on the network modeling on inputs

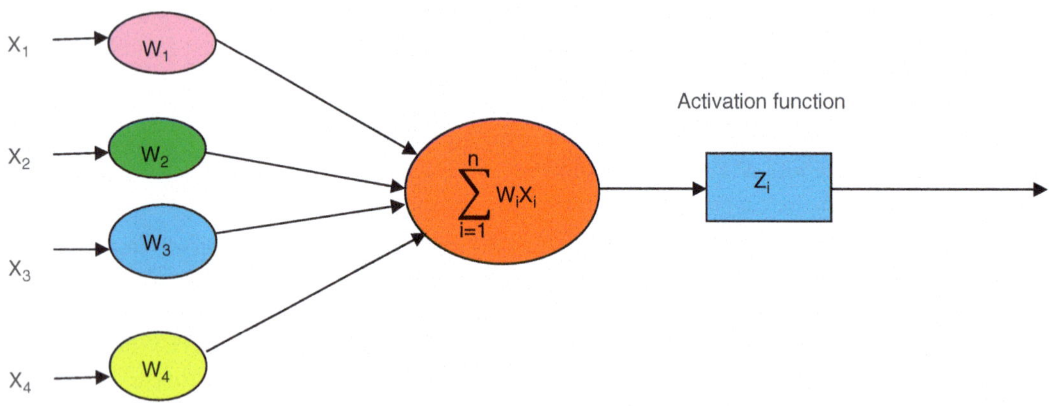

Fig. 4.4 Shows neural network linear model

Once we adding an intermediate layer with hidden neurons or layers, the artificial neural network (ANN) model will become a nonlinear. A simple example was shown in (Fig. 4.4); the chief architecture of the figure describes multilevel layers with hidden prospective (feed forward), in the above cited network model an each layer of parental nodes will receive input data from the previous layers (Spjotvoll 1977; Savran et al. 2008; Schapire and Freund 2012). The outputs of nodes in one layer are inputs to the next layer and vice versa. The inputs of each node are combined with weighted linear combinations of selected inputs. The fitted model results to derive the modified nonlinear function in the form of statistical approach before our output function or layers generated. For example, the inputs were converted into hidden neuron JJ, which were represented in Fig. 4.5; we generalized the linear regression model, i.e., combined with each layers

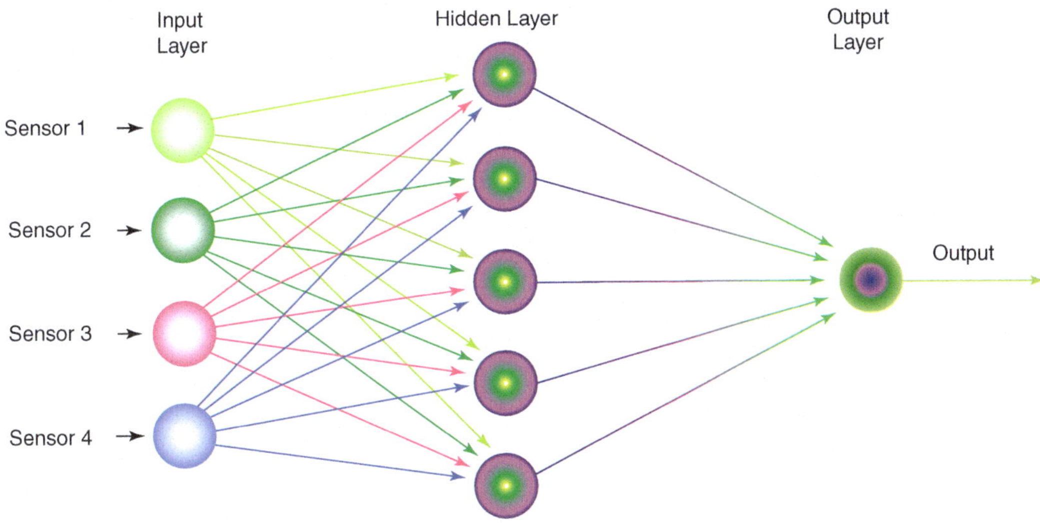

Fig. 4.5 Schematic diagram of neural network modeling

of inputs to provide the equation $Z_j = B_j + \sum X_i = W_i P_i Q_i$. In case of hidden layers, the modified form of network will produce non-linear combination of different layers formed a sigmoid equation $S(z) = L + e^{-z}$, where $L + e^{-z}$ gives input for the next layer. This equation seems to reduce the effect of extreme input values on real combination of various outputs; thus, we have smoothened the entire network from the statistical derivations (somewhat robust to the outliers). The parameters b_1, b_2, b_3, and $w_1 w_2$, w_k, are obtained from the Bayesian analytical approach (Bayesian analysis). The values of the assigned weights are often restricted for obtaining estimated values of output layers. On the other hand, the parameters were restricted; all assigned weights were shows "decay parameter," and it is often to set the values is equal to 0.1. The weights will be able to take any random values and begin to construct the network design. Consequently, the model will elaborately explain the elements of randomness from the parental and child nodes, respectively (produced by a neural network). Fitted ANN network is usually trained on the several times for producing outputs by considering different random starting points, the resulted starting points are averaged or summed for cleared and effective interpretation of the results or findings.

4.11 Application of Neural Network in Medical Science

The neural network model is a very good area to deal with most of the medical problems. It has been triggered with demonstration of many algorithms for classification, prediction, image processing, etc. The main objective of this research is to know the salient application of neural network techniques to classify the estimation of mortality and survivability. An artificial neural network (ANN) models can not only provide solution about the analytical research but also can improve the methodological aspects of highly active antiretroviral treatment (HAART). Practically, we have fitted ANN models considering a total of 110 people living with HIV/AID (PLHIVs) who had received treatment from 2004 to 2014. Ten years cohort data was extracted from CMIS data base, and we have fitted different neural network models from Thompson iteration method and back propagation. A separate neural network algorithm was obtained from the model (radial basis function); the fitted model has more accurately predicted mortality and efficacy of the HAART treatment. It will evaluate estimated values with greater accuracy and less mean squared standard error (MSE). Two models were fitted to know the accuracy of the estimation of HAART, viz. hierarchical and nonhierarchical. As per the hierarchical neural network, the actual predicted mortality rate at the end of the 5-year cohort was 26.30% with relative standard error (RE) 0.994. The specificity and sensitivity of the model were 93.26% and 84.28%, respectively, and also the accuracy of the model was tested by using ROC analysis and Akanke information. The net PPV (positive predictive value) and (negative predictive value) NPV were 90.26% and 9.74%. In case of nonhierarchical models, trainer set values had more epochs rather than hierarchical model, an actual predicted mortality rate was (18.63%). The specificity and true negative rate of the nonhierarchical model at this level were very less superior because the results were generated inaccurately and inconsistently (akaike information <10; AUC was 0.52), whereas the pattern of frequencies differs in both the model. The comparison of two-neural network models for the estimation of survival analysis was done; the estimation rate was 0.76. Summing of the model results concludes that the hierarchical neural network models for the estimation of survival analysis will provide efficient patterns of values with more epochs when compared to nonhierarchical model, also it will maintain greater accuracy and more reliable for predicting mortality rates consistently without any ambiguity. The HIV/AIDS is a chronic noncurable disease (scourge). Currently, 2.10 million people are HIV positive. However, new medications not only can slow down the progression of the infection rate, but also can suppress the virus, thereby restoring the body's immune function and permitting many HIV-infected individuals to lead a normal life in the society. Many research at national and global level are conducted and are ongoing to predict a better treatment for HIV patients, such as HIV drug prediction, various biomarkers for HIV diagnosis, drug resistance testing, and predicting biomarkers to know the side effects on certain regimens. In this herald, the prediction of accurate mortality and morbidity is a greatest challenge to disseminate the HIV research. Since all the patients are unique in their medical history, side effects, and allergic in particular drugs, the physician abstains from treating all patients in different ways, and it is very difficult to determine the efficacy of HAART regimen or treatment at a single point. In this pedagogy, the statistical tool is very important for the benefit of social cause and decision-making problems. In other aspects, the clinical decision is very common; if a patient with a set of certain symptoms consults the physician, the patient may get different opinions regarding the type of the underlying disease. Since the physician's judgment plays an important role in this regard for taking care of well-being of HIV-infected population. The modeling techniques or building of model research will greatly help us to narrate the novelty and computational intelligence at larger extent (widely). In the present scenario, the ANNs have been widely used in the medical diagnosis to solve the complex problems by developing decision support system with the application of neural network various algorithms (Rao 1965). The neural network is very prospective and receptive area in medical science to practice and prove medical problems with reliable solutions at population level. A proper utilization of a neural network technique to impart and implement large-scale health services research at global level, and it can facilitate full-blown information to the researcher for assimilating decision supports for physicians and policy makers at national and global level (Palmer and Faloutsos 2003).

4.12 Model Formulation

In the present research work conducted at the center of excellence of HIV care (NACO), Bowring and Lady Curzon Hospitals, Bangalore, a retrospective 5-year cohort data set of 110PLHIVs (patients who are initiated on HAART during 2004–2014) was extracted from the CMIS data base. The demographical profile, medical history, WHO-clinical stage, CD_4 count at inception of ART, and serial CD_4 counts and clinical outcomes of the HIV cases were collected, pretested, and structured questionnaires through direct and indirect interview. The collected CMIS data was modeled to know or predict the appropriate mortality and survivability of 5 year, the regimen specification were recorded systematically which will help the physician for estimation of efficacy of HAART drug. The ANN model was demonstrated by Thompson iteration and back propagation simulation techniques (Pilz 1991; Mentre et al. 1997). Two artificial neural networks, namely hierarchical and nonhierarchical models, were smoothened by the above simulation techniques and algorithms that were obtained from the radial basis function. Usually, an algorithm is used for classification and prediction of mortality rate of PLHIVs, and also we demonstrate massive non-transformed data (nonscalable) sets besides various iteration methods (obtained at multiple points). Two functions (survival and nonsurvival) were considered for model building (Aharonian et al. 2008; Aeberhard et al. 1992). The survivor function is defined as the probability that an individual survives at least up to a certain time. The hazard function represents the probability that an individual will die at a certain time; the parametric methods of survival analysis require some specification of a probability density function that will be required for estimating function (*f*). Nonparametric models do not require this specification and predominantly generate estimated values without any error. Many researchers have recently applied new nonparametric models for survival analysis, such as regression trees, Timpson iteration, and back propagation. Various concepts were used commonly in classical model fitting for survival analysis; these models will also be employed in neural network applications inclusion with actuarial life tables and product-limit estimation theory for estimation of survivor functions. It is the most complex model that would help researchers to summarize survival rate at larger extent. Both types of models will involve certain assumption, i.e., survival of an individual at time "t" and patients retain the mean survival rate at time (t − 1). The survivor function of actuarial life table and product-limit estimation was modeled for the estimation of hazard rate and survival function from the equation $\left[S(t) = \pi\left(\frac{n_j - d_j}{n_j}\right)\right]$, where '$d_j$' is the number of deaths at interval jth period and 'n_j' is the number of individuals at risk. In the actuarial method, 'n_j' is the average number of individuals who bears at risk constrains with higher hazard rate. An actuarial life table and product-limit estimator will differ in so many ways, i.e., time intervals and accuracy. The fitted models are presumably defined at certain equal time intervals and duration of highly active antiretroviral therapy (HAART) (death and survival). The latter part of the model was fitted one interval for each death without any cause of time loss and information which is extracted from the patient case history. Both models were allowed for making censoring and noncensoring data (censored data). After obtaining censored data, Kaplan–Meier survival model is substituted with hierarchical and nonhierarchical simulation models; after model building, different primary nodes have been generated composed with smoothening of data sets; awesome predicted values were generated from the fitted models in the form of trainer sets of various child and parental nodes (Mallet 1986; Lindstrom and Bates 1990). Finally, the Cox proportional hazards model was frequently used to know the importance of covariates for survival function estimation and extraction of akaike information criteria. The Cox model will support the reissuance of multiple regressions, semi-parametric model construction, which can allow for propagating various continuous covariates. The fitted model requires inbuilt assumptions (author decisions) that there is a simplified transformed data without fluctuating output (more information).

4.13 Model Results (Fig. 4.6)

4.14 Baseline Characteristics

Tables 4.2 and 4.3 depicted baseline characteristics; as per the results, the mean age of the patients was 30.76 ± 9.08 years with baseline CD_4 count 119.07 ± 74.11 μ/dL. After inception of highly active antiretroviral therapy (HAART), the serial CD_4 count was drew up (>65%), as per the findings of the research study we have seen that the CD_4 count at the end of the 5-year cohort was drastically increased at the mean rate of 558.86 ± 144.25 μ/dL. A total of 99.0% cases

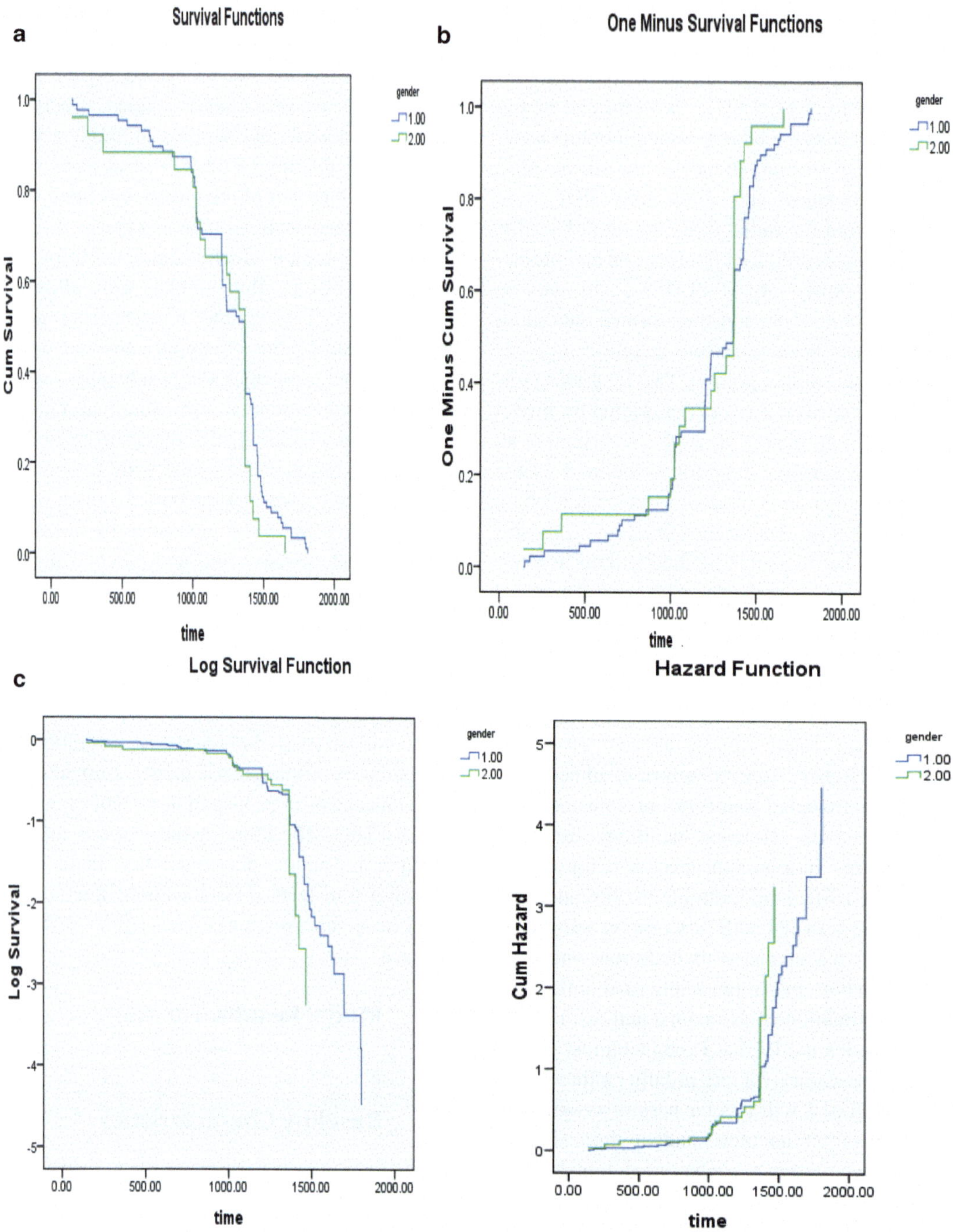

Fig. 4.6 (**a**) Survivability at 5 years. (**b**) Survivability function at 5 years. (**c**) Log survival function and Hazard function. (**d**) Cohort survivability and survival function among PLHA with different age class. (**e**) Log survival function and hazard function with different age class. (**f**) Multilayer neural network output and hidden layer. (**g**) Radial basis function neural network output and hidden layer. (**h**) Genderwise relation with survivability. Training (85.80%), testing (14.20%)

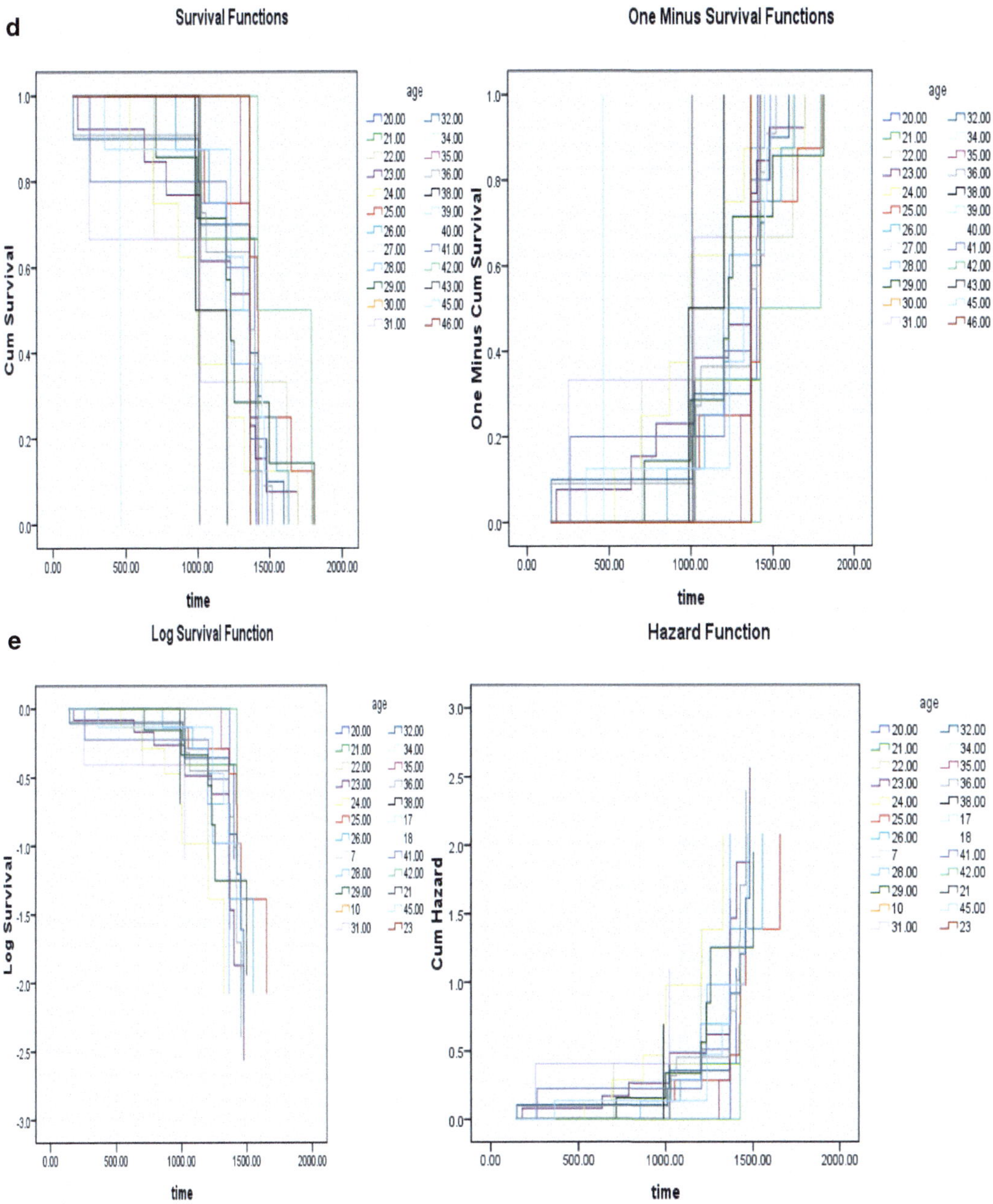

Fig. 4.6 (continued)

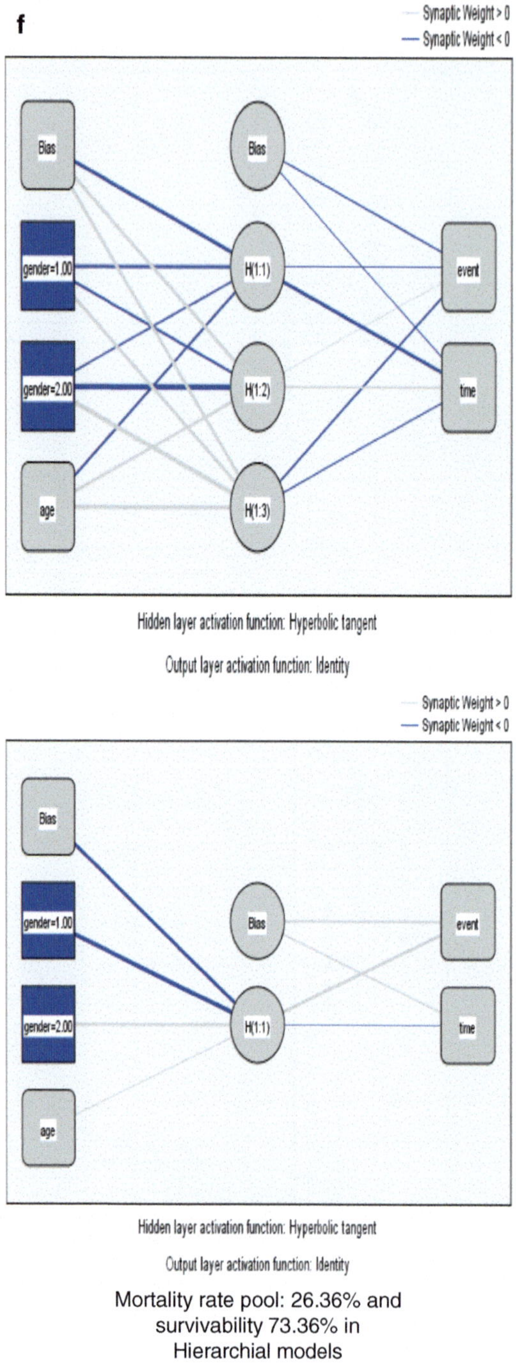

Fig. 4.6 (continued)

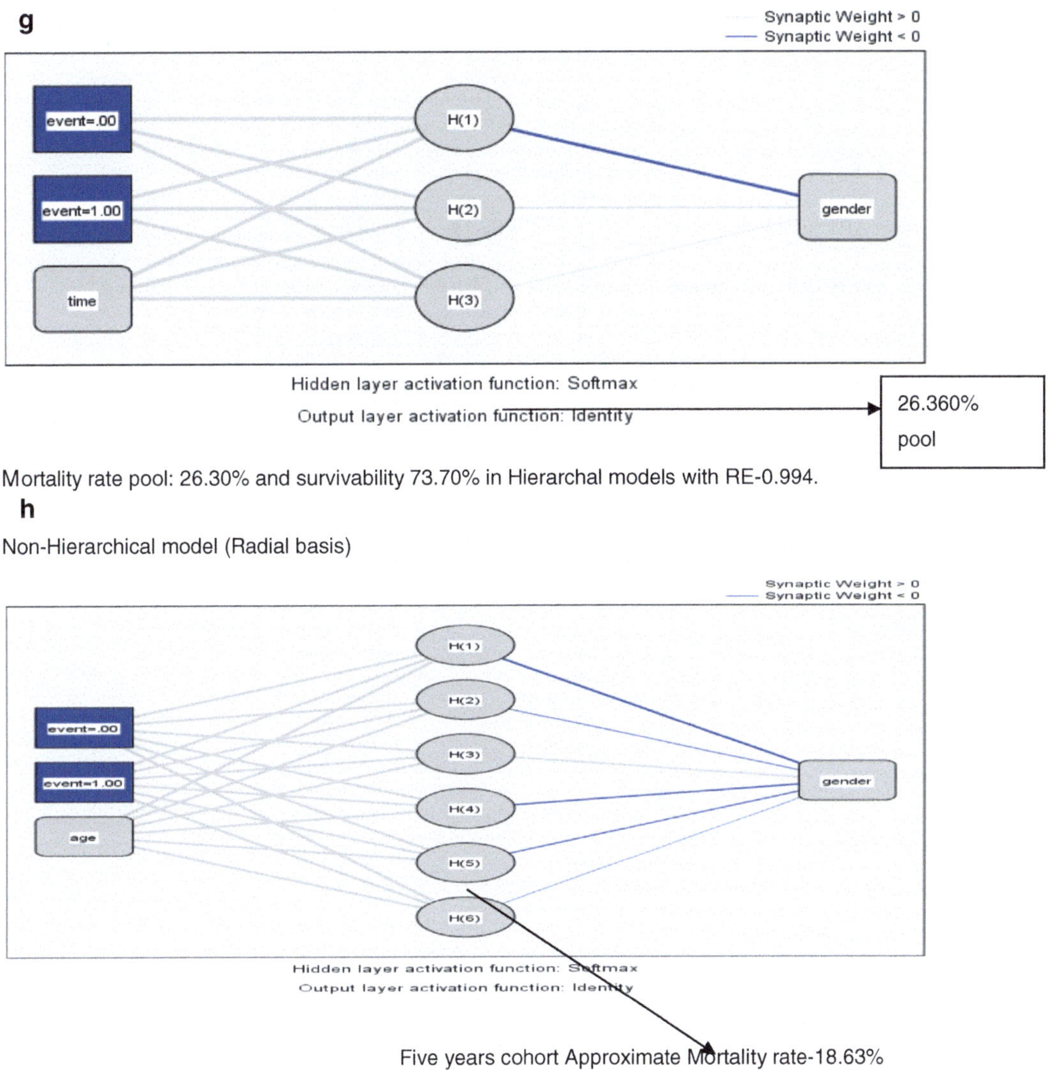

Fig. 4.6 (continued)

were initiated "HAART" treatment, whose clinical stage was (vi). Approximately 26.36% patients were suffering from TB-HIV co-infection initiated with HAART at lower baseline CD_4 counts (81.28 ± 136.99 μ/dL). The comorbidity was recorded and it was expressed as 7.27% of HIV TB co-infection and rest of the population as 1.22%. Survival function was estimated by Kaplan–Meier product-limit model; as per the model, the mean survivability of the 5-year cohort was 13.51 years with SEM 2.16 years and the CI 95% lower boundary of the survival rate of males was 1159.51 days followed by 1299.85 days upper boundary. In case of female PLHIVs, we observed that the efficacy and drug response was significantly associated with duration of the treatment (duration 5.12 with SD 1.25 years) $p < 0.01$. Both genders responded well to the HAART treatment with estimated values of lower boundary survivability recorded (1017.58 days) and upper boundary (2396.25 days). We conclude that younger the age group (20–35 years) without morbidity of PLHIVs will survive longer duration when compared to older age group ($p < 0.001$); this was found to be statistically significant ($p < 0.01$).

Table 4.2 Descriptive statistics of PLHIVs on the 5-year cohort data

Characteristic variables	Adult-Male Mean ± SD	Adult-Female Mean ± SD	Pool Mean ± SD
Age (year)	32.00 ± 9.20 (76)	26.52 ± 8.96 (34)	30.76 ± 9.08 (110)
Initial body weight (Kg)	52.35 ± 11.71 (76)	46.30 ± 13.22 (34)	48.02 ± 12.17 (110)
CD_4 at inception of ART (μ/dL)	120.12 ± 73.14 (76)	118.02 ± 76.28 (34)	119.07 ± 74.11 (110)
CD_4 at 6 months after HAART inception (μ/dL)	311.11 ± 120.62 (74)	336.58 ± 207.69 (28)	319.08 ± 15.07 (102)
CD_4 at 1-year cohort (μ/dL)	383.12 ± 160.31 (70)	379.00 ± 260.50 (26)	381.82 ± 19.37 (96)
CD_4 at 2-year cohort (μ/dL)	407.30 ± 207.38 (69)	452.58 ± 252.40 (24)	421.47 ± 22.46 (93)
CD_4 at 3-year cohort(μ/dL)	471.53 ± 217.58 (65)	507.77 ± 283.51 (21)	483.06 ± 239.85 (86)
CD_4 at 4-year cohort (μ/dL)	523.08 ± 203.36 (63)	481.72 ± 180.99 (20)	510.02 ± 199.03 (83)
CD_4 at 5-year cohort (μ/dL)	636 ± 110.25 (62)	585 ± 178.26 (19)	558.86 ± 144.25 (81)
WHO-Clinical staging			
WHOStage-I	Nil	Nil	Nil
WHOStage-II	Nil	Nil	Nil
WHOStage-III	8(10.52%)	03(8.82%)	11(10.00%)
WHOStage-IV	68(89.47%)	31(91.17%)	99(90.00%)
TB-HIV Co-infection			
Yes	21(27.63)	08(23.52)	29(26.36%)
Comorbidity			
Yes	6(7.89%)	2(5.88%)	8(7.27%)

4.15 Hierarchical Neural Networks for Survival Analysis

The model was fitted to know the relative differences observed in the pattern of CD_4 distribution and behavior of network; it was demonstrated in terms of time and relative effect of HAART treatment. We fitted ANN network models to identify rare events of PLHIVs. As we designed the following experimentation on demonstration of three systems of neural networks (hierarchical, nonhierarchical, and nonhierarchical with random process), new models were performed for the estimation of survival function "*f*". The results relatively express the model outputs. In case of nonhierarchical system, an output node will correspond to the probability that an individual will die during the first-year cohort, second-year cohort, followed by third, fourth, and so on (output codes are mutually exclusive and independent in nature). Training data was obtained at greater accuracy and reliability, resulted model training data has comprises numerical values and relative to an individual observed data sets (obtained from case history) who followed HAART treatment with dependent time and varied CD_4 counts at regular intervals. As there are output categories, we estimated the survival function "*f*" in the form of "alive" death in 1 year, 2 years, etc. All the mortality rate and incumbent biological variables were modeled by using survival function analysis (FA). The model results shows nonhierarchical with random process methods was showed lesser consistent when compared to

Table 4.3 Confidence interval of mean survivability with genderwise and different age class

Sl.	Variables	Lower bound CI-95%	Upper bound CI-95%	SE	*P*-value
I.	Genderwise				
01.	Males	1159.51	1299.85	44.45	$p < 0.05$
02.	Females	1017.58	1309.26	27.70	$p < 0.05$
II.	Agewise				
01.	20 years	1369.138	1416.196	26.128	$p < 0.05$
02.	21 years	1030.318	1551.682	324.966	$p < 0.05$
03.	22 years	651.492	1697.175	408.248	$p < 0.05$
04.	23 years	923.559	1371.210	142.281	$p < 0.05$
05.	24 years	782.552	1292.198	92.631	$p < 0.05$
06.	25 years	1214.613	1582.887	42.426	$p < 0.05$
07.	26 years	1112.925	1460.325	113.137	$p < 0.05$
08.	27 years	1365.000	1365.000	.	$p < 0.05$
09.	28 years	1126.297	1341.953	96.167	$p < 0.05$
10.	29 years	986.837	1503.163	37.970	$p < 0.05$
11.	30 years	1365.000	1365.000	.	$p < 0.05$
12.	31 years	257.417	1393.916	626.253	$p < 0.05$
13.	32 years	962.038	1485.562	183.412	$p < 0.05$
14.	34 years	881.800	1303.200	.	$p < 0.05$
15.	35 years	1314.862	1410.138	31.500	$p < 0.05$
16.	36 years	966.788	1433.576	187.164	$p < 0.05$
17.	38 years	884.320	1307.680	.	$p < 0.05$
18.	39 years	468.000	468.000	.	$p > 0.05$
19.	40 years	1456.000	1456.000	.	$p > 0.05$
20.	41 years	700.039	1574.361	175.271	$p > 0.05$
21.	42 years	1247.400	1972.600	.	$p > 0.05$
22.	43 years	1012.000	1012.000	.	$p > 0.05$
23.	45 years	985.301	1495.199	89.095	$p > 0.05$
24.	46 years	1365.000	1365.000	.	$p > 0.05$
25.	Overall	1151.125	1278.051	29.924	$p > 0.05$

hierarchical model ($R^2 = 0.56$, akaike information lesser than the reference range). Type-I censored data (data from patients followed for a short interval) are not used since the status of the patient during the last intervals is not known. Figure 4.2a–h depicted a nonhierarchical model variation (Lavine 1991; Lindstrom and Bates 1988; Li 2018; Kiefer and Wolfowitz 1956). Utilizing noise training data corresponds to individuals who have been followed at least the same number of days as that of the interval prediction was showed to be inconsistent results. Data from censored individuals are used forz model fitting; obtained data sets were presented to the network model building only up to the point where the data are confirmed. Therefore, the neural networks that are higher in the hierarchy (those predicting the event in the first intervals) will receive more input patterns than the ones that are generated trainer data is consistent. Each of the component network analysis may receive varied numerical values for time-dependent variables for the same individuals (Johnson 1980; Jennrich and Schluchter 1986; James et al. 2014). The present fitted neural network systems can predict accurate values of mortality rate in association with nonlinear relationships between continuous covariates and outcomes of the events. The hierarchical neural network systems are able to use Type-I censored data and can potentially and efficiently deal with time-dependent variables at a single point of time. We learnt from the observed resulted model findings that the present fitted model (hierarchical) is the ability to demonstrate censored data with higher precision and lower standard error (SE) of estimates (ignorable errors) and also it can obtain generalized scientific evidence-based results for estimation of mortality and survival function of PLHIVs. Similar models that were demonstrated by James et al. (2014) compared the various diagnostic markers of HIV at early inception of HAART.

4.16 Nonhierarchical Neural Networks for Survival Analysis

The nonhierarchical model that predicted absolute (or unconditional) survival was even better for detecting deaths in the second and third years than the nonhierarchical model because for these intervals the cumulative percentage of deaths (Fig. 4.1) made this category of patterns more easily identifiable. These preliminary results support our hypothesis that neural network systems are able to recognize infrequent patterns after a number of training cycles that are inversely proportional to the frequency of those patterns. The overall sensitivities and specificities of the hierarchical models, although superior to those of the nonhierarchical models, were small (Javadi and Mirroshandel 2019; Harville 2010; Gladitz and Pilz 1982; Grgic and Delac 2011). The limited use of data and the small number of patients may have caused the poor prognosis prediction in this preliminary experiment. The hierarchical systems of neural networks, by increasing the relative frequency of the outcome being sought, can greatly increase the speed of learning, whereas they do not hinder accuracy performance, when compared to nonhierarchical neural network systems. Figure denotes the neural network algorithm that is used to classify the patients into two groups, active and inactive, based on their regimen specification, and the radial basis neural network is also used to predict the regimen specification. All these three algorithms are used in this work to predict better regimen specification for HIV/AIDS patients.

4.17 Salient Findings of Neural Network Model Fitting

Each network of the hierarchical system was composed of demographic profile, clinical findings, laboratory parameters like CD_4 Count, hemoglobin (HB), LFT, RFT, CBC, etc.. Regimen specification is non-nucleoside reverse transcriptase inhibitors (NNRTI) with boosted protease inhibitor (NRTI + 2NNRTI and NtRTI + PI), duration of the HAART, comorbidities and drug toxicities parameters of input nodes was consider for model settings, nine hidden nodes, and three output nodes, whereas input values for gender, place of living urban or semi-urban, risk behavior, educational level, AIDS-defining diagnoses, and outputs for alive or death at each interval were coded by dummy variables (Fedorov et al. 2002; Fedorov and Leonov 2004). The hierarchical model had six input nodes, five hidden nodes, and four output nodes. Both systems used the back propagation algorithm for estimating the weights. The learning rate for both systems was 0.05, and the entropy error function was used. Output values corresponded to the probability of a given category (e.g., dead in 1 year, alive) and always summed to 1.0. We studied the ability of our networks to learn the death patterns using the training set, the training expressed (85.80%) with corresponded testing (14.20%) and actual predicted mortality rate was (26.30%) Refractive error (−0.994) (Sanchez et al. 2014). Specificity and sensitivity of the model are 93.26% and 84.28%, respectively, and the accuracy of the model was tested using positive predictive value (PPV) and negative predictive value (NPV). The PPV expressed 90.26% with rate of NPV 9.74%. The nonhierarchical models took approximately more epochs. Since the time required per epoch in the hierarchical system is smaller than that of the nonhierarchical system, this difference showed that the nonhierarchical models could learn the same patterns in more than half of the time that required by the hierarchical model (Fedorov et al. 1993; Friedman et al. 2000; Friedman 2001). We believe that this difference is primarily due to the different frequencies, and more clinical variables had involved in the input data for each system. For example, this hierarchical system could correctly identify 11 patients out of 30 who died in 5 years, whereas the nonhierarchical model could recognize only six. The training expressed 71.80% with corresponded testing 28.20% with RE −3.65. Actual predicted mortality rate was 18.63%.The specificity, or true negative rate, of the nonhierarchical model at this level was less superior, specificity (83.21%), sensitivity (76.28%), PPV (64.36%) with actual rate of NPV (25.64%). The pattern of frequencies has differed in both systems

4.18 Conclusion

The neural network model can be considered as a tool for HIV-clinical data analysis and interpretation. Analysis by neural networks improves the classification, accuracy, and data quantification and reduces the number of unwanted analogs. NN-model as a new modeling method can predict actual rate of mortality, survivability of PLHIV who are experiencing HAART lifelong. It can also be helpful for drug design, discovery of structure, bio-active structures, and can predict the chemotherapeutic response from PLHIVS who are on HAART. In conclusion, the comparison of two neural network models for survival analysis is done. For a cohort of 110 PLHIV patients, the hierarchical neural network models for survival analysis could provide efficient patterns faster than a nonhierarchical model. The hierarchical models also provide greater accuracy and more reliability in predicting mortality rates.

References

Aeberhard S et al (1992) Comparison of classifiers in high dimensional settings. Dept. Math. Statist., James Cook Univ., North Queensland, Australia, Tech Rep, p 92

Aharonian F et al (2008) Energy spectrum of cosmic-ray electrons at TeV energies. Phys Rev Lett 101(26):261104

Ahmed MM et al (2015) Protein dynamics associated with failed and rescued learning in the Ts65Dn mouse model of Down syndrome. PLoS One 10(3):96–98

Bacciu D et al (2014) An experimental characterization of reservoir computing in ambient assisted living applications. Neural Comput Appl 24(6):1451–1464

Bagirov AM et al (2003) Unsupervised and supervised data classification via nonsmooth and global optimization. Top 11(1):1–75

Baldi P et al (2015) Enhanced Higgs Boson to τ+ τ− search with deep learning. Phys Rev Lett 114(11):111801

Banos O et al (2014) Dealing with the effects of sensor displacement in wearable activity recognition. Sensors 14(6):9995–10023

Beumier C, Acheroy M (2001) Face verification from 3D and grey level clues. Pattern Recogn Lett 22(12):1321–1329

Bowyer KW, Chang K, Flynn P (2006) A survey of approaches and challenges in 3D and multi-modal 3D+ 2D face recognition. Comput Vis Image Underst 101(1):1–15

Demidenko E (2004) Mixed models. Wiley, New York

Demir C, Yener B (2005) Automated cancer diagnosis based on histopathological images: a systematic survey. Rensselaer Polytechnic Institute, Tech. Rep.

Donchin E, Spencer KM, Wijesinghe R (2000) The mental prosthesis: assessing the speed of a P300-based brain-computer interface. IEEE Trans Rehabil Eng 8(2):174–179

Dragalin V, Fedorov V (2006) Design of multi-centre trials with binary response. Stat Med 25:2701–2719

Fedorov V, Leonov S (2004) Parameter estimation for models with unknown parameters in variance. Commun Stat 33(11):2627–2657

Fedorov V, Hackl P, Mueller W (1993) Estimation and experimental design for second kind regression models, Informatik. Biometr Epidemiol Medizin Biol 24:134–151

Fedorov V, Gagnon R, Leonov S (2002) Design of experiments with unknown parameters in variance. Appl Stoch Model Bus Ind 18:207–218

Friedman JH (2001) Greedy function approximation: a gradient boosting machine. Ann Stat 1189–1232

Friedman J, Hastie T, Tibshirani R (2000) Special invited paper. Additive logistic regression: a statistical view of boosting. Ann Stat 28(2):337–374

Gladitz J, Pilz J (1982) Construction of optimal designs in random coefficient regression models. Statistic 13:371–385

Grgic M, Delac K (2011) GrgicSonja Cface–surveillance cameras face database. Multimed Tools Appl 51(3):863–879

Harville D (2010) ML approaches to variance component estimation and related problems. JASA 72:320–340

James G, Witten D, Hastie T, Tibshirani R (2014) An introduction to statistical learning: with applications in R. Springer Publishing Company, Incorporated

Javadi S, Mirroshandel SA (2019) A novel deep learning method for automatic assessment of human sperm images. Comput Biol Med 109:182–194

Jennrich R, Schluchter M (1986) Unbalanced repeated measures models with structured covariance matrices. Biometrics 42:805–820

Johnson L (1980) Stochastic parameter regression: an annotated bibliography. Int Stat Rev 1977;45:257–272; 48, 95–102

Kiefer J, Wolfowitz J (1956) Consistency of the MLE in the presence of infinitely many incidental parameters. AMS 27:887–906
Lavine M (1991) Problems in extrapolation illustrated with space shuttle O-ring data. J Am Stat Assoc 86(416):919–921
Li MH, Mestre TA, Fox SH, Taati B (2018) Automated assessment of levodopa-induced dyskinesia: evaluating the responsiveness of video-based features. Parkinsonism Relat Disord 53:42–45
Lindstrom M, Bates D (1988) N-R and EM algorithms for linear mixed-effects model. JASA 83:1014–1022
Lindstrom MJ, Bates DM (1990) Nonlinear mixed effects models for repeated measures data. Biometrics 46:673–687
Mallet A (1986) A MLE method for random coefficient regression models. Biometrika 73:645–656
Mentre F, Mallet A, Baccar D (1997) Optimal design in random-effects regression models. Biometrika 84:429–442
Palmer CR, Faloutsos C (2003) Electricity based external similarity of categorical attributes. Advances in knowledge discovery and data mining. Springer, Berlin Heidelberg, pp 486–500
Pilz J (1991) Bayesian estimation and experimental design in linear regression models. Wiley, New York
Rao CR (1965) The theory of least squares when parameters are stochastic. Biometrika 52:447–458
Sanchez MA et al (2014) Fuzzy granular gravitational clustering algorithm for multivariate data. Inf Sci 279:498–511
Savran A et al (2008) Bosphorus database for 3D face analysis. Biometrics and identity management. Springer, Berlin Heidelberg, pp 47–56
Schapire RE, Freund Y (2012) Boosting: foundations and algorithms. MIT Press, Cambridge
Spjotvoll E (1977) Random coefficients regression models. A review. Statistics 8:69–93
Wang Y, Liu J, Tang X (2010) Robust 3D face recognition by local shape difference boosting. IEEE Trans Pattern Anal Mach Intell 32(10):1858–1870
Weiss GM, Provost F (2003) Learning when training data are costly: the effect of class distribution on tree induction. J Artif Intell Res 315–354

5 Statistical Genetics and Its Application in Drug Trail

5.1 Introduction

The discovery of the Hardy–Weinberg law (HWL) is here marked for the research beginning in the field of population genetics (Abney et al. 2000; Abecasis 2000; Almasy and Blangero 1998; Aulchenko et al. 2007; Anderson 1936). In the last few decades, research findings have provided a starting point for extending advanced research intervention for many population geneticists or investigators. In this vein the Hardy–Weinberg principle is the fundamental law for extrapolating various quantitative attributes at panmictic population; eventually the HW law has driven various modern statistical approaches for solving the medical and clinical research (statistical testing, and several of its applications in various modern population genetic research areas). In 1908, the mathematician G H Hardy in England and the physician W- Weinberg in Germany independently developed a quantitative theory for defining the genetic structure of panmictic population. The Hardy–Weinberg law provides basic algorithms for describing the expected frequencies of various genotypes in a population. The similarity of their work, however, remained unnoticed until Stern (1943) drew attention to both papers and recommended that names of both discoverers were attached to the population formula. The Law states that gene frequencies in a population remain constant from generation to generation if no evolutionary processes like migration, mutation, selection, and genetic drift are operating. Thus, if mating are random, and no other factors disturb the reproductive abilities of any genotype, the equilibrium genotypic frequencies are given by the square of the allelic frequencies. Similar research findings were reported in biomedical, human and environmental genetics research often requires characteristics will be examined individuals genotype of each individual locus provides the basic knowledge of its morphological, physiological, and biochemical traits. This view is contrary to the aims of critical research findings, genetic information transferred from one individual to another through "DNA" and saved using genetic code or algorithms not only allow to specify the characteristics of organisms such as eye color of father is positively associated with son eyes, body composition, blood group of offspring as compared with paternal relations, etc. In human genetics heritable characters have determined the inheritance properties or allow the detection of susceptibility to certain genetic disorder or diseases (Boorman 1950; Boerjan and Vuylsteke 2009; Bernardo 1995; Bittner et al. 1999). The salient findings and understanding the genetic structure play a pivotal role in the prevention and therapeutic option of genetic-related diseases. However, estimation of parameter and current level of scientific and mathematical knowledge of genetics allows to

B. D. M., B. Narasimha Murthy, *Design of Experiments and Advanced Statistical Techniques in Clinical Research*, https://doi.org/10.1007/978-981-15-8210-3_5

accurately identifying the causes of many genetic diseases or disorder of hereditary origin. Many genetic have been experienced; there are already developed ways to treat genetic-inherited disease. Genetic screening is also conducted to identify persons, who are carrier of genetic diseases. The present research allows us to determine the risk of inheritance of disease by offspring or to predict how a disease, which develops in old age, will proceed and, thus, take appropriate remedial steps. Moreover, it is interesting to analyze the genetic structure of some species of organisms owing to paradigm on the ongoing ridiculous changes in cosine of time event. We have demonstrated real HIV therapy data, which factors had influence on the genetic composition of populations (*N*); it seems to be necessary to understand the course of evolution of genetic complexity of the selected population. It is worth noted the phenomena of dynamics shaping of various genetic variants or characteristics such as natural selection, mutation, migration, and genetic drift of the population at worldwide.

5.2 Random Mating or Panmixia Population

In any bisexual organisms, animal and plants, every individuals seems to mate at random or nearly so is called random mating population or panmixia. Furthermore, any one individual of one sex is equally likely to mate with any individual of opposite sex. In other words, the frequency of a certain type of mating is controlled by chance factor. That manner, if the mating is completely random in the population of AAXAA would be D^2 among all mating system. Assumed that, the genotypic proportion of both sexes are the same (shown in mating matrix Table 5.1).

Table 5.1 shows gene and genotypic frequencies. As per the resulted findings we noticed that the theoretical frequencies were realized only in very large population level. The term "panmixia" is sometimes used as a synonym of random mating and then the population is called as panmictic.

Table 5.1 Random mating frequencies

♂ ♀	AA	Aa	aa
AA	AA × AA $D \times D = D^2$	AA × Aa $D \times H$	AA × aa $D \times R$
Aa	Aa × AA $H \times D$	Aa × Aa $H \times \mathrm{H} = H^2$	Aa × aa $H \times R$
aa	aa × AA $R \times D$	aa × Aa $R \times H$	Aa × aa $R \times R = R^2$

5.3 Genetic Drift

The macro study was conducted at Department of Poultry Science, Veterinary College, Hebbal, Bangalore, during 2007–2009; the study aims to know the genetic drift of base population. The study has formulated genetic drift model without any other intervening forces, and also we demonstrated massive data sets of various quantitative traits of Punjab broiler PB_1 meat type flocks (nonoverlapping generation) (Churchill and Doerge 2008; Chen and Chen 2005; Castle 1903). The model was fitted to open web mathematical software. Later we would like to see if any genetic changes can affect the incumbent generation quantitative traits performance from genetic drift of the population (other forces). Further, the selection index was pooled into the massive data sets on each generation (Fig. 5.1). The genetic drift is practically determined from the following formula.

Genotypes	A_1A_1	A_1A_2	A_2A_2
Relative fitness	ω_{11}	ω_{12}	ω_{22}
Relative fitness in terms of *h* and *s*	$1 + s$	$1 + hs$	1

In this case we can find the frequency of the A_1 allele (p) after selection by using the following formula (s—effective selection, h: heritability s—selection difference p—varying population with diminishing numbers)

$$p' = \frac{p^2(1+s) + pq(1+hs)}{1 + 2pqhs + p^2 s}$$

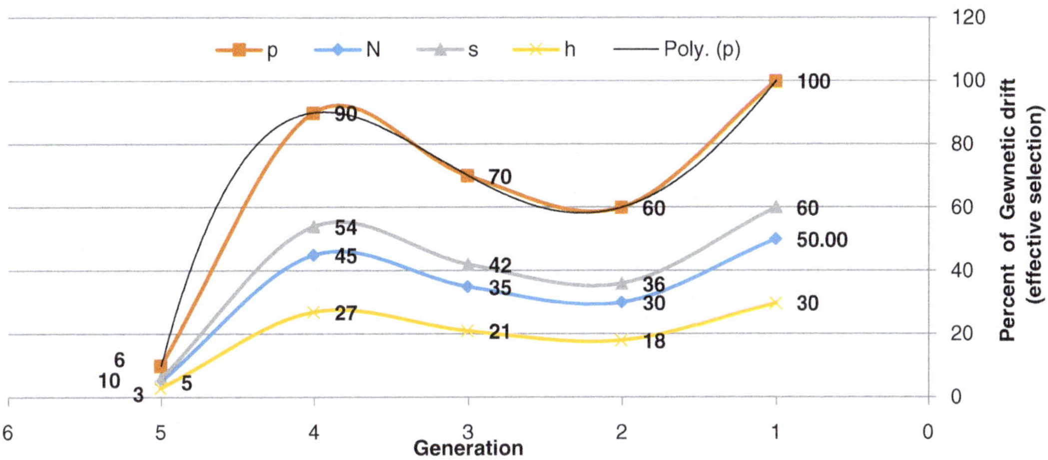

Fig. 5.1 Varying Genetic drift in association with relative fitness (*h*&*s*) in Poultry flocks

	Equation	*R*-square
Model	$y = -2.916x^4 + 22.5x^3 - 37.08x^2 - 42.5x + 160$	1 (100%)
Results	$y = -2.916 * 29 + 22.5 * 56 - 37.08 * 2.89 - 42.5 * 20 + 160$	378.25
Predicted	Δ_s = Traits mean score − Predicted score $\Delta_s = 378.25 - 256.22$ $\Delta_s = 122.03$ (100% accuracy was maintained during the process of flocks selection)	

X_1 = Age (20th week); X_2 = Body weight (2.89 kg); X_3 = Egg weight (56 g); X_4 = egg number at 40th week (29)

5.4 Gene Frequency

A population is a set of organisms that belong to the same species, live simultaneously in a particular environment, influence each other, and mate giving fertile offspring. These individuals have a certain set of alleles, which are forms of occurring genes. It is called the "gene pool." The characteristics of the population are mainly determined by its genetic composition, and thus the genotypes or allelic frequencies.

If the population consists of "*N*" individuals, and there occur "*n*" in different alleles of a particular gene, then the total number of possible genotypes will be

$$G' = \frac{n!}{2(n-2)} + n = \frac{n(n+1)}{2} \qquad (5.1)$$

To simplify the consideration, let us suppose that there is a population in which there are only two different alleles of a gene bearing dominant "A" and recessive "a." In accordance with formula (5.1) it is possible to obtain three genotypes: AA, Aa, and aa. Their cardinality in the population is denoted by N_{AA}, N_{Aa}, and N_{aa}. Then the frequency of each of them will be calculated as a share of a given genotype in *N*-individual population and

$$f_{AA} = \frac{N_{AA}}{N}, f_{Aa} = \frac{N_{Aa}}{N}, f_{aa} = \frac{N_{aa}}{N}. \qquad (5.2)$$

In addition to HW law the equation becomes

$$f_{AA}D + f_{Aa}H + f_{aa}R = 1 \qquad (5.3)$$

It is possible to determine the particular allelic frequencies in the gene pool. Nevertheless, it should be kept in mind that the population of "*N*" individuals are diploid and brings "2*N*" alleles while each homozygote will provide twice more alleles considered type than heterozygote. So, if we denote by "*p*" frequency of allele "A" and by *q* frequency of allele "a," we obtain the following relationships

$$p = \frac{2N_{AA} + N_{Aa}}{2N} = P_{AA} + \frac{1}{2}P_{Aa} \quad (5.4)$$

$$q = \frac{2N_{aa} + N_{Aa}}{2N} = P_{aa} + \frac{1}{2}P_{Aa} \quad (5.5)$$

$$p + q = 1 \quad (5.6)$$

5.5 Hardy–Weinberg Law (HWL)

Definition—In large random mating population, the gene and genotypic frequencies are the same from generation to generation without disturbing force of mutation, migration, and selection. A fundamental law, which is considered as the basis of population genetics, HW theorem was formulated independently by the eminent mathematician, Professor Godfrey Harold Hardy and German doctor Wilhelm Weinberg in 1908. It provides theoretical supports for the description of evolutionary phenomena. This law will be presented for a population of "*N*" individuals, where there are only two different alleles of a gene "A" and "a." Their proportion will be denoted as above (p, q). HW law holds good in the following criteria (Castle 1903; Cotterman 1941; Darvasi et al. 1993; Erhardt 2010; Foster et al. 2007.

1. Population is infinitely very large.
2. Organisms are diploid.
3. Organisms reproduce sexually.
4. In population, the mating is random—individuals do not have preference during mating; each male has equal chances of crossing with each female and vice versa.
5. Generation will not to be overlapping; therefore when the offspring matures into reproduction, the parental generation no longer has the ability to reproduce, and thus there is no intergenerational pairs.
6. Organisms do not migrate—population is isolated, there is no exchange of individuals between populations of the same species, so there is no flow of genes from one population to another.
7. In the population is no mutation—a swap genetic material is not observed, which can cause the transformation of existing alleles into a completely new form; in addition, there is no transformation of allele "A" to "a" and conversely.
8. The selection does not affect the tested locus—none of the combination of alleles has more than any other chances of surviving until give offspring.

So there is no difference in the adaptation between genotypes. Then the frequencies of individual alleles and genotypes in subsequent generations do not change. In addition, proportion of particular genotypes is in the form of $f_{AA} = p^2$, $f_{Aa} = 2pq$, $f_{aa} = q^2$ and they correspond to the distribution of binomial square $x_i \sim b(n, p)$.

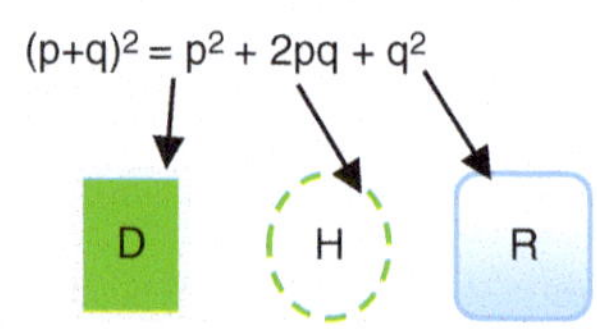

5.6 Binomial Distribution—HW Law

The binomial distribution is a discrete distribution that can describe the probability distribution of the number of successes in a sequence of "*n*" independent trials, each of them occurring with a probability of "*p*."

Definition of BD—If "*k*" is discrete random variable which can assume only non-negative values, the density function of binomial distribution is

$$P(k,n,p) = \binom{n}{k} p^k (1-p)^{k-1}, \text{ where} \binom{n}{k} = \frac{n!}{n-k!k!}$$

Since the "*k*" successes will occur anywhere among the n trials, we have to count all the possibilities. The number of ways to distribute the "*k*" successes in a defined sequences of n trials is given by the binomial coefficient $\binom{n}{k}$;

e.g., we consider a genetic sequence of length "n" (here $n = 10$) in which each nucleotide has a probability "p" success to be mutated (here $p = 0.5$). Then, the quotients are generating 10,000 sequences from the initial one (we called as mutation). A success of trail we called the distribution of occurrence of the number "k" of mutations (successes) may look like this.

5.7 Poisson Distribution

If the number of trial "n" is very large and the probability of success "p" is very small, the binomial distribution can fairly be approximated by a Poisson distribution. The Poisson distribution, sometimes referred to as the law of rare events, was first described by Simeon Denis Poisson (1781–1840).

Definition of BD—If "k" is discrete random variable which can assume only non-negative values, the density function of binomial distribution is

$$p(k,\lambda) = \frac{e^{-\lambda}\lambda^{k}}{k!}(k = 1\,\text{to}\,n)$$

Let us define $\lambda = np$ (with "n" very large and "p" very small), then the probability $p(k;\lambda)$ to observe "k" successes.

Parameter "λ" is the expected number of successes. It corresponds to the mean of the Poisson distribution. The Poisson distribution can be used to describe the probability distribution of the number of events occurring in a fixed period of time if these events occur with a known average rate and independently of the time since the last event. Example: the number of mRNA synthesized in a given period of time follows a Poisson distribution (PD). The PD can be obtained as the limiting form of binomial distribution when the number of trial "n" is very large and the probability of success "p" is very small, such as the product $\lambda = np$ will remain constant.

$$\lim_{n\to\infty} p(k, np) = \lim_{n\to\infty}\binom{n}{k}p^{k}(1-p)^{n-k}$$

$$= \lim_{n\to\infty}\left(\frac{n!}{n-k!k!}\right)\left(\frac{\lambda}{n}\right)^{k}\left(1-\left(\frac{\lambda}{n}\right)\right)^{n-k}$$

$$= \lim_{n\to\infty}\left(\frac{n}{k!}\right)\left(\frac{n}{k}\right)\left(\frac{n-1}{n}\right)\left(\frac{n-2}{n}\right)\ldots\ldots\left(\frac{n-k+1}{n}\right)\left(\frac{\lambda^{k}}{k!}\right)\ldots\left(1-\frac{\lambda}{n}\right)^{n}\left(1-\frac{\lambda}{n}\right)^{-k}$$

$$\lim_{n\to\infty} p(k, np) = \frac{e^{-\lambda}\lambda^{k}}{k!}$$

5.8 Normal Distribution

The binomial and passion distribution is nothing but discrete distribution because all the probability is concentrated at the positive integers, and all the discrete distribution have the property that the probability is concentrated at points between which there is no probability, the distribution is called as Gaussian distribution. The fundamental importance of the Gaussian distribution (GD) in the whole summarization of the statistical theory and its applications is presented in this section

Definition of ND—If "x" is continuous random variable which can assume only non-negative values, the density function of normal distribution is given by

$$P(X = x) = \frac{1}{\sqrt{2\pi\sigma}}\exp{-1/2}\left(\frac{x-\mu}{\sigma}\right)^{2} \quad (-\infty \le \text{ND} \le \infty)$$

The area under the whole curve (AUC) is unity corresponding to the fact that a random variable must be somewhere between $-\infty$ to $+\infty$.

The mean of the distribution is 'μ' and variance is 'σ^2', and the probability that the random variable takes a value less than "x" is equal to the area under curve (AUC) to the left of an ordinate erected at "x," many population in the real world appear to be normal distribution with respect to some characteristics (which is closely approximated by the normal distribution ND) presented in (Fig. 5.2).

It can be shown that in all certain mathematical sense most of the distribution tends in the form to a normal distribution at some parameter get large. The right tail and left tail of the curve does not touches the X-axis (Asymptotically normal), the population mean 'μ' and variance 'σ^2' are normally distributed. An error associated $e \sim N(\mu, \sigma^2)$ mean and variance of the population. Median and mode is always ordinates at the centermost point. The real population will be closely approximated to the normal distribution curve (Fig. 5.3).

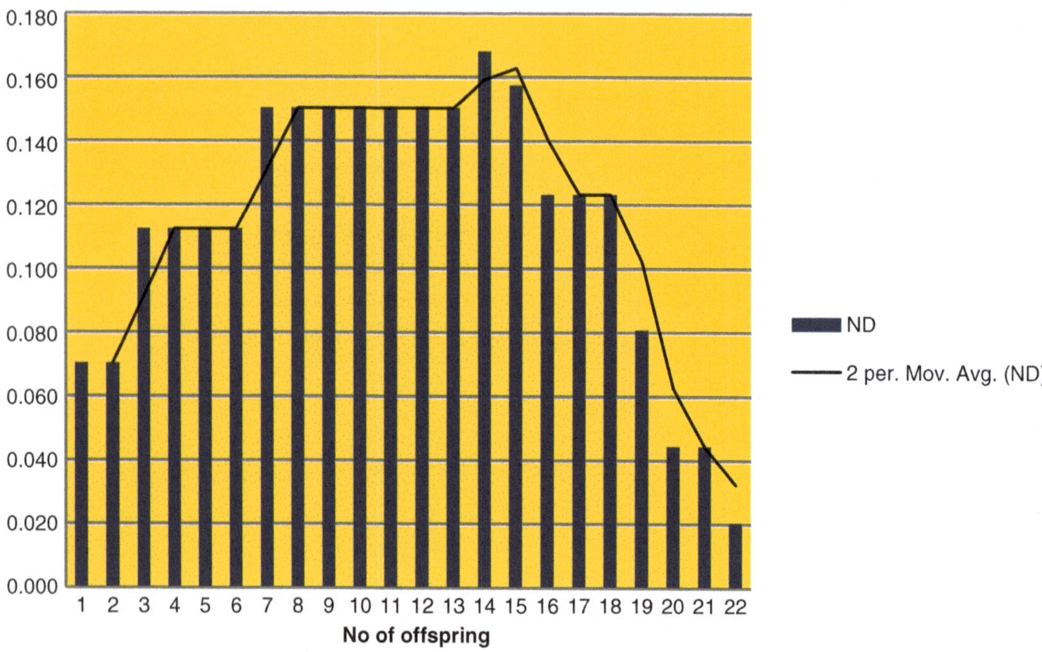

Fig. 5.2 Normal distribution curve showed no offspring produced in coupling phase

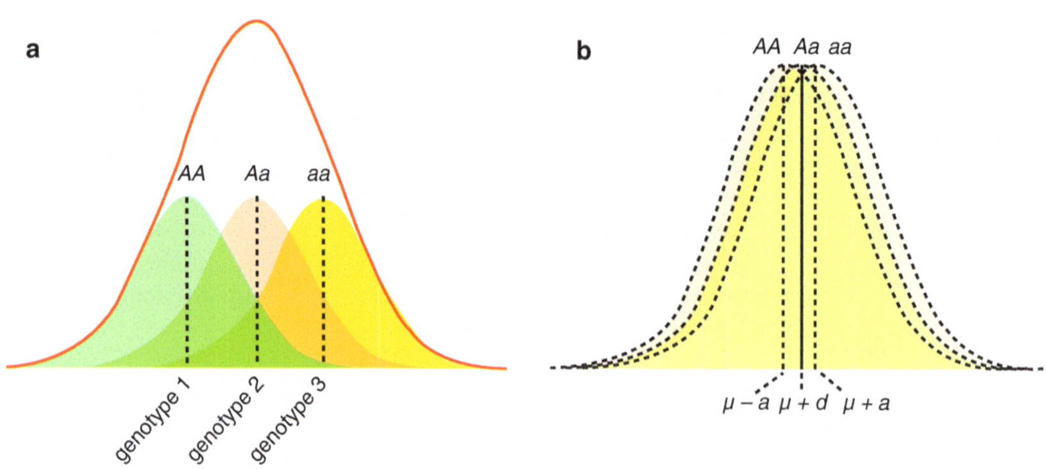

Fig. 5.3 Normal distribution of genotypes

5.8.1 Properties of Hardy–Weinberg Law (HWL)

1. In any diploid population the proportion of heterozygote is $H = 2pq$, the value of which never exceeds 0.50. Therefore the equation becomes $\frac{dH}{dq} = \frac{d}{dq}2q(21-q)$ Differentiation wrt to q. Normally we can see that the maximum value of H is 0.50 when $p = q = \frac{1}{2}$ H could be greater than either D or R as in the population, but never greater than twice of the other $p^2 > 2pq > q^2$.
2. The proportion of heterozygote is twice the square root of the product of the two homozygous proportion, i.e., $\frac{H}{\sqrt{DXR}} = 2$, $H = 2\sqrt{DXR}$. The relation between frequencies of genotypes in a population where a locus with two alleles is tested can be represented graphically. An excellent representation is the De Finetti diagram (Fig. 5.8). Any point inside the triangle illustrates a combination of the proportion of genotypes occurring in the population. For example, a point shown in figure represents a population, in which genotype frequencies are as follows:

$f_{AA} = 0.05$, $f_{Aa} = 0.60$, $f_{aa} = 0.35$. These values can be read by moving along the grid lines inside the triangle, which are routed perpendicular to the appropriate axis. The horizontal axis allows to determine the frequency of alleles occurring in the population. In the above example, you can read $p = 0.225$, which agree with expectation for the population in the Hardy–Weinberg Law (HWL).

$$p = f_{AA} + \frac{1}{2} f_{Aa} = 0.05 + 0.175 = 0.225$$

For each points inside the triangle, proportion of genotypes in the population, which it depicts, sums up to 1. Moreover the curve located in (Fig. 5.6) is the set of all those points that represent the populations in the genetic equilibrium state. Therefore, the De Finetti diagram makes it possible to determine whether the population meets Hardy–Weinberg Law (HWL) equation and allows to declare, how much should the proportion of genotypes be, at specified frequencies of particular alleles, for the population to be in a genetic equilibrium. The process is to identify a problem during clinical trials is usually to verify the distribution of alleles and genotype frequencies in the population in accordance with the chi-square test used. The value of chi-square statistics can be computed form the following formula

$$\chi^2 = \sum_{i=1}^{n} \left[\frac{(Oij - eij)^2}{eij} \right].$$

where Oij = observed value of ith row and jth column

E_{ij} = Expected value of ith row and jth column

The number of degrees of freedom (df) is equal to the number of possible genotypes of the tested locus minus the number of parameters estimated on the basis of data plus one. This test statistics is sometimes unreliable, especially when the checked gene has numerous alleles or if the alleles are rare. Then it is proposed to perform an exact test, for example, exact test analogous we obtained from Fisher test performed by the Monte Carlo simulation method. In addition, HW law is worth recalling the inheritance properties of two different alleles of one locus formulated by Mendel law of inheritance. He has illustrated on the so-called Punnett square (Table 5.2) which represents the possible combinations of gametes during the time of procreation.

All possible situations during reproduction in "N" individual population with two alleles of

Table 5.2 Punnett square of crossing of male and female genotypes with respect to hereditary disease

	Has the diseases	Does not have the diseases	
♂	A	a	
♀			Total
A	AA ¼ A	Aa ¼ B	AA + Aa ¼ + 1/4 $A + B$
a	Aa ¼ C	Aa ¼ D	Aa + aa ¼ + 1/4 $C + D$
Total	(AA + Aa) ¼ + 1/4 $A + C$	Aa + aa ¼ + 1/4 $B + D$	N

tested gene present (Table 5.2). It shows how often offsprings members of a certain genotypes is crossed and gives the probability of formation of a perpendicular genotype in the new offsprings

(a) Percent of patients with the disease that receive the positive results $= \frac{A}{A+C} \times 100$

(b) Percent of patients without the disease that receive the negative results $= \frac{B}{B+D} \times 100$

(c) Positive predicted value of both genotypes *wrt* disease transfer $= \frac{A}{A+B} \times 100$

(d) Negative predicted value of both genotypes wrt disease transfer $= \frac{D}{C+D} \times 100$

$$\mathrm{LR}^+ = \frac{\text{Sensitivity}}{1-\text{Specificity}} \quad \mathrm{LR}^- = \frac{1-\text{Sensitivity}}{\text{Specificity}}$$

$$\text{Odd ratio of the population} = \frac{\mathrm{LR}^+}{\mathrm{LR}^-} \quad \text{Logit odd} = \log\left(\frac{P}{1-P}\right)$$

The proportion of genotypes, which may occur in the offspring, is calculated as follows

$$f'_{AA} = 1f_{AA}{}^2 + \frac{1}{2}f_{AA}f_{Aa} + \frac{1}{2}f_{Aa}f_{AA} + \frac{1}{4}f_{Aa}{}^2 = \left(f_{AA} + \frac{1}{2}f_{Aa}\right)^2 = p^2$$

$$f'_{Aa} = \frac{1}{2}.f_{AA}f_{Aa} + 1.f_{AA}f_{Aa} + \frac{1}{2}f_{Aa}f_{AA} + \frac{1}{2}f_{Aa}{}^2 + \frac{1}{2}f_{Aa}f_{aa} + 1.f_{aa}f_{AA} + \frac{1}{2}.f_{aa}f_{Aa}$$

$$= 2\left(f_{aa} + \frac{1}{2}f_{Aa}\right)\left(f_{AA} + \frac{1}{2}f_{Aa}\right) = 2pq$$

$$f'_{aa} = \frac{1}{4}.f^2{}_{Aa} + \frac{1}{2}.f_{Aa}f_{aa} + \frac{1}{2}.f_{aa}f_{Aa} + 1.f^2{}_{aa} = \left(f_{aa} + \frac{1}{2}f_{Aa}\right)^2 = q^2$$

(Table 5.3) shows that frequencies of particular genotypes in the offspring generation can also be calculated directly from the available proportion of alleles in the parental population. Due to certain assumption of random mating frequency with which male gametes congaing allele "A" fuse in the process of reproduction with female gametes containing allele A, and create offspring with genotype AA is $f_{AA} = pxp = p^2$. Similarly, according to the probability theory, the frequency of homozygote "aa" can be determined as $f_{aa} = qxq = q^2$. Whereas setting a proportion of heterozygote "Aa" in offspring requires taking into account the fact that they arise from the merger of gametes carrying different alleles. It should be noted that under the assumptions of the HWL, allelic frequencies in the population remain constant from generation to generation. If the $p'q'$ denote the frequencies of allele A and a in the offspring, they can be calculated using the formulas

Table 5.3 Frequencies and probabilities of offspring genotypes in biallelic population

Genotype			The probability of genotypes in offspring		
Female	Male	Frequency	AA	Aa	aa
AA	AA	f^2_{AA}	1	0	0
AA	Aa	$f_{AA}f_{Aa}$	½	½	0
AA	aa	$f_{AA}f_{aa}$	0	1	0
Aa	AA	$f_{Aa}f_{AA}$	½	½	0
Aa	Aa	f^2_{Aa}	¼	½	¼
Aa	aa	$f_{Aa}f_{aa}$	0	½	½
aa	AA	$f_{aa}f_{AA}$	0	1	0
aa	Aa	$f_{aa}f_{Aa}$	0	½	½
aa	aa	f^2_{aa}	0	0	1

$$p' = f'_{AA} + \frac{1}{2} f_{Aa}' = p^2 + \frac{1}{2}.2pq = p^2 + p(1-p) = p$$

$$q' = f'_{aa} + \frac{1}{2} f_{Aa}' = q^2 + \frac{1}{2}.2pq = q^2 + q(1-q) = q$$

This allows concluding that, the frequency of genotypes also remains unchanged over time. They, depend only on frequencies of alleles in the parental population which, as has shown, are the same in the subsequent generations. If there are only two alleles A and a with frequencies p and q, respectively, the frequencies of the three possible genotypes are $(p + q)^2 = p^2 + 2pq + q^2$. If there are three alleles say A_1, A_2, and A_3 with frequencies p, q, and r, the genotypic frequencies would be: $(p + q + r)^2 = p^2 + q^2 + r^2 + 2pq + 2pr + 2qr$.

This square expansion will be used to obtain the equilibrium genotypic frequencies for any number of alleles. It must also be noted that the sum of all the allelic frequencies and of all the genotypic frequencies must always be one (unity). If there are only two alleles p and q, then $p + q = 1$, and therefore $p^2 + 2pq + q^2 = (p + q)^2 = 1$. If there are three alleles with frequencies p, q, and r, then $p + q + r = 1$, as well as $(p + q + r)^2 = 1$. The time required for attaining equilibrium frequencies has been determined. If a certain population of individuals with one set of allele frequencies mixes with another set and complete panmixis occurs (*i.e.*, random mating), then the genotypes of the next generation will be found in the proportion $p^2 + 2pq + q^2$, where "p" and "q" are allele frequencies in the new mixed population. Thus, it takes only one generation to reach Hardy–Weinberg equilibrium (HWL) provided the allelic frequencies are the same in males and females. If the allelic frequencies are different in the two sexes, then they will become the same in one generation in the case of alleles on autosomes, and genotypic frequencies will reach equilibrium in two generations. In general, equilibrium is arrived at within one or at the most a few generations. Once equilibrium is attained, it will be repeated in each subsequent generation with the same frequencies of alleles and of genotypes. The Hardy–Weinberg law is applicable when there is random mating. Random mating occurs in a population when the probability of mating between individuals is independent of their genetic constitution. Such a population is said to be panmictic or to undergo panmixis (George et al. 2000; Goffinet and Gerber 2000; Hernandez and Knott 2009). The mating between the genotypes occurs according to the proportions in which the genotypes are present. The probability of a given type of mating can be found out by multiplying the frequencies of the two genotypes that are involved in the mating. Mating are not random for instance when a population consists of different phenotypic characteristics or different communities as in India as there are preferred mating between members of the same racial or communal groups. In human genetics identification of genes underlying human traits including diseases is crucial to our understanding of their etiology and is an important prerequisite for clinical diagnosis and therapeutic options. We have seen in real world problem of coronary heart diseases or cardiovascular problems triggered by the genetic inheritance; many studies have reported that the gene can passes the risk of cardiovascular event, and they can also be responsible for passing on other conditions such as high blood pressure or high cholesterol levels, etc. There is no single gene that increases risk of getting heart disease. It is likely that several genes are responsible for expression of "CVD" risk of elderly population, and also lifestyle, such as smoking or poor diet, passed on from one generation to the next can also increase the risk of CVD (Fig. 5.2).

5.9 Inbreeding

Inbreeding results in increased homozygosity of alleles that are identical by descent (IBD). Define "f" (the inbreeding coefficient) as the probability that two homologous alleles in an individual are IBD. Let "*p*" represent the frequency of allele "A." Homozygosity from alleles that are identical by descent (IBD) and alleles that are identical in state. Combining these probabilities, the frequency of A_1A_1 is

$$P(A_1A_1) = \frac{p(\text{Identity by descent})}{pf} + \frac{P(\text{Identity in state})}{p^2(1-f)}$$

$$= pf + p^2(1-f) = pf + p^2 - p^2 f = f(p - p^2) + p^2 + fp(1-p) + p^2$$

$$P(A_1A_1) = p^2 + fpq$$

$$H(A_1A_2) = 2pq - 2fpq$$

$$P(A_2A_2) = q^2 + fpq$$

$$\text{if } f = 0, P(A_1A_1) = p^2 + 0\,pq = p^2$$

$$\text{if } f = 1, P(A_1A_2) = p^2 + 1\,pq = p^2 + p(1-p) = p^2 + p - p^2$$

Non-random mating and inbreeding; Thus, inbreeding and random mating terms are summarized as follows:

Frequency	$f = 0$	$f = 1$
$P(A_1A_1)$	p^2	p
$H(A_1A_2)$	$2pq$	0
$P(A_2A_2)$	q^2	q

Inbreeding changes genotypic frequencies, but not allelic frequencies. Therefore, the frequency of heterozygote would be calculated by $H = 2pq - 2fpq$; $H = 2pq(1 - f)$, $\frac{H}{2pq} = (1-f).f = 1 - \frac{H}{2pq}$. Analogous reasoning can be applied for the population, in which there is clear preference for individuals of the opposite genotype. Then the number of heterozygotes will be increased. This is caused by the fact that individuals with genotype 'AA' crossing with those of genotype "aa" can only beget heterozygote 'Aa'. It is possible to find suitable examples of non-random mating both in the real world (human and animal). An experiment factor influencing the choice of partner is the appearance; for instance, all individuals generally choose tall partners, Whereas in the case of livestock, animal husbandry inbreeding is often practiced. It is the reproduction from the mating of two genetically related parents which consolidates the desired trait to cumulate particularly valuable genes. In nature, this phenomenon is not preferred. It often contributes to the disclose of unfavorable recessive alleles due to increased homozygosity in the population, e.g., inbreeding takes place in the population of cheetahs. It is the result of isolation of areas, where these predators live due to human activities.

5.10 Weibull Distribution Model

Weibull distribution is an important continuous distribution model, widely used in population genetics, human genetics, genetics engineering, etc. As it could be outlined that the application of Weibull distribution model approach to determine the effect of AA, Aa, and aa in large random mating population in accordance with statement of HW-Law, the failure rate of dominant genotypic genetic carrier was derived by using shape, scale, and location parameters ($0 < \beta < 1$). The density function of Weibull distribution is

$$f(T) = \frac{\beta}{\eta}\left(\frac{T-\gamma}{\eta}\right)^{\beta-1} e^{-\left(\frac{T-\gamma}{n}\right)^{\beta}}$$

$$f(T) \geq 0, T \geq 0 \, or \, \gamma, \beta > 0, \eta > 0, -\infty < \gamma < \infty$$

β = Shapeparameters; η = Scaleparameter and γ = Locationparameter

Let us we arbitrarily assume that the genotypic AA, Aa, and aa's offspring distribution data sets on different parameters is considered. In Weibull distribution we can able to quantify the findings on the effect of dominant gene to carry

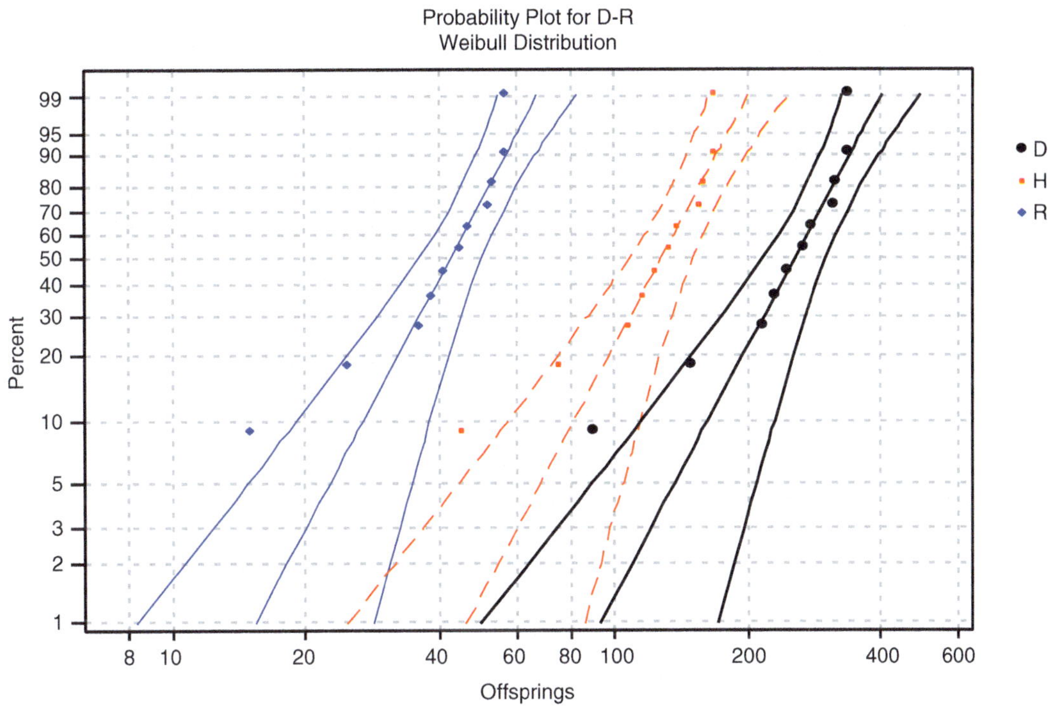

Fig. 5.4 Weibull distribution Curve on three genotypes (D,H,R). Shape: 4.16619, Scale: 46.5636, Char. Life: 46.5636

the hereditary character to the succeeding generation from the ancestors by using the values of shape parameter β, scale parameter η. The PDF of distribution characteristics depends on the values of shape, location, and scale parameters. The reliability and precision of HWL (increase on the effect of dominant gene effect) could be evaluated by the graph of Weibull distribution consideration with varied values of β, γ parameters ($0 < \beta < 1$). The Weibull distribution shape parameters "β" is also known as the slope of the curve. This is because the value of "β" is equal to the slope of the line in a probability plot. Different values of the shape parameter can have marked effect on the behavior of the distribution presented in (Fig. 5.4). Furthermore, another important aspect of "β" in case of non-random mating population that the cumulative graph has clearly depicted is that the increased trend of homozygosity (H = near to 0) over a period of time (generation effect) was assessed by the shape and scale parameters at zero and one. If the shape parameter $\beta < 1$, it has indicted that the failure rate of effect of dominant gene AA's could be apparently expressed at infantile or early stage failure. In case if $\beta = 1$ have a failure rate constant effect of dominant genotyped (D), it is indicative of useful life or random failures. Weibull distribution with $\beta > 1$ have a failure rate that increases with time, also known as wear out failure of AA's dominant effect. These comprise the three sections of the classic "bathtub curve." A mixed Weibull distribution with one subpopulation with <1, subpopulation $\beta = 1$, and one more subpopulation $\beta > 1$ as triggered by the offsprings has shown the failure rate plot that was identical to the "bathtub curve." That is, the effect of dominant genotype (D) is completely failure to the transfer of hereditary character to the next generation, e.g., malignancy or cancer carrier dominant gene

5.11 Exponential Model

While the exponential equation is a useful model to know the population dynamics in population genetics (i.e., changes in genotypic values over time on statement of HW-Law), in the real world we are not swimming in bacteria or paramecium or slime molds, That is, something happens to stop the growth of organisms, be they cells in the body, ciliates in ponds, or lions in the forest. That something else referred to as intraspecific competition, which means that the performance of the individuals in the population depends on how many individuals are in it, more usually referred to as density dependence (Henshalla and Goddard 1999; Haldane and Waddington 1931; Jeffery 2010). This is a complicated issue, one that has inspired much and acrimony in the past, and one that still forms an important base for more modern developments in the evolutionary. The idea was originally associated with the human population, and was brought to public attention as the eighteenth century by Sir Thomas Malthus. His writing influences Darwin's thinking and formed an important component of the development of the idea of evolution by natural selection (Figs. 5.5 and 5.6).

$Y_t = \dfrac{1}{1+e^{a+\beta X'}}$, where Y_t = Change in the genotypic value wrt. AA, Aa, and aa's

a = Intercept or line joining to the Y variable

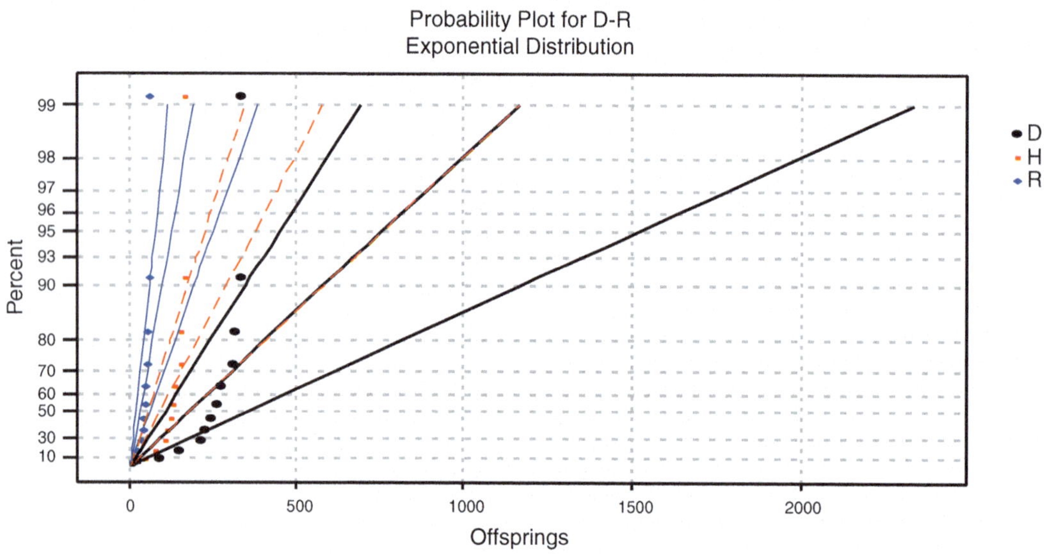

Fig. 5.5 Exponential distribution curve

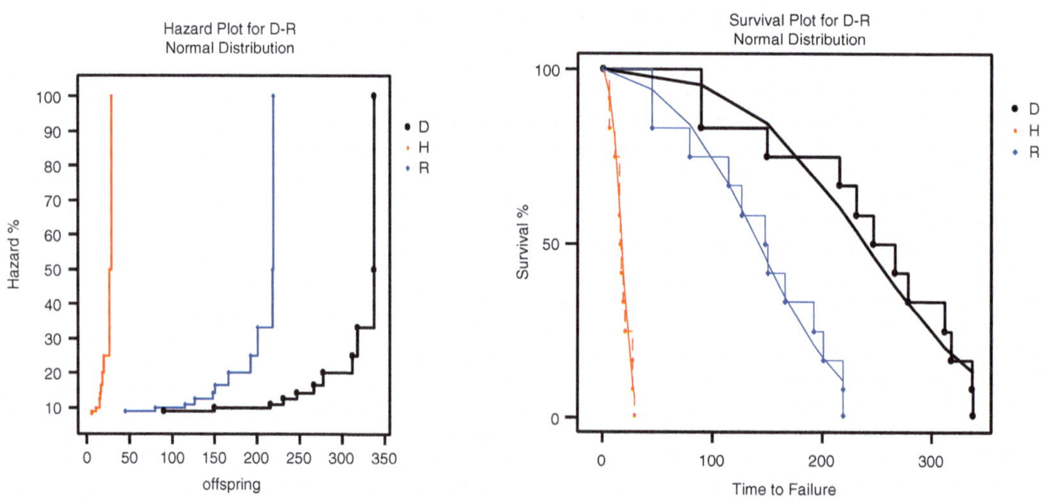

Fig. 5.6 Hz plot for dominant and recessive

β = Slope of the curve $\frac{\Delta Y}{\Delta X} a = \overline{Y} - \beta\overline{X}$;

$$\beta\left(\text{Slope of the curve}\right) = \frac{n\sum XY - \sum X \sum Y}{n\sum X^2 - \left(\sum X\right)^2}$$

Genotypic frequency	Offspring (No)	Traits Body weight (kg)
f^2_{AA}	20	2.85
$f_{AA}f_{Aa}$	23	3.10
$f_{AA}f_{aa}$	26	3.22
$f_{Aa}f_{AA}$	23	2.63
f^2_{Aa}	22	2.88
$f_{Aa}f_{aa}$	21	2.93
$f_{aa}f_{AA}$	23	2.85
$f_{aa}f_{Aa}$	20	2.96
f^2_{aa}	18	2.93

$X_t = \frac{1}{1 + e^{a + \beta Y'}}$, where Y_t = Change in the genotypic value wrt. AA, Aa, and aa's

a = Intercept or line joining to the X variable

β = Slope of the curve $\frac{\Delta X}{\Delta Y} a = \overline{X} - b\overline{Y}$

$$\beta\left(\text{Slope of the curve}\right) = \frac{n\sum XY - \sum X \sum Y}{n\sum Y^2 - \left(\sum Y\right)^2}$$

5.12 Design Approach to Human Genetics

Genetics is the study of hereditary, i.e., how the plausible variations have been precluded from generation to generation without any overlapping population. Practically, each of us have two entire sets of chromosomes: one set inherited from mother, and one set received from the father. These chromosomes carry genes, the unit of genetic material that "codes" for proteins and ultimately, through complicated biochemistry and molecular biology, determine all of our physical traits. Practically, we will investigate how a single gene (with two "favors", called alleles) is passed from one generation to the next. We will consider a particularly simple situation, when the single gene determines some physical trait (such as eye color of son and father). The trait (say blue or green eyes) will be denoted as the phenotype and the actual pair of genes (one on each parentally derived chromosome) will be called the genotypes. Suppose that the gene for eye color comes in two forms that will be referred to as A and a. For example, "A" might be an allele for blue eyes, whereas "a" could be an allele for brown eyes. Then each individual must have one of the following pairs of combinations: AA, Aa, or aa (note that aA and Aa will be considered to be equivalent). Suppose, we know that the fraction of all genes for eye color of type A in the population is p, and the fraction of all genes for eye color of type a is q, where $p + q = 1$

Genotypes	Aa	AA	aa	Aa
Probabilities	Pq	p^2	q^2	pq

o∕ +°	P	q	Total
P	$p * p = p^2$	$p * q = pq$	$P^2 + pq$
Q	$q * p = qp$	$q * q = q^2$	$qp + q^2$
Total	$p^2 + qp$	$pq + q^2$	N

Then we can interpret p and q as probabilities that a gene selected at random from the population will turn out to be type a (respectively A), i.e., (A) = p, P(a) = q. Now suppose we draw at random two alleles out of the (large) population. (This is like tossing a coin twice) (Jansen and Stam 1994; Moree 1950; Rife 1951). We get the following cases with given probabilities (computed with the second multiplication principle). The probability of finding the genotypes "aA" (or the equivalent Aa) is the same as the probability of a and A, the probability of any genotype (aa, aA, AA, or Aa) is then the same as the product of probabilities as follows; we do not distinguish between genotypes aA and Aa, since the "order" of the alleles does not matter. Thus, the probability of having a genotype which includes "a" and "A" (aA or Aa) is $2pq$. If the population size is "N," then, on average we would expect "Np^2" individuals of type "AA" $Nq^2$of type "aa" and $2N$ pq individuals of the mixed type. The total probability of any of the genotypes is $(p + q)^2 = p^2 + q^2 + 2pq = 1$.

5.13 Multinomial Distribution in Clinical Trial

Let us consider the simple situation of genetic experiments conducted in different geographical locations. We assume "n" trial of experimentation and there are "t" possible results. *viz.*, a_1, a_2, a_3,……a_t with probability that we shall get n_1a_1's n_2a_2's..a_n. Again the matter is solved by the permutation and combination for any possible arrangements of n_1a_1's, n_2a_2's …and so on, the probability of experimental trial is equal to: p_1^{n1}, p_2^{n2}, p_3^{n3}……. p_n^{nt}.

Then, the cumulative probability for pooled trial is calculated by the following density function

$$p(Xi = x) = \frac{n!}{n_1!n_2!n_3!n_4!}(p_1)^{n1}(p_2)^{n2}(p_3)^{n3}(p_4)^{n4}\ldots(p_n)^{nt}.$$

For example, the "OAB" blood groups in human being, the multinomial distribution model is as follows.

Blood groups	Gene frequency	Population size
A-Codes P	$p^2 + 2pr$	n_{11}
B-Coded q	$q^2 + 2qr$	n_{21}
AB	$2pq$	n_{31}
O-Coded r	r^2	n_{41}

The multinomial distribution becomes

$$p(Xi = x) = \frac{n!}{n_{11}!n_{n21}!n_{31}!n_{41}!}(p2 + 2pr)^{n11}(q2 + 2qr)^{n21}(2pq)^{n31}(r2)^{n41}\ldots(p_n)^{nk}$$

In our initial examples we have been observing that 3AA 5Aa 2aa, the above MN–distribution becomes $p(X = xi) = \frac{10!}{3!5!2!}(1/4)^3(2/4)^5(1/4)^2$. As per the Hardy–Weinberg equilibrium (HW-law) the "OAB" blood groups are dealt with

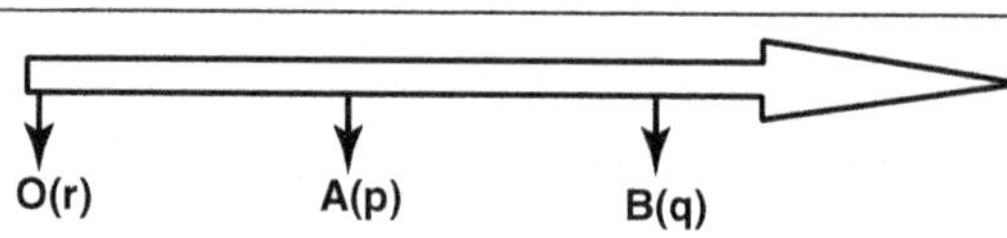

$$(p + q + r)^2 = p^2 + q^2 + r^2 + 2pr + 2qr + 2pq = 1$$

Suppose we noted observed and theoretical frequencies, should use the chi square large sample test for testing the hypothesis.

Genotypes o↗ +o	r^2	$p^2 + 2pr$	$q^2 + 2qr$	$2pq$	Column total
r^2	1	$r^2xp^2 + 2pr$	$r^2xq^2 + 2qr$	r^2x2pq	$\sum_{i=1}^{r} r^2$
$p^2 + 2pr$	$p^2 + 2prxr^2$	1	$p^2 + 2prxq^2 + 2qr$	$p^2 + 2prx2pq$	$\sum_{i=1}^{p} p^2 + 2pr$
$q^2 + 2qr$	$q^2 + 2qrxr^2$	$q^2 + 2qr\ xp^2 + 2pr$	1	$q^2 + 2qrx2pq$	$\sum_{i=1}^{q} q^2 + 2qr$
$2pq$	$2pqxr^2$	$2pqxp^2 + 2pr$	$2pqxq^2 + 2qr$	1	$\sum_{i=1}^{pq} 2pq$
Row total	$\sum_{i=1}^{r} r^2$	$\sum_{i=1}^{p} p^2 + 2pr$	$\sum_{i=1}^{q} q^2 + 2qr$	$\sum_{i=1}^{pq} 2pq$	Grand total

Expected values of reference cell frequency $(Eij) = \frac{\sum_{i=1}^{n} R_i x \sum_{i=1}^{n} C_j}{\text{Grandtotal}}$

Chi-square value $(\chi^2) = \frac{\sum_{i=1}^{n}(O_{ij} - E_{ij})^2}{E_{ij}}$, $(\chi^2) \sim N(n-1)df\,\chi^2$; df = (Row-1) (Column-1)

Hypothesis testing: $H_0 = \mu_1$ and $H_1 \neq \mu_1$. In general Xi (where $i = 1,2,3..n$) are "n" independent rv's with mean μ_i and common variance σ_i^2, then

$$\chi^2 = \sum_{i=1}^{n}\left(\frac{x_i - \mu_i}{\sigma_i}\right)^2 = \sum_{i=1}^{n} u_i^2 = \text{where } u_i = z_i = \frac{x_i - \mu_i}{\sigma_i} \sim N(0,1)$$

Since X_i's (rv) is crossing of genotypes with respect to males and females, the above cited formula will becomes standard normal distribution which leads to have independent predictors; therefore when there is increase of population size with undefined population, the estimation of probability values has been determined by normal or Gaussian distribution and the density function is given by

$$f(x) = \frac{1}{\sqrt{2\pi\sigma}}\text{expo} - \frac{1}{2}\sum_{i=1}^{n}\left(\frac{X_i - \mu_i}{\sigma_i}\right)^2$$

5.14 Effect of Genetic Inheritance on New Drug Trial

Randomized clinical trials are conducted either with single or blinded placebo. The newly administered drugs depend on multifarious genetic and environmental factors (more sensitive). However, the drug could cause itching, irritation, rashes, drossiness, *etc.* Say for example in Indian geographical condition different races and subpopulation have not responded to the particular drug (Rife 1951; Schneider et al. 2007; Sen and Churchill 2001; Stevens 1950). Eventhough, the genetic inheritance factors in the sense that the value observed for individual depends solely on the various genotypes (hereditary factors) of an individual respondents. For simplicity we take first the case when there are two alleles at locus at RCT selected population level. Let us consider three genotypes of selected population, AA—Dominant, Aa—Heterozygous, and aa—recessive characters.

Genotypes	Frequency	Genotypic value	Coded Genotypic value deviation taken from mean value
AA	p^2	D	$d - \mu = i$
Aa	$2pq$	H	$h - \mu = j$
Aa	q^2	R	$r - \mu = k$

Where μ = the population mean. In another example let us consider the following parameters of drug intervention.

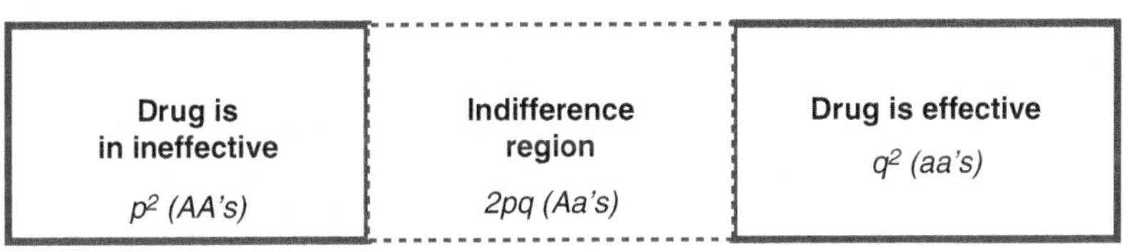

The genotypic value is the constant value given by an individual with the genotype. The mean effect of the drug at the population level is denoted by μ, where $\mu = p^2d + 2pqh + q^2r$. And the deviation from the mean genotypic values are denoted by I, j, and k, respectively, which therefore satisfy $p_i^2 + 2pq_j + q_k^2 = 0$. Now we wish to determine the extent to which the coded genetic values are denoted by i, j, and k, $i = 2\alpha$, $j = \alpha + \beta$ $k = 2\beta$ as in the general case of regression we obtain the values for α and β minimizing. Therefore, $Q = p^2(i - 2\alpha)^2 + 2pq(j - \alpha - \beta)^2 + q^2 (k - 2\beta)^2$. The normal equations as usual are

$$\frac{1}{2}\frac{\partial Q}{\partial \alpha} = 0 \quad \frac{1}{2}\frac{\partial Q}{\partial \beta} = 0 \text{ or in this case}$$

$$2p^2(i - 2\alpha) + 2pq(j - \alpha - \beta) = 0 \quad (5.7)$$

$$2pq(j - \alpha - \beta) + 2q^2(k - 2\beta) = 0 \quad (5.8)$$

Adding (5.7) and (5.8) equation we get

$$(4p^2 + 4pq)\alpha + (4q^2 + 4pq)\beta$$

$$= 2(p_i^2 + 2pq_j + q^2k) = 0$$

So that, $4p\alpha + 4q\beta = 0$

$$p\alpha = -q\beta \quad (5.9)$$

Let $P_x = \gamma$ so that $\alpha = \frac{\gamma}{p}\ \beta = \frac{-\gamma}{q}$ then

$$4p\gamma + 2pq\left(\frac{\gamma}{p} - \frac{\gamma}{q}\right)$$

$$= 2p\gamma + 2q\gamma = p_i^2 + 2pq_j$$

$$\gamma = p^2{}_i + pq_j$$

Hence, $\frac{p^2 + pq_j}{p}\ \beta = \frac{p_i^2 + pq_j}{q} = \frac{pq_j + q_k^2}{q}$

$$\alpha = p_i + q_j \beta = p_j + q_k$$

The effect of change gene 'a' in to 'A' then formula is equal to $(\alpha - \beta)$

$$(p_i + q_j) - (p_j + q_k) \text{ or } p(1 - j) + q(j - k)$$

5.15 Additive Effect of Gene on New Drug

We consider an example of the population genotypes

Genotypes	Frequency	Genotypic value coded
AA's	p^2	2
Aa's	$2pq$	1
Aa's	q^2	0

Here the mean is $2p^2 + 2pq$ which is equal to $2p$. The average effect of substituting the "A" gene for the "a" gene is $p(1 - j) + q(j - k)$ which is equal to $p(d - h) + q(h - r)$ so that we get $p(2 - 1) + q(1 - 01) = p + q = 1$ $\sigma_A = 2pq$ (additive genetic effect). Therefore the total variance in the population is equal to $p^2 \times 4 + 2pq \times 1 - (2p)^2$ which is equal $2pq$, so that is the present case additive genetic variance comprises the whole of the genotypic variance.

5.16 Model Application in AIDS Therapy

AIDS stands for Acquired human Immuno deficiency Syndrome. It is the end stage of infection with Human Immunodeficiency Virus (HIV), characterized by a cluster of life-threatening illnesses. The structural model of HIV. AIDS can be described as the worst plague in the present century. There is a multitude of problems arising from AIDS. Apart from being a public health hazard it has many social, ethical, legal, moral, behavioral, psychological, demographic, economic, and statistical implications. AIDS has serious impact on society by way of hindering all round development both at family and national levels. The HIV pandemic has undergone four main phases of evolution: emergence, dissemination, escalation, and stabilization. The first sign that a new disease was a foot was the appearance of a rare cancer known as Kaposi's sarcoma. It is a tumor of blood vessel tissue in the skin or internal organs that had been known mainly among older Italian and Jewish men and in Africa. In the late 1970s a more aggressive form of the same began to appear among young white middle class males. Many of these patients turned out to have a history of homosexuality and these men provided the basis for the first reports of a new syndrome, which was diagnosed in 1981. Since the first cases of AIDS were identified in the Red Corridor of Chennai (India 1983) nearly four decades ago, HIV/AIDS has emerged as one of the leading challenges for national and Global public health. Particularly in South Asian Countries, where the overwhelming majority of HIV/AIDS cases appear, the epidemic continues to takes a massive human toll. Present Scenario in Indian condition, the epidemic till epitome and suboptimal deviation taken from HIV-infected population. An understating from HIV/AIDS life data sets, the magnitude and trajectory points of the HIV/AIDS epidemic is alarming stage of addressing the high risk quality of life of people living with HIV/AIDS (HRQOL), as well as the uncertainty around these parameters, is critically important both for health policy, planning and evaluating control strategies and for preparing for vaccine trails based on the newer analytical tool and algorithms. The world health organization is flagging four important challenges as the prevention of HIV/AIDS (International AIDS conference, Durban, 2016). The organization is highlighting the need to renew attention to HIV prevention, while maintaining momentum on scaling up access to HIV comprehensive treatment. It is also signalling the growing emergency of HAART drug resistance and need for sustainable financing of the global response. The enormous progress on HIV particularly on treatment aspects is one of the big public health challenges for the forthcoming days but this is no time for compliancy. If the world is to achieve its goal of ending by 2030, it would rapidly expand and intensify the efforts of the salient goals of present control measures at global level. Globally, progress on HIV prevention has stalled. In 2015–2016 there were 2.10 million new HIV infections, marginally fewer than the 2.2 million in 2009–2010. In some regions, and among some groups, infections are arising. On the basis of geographical mapping where the epidemic had been under control, for example, in some urban population of men who have sex with men, it is re-emerging (UNAIDS2019). In 2014, 35% of new infections worldwide occurred among men who have sex with men; sex workers and their clients, transgender, inject drugs and prisons population. In India, women aged between 19 and 26 years remain particularly vulnerable and affected (UNAIDS). Reducing new infections means addressing the social and legal barriers that impede many people from accessing HIV services. It means tailoring prevention programs so that right services reach the groups that are most vulnerable and affected, ensuring that individuals have easy access to approach that work, and work for them. Although, the WHO notes that better prevention will happen if countries invest strategically in approach with greatest impact, for example, by exploiting new interventions, such as post-exposure prophylaxis (PEP) where ARV drugs are used to protect people at high risk of becoming infected with HIV. HAART Treatment aspects; Since 2015, WHO has recommend that all PLHIVs start ART as soon as possible to prevent illness and death. The uptake of WHO's treat all policy has been rapid, the implementation has been facilitated by recent dramatic improvements in ART being used with one novel regime a day which is safe and well tolerated. The HAART saves lives of PLHIVs and AIDS-related deaths have fallen (45%) since their peak in 2005 and (26%) since 2010. Expanding HIV HAART also helps reduce transmission as the level of the virus drops in a person, so does the risk of transmission. But many challenges remain unaltered. More than (40%) of PLHIVs still do not know they are infected, highlighting the need for ready access to simple and affordable testing services. Self testing provides an opportunity for more people to be tested, particularly those who are reluctant to use effective health services. Drug resistance; WHO pointed out that HIV-related drug resistance showed that only 5% of PLHIVs on HAART were resistant to at least one ARV drug. The individual organization is monitoring the trends and notes worrisome indications that drug resistance is emerging as a more significant threat in some countries and set of populations. As treatment continues to expand, countries will need to vigilant to ensure that the quality of HAART treatment services is assured to minimize the emergence of drug resistance. To address this threat, WHO is developing a Global action plan on HIV drug resistance calling on countries to continue surveillance to ensure rapid action. Lastly financing for a sustainable repose—the ever expanding, changing donor priorities and continuing threats to global economy all pose challenges to financing efforts end AIDS. It will be important to ensure full replenishment of the global fund to fight AIDS. The middle income countries will face particular challenges as they transition from external to predominantly domestic funding of their HIV and broader health services. A slow-acting virus: Most epidemic viruses have an impact in a matter of days or weeks. However, the deceptive feature of AIDS is that it is latent in infected person for a very long period. HIV-infected people have no symptoms of AIDS for about 10 years. Further, they appear healthy and right from seroconversion they can transmit the virus to the susceptible. At present there is no proven cure for AIDS and development of the disease is such that almost all HIV-infected cases will turn to AIDS and hence to death. In 1984, researchers isolated another AIDS virus, HIV-2, which appears to be slightly different in genetic makeup and has slower progress towards AIDS (Fig. 5.7).

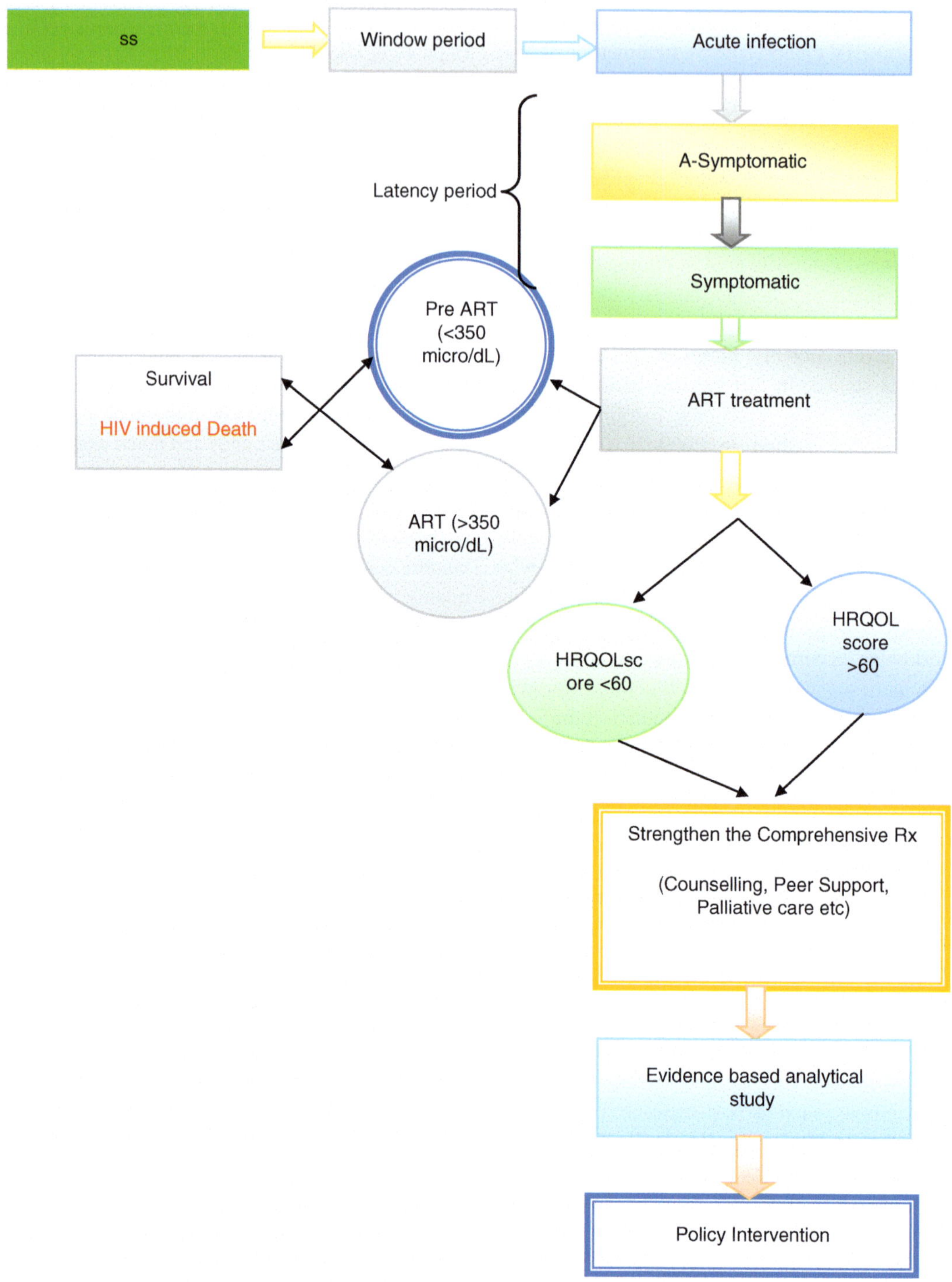

Fig. 5.7 Displays HIV disease process

Window period

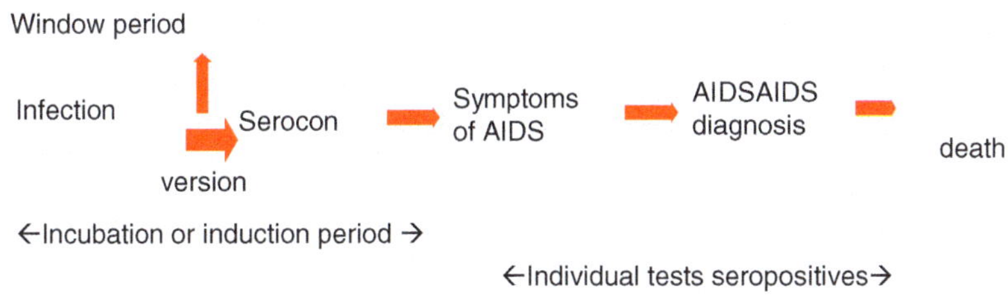

5.17 Statistical Implications

AIDS endemic is expected to place enormous demands on health care facilities. Statistical modelling of the disease is essential for estimation of current and future numbers of HIV seropositives and forecasting health care needs. AIDS endemiology is highly interdisciplinary and it calls for coordinated scientific effort across a wide range of disciplines. To this end, there must be an effective mechanism to share the data and to answer the following crucial questions:

1. How does HIV transmissibility vary with time after infection and with disease stage?
2. What is responsible for the large variation in incubation time?
3. What are the co-factors affecting infectivity?
4. What is the time between infection and transmission?
5. Will current trends in the spread of the virus continue?
6. Can we explain the past rate of growth of the endemic?
7. Can we predict the future size of the endemic precisely?

It is to be noted that information of HIV/AIDS is surrounded by sensitive, social, legal, and ethical issues. Researchers attempting to answer the above questions do not have access to the important elements of raw data. Identifying the sources and availability of such data itself is the beginning. Statisticians have to evaluate the available data sources and develop estimation and projection methods based on such data. Issues that are essential to the understanding and management of the disease have generated numerous statistical challenges. Some of these are as follows:

8. Estimation of incubation distribution.
9. Choosing proper infection density.
10. Projection of the course of the endemic.
11. Dealing with confidentiality and analysis of incomplete data.
12. Inadequacy of data on HIV/AIDS for assessing the size and progression of endemic.

Statistical methods have played an important role in understanding of HIV infection and its manifestation of AIDS. Statistical ideas and methods enter naturally in these studies in view of the considerable amount of uncertainty in disease phenomenon. Further, data from AIDS studies have many new features which need development of special types of statistical models and methodology. For a review of these methods. In Chaps. 3 and 4 we propose a new model under each mode of HIV transmission to estimate the number infected and suggest stochastic models for incubation period and HIV disease progression.

5.18 Data Availability

Data form the backbone of many statistical studies. But, data relating to HIV endemic are notoriously incomplete with missing information and delayed reporting and are subject to complex censoring and truncation mechanisms. This is mainly due to faulty reporting system. Also, there is a random time interval between infection and diagnosis. All these aspects result in incompleteness of data. Moreover, HIV infection is a delicate issue involving sensitivity in its spread. The associated social stigma makes the problem further complicated. As a result, it is difficult to gather reliable and truthful responses from individuals and organizations. In order to tackle this problem, Randomized Response Technique (RRT) and its variants have been shown to be useful. As the endemiology of AIDS is multidisciplinary, the compiled data should be made available for researchers, organizations, and policy makers. With advances in information technology, it is possible to have easy access to such data at different places and at different levels through a fully fledged central database. The statistical and mathematical modelling is a newer tool and very extensively used in the field of HIV medicine, drug trail, and clinical research. The modelling can be time consuming, particularly if the researcher is interested in measuring the long-term effects of disease process at population level. Any kind of (Quantitative and qualitative) research is very difficult to layout or administer at an early stage without applying advance statistical measures for testing the hypothetical statements. If the statistical measures have not been formulated properly in prior, the whole research findings will be given unrealistic conclusion about the HIV-infected population and comprehensive HAART treatment at long term due to faulty selection of statistical measures, study subjects, duration of the research etc. In latter part of the HIV research, it is too erroneous task to control the extraneous effects on the different variables and their magnitudinal differences from the HIV life data sets. Overwhelmingly, the entire resulted part will become false and not to produce any further HIV research hypothetical statements at population level. Particularly in the field of HIV medicine, clinical and drug development process, so many confounders would be aroused from the annotated HIV research, the effect of confounders will greatly increase the standard error (SE) in the experimental results and also researcher may deliberately contaminate the result part during the study period. In this practical insight of the HIV research, present study attempt to demonstrate various types of advanced statistical and mathematical modelling (particularly it is more applicable to HIV research) by using real data sets and also explore newer analytical techniques for formulating the various types of statistical measures (SM) to be capable for examining the casual relationship between the different independent variables. The present thesis saliently attributed high degree of control of extraneous and exogenous variables explicitly with direct and indirect control of errors. The following objectives were considered for the present research:

1. To explore new technologies for constructing the various statistical measures approach to real-time data sets of HIV/AIDS.
2. To develop a basic understanding of various attributes of HIV infection, transmission and treatment mechanism through theoretical and practical approach.
3. To build newer genetics and statistical measures that are superior to existing technologies for improvement of HIV research, drug development process, and HIV-related survey-based research (clinical and Biomarkers).
4. To demonstrate various genetic models to know the complexity of HIV transmission effects by using various attributes and also extrapolate any genetic variants for association between the selected factors in the HIV research.
5. To derive different analytical intervention of transmission mechanism and efficacy of HAART treatment through cascade linkage model at various levels for the benefit of end users (clinicians, research beginners, drug developers, academicians, etc.).

Mother to child transmission (MTCT) is the most critiqued and significant route of HIV transmission in children below the age of 15 years and neonatal baby. The National AIDS control organization (NACO 2014) reported that in India perinatal HIV transmission, even after HAART therapy, accounts for 5.40% of HIV cases which drew up and became alarming stage. An increasing data support host genetic factors as an important determinants of human immunodeficiency virus type-1 (HIV-I) is very susceptible and routed for mother to child transmission (MTCT). Of these genetic confounders, those impacting innate and adaptive immune responses would be distilled to instigate a critical role in viral infectivity and pitched for HIV progression rate among children. Many research have proved CD4 T-lymphocytes count and plasma RNA-viral load are considered as one of the genetic confounders for the transmission of HIV from mother to child.

The highly active antiretroviral therapy (HAART) has been harnessed as one of the key interventions in mitigating the HIV epidemics at global level. The primary goal of HAART is to decrease HIV-related morbidity and mortality. While patient on HAART, it was expected that the patient experience fewer HIV-related illnesses. However, when the CD_4 count reached threshold level the viral load should become undetectable (<47 copies/mL). Our main aim was to study the virological suppression (HIV viral load ≤47 copies/mL) and immunological functions (CD_4 Count >500 μ/dL) at 24, 48 weeks follow-up intervals from inception of HAART with NNRTI + PI's based regimen. Secondary: determination of baseline variables associated with virological suppression. The study aims to fit genetic model for high-dimensional data and evaluate the efficacy of the fitted model on the basis of theoretical and practical approach.

5.18.1 Methods: Model Formulation

According to the cohort data extracted (March, 2009) from Government hospitals of Bangalore city, 168 children had been initiated on HAART. Patients had to meet the inclusion criteria between age group 5 and <16 years at the time of HAART initiation. At least 12 months of follow-up data or one known viral load measurement and CD_4 count were available after initiation of HAART. No known prior exposure to HAART except exposure through prevention of mother to child transmission (PMTCT) was expected.

$$Y_{ijk} = \mu + \alpha_i + \varepsilon_{ijkl}$$

Y_{ijkl} = Observed value for *i*th mother *j*th period *k*th baby

μ = General mean

α_i = Effect of *i*th mother – HIV infected

β_{ij} = Effect of *i*th HIV-infected mother and *j*th period

ε_{ijkl} = Error associated with *i*th mother *j*th period *k*th baby CD_4—adjusted factor.

5.18.2 Assumption of the Model

(Table 5.4) observations are independent and identical, each CD_4 and viral load testing follow-up period is mutually exclusive test. Experimental error for each follow-up period are normally distributed with μ, common variance $\sigma^2\varepsilon_{ijkl}\sim N(\mu, \sigma^2)$. All possible CD_4 and viral load pairs of means are compared with the same precision even though differences between may be large.

Analytical procedure or methods

$$\text{Correction factor} = \frac{\left(\Sigma Y_{Yij}\right)^2}{N} \text{ or}$$

$$\text{TSS} = \Sigma Y_{ij}^2 - \text{CF}$$

$$\text{Group SS} = \frac{Y_{1.}^2 + Y_{2.}^2 + Y_{t.}^2}{r} - \text{CF}$$

Error SS = TSS − Group − SSB

Genetic correlation ($-1 \le r^2 \le 1$)

The genetic correlation is derived to know the resemblances between mother CD_4 count and

Table 5.4 Analysis of variance table for estimation of heritability

Source of variation	*df*	SS	MSS	EMS	Variance ratio "*F*" @1% level
Between groups (mothers)	$(M-1)$	S_B^2	$\text{MSB} = \frac{S_B^2}{M-1}$	$\sigma_W^2 + K_1\sigma_M^2$	$F = \frac{\text{MSB}}{\text{MSW}}$
Within groups (CD_4 count)	$(K-M)$	S_W^2	$\text{MSW} = \frac{S_W^2}{K-M}$	σ_W^2	
Total	$(N-1)$	TSS			

RNA plasma viral load for HIV transmission rate (Basavarajaiah et al. 2012). He pointed out that the lower CD_4 count and high plasma viral load was strongly associated with *in utero* transmission and similar studies were conducted by Basavarajaiah et al. and European collaborative study on MTCT (1999). In this proximity of the research, present hypothesis has fitted different genetic models approach to know the transmission rate of HIV-MTCT. Let X_1 be the variable considered as mother CD_4 count or RNA Plasma viral load at inception of HAART and $X_2, X_3 \ldots \ldots X_n$ be considered as follow-up CD_4 count or RNA plasma viral load at different intervals like 6, 12, 24 months, etc. The resemblance of the CD_4 count and RNA viral load is modelled as below:

The genetic correlation obtained by using the following theoretical approach

$$r_g = \frac{\sigma_{gX1Xn}}{\sqrt{\sigma^2_{gx1}\sigma^2_{gxn}}} \tag{5.10a}$$

$$r_p = \frac{\sigma_{gX1Xn} + \sigma_{eX1Xn}}{\sqrt{\sigma^2_{gx1} + \sigma^2_{gxn} + \sigma^2_{ex1} + \sigma^2_{exn}}} \tag{5.10b}$$

$$r_e = \frac{\sigma_{eX1Xn}}{\sqrt{\sigma^2_{ex1}\sigma^2_{exn}}} \tag{5.10c}$$

Table 5.5 ANOVA and covariances of CD_4 count and RNA Viral load

Source of variation	df	Variance X_1	Variance $X_2 \ldots .Xn$	Covariance X_1,v/s $X_2 \ldots .Xn$
Between CD_4 count or RNA Viral load	$S - 1$	$\sigma_{gx1}{}^2$	$\sigma_{gxn}{}^2$	$\sigma_{gx1\ xn}$
Between CD_4 count or RNA Viral load	$N - S$	$\sigma_{ex1}{}^2$	$\sigma_{exn}{}^2$	$\sigma_{ex1\ xn}$

As per the above fitted model (5.10a), (5.10b), and (5.10c), the final equation of the model becomes

$r_p = r_g + r_e$

Phenotypic Correlation = Genotypic correlation + Environmental Correlation

Variance of $\sigma_p{}^2 = \sigma_W{}^2 + \sigma_M{}^2$

Estimation of heritability ($0 \le h^2 \le 1$), from Table 5.5 is derived the heritability estimation at population level

Heritability (h^2)—The rate of MTCT is determined by using heritability, it is denoted by h^2, heritability lies between $0 \le h^2 \le 1$

$$h^2 = \frac{\sigma_M{}^2}{\sigma_W{}^2 + \sigma_M{}^2}, k = \frac{1}{M-1}\left(N - \frac{\Sigma n_i{}^2}{N}\right)$$

where k' is the number of HIV-infected child produced from the mothers

$$t = \frac{\sigma_M{}^2}{\sigma_W{}^2 + \sigma_M{}^2} = h^2 = 4(t),\ \mathrm{SE}(h^2) = \frac{\sqrt[4]{2(1-t)^2\{1+(k-1)t\}2}}{k(k-1)(m-1)}$$

Numerical results of genetic models

(Table 5.6) depicted the genetic correlation matrix on various traits of HIV mother to child transmission, the matrix was demonstrated from Eqs. (5.10a), (5.10b), and (5.10c). The results showed that the CD_4 counts at inception bears with lower level, more chance of transmission of HIV from mother to child ($h^2 = 0.12$) followed by the very less CD_4 counts of mother at the time of delivery (very important predictive traits toll the transmission rate $h^2 = 0.16$). However, the HAART inception is the lengthiest process, it seems to derive the highest probability for infecting the young ones (from the mother), if mother HAART traits shows negative correlation with respect to duration of HAART, age, and other associated parameters (Table 5.7).

(Table 5.8) results depicted the CD_4 counts follow-up intervals demonstrated by predictive genetic model for the estimation of heritability and genetic correlation. The source data was collected from the ART center. ANOVA mixed effect model was demonstrated to extrapolate the various genetic parameters. The CD_4 counts have been arranged with respect to various follow-up time intervals. The results indicate that the CD_4 count with various time interval was found to be statistically significant ($p < 0.01$, Fisher F-5.09).

Table 5.6 Genetic correlation matrix of CD_4 count follow-up of infected mother who transfers HIV infection to her child

Follow-up	Inception HAART	6 months	12 months	24 months	36 months	48 months	At time of delivery
Inception HAART	1 **h^2 = 0.12***	0.04	0.39	0.74	0.75	−0.08	0.56
6 months	0.20 ± 0.16	1 h^2=0.36[a]	−0.25	0.74	0.44	0.73	0.31
12 months	0.21 ± 0.18	−0.36 + 0.11	1 h^2=0.55	0.49	0.23	0.37	−0.34
24 months	0.52 + 0.22	0.11+-0.63	−0.18 + 0.67	1 h^2 = 0.62	−0.05	0.75	0.48
36 months	0.62 ± 0.13	0.28 + 0.16	−0.19 + 0.42	−0.16 + 0.11	1 h^2 = 0.59	0.57	0.49
48 months	0.14 ± 0.22	0.11 + 0.62	−0.26 + 0.63	0.28 + 0.47	0.33 ± 0.24	1 h^2 = 0.68	−0.41
At time of delivery	0.18 ± 0.38	−0.32 + 0.63	0.10 ± 0.44	0.63 ±[a] 0.15	0.63 ± 0.14	0.22 ± 0.63	1 h^2 = 0.16[a]

[a]Diagonal elements denoted heritability (h^2) lies between $0 \le h^2 \le 1$, above diagonal elements denoted phenotypic correlation r_p, below diagonal elements denoted genotypic and environmental correlation $r_g + r_e$

Table 5.7 Genetic correlation matrix of RNA Plasma viral load of infected mother who transfers HIV infection to her child

Follow-up	Inception HAART	6 months	12 months	24 months	At time of delivery
Inception HAART	1 h^2 = 18*	0.61	0.37	0.78	−0.55
6 months	0.23 + 0.38	1 h^2 = 0.12[a]	0.35	0.48	−0.23
12 months	0.11 + 0.26	−0.21 + 0.56	1 h^2 = 0.23	−0.26	−0.38
24 months	0.26 + 0.52	−0.24 ± 0.72	0.26 + 0.52	1 h^2 = 0.44	0.14
At time of delivery	−0.13 ± 0.42	−0.42 + 0.19	0.18 ± 0.56	−0.32 + [a]0.46	1 h^2 = 0.13[a]

[a]Diagonal elements denoted heritability (h^2) lies between $0 \le h^2 \le 1$. Above diagonal elements denoted phenotypic correlation r_p, below diagonal elements denoted genotypic and environmental correlation $r_g + r_e$

Table 5.8 Analysis of variance of CD_4 count (micro/dL) follow-up from inception of HAART to till baby delivery of HIV-infected mother who does not transfer infection to her child

Summary of data						
	Treatments					
	1	2	3	4	5	Total
N	21	21	21	21	21	105
$\sum X$	7395	7618	7722	7590	6788	37,113
Mean	352.1429	362.7619	367.7143	361.4286	323.2381	353.457
$\sum X^2$	2,607,223	2,770,638	2,846,540	2,748,834	2,301,894	13,275,129
Std. dev.	12.5031	18.8651	18.7754	16.72	73.4009	38.8877
Result details						
Source		SS	*df*	MS		
Between-treatments		26,634.4381	4	6658.6095	*F* = 5.09693**	(2.46,3.61)
Within-treatments		130,639.619	100	1306.3962		
Total		157,274.0571	104			

$F_{\text{calculated Value}} > F_{\text{Table Value}}$ at 5% level

ANOVA of ARV received mother

Source	*df*	SS	MSS	*F*	*P*
Follow-up period (Rows)	3	723,377.61	241,125.87	325.7	<0.001
Columns	3	107,174.18	35,724.73	48.26	<0.001
RXC	9	277,800.75	30,866.75	41.69	<0.001
Error	96	71,071.14	740.32		
Total	111	1,179,423.68			

Table 5.9 results depicted that CD_4 counts at the time of delivery was demonstrated by predictive genetic model for the estimation of heritability and genetic correlation. The source data was collected from the ART center. ANOVA fixed effect model was demonstrated to extrapolate the various genetic parameters. The results demonstrated that the CD_4 counts at the time of delivery were found to be statistically significant ($p < 0.01$, Fisher *F*-37.09). In this study intervention we aimed to assess immunological status ($CD_4 > 350$ micro/dL) at the start of ANCs service and childbirth, comparing HIV positive women with HAART. We then examined predictors of starting ANC with suppressed VL among women received the HAART prolonged duration until childbirth. The results indicated that nearly half of the HIV positive women had lower CD_4 count at the time of delivery, this increased fertility intention among women who started ART before pregnancy.

Table 5.10 results depicted that CD_4 counts at the time of delivery was demonstrated by predictive genetic model for the estimation of heritability and genetic correlation. The source data was collected from the ART center. ANOVA fixed effect model was demonstrated to extrapolate the various genetic parameters. The results indicated that the CD4 counts at the time of delivery were found to be statistically significant ($p < 0.01$, Fisher *F*-5.09).

Despite the success of prevention of mother to child transmission program in Indian context, the (25–38%) HIV prevalence among women of child bearing age requires the PMTCT program to be maximally efficient to sustain gains in the prevention of vertical HIV transmission. We aimed to determine the immunological and virological status at entry (inception) into antenatal care and at childbirth among HIV positive women who conceived under the lower CD_4 count (<350 micro/dL). ART eligibility threshold and universal test

Table 5.9 ANOVA of ARV received mother CD_4 Count at the time of delivery

Source of variation	*df*	Sum of square (SS)	Mean sum of square (MSS)	*F*-variance ratio	Fisher Value @1% level	Fisher value @5% level
CD_4 count follow-up period	6	5,647,864	941,311	37.19** ($P = 0.000$)	2.09	2.80
Error	252	6,377,512	25,308			
Total	258	12,025,376				

Table 5.10 Analysis of variance of CD_4 count (micro/dL) follow-up from inception of HAART to till baby delivery of HIV-infected mother who transfers infection to her child

Source of variation	*df*	Sum of square (SS)	Mean sum of square (MSS)	*F*-variance ratio	Fisher value @1% level	Fisher value @1% level
CD_4 count follow-up period	6	3,291,554	548,592	24.89* ($p = 0.002$)	2.16	2.92
Error	147	3,253,381	22,132			
Total	153	6,544,934				

and treat policies at Global level (Fig. 5.8) show that the inception of HAART mean CD_4 count just <250 micro/dL marginally 60% is less than the global average. The infectivity of MTCT will be drastically increased and pooled with fraction of total proportion estimated by (Basavarajaiah et al. 2012). The detailed analytical intervention is presented in (Figs. 5.8 and 5.9).

Various risk factors of HIV MTCT genetically estimated by the Heritability tool (Table 5.11)

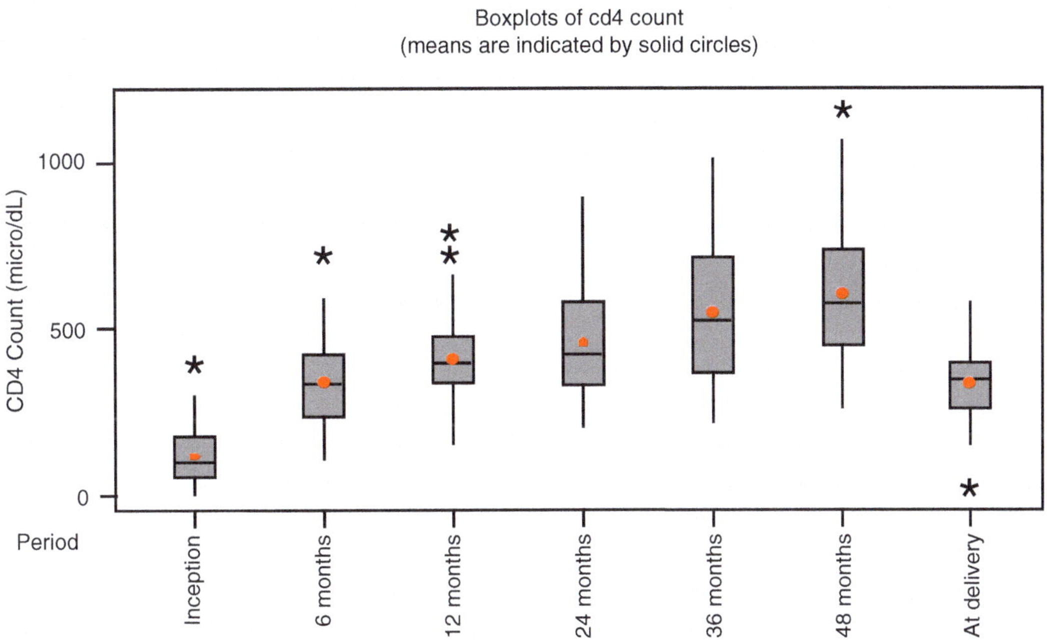

Fig. 5.8 CD_4 mean box plot on HIV-infected mother who does not transfer HIV infection to her child

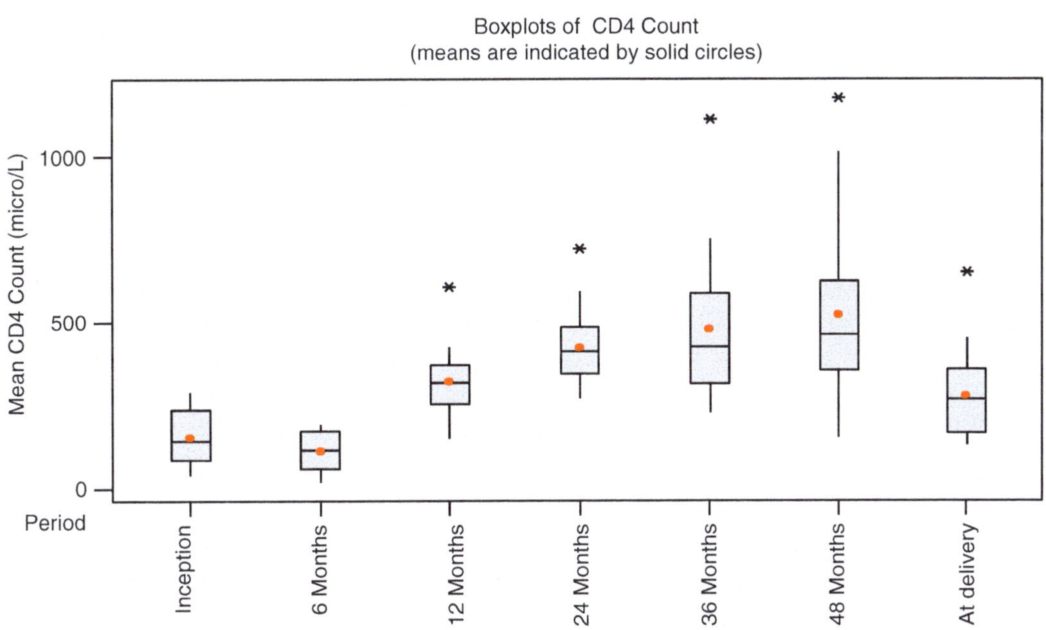

Fig. 5.9 CD_4 mean box plot on HIV-infected mother who transfers HIV infection to her child

Table 5.11 Heritability of risk factors of HIV mother to child transmission (HIVMTCT)

Risk factors	$h^2 \pm$ SE	*P*-value	Augmentation
High Maternal RNA Plasma VL (2.5 × 10^5 copies per mL)	0.36 ± 0.01	≤0.001	Strong
Genital tract VL	0.44 ± 0.00	≤0.001	Medium
Low CD_4Count (<250 micro/dL)	0.12 ± 0.06	≤0.001	Strong
Clinical stage of HIV WHO IV	0.26 ± 0.01	≤0.001	Strong
Unprotected sex with multiple partners	0.23 ± 0.00	≤0.001	Medium
Smoking and substance abuse	0.28 ± 0.03	≤0.001	Medium
Vitamin A	0.39 ± 0.01	≤0.001	Medium
STD's other co-infections	0.17 ± 0.09	≤0.001	Strong
Preterm delivery	0.12 ± 0.00	≤0.001	Strong
Placental disruption	0.33 ± 0.07	≤0.001	Medium
Invasive fetal monitoring	0.39 ± 0.02	≤0.001	Low to Medium
Duration of membrane rapture	0.74 ± 0.09	≥0.001	Low to medium
Vaginal v/s cesarean delivery	0.48 ± 0.03	≤0.001	Medium to strong
Prolonged breast feeding	0.14 ± 0.04	≤0.001	Strong
Breast health	0.69 ± 0.00	≥0.001	Strong
Genetic susceptibility			
HLA genotype	0.11 ± 0.00	≤0.001	Strong
CCR_5 karyotype deletion	0.16 ± 0.01	≤0.001	Strong
Provirus integrated in host genome	0.12 ± 0.00	≤0.001	Strong
HTL V 1-PVL in blood	0.22 ± 0.01	≤0.001	Strong
HTL V 1-PVL in milk	0.26 ± 0.00	≤0.001	Strong
HLA concordance	0.28 ± 0.00	≤0.001	Medium

Table 5.12 Heritability of risk factors of HIV MTCT

Risk factors	$h^2 \pm$ SE	*P*-value	Augmentation
Unplanned pregnancy	0.75 ± 0.0.25	<0.17	Strong
<=11–12 Years of formal education	0.116 ± 0.00	≤0.002	Moderate
First ANC's visit after 20 weeks	0.36 ± 0.03	≤0.00	Moderate
Unknown HIV status prior to index pregnancy	0.20 ± 0.01	≤0.00	Moderate to strong
Lack of literacy	0.85 ± 0.02	≥0.21	Strong
Low income	0.77 ± 0.22	≥0.33	Strong

showed that the risk factors were modelled by mixed effect ANOVA. Heritability was estimated in accordance with SOP, the results of various traits like High Maternal RNA Plasma VL ($h^2 = 0.36 \pm 0.01$) $p < 0.01$; Low CD_4Count (<250 micro/dL) ($h^2 = 0.12 \pm 0.06$) $p < 0.01$; STD's other co-infections ($h^2 = 0.17 \pm 0.09$) $p < 0.01$; Preterm delivery ($h^2 = 0.12 \pm 0.00$) $p < 0.01$; Prolonged Breast feeding ($h^2 = 0.14 \pm 0.04$) $p < 0.01$; Breast health ($h^2 = 0.69 \pm 0.00$) $p < 0.01$; Genetic Susceptibility-HLA genotype; CCR_5 Karyotype deletion $p < 0.01$; Provirus integrated in host Genome $p < 0.01$; HTL V 1-PVL in blood $p < 0.01$; HTL V 1-PVL in milk $p < 0.01$ and HLA Concordance $p < 0.01$ were strongly augmented for HIV mother to child transmission. From Table 5.12 Unplanned pregnancy ($h^2 = 0.75 \pm 0.0.25$) $p = 0.17$; Lack of literacy ($h^2 = 0.85 \pm 0.02$) $p = 0.21$, and low family Income ($h^2 = 0.77 \pm 0.22$) $p = 0.33$ were strongly associated with HIV MTCT, the driven results (Table 5.12) were estimated by the ANOVA fixed effect model.

$$\text{Predicted model for estimation} = \left[11 + \text{expo}^{-(1.66 - 0.0067\times 1 + 0.350\times 2 + 0.21\times 3)}\right]$$

Table 5.13 Matrix of CCR_5 in relation to Progression of HIV

	Progression of HIV			
CCR_5	Rapid	Moderate	Slow	Total
Aa homozygous wild types	20(29.85%)	32(47.76%)	8(11.94%)	60(89.55%)
Aa heterozygous	03(4.47%)	02(2.98%)	1(1.49%)	06(8.95%)
aa homozygous mutant types	00(0.00%)	01(1.49%)	0(0.00%)	01(1.49%)
Total	23(34.32%)	35(52.23%)	09(13.43%)	67(100%)

Table 5.14 CCR_5 in relation to Progression of HIV with various blood group (three-way ANOVA)

	Human blood group			
CCR_5	A	B	AB	O
Aa homozygous wild types	0.32 ± 0.21	0.22 ± 0.00	0.26 ± 0.011	0.48 ± 0.02
Aa heterozygous	0.45 ± 0.12	0.33 ± 0.013	0.17 ± 0.02	0.36 ± 0.00
aa homozygous mutant types	0.32 ± 0.16	0.41 ± 0.036	0.16 ± 0.036	0.22 ± 0.036

A genetic mutation known as CCR_5 delta 32 is responsible for the two types of HIV resistance that exist (Tables 5.13 and 5.14). CCR_5 delta 32 hampers HIVs ability to infiltrate immune cells. The mutation causes the CCR_5 co-receptors on the outside of cells to develop smaller than usual and no longer sit outside of the wall. In this present study intervention, we demonstrate the CCR_5 relation with human blood group OAB. As per the analysis, Aa homozygous wild types were genetically mutant with O blood group ($h^2 = 0.48$) $p < 0.001$ when compared to Aa heterozygous ($h^2 = 0.36$) and aa Homozygous mutant types ($h^2 = 0.22$)

Variable	Coefficient	Standard error	Predicted *P*-value	Odds ratio	95% confidence interval
CD_4 (micro/dL)	−0.0067	0.0033	0.0459	0.9934	(0.9869,0.9999)(0.9869,0.9999)
VL (copies/mL)	0.3503	0.4632	0.4495	1.4195	(0.5726,3.5192)(0.5726,3.5192)
Constant	1.6622	2.1320	0.4356		

HIV virus cell entry relies on binding to the CD_4 receptors and at least one of two possible chemokine co-receptors CCR_5 and RNA plasma viral load is the ability of the virus to bind to a specific co-receptor. The HIV strains that bind to CCR_5 are called R_5 tropic and those that bind $CxCR_4$ and X_4 tropic, dual tropic strains are capable of using either CCR_5 or $CXCR_4$. The CCR_5 is the predominant receptors for HIV cell entry. It is important to note that CD_4 count and RNA plasma viral traits correlating factors in association with CCR_5, transmitted HIV and are predominant during early stage of infection, while HAART history found to be negatively related with CCR_5 receptors. The concept of CCR_5 depleted HIV cells therapy was given credence by the first successful allogenic transplantation with a perfect HLA match from a donor homozygous for the CCR_5 d32 deletion. In this study we demonstrated any significant changes between CCR_5 with respect to cluster differential cell counts and RNA plasma viral load at the time of HIV transmission from mother to child. The serial CD_4 count and RNA plasma VL was demonstrated by using genetic predictive model. The model results showed that negative coefficient between CD_4 (micro/dL) and RNA plasma viral load when CCR_5 predominately binding with R_5 tropic. The serial CD_4 counts range between 356 and >450 microl/dL and VL in correlation with CCR_5 binding with R_5 tropic predictive probability and CI-95% presented in (Table 5.15).

The predicted variable "***y***" errors were estimated based on the sum of the deviation of average ratio to the total errors (in a perfect fit the curve will go right through every Data point: zero deviation). The deviation errors were observed from chi-square distribution (sum of the square of each data point's ratio of deviation to error).

$$\chi^2 = \left(\frac{\Delta_1}{\sigma_1}\right)^2 + \left(\frac{\Delta_2}{\sigma_2}\right)^2 + \left(\frac{\Delta_3}{\sigma_3}\right)^2 + \ldots.. \left(\frac{\Delta_N}{\sigma_N}\right)^2$$

Table 5.15 Probabilities Predicted by the Model

CD_4	VL (log scale)	CCR_5	PP	95% confidence interval
356.0000	3.2000	1	0.6013	(0.3980,0.7747)(0.3980,0.7747)
365.0000	4.4000	1	0.6838	(0.4647,0.8434)(0.4647,0.8434)
347.0000	3.6000	1	0.6481	(0.4697,0.7930)(0.4697,0.7930)
665.0000	3.2000	1	0.1613	(0.0305,0.5402)(0.0305,0.5402)
363.0000	3.3000	1	0.5985	(0.4114,0.7607)(0.4114,0.7607)
458.0000	1.2000	1	0.2750	(0.0329,0.8089)(0.0329,0.8089)
456.0000	3.2000	1	0.4364	(0.2600,0.6306)(0.2600,0.6306)
556.0000	3.6000	0	0.3139	(0.1364,0.5699)(0.1364,0.5699)
365.0000	3.5000	0	0.6120	(0.4437,0.7573)(0.4437,0.7573)
366.0000	3.9000	1	0.6432	(0.4780,0.7802)(0.4780,0.7802)
458.0000	3.8000	0	0.4853	(0.3406,0.6325)(0.3406,0.6325)
566.0000	4.1000	0	0.3377	(0.1429,0.6093)(0.1429,0.6093)
655.0000	4.2300	0	0.2278	(0.0538,0.6048)(0.0538,0.6048)
623.0000	4.6300	0	0.2958	(0.0800,0.6699)(0.0800,0.6699)
354.0000	4.4700	1	0.7045	(0.4692,0.8654)(0.4692,0.8654)
322.0000	4.9600	1	0.7780	(0.4528,0.9369)(0.4528,0.9369)
455.0000	4.4700	0	0.5488	(0.3378,0.7437)(0.3378,0.7437)
456.0000	4.3200	1	0.5341	(0.3452,0.7137)(0.3452,0.7137)
452.0000	4.4400	1	0.5512	(0.3451,0.7410)(0.3451,0.7410)
411.0000	4.3900	0	0.6133	(0.4136,0.7810)(0.4136,0.7810)
436.0000	4.3600	1	0.5705	(0.3779,0.7439)(0.3779,0.7439)
436.0000	4.6300	1	0.5935	(0.3563,0.7939)(0.3563,0.7939)
436.0000	4.4700	1	0.5799	(0.3698,0.7646)(0.3698,0.7646)
444.0000	4.6300	1	0.5806	(0.3436,0.7855)(0.3436,0.7855)
456.0000	3.8900	1	0.4965	(0.3498,0.6438)(0.3498,0.6438)
456.0000	3.8500	1	0.4930	(0.3479,0.6393)(0.3479,0.6393)
456.0000	3.6300	1	0.4738	(0.3285,0.6236)(0.3285,0.6236)
655.0000	3.6400	0	0.1935	(0.0443,0.5536)(0.0443,0.5536)
632.0000	3.3200	0	0.2000	(0.0492,0.5470)(0.0492,0.5470)
558.0000	3.3200	0	0.2904	(0.1142,0.5651)(0.1142,0.5651)
547.0000	3.1400	0	0.2925	(0.1130,0.5729)(0.1130,0.5729)
475.0000	3.1400	0	0.4005	(0.2172,0.6166)(0.2172,0.6166)
365.0000	3.6200	0	0.6220	(0.4593,0.7612)(0.4593,0.7612)
363.0000	3.2000	0	0.5900	(0.3915,0.7630)(0.3915,0.7630)
352.0000	3.1400	0	0.6026	(0.3892,0.7830)(0.3892,0.7830)
341.0000	3.6300	0	0.6596	(0.4764,0.8049)(0.4764,0.8049)
326.0000	3.4700	0	0.6694	(0.4653,0.8249)(0.4653,0.8249)
363.0000	3.6300	0	0.6259	(0.4619,0.7653)(0.4619,0.7653)
341.0000	3.2100	0	0.6258	(0.4124,0.7994)(0.4124,0.7994)
362.0000	3.3300	1	0.6026	(0.4179,0.7621)(0.4179,0.7621)
363.0000	3.4700	1	0.6127	(0.4408,0.7605)(0.4408,0.7605)
363.0000	3.6800	1	0.6300	(0.4670,0.7679)(0.4670,0.7679)
366.0000	3.1700	0	0.5826	(0.3823,0.7589)(0.3823,0.7589)
347.0000	3.6900	1	0.6553	(0.4787,0.7974)(0.4787,0.7974)
342.0000	3.4100	0	0.6405	(0.4471,0.7970)(0.4471,0.7970)
312.0000	3.5200	1	0.6934	(0.4782,0.8480)(0.4782,0.8480)
336.0000	3.6600	1	0.6693	(0.4821,0.8149)(0.4821,0.8149)
385.0000	3.4700	0	0.5774	(0.4196,0.7209)(0.4196,0.7209)
396.0000	3.2300	1	0.5386	(0.3605,0.7073)(0.3605,0.7073)

Table 5.15 (continued)

CD_4	VL (log scale)	CCR_5	PP	95% confidence interval
347.0000	3.5800	1	0.6465	(0.4674,0.7922)(0.4674,0.7922)
363.0000	3.6900	1	0.6308	(0.4679,0.7685)(0.4679,0.7685)
385.0000	3.4700	1	0.5774	(0.4196,0.7209)(0.4196,0.7209)
410.0000	3.2100	0	0.5136	(0.3369,0.6869)(0.3369,0.6869)
411.0000	4.5200	0	0.6240	(0.4029,0.8033)(0.4029,0.8033)
416.0000	4.6300	1	0.6252	(0.3859,0.8158)(0.3859,0.8158)
458.0000	4.7700	0	0.5698	(0.3088,0.7970)

On average we expect each term in the sum to be about unity, so that the total chi-square should be about equal to the number of data points. However, by selecting a fitting-curve with as many adjustable parameters as data points (age, BMI, duration of therapy, etc.), you can usually force the curve to exactly hit every data point to become perfect fit but probably of no significance. Approximately, each adjustable parameter of the curve should allow us to extrapolate on exactly hit one data point. The number of effective data points, i.e., those that could not be automatically hit by the curve, is called the number of degrees of freedom (*df*). Degrees of freedom (*df*) = number of data points − number of adjustable parameters. Above cited data points are exactly fitted by a polynomial with eight adjustable parameters. For example, researcher attempt to know the level of chemical concentration by fitting linear model, fitted model had chemical concentration and absorbance, he would expect a linear relationship between these two variables: that's the Beer-Lambert law. If you were measuring the rate of reaction and the substrate concentration in a simple process catalyzed by an enzyme, we would expect an inverse-inverse relationship between two variables, i.e., the Michaelis–Menten law (Yandell et al. 2007; Zhang et al. 2007; Zou et al. 2007). Based on the Michaelis Menten Law assumption we fitted linear models of various novel regimens of HIV. The following numerical simulation presented in the table matrix.

			Parameter values		
Model	Eqn	Reduced chi-square	*a*	*b*	*c*
Linear	$y = a + bX$	0.93	2.11	157	0
Power	$y = aX^b$	0.85	153	0.911	0
Inverse	$\frac{1}{y} = a + \frac{b}{x}$	0.77	0.002	0.0050	0
Quadratic	$y = a + bx + cx^2$	0.73	−3.7	215	−88

Quadratic model was formulated to know the reduction percentage of CD_4 count responsible for HIV MTCT with various time intervals and follow-up period. The constructed model clearly depicted that X = gestational weeks and $Y = CD_4$ counts. As per the model results, the maximum reduction of cd4 counts was seen in 19th week of gestation followed by 22, 23, and 26th week with mean CD_4 count (356.55 ± 10.25 micro/dL) (Fig. 5.10).

(Table 5.16) showed that the ARV prophylaxis with respect to ANCs eligible for ART was modelled by hierarchical fixed effect model, the HAART drug, namely AZT + 3TC + NVP ($h^2 = 0.44$) $p < 0.01$; AZT + 3TC + EFV ($h^2 = 0.56$) $p < 0.01$; TDF + XTC + NVP ($h^2 = 0.22$) $p < 0.01$; TDF + XTC + NVP ($h^2 = 0.23$) $p < 0.01$; BF population ($h^2 = 0.29$) $p < 0.01$; Daily NVP from birth to 6 weeks ($h^2 = 0.32$) $p < 0.01$; Non BF population ($h^2 = 0.38$) $p < 0.01$; AZT for 6 weeks ($h^2 = 0.18$) $p < 0.01$; NVP for 6 weeks ($h^2 = 0.16$) $p < 0.01$; ddi + ABC ($h^2 = 0.13$) $p < 0.01$, and TDF + 3TC(AZT) ($h^2 = 0.16$) $p < 0.01$, was found to be statistically significant with HIV MTCT, if the mother HAART start at very low CD_4 counts (350 micro/dL) and high RNA plasma VL.

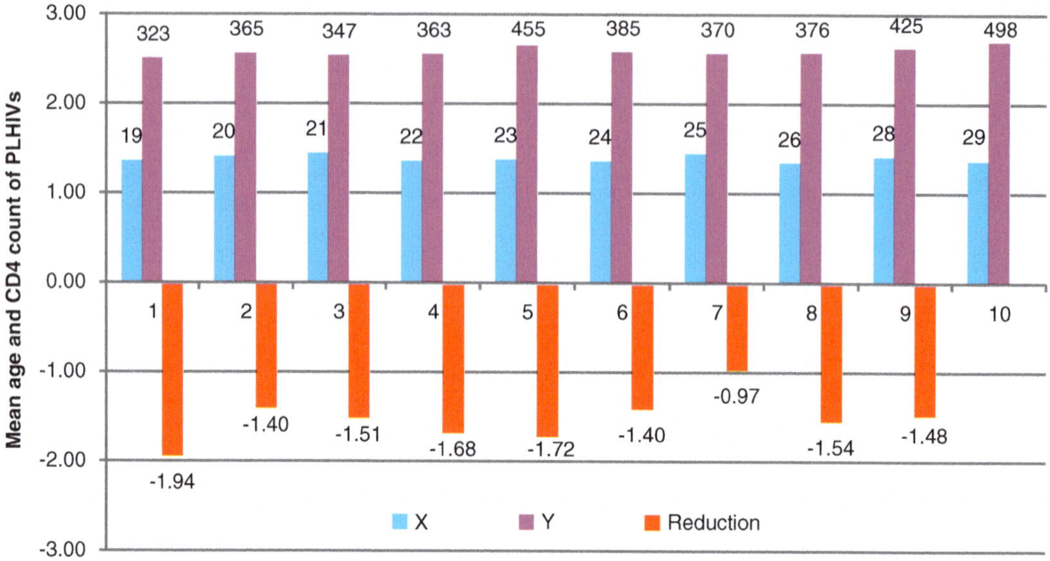

Fig. 5.10 Quadratic model shows error reduction techniques

Table 5.16 ARV prophylaxis ANCs eligible for ART

Mother (regimen)	h^2 (V_A/V_P)	*P*-value
AZT + 3TC + NVP	0.44	≥0.01
AZT + 3TC + EFV	0.56	≥0.01
TDF + XTC + NVP	0.22	≥0.01
TDF + XTC + NVP	0.23	≥0.01
Infants	0.16	≤0.01
BF population	0.29	≥0.01
Daily NVP from birth to 6 weeks	0.32	≥0.01
Non BF population	0.38	≥0.01
AZT for 6 weeks	0.18	≤0.01
NVP for 6 weeks	0.16	≤0.01
II line regimen	0.11	≤0.01
ddi + ABC Or TDF + ABC	0.13	≤0.01
TDF + 3TC(AZT) ddi + ABC ddi + 3 TC	0.16	≤0.01

5.19 Model Discussion

Global rate of mother to child HIV-1 transmission are heterogeneous; estimates range from 14 to 48%. In non-breast feeding population with fewer viral loads, the risk of perinatal transmission rate between 15 and 25%. The variations of transmission may be due to risk factors or to CD_4 and viral load characteristics in specific populations and also to differences in timing of transmission. Although many factors have been associated with an overall increased risk of MTCT, including increased maternal RNA plasma viral load (>3.26 $\log_e 10^4$), CD_4 + T Lymphocyte count, decreased maternal cell mediated immunity, vaginal delivery, prolonged rupture of membrane, prematurity, low birth weight, prolonged breast feeding and prolonged labor were considered as creeping factors for HIV MTCT transmission rate (Strandskov, 1941; 1942; 1950). According to widely used hypothesis, the rate of transmission was determined by new intervened genetic models. The present fitted model revealed that the declined trend of CD_4 count and RNA plasma viral load was at more proximity for HIV transmission ($h^2 = 0.13^*$, $p < 0.001$). The genetic correlation (0.23) and environmental correlation ($h^2 = 0.38$) were found to be statistically significant ($p < 0.001$) with HIV transmission. At the time of inception of HAART, the viral load was relatively more and laid down by the immunity of the mother. In (Tables 5.8 and 5.9) it is depicted the follow-up CD_4 count and RNA plasma viral load and the heritability estimates expressed lower values and were found to be statistically significant ($p < 0.001$), when compared to transmission rate. (Schneider et al. 2007) reported that maternal lower CD_4 count (<250 micro/dL) and high plasma RNA viral load (3.80 $\log_e 10 \times 10^6$) at the time of delivery was a risk factor for HIV transmission and also decreased maternal cell mediated immunity was associated with perinatal transmission and hypothesized to be risk factors for in utero transmission. The present study concludes that the lower CD_4 cells at the time of inception of HAART was more significantly ($p < 0.05$) associated with increased risk of transmission ($h^2 = 0.18$, $p = 0.00$) which further supported the hypothesis that maternal immunosuppression at delivery was a risk factor for intrapartum transmission. This study confirmed that approximately (30–40%) of HIV-infected infants were infected by mother with lower CD_4 count and high RNA plasma viral load, this is because maternal viral load should be amenable to direct intervention. Similar study reported by (Schneider et al. 2007) concluded that the cell-mediated immunity was correlated with increased vertical transmission. The cell-mediated immunity may directly influence transmission or may be a surrogate marker for maternal viral load. As per his fitted logistic regression model prolonged breast feeding, lower CD_4 count and high plasma viral load, prematurity, low birth weight, maternal immunity, and deficiency of vitamin C were significantly ($p < 0.001$) associated with HIV transmission. Another European collaborative study (2009) suggested that HIV–RNA dynamics over pregnancy differs by time, type of HAART therapy, drug adherence, and WHO clinical stage.

5.20 Robustness of Genetic Model

The model robustness was tested by using maximum likelihoods (MLEs). Fitted model in the present study was found to be more MLEs (−2loglikelihood was 120.16), it signifies the new intervened and the fitted model was considered as best fit ($R^2 = 90.63\%$). The fitted model was showed to be more positivity for estimation of heritability (h^2) and genetic correlation. The assumption of the model can be easy to estimate the interaction effects with respect to different biological and laboratory parameters. The homogeneity of both variables, CD_4 count and RNA plasma viral load were tested with analysis of Variance (ANOVA) was statistically significant ($p < 0.001$) and observations were normally distributed.

5.21 Modelling on RNA Plasma Viral Load and CD_4 Count (micro/dL)

5.21.1 Linear Model

CD_4 count and RNA plasma viral load were varied parameters. The series of data matrix was not always stationeries instead, the parameters will make changes on ANC's population based on body condition, OI's and drug adherence. This pattern was observed by using linear model fitting:

$$Y_{t=0-56\,\text{months}} = \alpha + \beta^t,$$

where t = interval of time (Inception of HAART to 56 months)

α = intercept and β = Slope of the curve

5.21.2 Exponential Model

$$Y_{t=0-56\,\text{months}} = ce^{kt} \quad k > 0$$

where C = initial value increases without bound to asymptotic to Y

5.21.3 Logarithmic Model

The logarithmic model was developed to know the monotonicity of CD_4 count and RNA Plasma viral load.

$$Y_{t=0-56\,\text{months}} = a + b\ln(x)$$

where t = interval of time (Inception of HAART to 56 months)

α = intercept and β = Slope of the curve

5.21.4 Power Model

The power model used to know the strength of the relation between follow-up CD_4 count RNA plasma viral load. The model distributed a wide range of magnitude; these include size of the population and scale invariance.

$Y_{t=0-56\text{ months}} = \alpha X^{\beta}$, Take log on both sides

Log Yt = Log $\alpha + \beta$ log X, Finally, the power model becomes

$$Y_{t=0-56\,\text{months}} = e^{\alpha+\beta X}$$

5.22 Conclusion

This chapter is necessary to the subject of various statistical methods, formulated methods demonstrated with real data sets of clinical and medical research. The basic principles and practical applications of genetic statistics is briefly explained with suitable illustrations and mathematical derivations. Demonstrated models are very useful for derivations of new genetic algorithms of therapeutic, study and state space of drug development process and is also very suitable for early identification of rare genetic disorder, evidence based medicine for cancer and life threatened diseases line HIV/AIDS, Azimer, etc. Newer simulation techniques were also derived to extrapolate the genetic complexity of drug to drug, drug to food, and drug to environmental interactions. The subjective of interactive effects of Hardy–Weinberg equilibrium law is determined to know the threshold level, heritability and repeatability by using Gauss Markova optimization technique. The drive demonstrated that newer methods or models are very useful for the human geneticists, drug developers, and research beginners for the formulation of new research hypothesis in medical, clinical, and interdisciplinary life science.

References

Abecasis GR (2000) GOLD—graphical overview of linkage disequilibrium. Bioinformatics 16:182–183
Abney M, McPeek MS, Ober C (2000) Estimation of variance components of quantitative traits in inbred populations. Am J Hum Genet 66:62
Almasy L, Blangero J (1998) Multipoint quantitative-trait linkage analysis in general pedigrees. Am J Hum Genet 62:1198–1211
Anderson E (1936) The species problem in Iris. Ann Missouri Bot Garden 23:457–509
Aulchenko YS, De Koning DJ, Haley C (2007) Genomewide rapid association using mixed model and regression: a fast and simple method for genome-wide pedigree-based quantitative trait loci association analysis. Genetics 177:577–585
Basavarajaiah D M, Leelavathy B, Narasimhamurthy B, Maheshappa K, Shetty I J. Prevalence of Smoking and Health Consequences of Tobacco Use in HIV – Positive Clients in Karnataka State. Int.J. Engineering Science and Innovative Technology 2012;1(6):67–72
Basavarajaiah D DM,Leelavathy B, Prabhakar B,Chandrashekar P. Neural Network Modeling in HIV/AIDS –Five Years Survival Cohort Data. In.J. Engineering Science and Innovative Technology 2012;1(2):86–94
Basavarajaiah D M, Narasimhamurthy B, Leelavathy B. Comparative analysis of Survival and Growth Model approach in Relation to CD4 Count in HIV Positive Pregnant Women.Int.J.General Medicine and Pharmacy 2013;2(2):1–10
Bernardo R (1995) Genetic models for predicting maize single-cross performance in unbalanced yield trial data. Crop Sci 35:141–147
Bittner M, Meltzer P, Trent J (1999) Data analysis and integration: of steps and arrows. Nat Genet 22:213–215
Boerjan W, Vuylsteke M (2009) Integrative genetical genomics in Arabidopsis. Nat Genet 41:144–145
Boorman KE (1950) An analysis of the blood types and clinical conditions 2000 consecutive mothers and their infants. Ann Eugenics 15:120–134
Castle WE (1903) The law of heredity of Galton and Mendel and some laws governing race improvements by selection. Proc Am Acad Arts Sci 39:223–242
Chen Z, Chen H (2005) On some statistical aspects of the interval mapping for QTL detection. Stat Sin 157:909–925
Churchill GA, Doerge RW (2008) Naive application of permutation testing leads to inflated type I error rates. Genetics 178:609–610
Cotterman CW (1941) Relatives and human genetic analysis. Sci Mon 53:227–234
Darvasi A, Weinreb A, Minke V, Weller JI, Soller M (1993) Detecting marker-QTL linkage and estimating QTL gene effect and map location using a saturated genetic map. Genetics 134:943–951
Erhardt V (2010) Locating multiple interacting quantitative trait loci with the zero-inflated generalized Poisson regression. Stat Appl Genet Mol Biol 3:48–51
Foster SD, Verbyla ADP, Pitchford WS (2007) Incorporating LASSO effects into a mixed model for quantitative trait loci detection. J Agric Biol Environ Stat 12:300–314
George AW, Mengersen KL, Davis GP (2000) Localization of a quantitative trait locus via a Bayesian approach. Biometrics 56:40–51
Goffinet B, Gerber S (2000) Quantitative trait loci: a meta-analysis. Genetics 155:463–473

Haldane JBS, Waddington CH (1931) Inbreeding and linkage. Genetics 16:357

Henshalla JM, Goddard ME (1999) Multiple-trait mapping of quantitative trait loci after selective genotyping using logistic regression. Genetics 151:885–894

Hernandez J, Knott S (2009) Haplotyping via minimum recombinant paradigm. BMC Proc 3:S7

Jansen RC, Stam P (1994) High resolution of quantitative traits into multiple loci via interval mapping. Genetics 136:1447–1455

Jeffery WR (2010) Pleiotropy and eye degeneration in cavefish. Heredity 3:98–91. https://doi.org/10.1038/hdy.2010.7

Moree R (1950) A modification of the Hardy Weinberg law. Science 111:691–692

Rife DC (1951) A method of gene frequency analysis to the interpretation of data from twins. Hum Biol 22:136–145

Schneider A, Dessimoz C, Gonnet GH (2007) OMA Browser—exploring orthologous relations across 352 complete genomes. Bioinformatics (Oxford, England) 23:2180–2182

Sen S, Churchill GA (2001) A statistical framework for quantitative trait mapping. Genetics 159:371–387

Stern C (1943) The Hardy Weinberg law. Science 97:137–138

Stevens WL (1938) Estimation of blood groups gene frequencies. Ann Eugen 8:362–375

Stevens WL (1950) Statistical analysis of the ABO blood groups. Hum Biol 22:191–217

Strandskov HH (1941) The distribution of human genes. Sci Mon 52:203–215

Strandskov HH (1942) The genetic of human population. Am Nat 76:156–164

Strandskov HH (1950) Genetics and the origin and evolution of man. Cold Spring Harb Symp Quant Biol 15:1–11

Yandell BS, Mehta T, Banerjee S, Shriner D, Venkataraman R, Moon JY, Neely WW, Wu H, von Smith R (2007) Yi R/qtlbim: QTL with Bayesian Interval Mapping in experimental crosses. Bioinformatics (Oxford, England) 23:641–643

Zhang Z, Todhunter RJ, Buckler ES, Van Vleck LD (2007) Technical note: use of marker-based relationships with multiple-trait derivative-free restricted maximal likelihood. J Anim Sci 85:881–885

Zou W, Aylor DL, Zeng ZB (2007) eQTL Viewer: visualizing how sequence variation affects genome-wide transcription. BMC Bioinformatics 8:7

6 Statistical Implications for Estimation of Genetic Traits in Human Vaccine Trials

6.1 Introduction

In most of the developing countries, substantially large proportion of subjects are infected with tubercle bacilli or leprosy bacilli, but of those infected, less than (10%) develop overt disease during their life time (Altman 2012; Childs and Der Kaloustian 1968a, b; Curnow and Smith 1975). This is because of the inherent immunity in the host, which is more likely to be influenced by genetic traits, socioeconomic and cultural factors, etc. (Daum 1987). Though almost all illnesses or diseases are genetically influenced or determined, the diseases such as schizophrenia, asthma, cleft lip and cleft palate, pyloric stenosis (congenital), ankle lowering spondylitis, clubfoot, coronary artery, hypertension, dislocation of hip, anencephaly of spina bifida, peptic ulcer, and congenital heart disorders. The infections are already listed as affected by genetic or hereditary traits and environmental factors (Ederer and Mantel 1974). The interface of genetics and epidemiology is very important to examine how epidemiologists and geneticists envision the role of genetic factors in disease causation (Khoury et al. 1986). More number of research intervention in this direction is warranted, particularly in the context of malaria where there are reports suggesting that the genetic marker (Duffy-negative antigen) will prevent protection against P. vivax infection in American Blacks and Africans, approximately 70–90% of them have this antigen (Spencer et al. 1978) and several studies reported that the malaria vaccine is in the offing. Some genetic markers were associated with malaria, and they have also been reported in tribal population in India, but the evidence is 0 and 12% (Vasantha et al. 1982). On the other hand, there is evidence to suggest that genetically distinct serotypes produce human papillomavirus infection, a significant risk factor for cervical cancer (Katz et al. 1978; Musser et al. 1990). In this context, both preventive and therapeutic vaccines are being targeted (Vasantha et al. 1982). Evaluation of protective vaccine efficacy (VE) in the field for diseases affected partially by hereditary or genetic traits will be tricky. The study designs, viz. cohort and case-control for field evaluation of vaccine efficacy suggested earlier by (Marks et al. 1982) results shows hold good they will not take care of the cases that can be considered as partly due to genetic traits and the rest due to environmental factors. The incidence due to environmental factors could be manipulated by vaccination. In this situation, one is interested to estimate the protective vaccine efficacy with a predetermined narrow confidence interval for the estimated vaccine efficacy. Further, the statistical implications on determining the sample size for estimating at 95% confidence interval (CI) to demonstrate estimated vaccine efficacy in given length of time and relative standards to

B. D. M., B. Narasimha Murthy, *Design of Experiments and Advanced Statistical Techniques in Clinical Research*, https://doi.org/10.1007/978-981-15-8210-3_6

itself need to be solved. In this chapter, we suggested that the method for the estimation of vaccine efficacy and its 95% CI in the presence of genetic traits causing the specific disease in the community. Simultaneously, we compared the computed variance in association with assumed values of VE ranging from 40 to 80%. We also formulated a method for the computation of sample size required to estimate at 95% CI for vaccine efficacy with a pre-specified degree of relative precision. The conclusion of the resulting sample sizes to those required for conducting vaccine trials in the communities with no genetic traits. Taking the range of reported frequencies of genetic marker in the community of malaria, extrapolate the results and implications on the estimated variance with defined sample size. In case of vaccine trials with assumed levels of VE ranging from 40 to 80%. In real-life example, we estimated efficacy of haemophilus influenzae type B of polysaccharide vaccine in Finnish children aged between 24 and 35 months as 79.9% with the reported variation of human influenza due to genetic diversity ranging from 0 to 64% considered for model settings.

6.2 Estimation of Vaccine Efficacy in the Presence of Genetic Traits

Before conducting the vaccine trial at community level, we screened the entire population to know the disease condition. The disease-free population was grouped randomly into two or more groups depending upon the number of vaccines to be tested for their efficacy in the field and the effective duration of the trial. The number of patients to be recruited in each group into the trial depends heavily on the time period of the study. In this research intervention, we assumed two groups, viz. vaccinated and unvaccinated, which are to be observed for fixed time of equal intervals. Let I_u and I_ϑ be the probabilities of experiencing disease in the sample cohorts of "unvaccinated" and "vaccinated" group, respectively. Let "M" be the number of cases due to genetic traits in the community. Let the relative risk be $RR = I_\vartheta \div I_u$ so that the vaccine efficacy (VE) is defined as $(1 - RR)$. Let $\beta = \ln RR$. Let "ψ" be the RR in the absence of genetic traits (Orenstein et al. 1985; Orenstein et al. 1985; O'Neill et al. 1985).

6.3 Formulation of the Model

We consider n_1 and n_2 to be the individuals in the sample cohorts of "vaccinated" and "unvaccinated" groups, respectively. Each case of disease due to genetic and nongenetic traits was observed separately. The cases in "vaccinated" and "unvaccinated" sample cohorts were displayed in Table 6.1; "m_1" and "m_2" were the observed number of cases in the sample cohorts of "vaccinated" and "unvaccinated" groups, respectively. It was observed from (Table 6.1) that the number of cases $(y - m_2)$ in the unvaccinated cohort has reduced to $(x - m_1)$ due to vaccination.

6.4 Estimation of VE (σ^2) in the Presence of Genetic Traits

The estimation of relative risk (RR) in the presence of genetic traits was modeled in the following manner:

$$R\hat{R} = \frac{\hat{I}_\upsilon}{\hat{I}_u} = \frac{(x - m_1) \div n_1}{(y - m_2) \div n_2} \tag{6.1}$$

Table 6.1 Model formulation metrics cases and control (cohort study)

Group	Cases	Non-cases		Total
Vaccinated	m_1	$x - m_1$	$n_1 - x$	n_1
Unvaccinated	m_2	$y - m_2$	$n_2 - y$	n_2
Total	$m_1 + m_2$	$x + y - m_1 - m_2$	$n_1 + n_2 - x - y$	n

The estimated VE in the presence of genetic traits VE = (1 − *RR*)

$$\mathrm{VE} = 1 - \frac{\left(x-\hat{M}\right)/n_1}{\left(y-\hat{M}\right)/n_2} \tag{6.2}$$

Usually, the sample sizes n_1 and n_2 in RCTs are nearly equal. Without loss of generality, *I* assume $n_1 = n_2$.

$$\mathrm{VE} = \frac{y-x}{y-\hat{M}} = \frac{1-\hat{\psi}}{1-\hat{\theta}} \text{ where } \hat{\theta} = \frac{\hat{M}}{y} = \left(1-\hat{\psi}\right)\left(1-\hat{\theta}\right)^{-1} > \left(1-\hat{\psi}\right) \tag{6.3}$$

If $Y = f\ (X_i,\ Y_i)$, the estimated unknown parameters become $Y \sim N(\theta, X)$, where θ is unknown parameters and X is the random variable subjected to normally distributed with mean μ and σ^2

$$\sigma^2 = \frac{1}{n}\sum_{i=1}^{n}\left(X_i - \bar{X}_i\right)^2, \mu = \frac{\sum_{i=1}^{n} X_i}{N}.$$

The correlation between dependent and independent variable at massive data sets, the equation becomes

$$r_{xy} = \frac{\mathrm{cov}(x,y)}{v(x)v(y)}, -1 \le rxy \le 1,$$

where $r_{xy} = \theta\ r_{xy} = 0$. There is no correlation between dependent and independent variables.

If $\hat{\theta} = 0$, then $VE = 1 - \hat{\psi}$ original vaccine efficacy in the absence of genetic traits.

Since $0 \le \sigma^2 \le 1$, $1 - \psi \le 1 - \theta \Rightarrow \psi \ge \theta$.

It is clear from the above relationship that θ can be 0 but cannot be 1 while evaluating vaccine efficacy.

95% confidence interval (CI) for the VE is estimated as follows:

The estimate of β, i.e.,

$$\hat{\beta} = \ln(RR) = \ln\left[\frac{\hat{\psi}-\hat{\theta}}{1-\hat{\theta}}\right] = \ln(\psi - \theta) - \ln(1-\theta).$$

By Taylor's expansion

$$\beta = \ln\psi - \theta \div \psi - \ln(1-\theta)\ln\psi - \frac{\hat{\theta}}{\psi} - \ln(1-\theta), \tag{6.4}$$

vaccine trials usually involve large sample sizes and for large samples, $\hat{\beta}$ is asymptotically normally distributed with variance given by

$$\text{Variance} = \frac{n_1-(x-m_1)}{n_1(x-m_1)} + \frac{n_2-(y-m_2)}{n_2(y-m_2)} - \frac{1}{x-m_1} - \frac{1}{n_1} + \frac{1}{y-m_2} - \frac{1}{n_2}$$
$$\frac{1}{x-m_1} + \frac{1}{y-m_2} = \frac{1}{x} + \frac{m_1}{x(x-m_1)} + \frac{1}{y} + \frac{m_2}{y(y-m_2)} > \frac{1}{x} + \frac{1}{y} \tag{6.5}$$

σ^2 in the presence of genetic traits is more than the variance in the absence of genetic traits by a quantity equal to $\frac{m_1}{x(x-m_1)} + \frac{m_2}{y(y-m_2)}$.

Though there are several methods for the computation of the confidence intervals for the ratio of two binomial outcomes, we have chosen the procedure for the estimation of the 95% CI based on the log of the ratio of two binomial variables as suggested by Katz et al. (1978) because it is simple and the resulting confidence intervals are symmetrical in the log scale. This procedure can also be approximated to the procedure based on the assumption that counts follow a Poisson distribution as proposed by Ederer and Mantel (1974). The 95% CI for VE can be obtained by deriving first the 95% CI for *RR* and then subtract these limits of *RR* from 1. The 95% CI for β will be $\hat{\beta} \pm z\hat{\sigma}$, where z is the normal deviate corresponding to $(1 - \alpha)$ percentage point.

95% CI for $RR = \exp\left(\widehat{\beta} \pm z\widehat{\sigma}\right)$

95% CI for VE is

$$\left[1-\exp\left(\widehat{\beta}+z\widehat{\sigma}\right) \& 1-\exp\left(\widehat{\beta}-z\widehat{\sigma}\right)\right] \quad (6.6)$$

The 95% CI for VE is asymmetric about the point estimate of VE, the lower and upper limits being 1-exp (β + $z\sigma$) and 1 − exp (β − $z\sigma$), respectively.

6.4.1 Absolute Width

The absolute width of the 95% CI for VE is the difference between the upper and lower limits, viz.

$$\exp\left(\widehat{\beta}+z\widehat{\sigma}\right)-\exp\left(\widehat{\beta}-z\widehat{\sigma}\right)=\exp\widehat{\beta}\left\{\exp z\widehat{\sigma}-\exp\left(-z\widehat{\sigma}\right)\right\}=\exp\widehat{\beta}\,\left(e^{\hat{d}}-\overline{e}^{\hat{d}}\right), \quad (6.7)$$

where $d = z\widehat{\sigma}$

6.4.2 Relative Width (*R*)

The relative width is the ratio of absolute width of the 95% CI of VE to itself. For example, relative width equal to *R*% means that the total width of the confidence interval for VE is *R*% of the magnitude of the point estimate of VE. The detailed description of the concept of relative width for VE is given in the paper by O'Neill and is omitted here.

Therefore,

$$R=\frac{\exp\widehat{\beta}\,\left\{e^{\hat{d}}-\overline{e}^{\hat{d}}\right\}}{1-\exp\widehat{\beta}}=\frac{\left(\widehat{\psi}-\hat{\theta}\right)\left(e^{\hat{d}}-\overline{e}^{\hat{d}}\right)}{1-\widehat{\psi}}, \quad (6.8)$$

where $e^{\hat{d}}=\dfrac{R\left(1-\hat{\psi}\right)\pm\sqrt{R^2\left(1-\hat{\psi}\right)^2+4\left(\hat{\psi}-\hat{\theta}\right)^2}}{2\left(\hat{\psi}-\hat{\theta}\right)}$

Since $e^{\hat{d}}$ should always be positive, the above expression can be written as

$$e^{\hat{d}}=\frac{R\left(1-\hat{\psi}\right)+\sqrt{R^2\left(1-\hat{\psi}\right)^2+4\left(\hat{\psi}-\hat{\theta}\right)^2}}{2\left(\hat{\psi}-\hat{\theta}\right)} \quad (6.9)$$

$R = 0.5$ for VE = 0.8 means that 95% CI of VE has width 0.40.

6.4.3 Sample Size Required to Estimate 95% CI of a Given Relative Width for VE

Assume equal numbers in each of the vaccinated and unvaccinated cohorts. Solving for "*n*" from equations given by Eq. (6.2) and $d = z\sigma$, the expression for computation of sample size is given by

$$n=\left(\frac{Z}{\hat{d}}\right)^2\left\{\frac{1}{\hat{I}_\vartheta}+\frac{1}{\hat{I}_{\text{u}}}-2\right\}$$

$$=\left(\frac{Z}{\hat{d}}\right)^2\left\{1+\frac{1-\hat{\theta}}{\left(\hat{\psi}-\hat{\theta}\right)\hat{I}_{\text{u}}}+\frac{1}{\hat{I}_{\text{u}}}-2\right\}$$

$$\left(\frac{Z}{\hat{d}}\right)^2\left\{\left(1+\frac{1-\hat{\theta}}{\hat{\psi}-\hat{\theta}}\right)\div\hat{I}_{\text{u}}-2\right\}$$

In the absence of genetic traits for the disease occurrence, the above expression (ϑ) for the computation of required sample size will reduce to

$$=\frac{z^2}{\hat{d}^2}\left[\frac{\left(1+{}^{1}\!/\!_{\hat{\psi}}\right)}{\hat{I}_{\text{u}}}-2\right]$$

6.5 Estimation of VE in the Presence of Genetic Traits

Suppose the true VE is 80%. If the disease is not influenced by genetic traits, i.e., $\theta = 0$, then the resulting VE is same as 80%, from expression (6.3). On the other hand, if $\theta = 10\%$ (since $\psi = 0.2$ should be greater than θ), the VE = 0.80 ÷ 0.90 = 0.89 or 89%.

If $\theta = 5\%$, then VE = 0.80 ÷ 0.95 = 0.84 or 84%.

If $\theta = 20\%$, then VE = 0.8 ÷ 0.8 = 100%. Similarly, the resulting estimates of VE for θ ranging from 0 to 40% for assumed levels of VE can be worked out. To estimate from Eq. (6.3), the vaccine efficacy in the presence of genetic traits, an investigator must specify the assumed values of the vaccine efficacy with which the trial is initiated and the estimate of θ. The estimated value of θ is determined by conducting literature survey on the extent of genetic markers/genetic structure in the disease of interest. The estimated vaccine efficacy in the presence of genetic traits for assumed levels of vaccine efficacy ranging from 40 to 80% and possible values of the genetic component (θ) ranging from 0 to 60% were worked out. The estimated VE can change dramatically as a function of θ. The estimated VE increases in the presence of genetic traits (Tindle et al. 1987). The extent of escalation is dependent upon the estimated value of θ and the absolute value of the assumed VE. The 95% CI for the estimated VE in the presence of genetic traits for a given relative width (R) can be estimated from the equation. To comprehend better the concept of 95% CI of the estimated VE, the widths of the 95% CI for assumed values of VE = 50% and 80%, for $R = 1$ and 0.1 and for possible values of $\theta = 0$, 0.05, 0.1, 0.2, 0.3, and 0.4 were observed. It was evident that there exists change in the location as well as asymmetry of the 95% CI over the point estimate of VE. The extent of asymmetry depends upon the level of relative width, the level of assumed VE, and the possible value of θ. The investigator needs to specify (1) the level of significance, (2) the assumed incidence rate in the unvaccinated cohort (I_u), the assumed level of VE, the desired width "w" of the CI, and the possible value of genetic component. The value of "d" for a given relative width, assumed level of VE, and for a given θ is obtained by solving equation when the expected value is substituted for the observed value. The sample size can be estimated using either absolute width or relative width. The sample size required for each of the unvaccinated and vaccinated cohorts for estimating 95% CI of assumed VE (40, 50, 60, 70, and 80%) with disease incidence $I_u = 0.005$, relative width (R) = 0.5 for possible values of θ were worked out. The sample size required to achieve a confidence interval of a fixed pre-specified width and for a given incidence rate in the control cohort can change substantially as a function of the genetic component (θ) and the level of VE. It was observed that as the assumed level of VE increases the sample required for vaccinated and unvaccinated cohort decreases. Further, for assumed level of vaccine efficacy the sample required for each of the vaccinated and unvaccinated cohorts also decreases as the value of genetic component increases. The extent of decrease in the numbers depends upon the value of genetic component θ. Consideration of the genetic component while planning the trials results in savings in sample size for each of the vaccinated and unvaccinated cohorts (Rabinovich et al. 1999; Segre et al. 2005). Sample sizes required for each of the vaccinated and unvaccinated cohorts for 95% confidence intervals for VE for an assumed VE of 50%, for a specified relative width of 0.5, for selected assumed values of incidence rates in the unvaccinated cohort, and for possible values of θ, the lower the incidence rate the larger the sample size for all possible values of θ. However, whatever be the value of θ, the percentage increase is same. On the other hand, for a given incidence rate in the unvaccinated cohort the required sample size for each of the unvaccinated and vaccinated cohort decreases as the genetic component θ increases. Again, the percentage decrease is same for all values of I_u. Sample sizes required for estimating 95% CI of VE = 50% for selected pre-specified relative widths are observed. It was noticed that the less the relative width the more the sample size and more the genetic component the lesser the required sample size.

6.6 Components of Genetic Variance

The total genetic variance for a character V_g is function of Additive genetic variance + Dominant genetic variance + epistatic variance

$$V_G = V_A + V_D + V_E.$$

6.7 Additive Genetic Variation

The genetic variance is defined as the genetic character which can be transferred from generation to generation without cause of mutation, e.g., Father's eye is highly correlated to son's eye. Certain diseases like cancer and Huntington genetic disorder are the best examples for genetic variance. Genetic variance (Vg) is controlled by drug trial experimentation in evidence based medicine for treating the exposed population at an early stage. The additive variation is caused due to additive factors or (Va) variations, and so many examples are cited by the Genetist for deriving the additive effect (Va). In case of clinical trial experimentation, an additive effect is the most prime factor to control certain genetic characters, e.g., height, obesity, and skin texture of the person. Especially, the novel drug trial, drug is sensitivity is important rather than the dosage of formulation. Nevirapine drug is sensitive to the skin of HIV-infected patients. Even after drug trial, we have seen many incumbent side effects of the patients (long-term therapy). The side effects of HIV infected patients after drug trail which is being controlled by management of patients, and early screening of side effects and food intake is the key factor to control the additive genetic variance. It is associated with homozygosis, and therefore it is expected to be maximum in self-pollinating crops and minimum in cross-pollinating crops. The GCA governed by the effect of a parent is measured of additive gene effects. Additive genetic variance gets depleted proportionate to the improvement made by recruitment of respondents for drug trials.

6.8 Dominance Genetic Variation

It refers to the deviation from the additive scheme of a gene action resulting from intra-allelic interaction, i.e., interaction between alleles of the same gene or same locus. The relation of variation-related dominance among alleles is denoted as V_D. It refers to the deviation from the additive schemes of gene action, resulting from intra-allelic interaction. The feature of dominance variance is a measure of gene action. Such genes show incomplete dominance, complete dominance, or over dominance. Heterozygote does not effect the mean value of two parents of a particular characters. In case of clinical trial experimentation, certain characters or attributes do not correlate with dominance effect and also are closely approximated with recessive characters. The dominance variance is associated for controlling heterozygosity, and therefore it is expected to the maximum crossbreed population, for example, male or female married different religion and minimum in self-bred population, for example, the male and female married within the family. The dominance variance is the chief cause of heterosis or hybrid vigor (the progeny performance of offspring is more than the parents) (Parkhomenko E et al. 2009). The height of son is more than parent's height (hybrid vigor). The dominance variance is depleted through selfing or inbreeding. In natural breeding population, dominance variance is always lesser than the additive variance.

6.9 Epistatic Genetic Variation (V_I)

Variation is due to interaction among loci; it is a measure of epistatic gene action. Epistatic gene is of three types: AA, AD, and DD.

AA—is fixable; the interaction among two or more loci each exhibiting lack of dominance individually, e.g., the Stavudine normal regimen has delirious effect on HIV-infected population in the form of rashes, Steven–Johnson syndrome, and depletion of cd4 counts.

AD—interaction among two or more loci is non-fixable.

DD—interaction of two or more loci each exhibiting dominance individually is non-fixable.

The phenotypic variance is the component of genetic and environmental variance.

$$\sigma^2_{\mathrm{P}} = \sigma^2_{\mathrm{G}} + \sigma^2_{\mathrm{E}}$$

$$\sigma^2_{\mathrm{P}} = \sigma^2_{\mathrm{A}} + \sigma^2_{\mathrm{D}} + \sigma^2_{\mathrm{I}} + \sigma^2_{\mathrm{E.}}$$

σ^2_{P} = Phenotypic variance; σ^2_{A} = Additive genetic variance

$\sigma^2_{\mathrm{D}} + \sigma^2_{\mathrm{I}}$ = Nonadditive genetic variance; σ^2_{E} = Environmental variance

The genetic parameter of heritability was estimated by the quotient of V_g and V_p

$$h^2 = \frac{V_g}{V_p} = \frac{\hat{\sigma}^2_{\text{genetic}}}{\hat{\sigma}^2_{\text{genetic}} + \hat{\sigma}^2_{\text{Environmental}}}$$

In case of homoscedasticity data sets, the ANOVA tabulation was calculated as σ^2_g

$\sigma^2_g = \frac{(\mathrm{MSG} - \mathrm{MSE})}{r}$, where MSG is the mean square with respect to genetic component, MSE is mean square error, and r is the number of replication.

$$\sigma^2_p = \frac{(\mathrm{MSG})}{r}, \sigma^2_e = \frac{(\mathrm{MSE})}{r}$$

$$h^2 = \frac{\sigma^2_g}{\sigma^2_p}; \mathrm{PCV} = \frac{\sqrt{\sigma^2_p}}{\overline{X}} \times 100 \text{ and } \mathrm{GCV} = \frac{\sqrt{\sigma^2_g}}{\overline{X}} \times 100\,;$$

One of the most important questions we can put to the reader to understand evolutionary, climatic changes is how the phenotypes of parents and their offsprings are related (Tables 6.2 and 6.3). We already described the phenotypic effect on drug trial experimentation and how to deal with genetic variation when each generation or with varied population structure, phenotypic variance is deleterious effect of quotient of environmental and nonadditive genetic effects, when each generation there is re assortment of the gene into new genotypes and how much of the phenotypes of a traits is heritable via transmission of gene. Many scientists classified the genetic variance into different ways

Authors	Types of V_g	Brief description
Fisher (1918)	Additive Dominance Epistatic	Average effect of genes on all segregating loci Deviation from mean value due to intra-allelic interaction Deviation from mean value due to nonallelic interaction. It is of three types: AA, AD, and DD
Wright (1935)	Additive and Nonadditive	Same as given by R.A. Fisher It includes dominance and epistatic variance
Mather (1949)	Heritable–Fixable Heritable–Non-Fixable	It includes dominance and AA component of epitasis Includes DD, AD, and AA

Table 6.2 Comparative genome sizes of organisms

Organisms	Size (BP)	Gene number	Average gene density	Chromosome number
Homosapiens	3.2 billion	–25,000	1 gene/100,000 bases	46[a]
Mus musculus (mouse)	2.6 billion	–25,000	1 gene/100,000 bases	40[a]
Drosophila melanogaster (Fruit fly)	137 billion	13,000	1 gene/9000 bases	8
Arabidopsis thaliana (plant)	100 billion	25,000	1 gene/4000 bases	10
Caenorhabditis elegans (roundworm)	97 billion	19,000	1 gene/5000 bases	12
Saccharomyces cerevisiae (yeast)	12.1 billion	6000	1 gene/2000 bases	32
Escherichia coli (bacteria)	4.6 billion	3200	1 gene/1400 bases	1
H. influenzae (Bacteria)	1.8 billion	1700	1 gene/1000 bases	1

[a]All vaccine trials were initially conducted on animal intervention in Mus musculus (mouse) population because the average gene density is similar to homosapiens (human)

Table 6.3 Maximum profit per head red cattle by leptin genotypes

Price	Genotype	Lot1 (Steers)	Lot2 (heifers)	Lot3 (heifers)
Low	CC	59	38	9
	CT	43	17	16
	TT	82	52	47
Medium	CC	125	101	70
	CT	109	79	75
	TT	153	117	106
High	CC	192	164	131
	CT	176	140	135
	TT	224	182	165

CT and TT genotypes are less variance and h^2 is 0.18 ± 0.001

6.10 Real-Life Illustration of Estimation of Variance in Human Trial

It was reported that the efficacy of *H.* influenzae type b polysaccharide vaccine efficacy was 80% with 95% CI was 7–95% replicated in randomized controlled trial of 8453 vaccinated and 8573 unvaccinated population (Finnish children aged between 24 and 35 months). (Musser et al. 1990) reported that the variation of *H.* influenzae it might occur due to genetic diversity ranging from 0 to 64%. The incidence rate of (I_u) derived from '*H*' influenzae in the unvaccinated Finnish children was estimated figure is 0.0012. In the presence of genetic traits in the order of (15%), the estimated vaccine efficacy would be (91.40%) from Eq. (6.3). We tested the hypothesis from fitted model; the results found that 95%-CI with relative width of the interval was 0.5 in the estimated variance (91.4%) and also by using fitted model we estimated θ and I_u. It was found to be 0.15 and 0.0012, respectively. The sample size of 13,131 as compared to 24,217 on each of the vaccinated and unvaccinated cohorts suffixed of our objective of interest.

6.10.1 Model Discussion

The possibility we escalated $\widehat{\sigma^2}$ component for given vaccinated and unvaccinated cohort population, the model was assumed desired level of significance that there exists genetic component in the community which causes/protects disease irrespective of the vaccination. With technological advances, genetic markers were identified for other diseases also, and the method developed to determine the proportion of the cases that is due to genetic markers would be near feasible. On parallel basis, we demonstrated our approach and the utility of analysis of covariance to reduce the residual error variance RE in the experimental design (by taking cognizance of the relationship between a covariate and the outcome measure), and thereby bring about a saving in the required sample size in given relative width of 95% CI. It is an adorable factor to adapt this analytical procedure in other situations also. For example, there may be several factors that are associated with an adverse outcome (e.g., infant mortality, low birth weight) and some of these (e.g., literacy rate, socioeconomic status); it may not be admitted that modification in the immediate future is due to tremendous resource constraints, while others can be improved readily by special intervention programs (e.g., immunization campaigns, delivery of better antenatal packages) (Khoury et al. 1986). If one wishes to test whether the intervention measures are found to be a statistically significant impact, and if the contribution of the "not so easily modifiable" factors were escalated from previous studies, it can be regarded as equivalent to the genetic components. The point of interest that emerges from the study is that substantial savings in sample size gained in the event of successful identification of genetic component in the community causes or protects the specified disease for which vaccine trial needs to be conducted. Most importantly, the VE can be estimated unbiasedly with a given relative precision. We considered only the cohort study design in the form of randomized controlled trial which is usually the recommended method to assess the protective efficacy of vaccine in the community level (Shifman et al. 2006; Sorensen et al. 2002; Spencer et al. 1978; Vasantha et al. 1982). The design assumed fixed interval of time in which the cases were exclusive under two binomial populations. The results of the trials in terms of cases come from two binomial populations, the methodology of our estimation of VE and the sample size required to estimate 95% CI extended to counts coming from Poisson populations for rare diseases. It may also be possible to have study designs with varying time intervals for the entry and follow-up of people resulting in varying incidences. One of the limitations of this study was the assumption of model that is the asymptotic normality of the variance on the basis of large sample sizes which may be true in most of the vaccine trials. Further, the proportion of cases that are due to genetic component depends heavily on the incidence of the disease (Koopman 1984). One should therefore be cautious while calculating the sample sizes when the incidence of the disease in the community is very small. We should consider the importance of genetic component in the community especially in situations, for example, malaria where there is near-complete protection against infection or for preventing cervical cancer in the community where there are efforts to develop vaccines or for preventing Haemophilus influenzae type b through an already developed vaccine.

6.11 Conclusion

The measure of variance component is very important to know the mechanism of genotypes and genotypic interaction with environmental conditions (micro level). Based on genetic variance, the researcher can draw a very conclusive inference at sampled level without any bias. The present study concludes that the estimated parameters were found to substantially reduce probable errors (PE) and also unknown genetic component "θ" restoring reasonably good sample size.

References

Altman R (2012) Translational bioinformatics Clinical Pharmacology & Therapeutics 91(6):994–1000. https://doi.org/10.1038/clpt.2012.49

Childs B, Der Kaloustian MV (1968a) Genetic heterogeneity. N Engl J Med 279:1205–1212

Childs B, Der Kaloustian MV (1968b) Genetic heterogeneity (Concluded). N Engl J Med 279:1267–1274

Curnow RN, Smith C (1975) Multifactorial models for familial diseases in man. J R Stat Soc Ser A 138:131–169

Daum R (1987) Immunization monitor. 1(1):3–7

Ederer F, Mantel N (1974) Confidence limits on the ratio of two Poisson variables. Am J Epidemiol 100:165–167

Katz D, Baptista J, Azen SP, Pike MC (1978) Obtaining confidence intervals for the risk ratio in cohort studies. Biometrics 34:469–474

Khoury MJ, Newill CA, Chase GA (1985) Epidemiologic evaluation of screening for risk factors: application to genetic screening. Am J Public Health 75:1204–1208

Khoury MJ, Beaty TH, Cohen BH (1986) The interface of genetics and epidemiology. J Chronic Dis 39:963–978

Koopman PAR (1984) Confidence intervals for the ratio of two binomial proportions. Biometrics 40:513–517

Marks JS, Hayden GF, Orenstein WA (1982) Methodological issues in the evaluation of vaccine effectiveness. Measles vaccine at 12 versus 15 months. Am J Epidemiol 116:510–523

Miller LH et al (1985) The resistance factor to Plasmodium vivax in blacks. The Duffy-blood-group genotype, FyFy. N Engl J Med 295:302–304

Musser JM, Simon Kroll J, Granoff DM, Richard Moxon E, Brodeur BR, Campos J, Dabernat H, Frederiksen W et al (1990) Global genetic structure and molecular epidemiology of encapsulated Haemophilus influenza. Rev Infect Dis 12:75–111

O'Neill RT et al (1985) On sample sizes to estimate the protective efficacy of a vaccine. Stat Med 7:1279–1288

Orenstein WA et al (1985) Field evaluation of vaccine efficacy. Bull World Health Organ 63:1055–1068

Parkhomenko E et al (2009) Sparse canonical correlation analysis with application to genomic data integration. Stat Appl Genet Mol Biol 8:Article1. https://doi.org/10.2202/1544-6115.1406

Rabinovich NR et al (1999) Overview. Epidemiol Rev 21:1–6

Segre D et al (2005) Modular epistasis in yeast metabolism. Nat Genet 37:77–83. https://doi.org/10.1038/ng1489

Shifman S et al (2006) A high-resolution single nucleotide polymorphism genetic map of the mouse genome. PLoS Biol 4:395. https://doi.org/10.1371/journal.pbio.0040395

Sorensen D et al (2002) Likelihood, Bayesian, and MCMC methods in quantitative genetics. Springer, p 739

Spencer HC et al (1978) The Duffy blood group and resistance to Plasmodium vivax in Honduras. Am J Trop Med Hyg 27:664–670

Tindle RW et al (1997) Vaccine against papillomavirus infections. In: Levine MM, Woodrow GC, Kaper JB et al (eds) New generation vaccines, 2nd edn. Marcel Dekker, New York, pp 767–781

Vasantha K et al (1982) Genetic markers in malaria endemic tribal populations of Dadra and Nagar Haveli. In: Proc. recent trends in immunohaematology, Institute of Haematology, ICMR, Bombay, pp 162–168

Statistical Implications and Its Practical Approach to Research Methodology

7

7.1 Introduction: Statistical Dealing with Success of Good Research

This note monologue, at a prior level, extensive postulates that apply to many different disciplines of research (Medical, Agriculture, Biological, and Veterinary Sciences). Anyone that has a research degree/empathy should be aware of them, whether or not they arise in their own research process. They give, also, pointers that may help in getting a clear view of where the researcher's project headed. Many researchers have successfully ventured to the research cascade itself and in the salient examples. They are several reasons why researchers should take interest in broad ranging multiple issues at the time of research planning and hypothesis concord. Many assumed hypotheses have been precluded that the following key points will narrate the story of research. The immediate research project may take twists and turns that are different from those for which earlier has been a preparation. This is especially likely for highly applied research projects, which typically demand a range of diverse skills and other variants affected during the study period (Food and Drug Administration, 1999). Those who acquire a wide range of research skills and knowledge are thereby better placed, after objective finalization to turn their hand to tasks different from those for which their immediate research training has equipped them. Broad-based research skills will best equip to nurture for the researchers to respond to changing the subject area, as they move from one task to another. The designing and planning of research is very important tool *or* indicator; the instrument panel of a research on large questioner domains may appear like multifaceted problems arise (Altman 2000; Alderson et al. 1996; Altman et al. 1996). It can really emphasize that the critical and questioning role of scientific ways of thinking is the best solution for obtaining trust worthy results. It does not matter much as to where you start practicing scientific thinking and project implementation, *etc*. Because its explanatory power is so great deal to maintain open pedagogy, once you get the hang of scientific reasoning you are bound to start applying it everywhere during the course of action.

Finally, the scientific criticism and questioning are in tension with the openness to imaginative insight that is equally important to the research continuum process. Data may be in tension with the theoretical and practical insight that generates their collection. Robert Langkjaer B fellow of Royal statistical Society (2019) has quoted that "data are not just numbers without meaning or context." The issue of evidence is central and there must be an assessment of the evidence in the literature that is the starting point for the research. There must be a research strategy that will bring together data sets that blissfully

B. D. M., B. Narasimha Murthy, *Design of Experiments and Advanced Statistical Techniques in Clinical Research*, https://doi.org/10.1007/978-981-15-8210-3_7

address the research questions and hypothesis. Statistical analysis will plausibly extract from the real data evidence that must be integrated into the body of the earlier knowledge, creating a coherent account that will assimilate in the insight of clinical research (Clark and Leaverton 1994; Chou and Owen 1986; Delaney 2000).

7.2 Research Perspectives in New Horizon

According to research prospective and ethical issues, there is an inherent frankness to new ideas and the ruthless criticism to which the scientific research process insists on extrapolating new ideas. In addition to research ethical issues, principles and methodological aspects to specify or describe the particular discipline, there are general statistical principles and methodologies, though avoiding any attempt at rigid prescription of an acceptable scientific procedure. In order to criticize or address the research planning we would establish a frame work that is broad enough for most of the research projects. The plan should include examination of an existing knowledge, a decision on a research question or hypothesis, a plan to follow in seeing answers, an analysis of the research data sets, and an eventual report formulation.

Many researchers have cited in the research methodological intervention certain elements that have been elucidating the pure objective of research hypothesis. Firstly, the generation of new ideas that would be considered for the assessment or evaluation of data set, eventually the researcher openness to new ideas for solving the realistic problems and approaches to the new scientific interventions and methodological aspects (Dixon et al. 1948; Dodge and Romig 1929; Emond 2000). R.A Fisher cited new approach for conducting research noteworthy way back in 1926, as proved and disproved the hypothesis based on existing data sets on hypothetical way. If the experimentation leads to have negativity (negative predictive value), we do not call it as failure of experimentation. The researchers quantify the reasons behind failure of the experimentation. Different types of studies have triggered the salient solution for manipulation of data sets through maximization of sample size and "SWOT" analysis at inception stage. The creativity is very important to make or draw right decision at right time based on the preliminary study and sample size. The Juxtapose of any project will begin with "SWOT" analysis (Fig. 7.1).

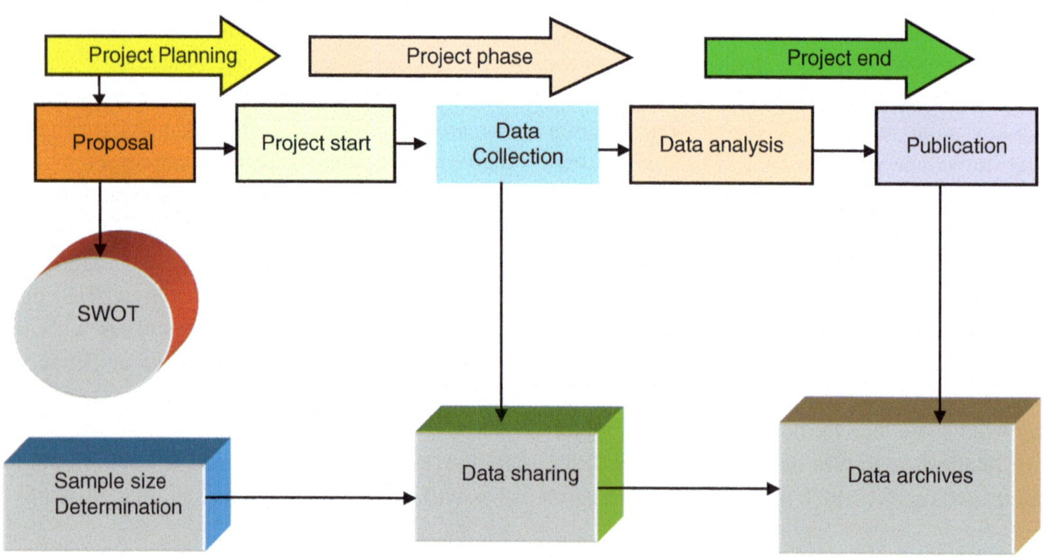

Fig. 7.1 Schematic diagram of research project flow

7.2.1 Strength

The ability to widely distribute the project information to vast audience.

7.2.2 Weakness

Lack of Knowledge on technical information which can lead to misinformation being disseminated, the exposure of information before formal announcement are made.

7.2.3 Opportunities

Promote communication and engagement through various types of media source.

7.2.4 Threats

Disgruntled environmentalists contracting the media.

7.3 Statistical Thinking on Thematic Research Area

In the design of data collection, and in interpreting results, subject area insights should mesh with statistical and data analysis insights in ways that will vary from study to study. The researcher's challenge is to put together all the evidence—evidence from the literature, from the analysis of the researcher's own data, and less formal evidence that may not be amenable to statistical analysis, in a manner that presents a coherent story (Edgington 1996). This demand for coherence will appear repeatedly in these notes. This section is written from the point of view of a practicing statistician who has often been involved in the research of others. A key emphasis is that there must be a correlation of statistical insights with application area insights. There must be shoe leather as well as statistical analysis. Careful planning will greatly increase the chances that, when your data analysis is complete, there will be a compelling story to tell. It is a fortunate researcher whose data tell a story that is as compelling as RA Fisher and Bayesian data, or as John Snow's data. Good planning of the project, and of the data collection, can greatly increase the chances of such good fortune.

7.4 Methods: Formulation and Frame Work of Research Project

The aim of any new research project is to develop a framework that will be helpful in the later discussion of research projects. Since, it is fragile to get started at all unless there is a research question, or at least the beginnings of research questions. It will be convenient to group the different components of a research project under the following headings:

1. Define the state variables—Assessment of the state of existing knowledge.
2. Implicit and explicit questions to presume your null hypothesis (Generation and honing of ideas).
3. Formulate proper design of experiment and execution of research that will explore or test specific ideas (Statistical methods for data analysis).
4. Analysis, interpretation, and presentation of the resulting data sets.

While statistical ideas may not have much role in idea generation, they are certainly important, viz., assessing existing knowledge, designing, executing research and data analysis and interpretation, etc. In case of Veterinary and Medical Science Research emphasis is put on the review of existing knowledge, an area where the insights of experienced statisticians are sorely needed for guiding the research projects and Interim analysis work. An assessment of how effectively earlier workers have designed their study, and of how compelling their results are, may rely heavily on statistical insights or fore thoughts. Even if the study design seems to stand up to critical scrutiny, the funding agency will ask whether the data interpretation is correct. Mistakes in the statistical analysis or in the interpretation of the analysis may lead to quite wrong conclusions, as in some of the examples that we give later. Sound statistical tool will curb the error of sample or population.

7.5 Sample Size Determination

Perhaps the most frequently asked question concerning sampling is, "What size sample do I need?" The answer to this question is influenced by a number of factors, including the purpose of the study, population size, the risk of selecting a "bad" sample, and the allowable sampling error. This section reviews criteria for specifying a sample size and presents several strategies for determining the sample size, *etc*. In very important criteria for sample size determination is level of precision, level of confidence or risk, and the degree of variability in the attributes being measured. Usually sample size determination has been following five basic approaches:

1. Arbitrary approach—Rules of thumb (10% of the population).
2. Conventional approach—Average of similar studies (what others have done).
3. Cost basis approach—Availability of resources.
4. Statistical approach—Statistical consideration (adequate for sub group analysis).
5. Confidence Interval approach—Concept of variability, sampling decision, and SE(x) (allows us to predetermine how precise our estimates are).

7.5.1 Different Approaches of Sample Size (Fig. 7.2)

Many pragmatic questions are most frequently posed from the clinical researcher or statistician "How a large sample size would be determined on the basis of scientific ethos." The cited question is somewhat relayed upon the subjective attributes; there is no universal answers for the

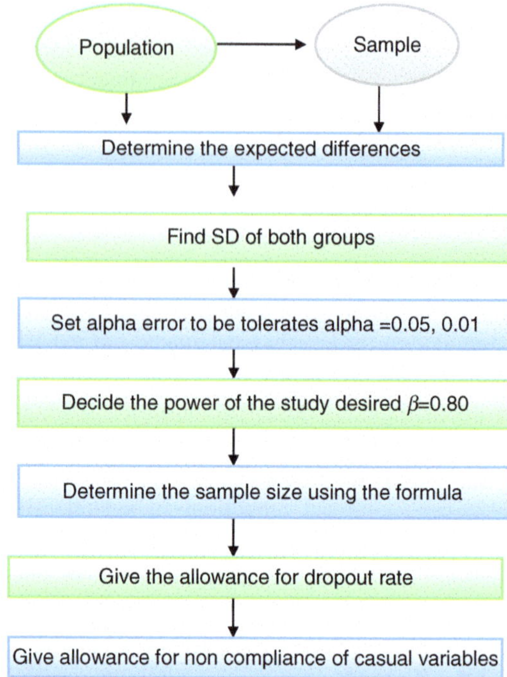

Fig. 7.2 Flow chart shows sample size determination wrt population and sample

cited question. The statistician will be provided an ample of information on subjective illustrations based on the realistic and practical approach (Flournoy and Olkin 1995; Fontana et al. 1991; Farewell and Angio 1981). They can opine that the required sample size will eagerly depend on the various underlying assumptions of type I-error, Power of the test (1-alpha), etc. In addition to that, some other important novel parameters have been considered for the determination of reliable sample size: (1) cost of the research, (2) time-frame, (3) feasibility and economic losses driven by nonresponse attributes, etc. As on the account of decision-making theory of the medical research, we should be conscious about the objectives of the study interest or with intervention of different subjects or cases. Finally, the researchers shall decide sample size (number of samples required for the study) before inception of the research. In other words, the sample size estimation has not been exclusively obtained, it is derived from mathematical or statistical exercise. It involves various assumptions and novelty of the study attributes which are drawn on the subjective approach, e.g., samples are drawn from the population considering experimental groups (estimated the variation between and within the observations). The investigator and the statistician are being necessary for some sort of exercise, they are drew up with meaningful and scientific pedagogy. The sample size determination has been considered for the following situations: (1) to demonstrate any significant difference between the two proportions or mean values (e.g., in a clinical trial or an observational study) and also significantly deviation from zero value, (2) attempt to demonstrate relative risk factors (e.g., in a case–control study) is significantly associated from the unit of observations, (3) estimation of proportion or mean values (e.g., in a sample survey) with pre-specified degree of precision, and finally (4) we estimated the magnitudinal differences between and within the parameters or variables (e.g., a difference between two proportions or two mean values drawn for prospective study design or interventional trial).

7.6 Demonstrating a Statistically Significant Difference Between Two Proportions

Suppose we consider a novel regimen with efficacy of 80% and a new regimen that has been evolved for the researcher interest with good efficacy (at least 10% more effective). The previous analytical methods highlight the known form of derivations aggravated with practical insight, the previous experience driven by the latter part of the decision is yet to be decided by the investigator, i.e., whether a 10, 15, or 20% differences was found in the practical interest. The magnificent of type I error (usually 0.05) will help us to accurate prediction of sample size and also describe whether the test is more reliable for testing the hypothesis. It would be considered as the possibility of the new treatment has been expressed as a short fall of potency or better than standard one when we compared to new regimen (better or worse). From the standard treatment we decided whether test is significantly feasible for determination of sample size (two-tail probability factor of 1.96 for 5% significance level) or a one-tail probability (factor of 1.645 for 5% significance level). The power of the test, i.e., the probability of obtaining a statistically significant results, if the difference exceeds a pre-specified amount, must also be specified by the investigator; it is often taken to be 90% but it could be less than 80%, 75%, etc. The trial size is presented in the following formula.

$$N = \frac{2\left(Z_\alpha + Z_\beta\right)^2 \left(P_1Q_1 + P_2Q_2\right)}{\left(P_1 - P_2\right)^2}$$

where P_1 is the proportion of successes in Group-I; Q_1 is the proportion of failures in Group-I ($q_1 = 1 - P_1$); P_2 is the proportion of successes in Group-II; Q_2 Proportion of failures in Group II ($q_2 = 1 - P_2$); S_o: Factor corresponding to Type I error of α^2 (usually α is taken as 5% and S_o is then 1.645 for one-tail test and 1.960 for two tailed test); Z_β: Factor corresponding to Type II error of β, i.e., Power of the test is $(1 - \beta)$ (usually $1 - \beta$ has taken to be 90% and Z_β is then 1.28). In the above-cited example, $P_1 = 0.8$ or 80%, $P_2 = 0.9$ or 90% (Z_α (one-tail): 1.645, $Z_\beta = 1.282$, and consequently).

$$N = \frac{2\left(1.64 + 1.28\right)^2 \left(80 * 20 + 90 * 10\right)}{\left(80 - 90\right)^2}$$

The sample size is determined based on the various combinations of P_1, P_2, Z_α and Z_β. It was determined that (a) as difference found in efficacy increases, the required sample size tends to decrease, (b) as the power of the test decreases, the required sample size decreases, and (c) as the significance level decreases (e.g., from 0.05 to 0.01), the required sample size increases. Finally, it should be noted that the sample size is also eagerly influenced by the absolute values of the two proportions for some sort of instance considering $\alpha = 0.05$, power – 90% and difference in efficacy is 10%, the required sample size is 300 when $P_1 = 0.95$; 428 when $P_1 = 0.90$; and 540 when $P_1 = 0.85$.

7.7 Pragmatic Approaches to Determining Sample Size

Sometimes, the number of patients available for the clinical study is very limited; we shall quantify the known values of sample size by using pragmatic approach (Fisher 1935; Flournoy 2000). An account of nonavailability of large number of eligible patients or because of the poor resource constraints (cost, time and staff) we employed the alternative method or design (pragmatic approach). In this new design we will be able to overcome the insight research problems at population and sample level for determination of sample size with desired level of significance and power of the test presented in Tables 7.1 and 7.2. Suppose we consider 300 CVD risk patients (recruited for conducting the clinical trial cited in the above situation described). One might we have rephrased the subjective questions or approach for calculation of effective sample size. Our questions is what is the smallest superiority value of sampled cases recruited for the study purpose. In this above vein we are able to detect the sample size in a desired level of significance and Power of test (90%) or we determine the sizes of sample 10% of superiority, it would be detected for the determination of unknown figure or sample size. With the above intervention we have computed the value of sample size based on the cited formula (table).

Table 7.1 Matrix of table shows total trail size α (1 – tail) = 0.05

Efficiency			Power of the design		
New	Standard (%)	Difference in efficacy (%)	90%	75%	50%
95%	85	10	300	188	94
	80	15	158	100	50
	75	20	100	64	32
90%	80	10	428	268	136
	75	15	212	132	66
	70	20	128	80	40
85%	75	10	540	338	170
	70	15	258	162	82
	65	20	152	96	48

Table 7.2 Matrix of table shows total trail size α (1 – tail) = 0.01

Efficiency			Power of the design		
New	Standard (%)	Difference in efficacy (%)	90%	75%	50%
95%	85	10	456	316	190
	80	15	240	166	100
	75	20	154	106	64
90%	80	10	652	450	270
	75	15	322	222	134
	70	20	196	136	82
85%	75	10	820	568	342
	70	15	390	270	162
	65	20	232	160	96

7.8 Demonstrating That a Relative Risk Is Significantly Different from Unity

In case we wish to conduct a case–control study at population level, the proportion of individuals who are exposed to risk factor and the relative risk (RR) factors were obtained in the practical interest; we should specify the values together with type I error and Power of the test for calculating the unknown sample size. For this particular instances, we consider a situation where the proportion of subjects or cases who have taken contaminated food is 0.3 (30%) and our interest for detecting relative risk (RR) of diarrhea at least 3 in cited subjects, when we compared to those who have not taken contaminated food. If P_2 is the proportion of diarrhea cases who have consumed contaminated food. The RR is calculated for the following metrics.

Consumed contaminated food	Cases (diarrhea)	Control (non-diarrhea)
Yes	P_2	0.3
No	$1 - P_2$	0.7

The relative Risk (RR) = $\dfrac{0.7P2}{0.3(1-P2)}$ is 3.0

from which P_2 is derived to be 0.56 and the our problem was delineated for comparing the two proportions 0.30 and 0.56, respectively; in this intervention the study size was found (from the formula) to be 140, i.e., 70 number for cases and rest of the 70 cases for control group (two-tailed test). If only 50 cases are available, the sample size determination questions would be reformulated by using above formula with substitution of form factor. In practical point of view we summarized the practical insight questions as What is the Power of detecting RR of 3 or what is the smallest RR that can be detected with power of 90%. Our cited answer to the above said question is 75%.

7.9 Demonstrating a Statistically Significant Difference Between Two Means

The proportion of two groups were demonstrated, and if any significant differences are found to address the situation of our research interest, the sample study size is denoted as "N" which is presented in the following formula,

$$N = \frac{2(Z_\alpha + Z_\beta)^2 (s_1^2 + s_2^2)}{(m_1 - m_2)^2}$$

where m_1 and m_2 are the mean values in the two groups and s_1^2 and s_2^2 are the variances. Suppose, we consider, the mean birth weight of baby was 3000 g, these data sets were obtained from one district with SD of 500 g, our interest is detecting 200 g, the difference will be expressed either way in another district where again the SD is 500 g. These practical constrains have to be substituted with the corresponding values of table Z (two-tailed), so that table Z is 1.96 with Power of 90% as before, Z_β is 1.28.

$$N = \frac{2(1.96 + 1.28)^2 (500^2 + 500^2)}{(3200 - 3000)^2} = 262 \text{ Required sample size}$$

From the above-cited formula we described how to determine the sample size with equal and unequal mean differences; with the resulted findings in the following manner we discusses the following salient points: (1) A larger the stipulated differences were seen in the two districts ($m_1 - m_2$) in another end, the larger values bears with denominator, consequently leading to smaller sample size, (2) The larger the SD in the two groups, larger value bears with numerator consequently which can yield larger sample size, (3) greater the Power, larger the value of Z_β expressed with numerator, and consequently greater the value of sample size, and finally (4) lower the significance level (Type I error), larger is the value of Z_α expressed with the numerator, with resulted factors yielding greater number of sample size.

7.10 Estimating a Proportion with a Pre-specified Degree of Precision

If "P" is the proportion of one attribute (estimated from the test of proportion formula) and Q is its complement (i.e., 1 − P) and the limit of accuracy (L) is necessary to define the wide terms of percentage of the estimates (e.g., 10% of P) and "Z" is the confidence limit factor (usually taken 1.96, corresponding to the 95% confidence limits), the number of subjects necessary to be included in the sample is given by the following formula

$$N = \frac{Z^2\alpha PQ}{L^2}$$

If the proportion of deaths due to diarrhea is believed to be the order of 2.0% and the limit of accuracy is 25% (of 2%, i.e., L = 0.5%) and the degree of confidence is 95% (i.e., Z_α = 1.96)

$$N = \frac{1.96^2 x2 * 98}{0.5^2}$$

It is clear that the sample size shows increased trend and P is found to be decreasing (e.g., 3012 for P −2% and 6085 for P −1%); it also increased the value of L (the limit of accuracy) and decreased values of less than 3012 (e.g., 3012 for L −25% and 18,824 for L −10%)

Mortality (%)	P	L (±25% of P)	N (Sample size)	L (±10% of P)	N (Sample size)
10	0.10	±0.0250	553	±0.010	3457
5	0.05	±0.0125	1168	±0.005	7299
2	0.02	±0.0050	3012	±0.002	18,824
1	0.01	±0.0025	6085	±0.001	38,032

The computation of values is pertaining to the above situation. We demonstrate the subjects on simple random sampling to select the study subjects. In practical approach, this technique is not feasible and convenient. An investigator will take recourse operationally by selecting feasible methods. Such method we called as cluster sampling or multi-stage sampling techniques. While latter part of alternative methods is very easy to implement at population level, we can estimates the values with larger sampling error. Consequently, the multiplication factors (usually called "design effect") were used to escalate the study size accurately. If cluster sampling was employed considering with the design effect 2, the required sample size roughly would be (3012 × 2 = 6024).

7.11 Estimating a Difference Between Two Proportions with a Pre-specified Degree of Precision

If the limit of accuracy required for estimating a difference between two proportions P_1 and P_2 is L, and X_α is the confidence factor (1.96 for 95% confidence), the reliable sample size (N) in each group is given by

$$N = \frac{Z_\propto^{\,2}\left(P_1Q_1 + P_2Q_2\right)}{L^2}$$

where P_1 = 30%, P_2 = 15%, L = 10%, and $Z_\alpha = 1.96$

$$N = \frac{1.96^2\left(30*70+15*85\right)}{10^2}$$

The study size is therefore 135 × 2 = 270

7.11.1 Estimation of Mean with Required Degree of Precision

If the standard deviation is "S" and the mean (m) is to be estimated with an accuracy of L% and the confidence factor is Z_α (1.96 for 95%).

$$N = \frac{Z_\propto^{\,2}s^2}{\left(L\%ofm\right)^2}$$

If m = 5000 g, s = 500 g, and L = 1%,

$$N = \frac{1.96^2 * 500^2}{\left(50\right)^2} = 384$$

7.11.2 Estimation of Difference Between Two Means with a Specified Degree of Precision

If m_1 and m_2 denote two means whose difference is to be estimated with a limit of accuracy of L% and a confidence factor of Z_α, the sample size in each group

$$N = \frac{2Z_\propto^{\,2}s^2}{\left(L\%\text{of}m_1 - m_2\right)^2}$$

If m_1 = 2000 g, m_2 = 3200 g and L = 50%, and s = 500 g and Z_α = 1.96

$N = \frac{2*1.96^2 500^2}{\left(100\right)^2} = 192$, study size = $2N$

= 2*192 = 384

Note: The following steps were constituted to know the pragmatic approach to the drawn decision-making solution for determination of sample size; we kindly ascertain the following: (1) remember that there is no stock answers for cited questions. The researcher has been initiating an early dialogue incumbent with applied statisticians; we narrate the entire pragmatic objective of the study interest (consider salient assumptions, data feasibility, accuracy, methodological intervention, etc.). We examined the feedback obtained from the statistician before inception of the research program. The researcher should kindly ensure and consider relevant factors such as availability of subjects, cost, time, etc. Finally, the researcher makes a balanced choice and try to extract the overall solution from the selected problem (concurrence with statistician), our frame work question or statement is as follows: (1) if the sample size number gives a reasonable prospective to draw useful and valid conclusions after completion of experimentation conducted by the researcher (if yes, proceed; if no, reformulate the problem for the study intervention), (2) Provided cost and conducive environment should supplement to the selected subjects or treatment. If a trial design is employed wherein each patient receives both the treatments (e.g., on two separate occasions to the same eye, with a wash-out period between them; or on the same occasion but with one treatment to each eye), the trial design will be more efficient, and the required trial size will be smaller; the gain will depend on the magnitudinal difference between the correlation of the same patient.

7.12 Comparison of Proportions

If the outcome measure is dichotomous (e.g., success/failure), the difference between the two treatments will be tested by a paired chi-square test (McNemar's test), which is essentially based on the pairs in which one treatment succeeds while the other fails (discordant pairs). One therefore needs to have an estimate of f, the proportion of such pairs. If $P_2 - P_1 = d$, the number of patients (N) required is given by the formula

$$N = \frac{\left[Z_{\alpha}\sqrt{f} + Z_{\beta}\sqrt{\left(f - d^2\right)}\right]^2}{d^2}$$

If $P_1 = 0.8$ and $P_2 = 0.9$, $d = 0.1$; f is unknown but it can be shown that its highest value will be $[(P_1 + P_2 - 2\ P_1 \times P_2) - d^2]$, i.e., 0.26–0.01 = 0.25; this is obtained when the findings for the two eyes are uncorrelated. Setting $d = 0.1$, $f = 0.25$, $Z_\alpha = 1.645$, and $Z_\beta = 1.282$, $N = 210$, i.e., 420 eyes are required. This is similar to the 428 patients (eyes) we would have required, had we administered only one treatment to each patient. However, if it takes a value lower than 0.25 because there is correlation between the results of the two treatments, there will be a decrease in sample size. For example, if $f = 0.2$, $N = 168$, i.e., 336 eyes.

7.12.1 Comparison of Mean Values

If the outcome measure is quantitative (e.g., IOP), the difference between the two treatments will be tested by a paired t-test, i.e., the mean of the differences between the two treatments in individual patients is tested to be equal to zero. If s_d^2 denotes the variance of this difference, the number of patients required is given by

$$N = \frac{S_d^{\,2}\left[Z_{\alpha} + Z_{\beta}\right]^2}{d^2}$$

If s_d^2 is unknown, it may be estimated by $2S^2(1 - r)$, where "r" is the estimated intraclass correlation coefficient and s is the estimated standard deviation for one of the treatments (e.g., Control).

7.12.2 Demonstrating That Two Treatments Are Equally Effective

Till now, sample sizes are estimated on the premise that new treatment is better than the standard treatment. However, there are situations where the interest is to demonstrate that two treatments are equally effective. For example, in breast cancer, one is interested to know whether simple mastectomy is as effective as radical mastectomy. Suppose the response is p with standard treatment. Then one chooses a value d such that the upper 95% confidence limit of the difference in the responses of the new and standard treatments should not exceed d with Power $(1 - \beta)$. Suppose $p = 90\%$, $d = 5\%$, α (Type 1 error) = 5%, and β (Type II error) = 10%, i.e., Power = 90%.

$$N = \frac{2\left[Z_{\alpha} + Z_{\beta}\right]^2 PQ}{d^2}$$

$$N = \frac{2\left[1.64 + 1.28\right]^2 90 * 10}{5^2} = 620$$

The sample size required in each group is 620. This illustrates that a substantial number of patients are required to establish the equivalence of two treatments.

7.12.3 Pragmatic Approaches with Modified Power Estimates

Sometimes the number of patients available for the study is limited, on account of nonavailability of large numbers of eligible patients or because of resource constraints (cost, time, and staff). In such situations, the problem of the sample size may be formulated in other ways. For instance, only 300 patients are available in the situation described in the beginning (Gow and Mutimer 2001). One might rephrase the question as "What is the Power with which a 10% superiority can be detected?". By use of the formula on page 2, it can be computed that the answer to the question is 80% Power. Suppose only 270 patients are available, then the Power is 75%. If only 100 patients are available, then the Power is 50%. Very large values of Type II error, say 50%, i.e., Power of 50% are not really acceptable because the chances of missing the true difference becomes too high. Realistic assessment of the sample size with corresponding Power has to be made. Many pragmatic questions are most frequently posed to clinical researcher or statistician, "How the large sample size would be calculated on scientific ethos?". The cited question is somewhat relayed on the subjective attributes, there is no universal answer for the cited questions. The statistician is able to provide ample amount of information on subjective illustrations based on the realistic and practical approach. He opined that the required sample size depends on the underlying assumptions and the investigator's requirements of type I error and Power of the test. In addition to that some other important parameters were considered for determination of reliable sample size, viz. cost, time-frame, feasibility, and economic losses driven by nonresponse. As an account of decision-making, we will be conscious about the objective of the study or intravenous of the subject or cases. Finally, the researcher decides sample size figures before inception of the research. In other words, the sample size estimation has not been exclusively mathematical or statistical exercise. It involves various assumptions and novelty of the study attributes on the subjective implications; therefore, close interactions that were found to be experimental group within the variations were seen. The investigator and the statisticians who are necessary for some sort of exercise drew up with meaningful and scientific pedagogy. The sample size determination has been considered for the following situations, *viz.*, (1) demonstrating that a difference between the two proportions or mean values (e.g., in a clinical trial or an observational study) significantly differs from zero, (2) demonstrating that the relative risk (e.g., in a case–control study) significantly differs from the unit, (3) estimating proportion or mean value (e.g., in a sample survey) with a pre-specified degree of precision, and (4) estimating the magnitudinal effect (e.g., a difference between two proportions or two mean values in a prospective study or intervention trial) with a pre-specified degree of precision.

7.12.4 Demonstrating a Statistically Significant Difference Between Two Proportions

Suppose we consider a novel regimen with an efficacy of 80% and a new regimen that has been evolved for the researcher interest with good efficacy (at least 10% more effective). The previous section highlights the previous experiences but the latter part of the decision is yet to be decided by the investigator, i.e., whether a 10, 15, or 20% differences are found in the practical interest. The magnificent of type I error (usually 0.05), whether the test would be considered as the possibility of new treatment is expressed as a short fall of potency or better when compared to the new regime (better or worse) or from the Standard treatment or only being better, i.e., whether we employed a two-tailed probability (factor of 1.96 for 5% significance level) or a first tailed probability (factor of 1.645 for 5% significance level). The power of the test, on probability for obtaining a statistically significant result, suppose if the difference exceeds with pre-specified amount, we must also be specified by the investigator; it is often obtained 90% of relevancy, but we could be less (80%, 75%, etc.) than the trial size

$$N = \frac{2\left(Z_{\alpha} + z_{\beta}\right)^{2}\left[P_{1}Q_{1} + P_{2}Q_{1}\right]}{\left(P_{1} - P_{2}\right)^{2}}$$

P_1: Proportion of successes in Group 1; Q_1: Proportion of failures in Group 1 (= 1 − P_1); P_2: Proportion of successes in Group II; Q_2: Proportion of failures in Group 2 (= 1 − P_2); Z_α: Factor corresponding to Type I error of α^2 (Usually α is taken as 5% and Z_α is then 1.645 for one-tail test and 1.960 for two-tail test); Z_β: Factor corresponding to Type II error of β, i.e., Power of $1-\beta$ (usually $1-\beta$ is taken to be 90% and Z_β is then 1.282). In the example above, $P_1 = 0.8$ or 80%, $P_2 = 0.9$ or 90% (Z_α (one-tail): 1.645, $Z_\beta = 1.282$, and consequently).

Table 7.3 Matrix of table shows total trail size α (1 − tail) = 0.05

Efficiency		Difference in efficacy	Power of the design		
New	Standard (%)	(%)	90%	75%	50%
95%	85	10	300	188	94
	80	15	158	100	50
	75	20	100	64	32
90%	80	10	428	268	136
	75	15	212	132	66
	70	20	128	80	40
85%	75	10	540	338	170
	70	15	258	162	82
	65	20	152	96	48

$$N = \frac{2\left(1.645 + 1.28\right)^{2}\left[80 * 20 + 90 * 10\right]}{\left(80 - 90\right)^{2}}$$

In Table 7.3, the sample size is set out for various combinations of P_1, P_2, Z_α, and Z_β. It may be seen that (above formula) (a) as the difference in efficacy increases, required sample size decreases; (b) as the power of the test decreases, the required sample size decreases simultaneously; and (c) as the significance level decreases (e.g., from 0.05 to 0.01), the required sample size increases. Finally, it should be noted that the sample size will be also influenced by the absolute values of the two proportions, for instance, in case $\alpha = 0.05$, power of test is 90% and difference in efficacy is 10%, the required sample size is 300 when $P_1 = 0.95$; 428 when $P_1 = 0.90$; and 540 when $P_1 = 0.85$.

7.12.5 Pragmatic Approaches to Determining Sample Size

Sometimes the number of patients available for the clinical study has been limited, in an account of nonavailability of large number of eligible patients or because of the resource constraints (cost, time, and staff) (Goldstein 1978; Gibbons 1990). In this prejudice, the problem of determination of sample size has been formulated in some other ways (Table 7.4). Suppose we consider 300 patients were available for conducting trail (situation described above). One might rephrase the

Table 7.4 Matrix of table shows total trail size α (1 – tail) = 0.01

Efficiency		Difference in efficacy	Power of the design		
New	Standard (%)	(%)	90%	75%	50%
95%	85	10	456	316	190
	80	15	240	166	100
	75	20	154	106	64
90%	80	10	652	450	270
	75	15	322	222	134
	70	20	196	136	82
85%	75	10	820	568	342
	70	15	390	270	162
	65	20	232	160	96

subjective questions, what is the smallest superiority that will be detected with a Power of 90% or what is the Power with which 10% superiority can be detected for determination of sample size. It would be computed based on the above-cited formula (Table 7.3).

7.12.6 Demonstrating That a Relative Risk Is Significantly Different from Unity

In case–control study, the proportion of individuals who are exposed to risk factor and the relative risk (RR) was obtained in the practical interest and must be specified together with Type I error and Power of the test for determining the sample size. For this above instance, we consider a situation where the proportion of subjects who have taken contaminated food is 0.3 (30%) and our interest for detecting relative risk (RR) of diarrhea at least 3 in cited subjects when compared to those who have not taken contaminated food. If P_2 is the proportion of diarrhea cases who have consumed contaminated food, the relative risk (RR) is calculated from the following phrase

Consumed contaminated food	Cases (diarrhea)	Control (non-diarrhea)
Yes	P_2	0.3
No	$1 - P_2$	0.7

The relative Risk $(\text{RR}) = \dfrac{0.7P_2}{0.3(1-P_2)} = 3$, from which P_2 can be derived to be 0.5625 and the problem was reduced to comparing two proportions 0.30 and 0.5625; in this intervention the study size can be found (from the formula) to be 140, i.e., 70 for cases and 70 for controls (two-tail test). If only 50 cases are available, the sample size question could be reformulated as "What is the Power of detecting RR of 3" or "What is the smallest RR that can be detected with a Power of (90%)." The answer to the former question is 75% and the latter it is an RR of 3.6, respectively.

7.12.7 Demonstrating a Statistically Significant Difference Between Two Means

The proportion of two groups demonstrating statistically significant differences was used to know the sample of interest, the study size can be denoted by "N" presented in the following formula

$$N = \frac{2(Z_\alpha + Z_\beta)^2 (S_1^2 + S_2^2)}{(m_1 - m_2)^2}$$

where m_1 and m_2 are the mean value of two groups, and s_1^2 and s_2^2 are the variances. Suppose we consider the mean birth weight of baby is 3000 g in one district with an SD of 500 g, of our interest, detecting 200 g difference either way in another district where again the SD is 500 g. This situation will be corresponded to a two-tailed test, so that Z is 1.96, with Power of 90% as before, $Z_\beta = 1.28$.

$$N = \frac{2(1.96+1.28)^2 (500^2 + 500^2)}{(3200-3000)^2} = 262$$

From the cited formula we described the resulted findings for the following manner: (1) the larger the stipulated difference between the two districts ($m_1 - m_2$), the larger is the denominator, and consequently the smaller is the study size; (2) larger the SD in the two groups, larger is the numerator and, consequently, larger is the study size; (3) greater the Power, larger is the value of Z_β and the numerator, and consequently greater is the study size; (4) lower the significance level (Type I error), larger is the value of Z_α and the numerator, and consequently greater is the study size.

7.12.8 Estimating a Proportion with a Pre-specified Degree of Precision

If P is the proportion to be estimated and Q is its complement (i.e., $1 - P$) and the limit of accuracy (L) required to define in terms of a percentage of the estimates (e.g., 10% of P) and Z is the confidence limit factor (usually taken 1.96, corresponding to the 95% confidence limits), the number of subjects necessary to be included in the sample is given by

$$N = \frac{Z^2 \alpha PQ}{L^2}$$

If the proportion of deaths due to diarrhea is believed to be the order of 2% and the limit of accuracy required is 25% (of 2%, i.e., $L = 0.5\%$) and the degree of confidence is 95% (i.e., $Z_\alpha = 1.96$)

$$N = \frac{1.96^2 x 2 * 98}{0.5^2}$$

It is clearly noted that the sample size shows increased trend and "P" was found to be decreased by (e.g., 3012 for P –2% and 6085 for P –1%); it has also increased value of L (the limit of accuracy) and resulted with decreased values of less than the central values (e.g., 3012 for L –25% and 18,824 for L –10%).

Mortality (%)	P	L (±25% of P)	N (Sample size)	L (±10% of P)	N (Sample size)
10%	0.10	±0.0250	553	±0.010	3457
5%	0.05	±0.0125	1168	±0.005	7299
2%	0.02	±0.0050	3012	±0.002	18,824
1%	0.01	±0.0025	6085	±0.001	38,032

The computation of values is pertaining to the above situation. We demonstrate the subjects on simple random sampling to select the study subjects. In practical approach, this technique is not being feasible and convenient, because an investigator will take recourse operationally by selecting feasible methods, such as cluster sampling or multistage sampling techniques. While the latter methods will be very easy to implement at field condition, and we estimate the values with larger sampling error (SE). Consequently, the multiplication factor (usually called "design effect") has been used to escalate the study sizes accurately. If cluster sampling was employed considering design effect of 2, the required sample size would be determined in the figure (3012 × 2 = 6024).

7.12.9 Estimating a Difference Between Two Proportions with a Pre-specified Degree of Precision

If the limit of accuracy required for estimating a difference between two proportions P_1 and P_2 is L, and X_α is the confidence factor (1.96 for 95% confidence), the reliable sample size (N) in each group is given by

$$N = \frac{z_\alpha{}^2 (P_1Q_1 + P_2Q_2)}{L^2}$$

If $P_1 = 30\%$, $P_2 = 15\%$, $L = 10\%$ and $Z_\alpha = 1.96$

$$N = \frac{1.96^2 (30 * 70 + 15 * 85)}{10^2} = 135$$

The study size is therefore 135 × 2 = 270

7.12.10 Estimation of Mean with Required Degree of Precision

If the standard deviation is s and the mean (m) is to be estimated with an accuracy of $L\%$ and the confidence factor is Z_α (1.96 for 95%).

$$N = \frac{Z_\alpha^2 s^2}{(L\% \text{of } m)^2}$$

If $m = 5000$ g, $s = 500$ g, and $L = 1\%$,

$$N = \frac{(1.96)^2\, 500^2}{50^2} = 384$$

7.12.11 Estimation of Difference Between Two Means with a Specified Degree of Precision

If m_1 and m_2 denote two means whose difference is to be estimated with a limit of accuracy of $L\%$ and a confidence factor of Z_α, the sample size in each group

$$N = \frac{2Z_\alpha^2 s^2}{(L\% \text{of } m_1 - m_2)^2}$$

If $m_1 = 2000$ g, $m_2 = 3200$ g and $L = 50\%$, and $s = 500$ g and $Z_\alpha = 1.96$

$$N = \frac{2(1.96)^2\, 500^2}{(100)^2} = 192$$

Study size = $2N = 2 \times 192 = 384$

Note: The following steps constitute a pragmatic approach to the drawn well decision for making solution for determination of sample size, we kindly ascertain the followings; analytical remarks, namely, (1) The researcher should be initiating an early dialogue with an applied statisticians, narrate the entire pragmatic objective of the study (assumptions, data feasibility, accuracy, and methodological intervention) (Gibbons 1987). Researcher should be examining the feedback which are obtained from the statistician before inducting research program and also kindly ensure and consider relevant factors such as availability of cases, cost, and time. Finally, the researcher will formulate a balanced choice and try to overcome the solution for the problems (concurrence with statistician). Finally frame the questions, if the sample size number gives reasonable prospective to draw useful and valid conclusions after completion of the entire experimentation (if yes, proceed; if no, reformulate your problem for the study intervention).

7.13 Comparison of Proportions

If a trial design is employed wherein each patient receives both the treatments (e.g., on two separate occasions to the same eye, with a wash-out period between them; or on the same occasion but with one treatment to each eye), the trial design will be more efficient, and the required trial size will be smaller; the gain will depend on the magnitude of the correlation between the results in the same patient (Kleiber 1999).

If the outcome measure is dichotomous (e.g., success/failure), the difference between the two treatments will be tested by a paired chi-square test (McNemar's test), which is essentially based on the pairs in which one treatment succeeds while the other fails (discordant pairs). Therefore, we need to estimate "f," the proportion of such pairs. If $P_2 - P_1 = d$, the number of patients (N) required for the intervention is determined by the following formula.

$$N = \frac{\left[Z_\alpha \sqrt{f} + Z_\beta \sqrt{f - d2}\right]^2}{d^2}$$

If $P_1 = 0.8$ and $P_2 = 0.9$, $d = 0.1$ and "f" is unknown but it can be shown that its highest value will be $[(P_1 + P_2 - 2\, P_1 \times P_2) - d^2]$, i.e., 0.26–0.01 = 0.25; this was obtained when the findings for the two eyes are uncorrelated. Setting $d = 0.1$, $f = 0.25$, $Z_\alpha = 1.645$, and $Z_\beta = 1.282$, $N = 210$, i.e., 420 eyes is required for the study. This is similar to the 428 patients determined based on the above-cited formula (eyes); we administered only one treatment for each patient. However, if takes a value lower than 0.25 because there is positive correlation between the resulted findings of our objective of interest of the two treatments, there will be a decrease in sample size as we mentioned in the above salient objectives. For example, if "$f = 0.2$," $N = 168$, i.e., 336 eyes is being necessary for the study intervention.

7.14 Comparison of Mean Values

If the outcome measure is quantitative (e.g., IOP), the difference between the two treatments will be tested by a paired t-test, i.e., the mean of the differences between the two treatments in individual patients is tested to be equal to zero. If s_d^2 denotes the variance of this difference, the number of patients required is given by

$$N = \frac{s_d^2\left[Z_\alpha + Z_\beta\right]^2}{d^2}$$

If s_d^2 is unknown, it may be estimated by $2s^2(1 - r)$, where r is the estimated intraclass correlation coefficient and s is the estimated standard deviation for one of the treatments (e.g., Control).

7.15 Demonstrating That Two Treatments Are Equally Effective

In the above-cited intervention, the sample sizes are estimated on the premise that new treatment is better than the standard treatment. However, we had varied situations, our experimental research interest will be demonstrating that if two treatments are equally effective. For example, in breast cancer, one is interested to know whether simple mastectomy is as effective as radical mastectomy. Suppose the response is p with standard treatment. Then one chooses a value d such that the upper 95% confidence limit of the difference in the responses of the new and standard treatments should not exceed d with Power $(1 - \beta)$. Suppose $p = 90\%$, $d = 5\%$, α (Type 1 error) = 5% and β (Type II error) = 10%, i.e., Power = 90%.

$$N = \frac{2\left(Z_\alpha + Z_\beta\right)^2 pq}{(d)^2} = \frac{2(1.645 + 1.282)^2 (90)(10)}{5^2} = 620$$

The sample size being required in each group is 620. This above illustrates that a substantial number of patients are required to establish the equivalence of two treatments.

Results (Tables 7.5, 7.6, 7.7, 7.8 and 7.9)

7.15.1 Merits of Sample Size Determination

(a) Low cost of sampling—Cost minimization (Reduced cost)
(b) Less consuming in Sampling—Consistency result
(c) Scope of sampling is high (Error of sample is very less)
(d) Maintain good accuracy and precision of the experiment
(e) Suitable in very limited resources *wrt* geographical location
(f) Better rapport of research insight

7.15.2 Demerits of Sample Size Determination

(a) Chance of bias at induction or end of the experiment
(b) Difficulties in selecting random true representative samples during the study period
(c) Need for subject expertization
(d) Changeability of sampling unit due to intrinsic and extrinsic factors
(e) Plausible changes of sampling unit due to accidental causes (bottle neck effect)

Table 7.5 Matrix shows various formulas to determine sample size

Types	Sample	Population
Proportion	$n = \frac{Z_\alpha^2 pq}{e^2}$ Z_α = Table value for ND p = Estimated proportion of sample $q = (1 - p)$ e = precision of the experiment (0.05)	$n = \frac{n_0}{1 + \frac{n_0 - 1}{N}}$ n = sample size n_0 = slected population small in size N = population
Mean	$n = \frac{Z_\alpha^2 \sigma^2}{e^2}$ Z_α = Table value for ND σ = SD of the sample e = precision of the experiment (0.05)	$n = \frac{Z_\alpha^2 \mu_\sigma^2}{\text{Me}^2}$ Z_α = Table value for ND μ_σ = SD of the population Me^2 = Marginal error
	$\text{ME} = Z_\alpha \sqrt{\frac{P(1-P)}{n}}$ $\text{ME} = 1.96\sqrt{\frac{P(1-P)}{n}}$ Formula based on t score $\text{ME} = t\left(\frac{\sigma}{\sqrt{n}}\right)$ $n = \left(\frac{\sigma t}{\text{ME}}\right)^2$	
	$N = \frac{N}{1 + Ne^2}$ n = the sample size, N = the Population size, e = the acceptable SE	
	$n = \frac{\left(\frac{\text{Range}}{2}\right)^2}{\left(\frac{\text{Accuracy}}{\text{Confidencelevel}}\right)^2}$ $\text{size} = \frac{\chi^2 np(1-p)}{d^2(n-1) + \chi^2 p(1-p)}$ where χ^2 = table value of chisquare N = population size P = population proportion d = degree of accuracy (expression as proportion)	

Table 7.5 (continued)

Types	Sample	Population
	Pocock sample size formula $$n = \frac{\left[P_1(1-P_1)+P_2(1-P_2)\right]\left(Z_\alpha + Z_\beta\right)^2}{\left(P_1 - P_2\right)/2}$$ n = required sample P_1 = estimated proportion of study outcome in the exposed group P_2 = estimated proportion of study outcome in the un exposed group Z_α = represents the desired level of significance 0.05 Z_β = represents the desired power 0.84	
	Calculating sample size for independent t test $$n = \frac{(M_1 - M_2)-(\mu_1 - \mu_2)}{(\mu_1 - \mu_2)^2}$$	
	$$n = \frac{N\Sigma N_h S_h^{\ 2}}{N^2 D^2 + \Sigma N_h S_h^{\ 2}} D = \frac{e^2}{t^2}$$ n = sample size N_h = Number of respondents in accessible population S_h = SD of each stratum D^2 = Desired variance e = Permitted error t = table t value	

Source: Kish, Leslie. 1965. *Survey Sampling*

Table 7.6 Sample size for ±5%, ±7%, and ±10% precision levels where confidence level is 95% and $P = 0.5$

Size of the population	±5%	±7%	±10%
100	81	67	51
125	66	78	56
150	110	86	61
175	122	94	64
200	134	101	67
225	144	107	70
250	154	112	72
275	163	117	74
300	172	121	76
325	180	125	77
350	187	129	78
375	194	132	80
400	201	135	81
425	207	138	82
450	212	140	82

7.16 Level of Precision

The level of precision, sometimes called sampling error (SE), is a range in which the true likelihood values of the population is estimated to be. This range is often expressed in percentage numerals (e.g., ±5, ±10%), in the same way that results for survey on QOL are reported by the Basavarajaiah et al. (2012). They Opined that total (60%) of the farmers who are rearing animal husbandry have adopted recommended scientific practices with precision rate of ±5%, and then they have concluded that between (55%) and (65%) of farmers have adopted the practice of animal husbandry services.

Table 7.7 Sample size for ±3%, ±5%, ±7%, and ±10% precision levels where confidence level is 95% and $P = 0.5$

	Sample size for precision "*e*"			
Size of the population	±3%	±5%	±7%	±10%
500	A	222	145	83
600	A	240	152	86
700	A	255	158	88
800	A	267	163	89
900	A	277	166	90
1000	A	286	169	91
2000	714	333	185	95
3000	811	353	191	97
4000	870	364	194	98
5000	909	370	196	98
6000	938	375	197	98
7000	959	378	198	99
8000	976	381	199	99
9000	989	383	200	99
10,000	1000	385	200	99
15,000	1034	390	201	99
20,000	1053	392	204	100
25,000	1064	394	204	100
50,000	1087	397	204	100
1,000,000	1099	398	204	100
>1,000,000	1111	400	204	100

A is assumption of normal distribution (ND) (Hauck et al. 1999). The entire population should be sampled

7.17 The Confidence Level

Central Limit Theorem clearly states that any state variables (quantitative/qualitative) can be normally distributed with parameters μ and common variance σ^2. If the variable is not normally distributed, the confidence boundary leads to be skewness (positive/negative). However, the researcher addressed the issues of variable of interest. As per the theorem the key idea encompassed in the Central Limit Theorem is that, when a large population is repeatedly sampled with large entries, the average value of the attributed data obtained by those samples is equal to the true population mean value μ. Furthermore, μ values obtained by these samples are distributed normally $N(\mu, \sigma^2)$ about the true value, with some samples having a higher value and some obtaining a lower score than the true population value is accord. In a normal distribution approximation, approximately (95%) of the sample values are within two standard deviations of the true population value (e.g., mean). In other words, this means that, if a 95% confidence level is selected, 95 out of 100 samples will have the true population value within the range of precision specified earlier (repetitions of the experimental

Table 7.8 Comparison of Independent sample groups based power (Group I and II)

	Percent of group I									
Percentage of group II	0	10	20	30	40	50	60	70	80	90
10	74									
20	34	199								
30	21	62	293							
40	15	32	81	356						
50	11	20	39	93	387					
60	8	13	23	42	97	387				
70	6	10	14	23	42	93	356			
80	5	7	10	15	23	39	81	293		
90	4	5	7	10	14	20	32	62	19	
100	2	4	5	6	8	11	15	21	34	74

Note: $\alpha = 0.05$, $\beta = 0.80$

Table 7.9 Matrix for medical/veterinary study for sample size determination

	CI-95%									
Population	10	20	30	40	50	60	70	80	90	95
60	37									
70	41	18								
80	44	19	19							
90	47	19	18	16						
100	49	20	20	17	16					
110	52	20	20	17	16	15				
120	54	20	20	17	16	14	14			
130	55	20	20	17	16	14	14	13		
140	57	21	20	17	16	14	14	12	10	
150	59	20	20	17	18	14	14	12	10	9
160	60	21	20	17	18	14	14	12	10	9
170	62	21	20	18	18	14	14	12	10	9
180	63	21	20	18	19	14	13	12	10	9
190	64	21	20	18	19	13	12	12	10	9
200	65	22	20	18	19	14	12	12	10	9
210	66	22	20	18	19	14	12	12	10	9
220	67	22	21	19	19	12	12	12	10	9
234	68	22	21	19	20	13	12	12	10	9
240	69	22	21	19	20	12	12	12	10	10
250	70	22	21	19	20	12	12	12	10	10
>250	71	24	22	19	20	12	12	12	10	11

value). There is always a chance that the sample you obtain does not represent the true population value. This risk is reduced for 99% confidence levels and increased for (90%) (or lower) confidence levels.

$$\text{CI}\,95\% = \bar{\mu} + Z_{\alpha 1/2} < \text{ND} < \bar{\mu} - Z_{\alpha 1/2}$$

7.18 Using a Sample Size of a Similar Study

Another salient approach is to use the sample size as those of studies similar to the one you plan. Without reviewing the procedures employed in these studies you may run the risk of repeating errors that were made in determining the sample size for another study. However, a review of the literature in your discipline can provide guidance about typical sample sizes which are used in the experimentation.

7.19 Degree of Variability

The important third criteria, the degree of variability in the attributes being measured refers to the distribution of attributes in the population. The more heterogeneous a population is, the larger is the sample size required to obtain a given level of precision. The less variable (more homogeneous) a population is, smaller the sample size is. The point to be noted is that the proportion of 50% indicates a greater level of variability than either 20 or 80%. This is because 20 and 80% indicate that a larger majority do not or do, respectively, have the attribute of interest. Because a proportion of population is necessary. The research study indicates the maximum variability in a population; it is often used in determining a more conservative sample size, *i.e.*, the sample size may be larger than if the true variability of the population attributes were used. A third way to determine sample size is to rely on published tables which provide the sample size for a given set of criteria. The sample size would be necessary for given combinations of precision; the confidence level and variability have been considered for determination of sample size; it is presented in Tables 7.1 and 7.2. The following note has been an inclusion for sample size reflect, viz., the number of obtained responses and not necessarily the number of surveys mailed or interview planned (this number is often increased to compensate for nonresponsive). Second, the sample sizes in Table 7.2 presume that the attributes being measured in various characteristics and also measurements are distributed normally or nearly so. If these assumptions cannot be met, then the entire population may need to be surveyed with cost minimization (Heyd et al. 1999; Kolata and Eichenwald 1999; Kpamegan et al. 2001). One approach is to use the entire population as the sample. Although cost considerations make this impossible for large populations, a census is attractive for small populations (e.g., 200 or less respondents) (Table 7.4). A census eliminates sampling error and provides data on all the individuals in the population. In addition, some costs such as questionnaires design and developing the sampling frame are fixed. They will be the same for samples of 50 or 200. Finally, virtually the entire population would have to be sampled in small populations to achieve a desirable level of precision of the experiments or research, *etc.*

7.20 Discussion

As per the previous studies, sample size is a very important domain for drawing correct decision about the population and solving the real-world problems at larger extent; the insight of study will describe the characteristics of parameters tested. Too small sample size is more likely to generate inconclusive, incorrect, or spurious results. This is because a smaller sample size will generate estimates which have higher variation. These estimates will then be less useful in modelling and understanding the real underlying hypothesis of interest. Secondly, studies which are more likely to fail are due to inadequate sample size are considered unethical. This is because exposing human subjects or lab animal/patients recruitment for the study to the possible risks associated with research is only justifiable if there is a realistic chance that the study will yield useful information (Kolata 1997; Matthews 1995; Thall et al. 1995). Additionally, a study which is too large faces the same ethical problem and will also waste scarce resources such as money, subject, and time. When conducting research, quality sampling may be characterized by the number and selection of subjects or observations. Obtaining sample size that is appropriate in both regards is critical for many reasons. Most importantly, a large sample size is more representative of the population, limiting the influence of outliers or extreme observations. Sufficiently large sample size is also necessary to introduce results among variables that are significantly different and for qualitative studies, where the goal is to reduce the chances of discovery failure. A large sample size broadens the range of possible data and forms a better picture for analysis (Kolata 1995; Kim and Demets 1995). Sample size is also very important for economic, physical, psychological, and ethical reasons. As Russell Length from the University of low explains "An undersized study can be a waste of resources for not having the capability to produce useful results, while an oversized one uses more resources than necessary." In an experiment involving human or animal subjects, sample size is a pivotal issue for ethical reasons. An undersized experiment exposes the subject to potentially harmful treatments without advancing knowledge. In an oversized experiment, an unnecessary number of subjects are exposed to a potentially harmful experiments or research of interest.

7.21 Conclusion

In designing experiments or study, sample size calculation is very important for methodological, ethical reasons, as well as for reasons on human and animal intervention and also financial resources. When conducting a research, the researcher should be alert to ascertain that, the study is subjected to sample size determination. In the absence of the sample size determination, the findings of the study should be interpreted with serious caution and elucidate with probable realistic threat. An appropriate sample size renders the research more efficiently, data generated are reliable, and resource investment is as limited as possible, while conforming to ethical and research perspectives. The use of sample size determination directly influences the research intuition and findings. Researcher would have confined to validate the samples at inception of research study, as a result, eliminate the biasness and hypothetical errors.

7.22 Remarks

The following steps constitute a pragmatic approach to decision-making on sample size.

1. Remember that there is no stock answer.
2. Initiate early dialogue with an applied statistician.
3. Discuss your assumptions with the statistician—consider various possibilities—for instance, a range of values if you are not too sure of your assumed estimates.
4. Examine feedback from the statistician.
5. Consider other factors also, e.g., availability of cases, cost, and time.
6. Make a balanced choice.
7. Ask if this number gives you a reasonable prospect of coming to useful conclusions.
8. If yes, proceed; if no, reformulate your problem for study.

References

Alderson P et al (1996) Equipoise as a means of managing uncertainty: personal, communal and proxy. J Med Ethics 22:135–139

Altman LK (2000) Ethical and patient information concerns: who goes first? Presentation to the Institute of Medicine Committee on Strategies for Small-Number-Participant Clinical Research Trials; September 28, Washington, DC

Altman LK et al (1996) Safety of catheter into the heart is questioned, startling doctors. The New York Times; September 18. p 1

Chou Y, Owen D (1986) One-sided distribution-free simultaneous prediction limits for *p* future samples. J Qual Technol 18:96–98

Clark PI, Leaverton PE (1994) Scientific and ethical issues in the use of placebo controls in clinical trials. Annu Rev Public Health 15:19–38

Delaney M (2000) Small clinical trials: tool or folly? Presentation to the Institute of Medicine Committee on Strategies for Small-Number-Participant Clinical Research Trials, September 28, Washington, DC

Dixon WJ et al (1948) A method for obtaining and analyzing sensitivity data. J Am Stat Assoc 43:109–126

Dodge HF, Romig HG (1929) A method for sampling inspection. Bell Syst Tech J 8:613–631

Edgington ES (1996) Randomized single-subject experimental designs. Behav Res Ther 34:567–574

Emond J (2000) Progress in surgery: innovation or research. Presentation to the Institute of Medicine Committee on Strategies for Small-Number-Participant Clinical Research Trials, September 28, Washington, DC

Farewell VT, Angio GJD (1981) A simulated study of historical controls using real data. Biometrics 37:169–176

Fisher RA (1935) The design of experiments. Oliver and Boyd, Edinburgh

Flournoy N (2000) Up-and-down designs. In: Encyclopedia of environmetrics. Wiley, London

Flournoy N, Olkin I (1995) Do small trials square with large ones? Lancet 345:741–742

Fontana RS, Sanderson DR, Woolner LB et al (1991) Screening for lung cancer: a critique of the Mayo Lung Project. J Cancer 67(Suppl 4):1155–1164

Food and Drug Administration (1999) International Conference on Harmonisation; E10 Choice of control group in clinical trials: draft guidance. Federal Register 1995 64:51767–51780

Gibbons RD (1987) Statistical prediction intervals for the evaluation of ground-water equality. Ground Water 25:455–465

Gibbons RD (1990) A general statistical procedure for ground-water detection monitoring at waste disposal facilities. Ground Water 28:235–243

Goldstein H (1978) Multilevel statistical models, 2nd edn. Halstead Press, New York

Gow PJ, Mutimer D (2001) Liver transplantation for an HIV-positive patient in the era of highly active antiretroviral therapy. AIDS 26:291–292

Hauck W et al (1999) Some issues in the design and analysis of equivalence trials. Drug Inf J 33:109–118

Heyd JM et al (1999) Adaptive design improvements in the continual reassessment method for phase I studies. Stat Med 18:1307–1321

Kim K, Demets DL (1995) Sample size determination for group sequential clinical trials with immediate response. Stat Med 11:1391–1399

Kleiber C (1999) Effects of distraction on children's pain and distress during medical procedures: a meta-analysis. Nurs Res 48:44–49

Kolata G (1995) Women resist trials to test marrow transplants. The New York Times; February 15. p C8

Kolata G (1997) Lack of volunteers thwarts research on prostate cancer. The New York Times; February 12. p 18

Kolata G, Eichenwald K (1999) Business thrives on unproven care, leaving science behind. The New York Times; October 3. p 1

Kpamegan E et al (2001) An optimizing up-and-down design. In: Optimum design. Kluwer, Boston

Matthews JNS (1995) Small clinical trials: are they all bad? Stat Med 14:115–126

Thall PF et al (1995) Bayesian sequential monitoring designs for single-arm clinical trials with multiple outcomes. Stat Med 14:357–379

Statistical Modelling for Life-Threatening Diseases

8

8.1 Introduction

The Pediatric HIV epidemic is a scourge, the incidence was derived based on the advance statistical modeling techniques, these modeling techniques are used to determine the various pragmatic factors associated with ANC (antenatal care women) for the estimation of HIV prevalence in infants (1 year) and children up to 15 years of age groups. The Pediatric HIV prevalence is significantly transferred from mother-to-child (PMTCT) from various risk factors, the HAART (highly active antiretroviral therapy) programs is one of the significant life domain factor to prevent or curb geometric progression of HIV and also aims to identify the effectiveness of therapy to know the survivability of PLHIVs at larger extent. Many HIV related research literatures cited at national and global level, described route of HIV transmission from mother to child has been solved on realistic problems from recent analytical techniques. The ARV drug and HAART therapy is a very useful indicator to control or prevent HIV transmission from mother to child. There is a paucity of literature on analytical intervention for the estimation of HIV prevalence in pediatrics population (based on the mathematical and statistical simulation techniques) coveted in various processes driven by the analytical research. In this proximity of the research gap, the present chapter aims to evaluate the impact of PMTCT and effectiveness of ARV drugs to prevent HIV transmission rate. Retrospective cohort data were collected from ART centers of Karnataka, India. Inclusion and exclusion criteria were used to describe the statistical model settings. A new statistical model for HIVMTCT incidence in children and their survival rate was created from the original HIV database (collected from ART center), the CMIS data extracted from main portal of national AIDS control organization (NACO) open source software. The model was formulated based on the size of the population (monthly intervals). Non-AIDS mortality rates and annual number of births to HIV-infected mothers (ANC) who are HIV-positive and HIV-negative data sets were obtained from the ASSA model. Since the rate of vertical transmission of HIV is considered as a dependent variable, the maternal follow-up or serial CD_4 counts, risk factors, clinical findings, demographic parameters, and HAART details (ARV drugs) were considered as independent variables. Recieving of HAART relative to short-course ARV prophylaxis, base line CD_4 count would be expected as relative comparative variables are substituted for model formulation. Based on a review of CD_4 distributions among pregnant women, we formulated separate models to know the relative risk of vertical transmission at lower CD_4 count at inception HAART.

B. D. M., B. Narasimha Murthy, *Design of Experiments and Advanced Statistical Techniques in Clinical Research*, https://doi.org/10.1007/978-981-15-8210-3_8

8.2 Model Description

The AIDS vertical transmission rate life data sets (neonates and children) were obtained from ASSA model. The model assumes the rate of incidence and is obtained from the various risk factors (RF). An estimation and incidence were determined by using ASSA model. An annual MTCT probability rate of children aged "*a*" (in years) in year "*t*" was extrapolated from CMIS softwares. The children aged between 1 year and older (2–15 years), the monthly transmission rate was assumed to be one-twelfth of the annual transmission rate ieat "*q*"

$$-\frac{1}{12}\ln\left(1-qat\right). \quad (8.1)$$

However, for children under the age of 1 year, the annual MTCT probability rate was shown arbitrarily high, and the mortality risk would be concentrated in the first month of HAART therapy. Therefore, the follow-up action is being taking place to know the exact incidence of HIV in different time intervals approached by newer techniques of ASSA model; this approach was derived (Bryk and Raudenbush 1987; Gibbons 1994, 1996, 2000) from Weibull distribution modeling techniques to evaluate the monthly incidence of MTCT. Transmission rate was also assumed ARV prophylaxis (the mother received single-dose nevirapine with or without after delivery is created from the ASSA model). Suppose *r* and *b* are the rate and shape parameters considered to know the trivial changes of incidence rate cited in Eq. (8.2). Further, Weibull distribution model was tested by ROC analysis (transmission of HIV from infected mother to child up to 18 months of age), i.e., from Eq. (8.1) the proportion of infants born from HIV-infected ANCs at the age "*a*" (in years) is as follows:

$$\exp\left(-rab\right). \quad (8.2)$$

Suppose that $q0t$ and $q01t$ represent infant and children (2–15 years) at age *a* and infection time '*t*', *i.e.*, the probabilities of HIV transmitted among infected mother to her child by 12 months and 1 month, the equation becomes

$$q0t = 1-\exp\left(-r\right), \quad (8.3)$$

$$q01t = 1-\exp[\left(-r\left(\frac{1}{12}\right)b\right]. \quad (8.4)$$

Equation (8.4) follows at various risk factors and incidence is formulated in Eq. (8.5)

$$r = -\ln\left(1-qot\right), \quad (8.5)$$

$$b = \ln\left[\frac{\ln\left(1-q01t\right)}{\ln\left(1-qot\right)}\right]\left[\ln\frac{1}{12}\right]^{-1}\leftarrow. \quad (8.6)$$

Substituting the values of $q0\ t$ and $q0\ t$ we have estimated "*b*" (Gibbons 1987, 2000; Gibbons and Hedeker 2000). Numerically the fitted model has generated various parametric values (0.0454 and 0.0198, respectively, for births in the preceding 5 years, gives $r = 0.0265$ and $b = 0.43$). For the sake of ease to ease convenience, we have substituted "*b*" in all estimated years (the parameters might be expected to vary over time). This makes it possible to estimate the monthly transmission probabilities in each year substituted (Hoel et al. 1972; Jones 1993; Johannessen 1991; Jennison and Turnbull 1983; James and Stein 1961; Krishnamurti et al. 2001). In contrary, we have estimated the average rate of transmission on or before birth, in the absence of PMTCT from Eqs. (8.5) and (8.6). As per the fitted model, the incidence or prevalence of HIVMTCT is 46.0%, if the mother has a CD_4 count between 100 and 200 μ/dL, and transmission rate expressed is 19.80% if the mother has a CD_4 count between 201 and <250 μ/dL; The prevalence expressed is 8.60%, if the mother has a CD_4 count of 251–350 μ/dL, and finally a prevalence accrued is 2.5% if the mother has a CD_4 count greater than >500 μ/dL. This present model suggests that the PMTCT program in India had a significant pediatric impact on HIV incidence, and that the recent adoption of new PMTCT protocols can be expected to lead about 75% reduction in Pediatric HIV incidence by 2015 and also there is no complexity to describe the HIV incidence in pediatric population at global level.

Several recent studies in India have suggested that a higher level of HIV prevalence among children was estimated by statistical models.

Numerous research litrature cited for HIV MTCT prevalence at national and global level, as per the research findings various factors including nosocomial transmission of HIV. The HIV transmission as a result of sexual abuse, false-positive reactions on HIV antibody tests, etc. Since the lower-than-expected rates of mortality accrued children infected with HIV as compared with higher incidence of mother-to-child transmission. The present chapter aims to characterize and estimate pediatric HIV epidemic in India by using advanced statistical modeling techniques, and also assesses the HAART effectiveness with respect to survivability. A further objective was to evaluate the prevalence and impact of the prevention of mother-to-child transmission (PMTCT) and to know the trend of pediatric antiretroviral treatment (ART) program in Karnataka state as to assess how the impact of these programs may change in the future. A statistical model of HIV incidence of children and their HIV survival has created, using ART Karnataka CMIS data source. The model determines the size of the population under the age of 15 and infants on monthly interval basis starting from 2005 to 2009. Non-AIDS and AIDS mortality rates, annual numbers of births to mothers who are HIV-positive as well as HIV-negative cases were extracted from ASSA-AIDS and Demographic transition model. Further, likelihood estimation values of HIV incidence were estimated by suitable statistical modeling. So our fitted model will allow for estimation of vertical transmission from mothers who seroconvert after their antenatal HIV screening visit. The model was driven to demonstrate two modes of HIV transmission in children under the age of 15 and children born from infected mothers at or before birth (Intrapartum or intrauterine transmission), transmission from infected mothers after birth, as a result of breastfeeding, etc. In the absence of PMTCT, women who are HIV-seropositive at the time of their first antenatal screening visit shall be assumed to have an average probability of transmitting the virus at delivery equal to 0.2, with the probability varying according to the mother's CD_4 counts. A higher transmission probability will apply if the mother becomes infected prior to delivery and seroconverts after her first antenatal visit. In the absence of PMTCT, women who are HIV-seropositive at the time of delivery is assumed to have a constant HIV transmission probability per month of breastfeeding (BF). If the woman acquires HIV while breastfeeding, a higher transmission probability was assumed to apply during the acute phase that follows HIV acquisition, it was assumed that (66.70%) of undiagnosed HIV-positive mothers breastfeed and the median duration of breastfeeding was 21 months (CI 18.65–23.54). The HIV transmission probability at birth was assumed to be reduced by 82% if the mother receives single-dose nevirapine during labor. Women who are initiated on highly active ART (HAART) during pregnancy are assumed to have a 0.03, the probability of transmitting the virus to their infants at birth. An approximately 50% of women who receive positive test results prefer formula feeds, (45.6%) initially practice exclusive breastfeeding (which is assumed to reduce the risk of transmission per month of breastfeeding), and the remaining population was preferred mixed feeding from birth with a median duration of 8–10 months. In women who know themselves to be positive and preferred exclusive breastfeeding (EBF), the median duration of EBF was 4 months. If women received HAART while breastfeeding, the monthly postnatal transmission risk was reduced by 86%. If the mother does not receive HAART while breastfeeding, but the infant receives extended nevirapine (NVP) prophylaxis, the rate of transmission was reduced by 60%.

8.3 Demographic Features of HIV-Infected Women

Over 18 years of pregnant women and children from 1 to 18 months infants to 15 years age group population were considered for the study. Of the studied population, 78% are illiterate, 63.35% in below poverty line, and 10.65% in high income group. The mean age of the pregnant women was 24.65 ± 4.8 years with (IQR 21.25–26.14). Twenty-five percent of pregnant women's families were migrated from other parts of the state for seasonal employment, 80% of the patients were heterosexual, primigravida 55.26%, Gravida-II 13.26%, and the remaining were Gravida-III and -IV. Discordant couples of 31.26% was recorded. 82.36% of patient's husbands had seroconversion. Mean base line CD_4 count was 116.35 ± 56.25 μ/dL (CI 102.23–123.65%) before initiation of HAARTCD_4 which showed decreased trend; after 1 year of completion of HAART and at the onset of pregnancy, CD_4 count mean was 289 ± 45.22 μ/dL (CI 265.20–301.28%), which showed very less values during the manifestation of opportunistic infections and non-AIDS-defining illnesses (Boers et al. 1998; Bryk and Raudenbush 1987; Cappelleri et al. 1996), and Found a CD_4 count of <100 μ/dL recorded at the inception of HAART (Tables 8.1 and 8.2).

Table 8.1 Probabilities of transmitting HIV, at of before birth by ASSA model (N = 100)

Antenatal care	Probability of transmission
HIV-seropositive at first antenatal visit, no prophylaxis	0.621
Receiving single-dose nevirapine	0.140
Receiving AZT from 28 weeks	0.338
Receiving single-dose nevirapine and AZT from 28 weeks	0.245
Receiving highly active HAART—Started during pregnancy	0.446
HIV seronegative at first ANC visit	0.743
Not receiving ARV prophylaxis	0.845

8.4 Intrauterine and Intrapartum Transmission

This section begins with a review of estimates of mother-to-child transmission at birth, in the absence of any intervention, and the effects of short-course antiretroviral prophylaxis, as well as antiretroviral treatment (ART) initiated for the mothers with CD_4 count >250 μ/dL. Evidence on the probability of vertical transmission from mothers who acquire HIV in late pregnancy is also reviewed. Single-dose NVP was given to the mothers after delivery in 1–6 h. The DBS and polymerase chain reaction test (PCR) was conducted at different intervals for screening of HIV.

8.5 Transmission Probability at or Before Birth, in the Absence of ARV Prophylaxis

Although there are several studies conducted in India, cited studies have estimated the proportion of pregnant women who transmit HIV to their children before or soon after birth, and it is difficult to estimate the proportion of children who are infected intrauterine/intrapartum on the basis of cited studies. This is because the PCR test typically does not yield a positive result until 18 months after HIV transmission has occurred. It is therefore necessary to wait for at least a month

Table 8.2 Probabilities of transmitting HIV of African infants infected at 4–6 weeks, after birth to mothers on HAART

Study	Location	Timing of HAART initiation	HAART initiation criteria	n	% HIV+
Coutsoudis et al. (1999)	Rwanda	28 weeks	None	532	1.1
	Uganda	Before conception	CD_4 < 250, WHO stage III/IV	218	0.0
Sperling et al.(1996)	Abidjan (Côte d"Ivoire)	During pregnancy	CD_4 < 200, WHO stage IV, CD_4 < 350 + stage III	250	1.0
Spira et al.(1999)	Mozambique, Malawi, Tanzania	During pregnancy	None	809	0.8
During pregnancy		None	341	1.28	
Bera et al. (2010)	East London (South Africa)	During pregnancy	CD_4 < 250, WHO stage IV	495	2.8
Before conception		172		1.24	
Average transmission rate if HAART initiated during pregnancy			2.13		
Average transmission rate if HAART initiated prior to conception			0.62		

before one can reliably identify almost all of the infants who have been infected on or before birth. However, some infants would have acquired HIV through breastfeeding, and might also be polymerase chian reaction (PCR) positive at the time of testing. This makes it difficult to identify the infants who were truly infected on or before birth. It is possible to estimate the proportion of children who become infected on or before birth, based on what is known about the rate of transmission through breast milk and the rate at which newly infected infants develop detectable virus. Suppose that $R(a)$ is the proportion of infants born to HIV-positive mothers, who test positive at age a (in months) on a PCR test, and further suppose that π is the proportion of infants, who acquire HIV at or before birth, in the absence of any antiretroviral prophylaxis (ARV), if f is the proportion of HIV-positive mothers, received formula-feed exclusively $\beta(a)$ and is the probability that a breastfed child acquires HIV postnatally and PCR-detectable virus by age a is as follows:

$$R(a) = \pi + (1-\pi)(1-f)\beta(a). \tag{8.7}$$

If it is assumed that all of the infants infected at or before birth have PCR-detectable virus by age a (this would generally be the case for $a \geq 1.5$ (Newell et al.)). From this it follows that

$$\pi = \frac{R(a)-(1-f)\beta(a)}{1-(1-f)\beta(a)}. \tag{8.8}$$

Suppose that breast-fed infants acquire HIV at rate h and newly infected infants develop PCR-detectable virus at rate γ. Then

$$\beta(a) = \int_0^a h\exp(-ht)(1-\exp(-\gamma(a-t))dt, \tag{8.9}$$

$$1-\left(\frac{\gamma\exp(-ha)-h\exp(-\gamma a)}{r-h}\right). \tag{8.10}$$

The parameters h and γ have been estimated to be 0.014 × 1/12 and 2.0 per month, respectively (see Sect. 8.3). In all of the studies considered here, a is 1.5 months, and hence is 0.012, relate only to women who were not receiving any antiretroviral prophylaxis. For all studies except Gibbons (2000), Finkelstei et al. (1996), and Faustman (2000), the results presented are based on a meta-analysis published by (Cappelleri et al. 1996) rather than the originally published results (Basavarajaiah et al. 2012). The average estimate of the proportion of infants who acquire HIV intrauterine or intrapartum is 19.7%, only fractionally lower than the proportion of infants who have detectable virus at the age of 4–6 weeks (Fig. 8.1).

Since the rate of vertical transmission of HIV solely depends on the maternal CD_4 count and uptake of HAART compared to short-course ARV prophylaxis also depends on the pregnant woman's CD_4 counts, it is necessary to estimate the rate of vertical transmission that would be expected in each CD_4 count follow-up period and to re-express the effect of the short-course of ARV regimens in terms of estimation of percentage reductions of HIV transmission. Based on a review of CD_4 distributions among pregnant HIV-positive women, the relative rate of vertical transmission varied CD_4 counts at different intervals (63.50%). The fitted model estimates an average rate of transmission on or before birth (14.0%) in the absence of PMTCT. An approximately 46.0% of transmission prevalence is driven by lower CD_4 count if the mother has a CD_4 count of <100–200 μ/dL, a total of 19.80% if the mother has a CD_4 count of 201 to <250 μ/dL, 8.60% if the mother has a CD_4 count of 251–350 μ/dL, 2.5% if the mother has a CD_4 count >500 μ/dL, and 1.4% if the mother has a CD_4 count >500 micro/dL. The proportions of HIV-positive women in CD_4 < 200, 200–349, 350–500, and >500 categories were estimated to be 14.0%, 24.9%, 24.5%, and 36.6%, respectively. Single-dose nevirapine will be assumed to reduce the transmission probability by 40%, and when combined with AZT from 28 weeks (previous guidelines NACO), it is assumed to reduce the probability by 80%. The efficacy of AZT alone is 35%. The percentage reduction due to short-course ARV prophylaxis is same regardless of the maternal lower CD_4 counts as there is little consistency seen in relation between efficacy and CD_4 counts (Chi et al. 1989; Bock 1989). In this chapter, a nonlinear statistical model was proposed to know the transmission of HIV/AIDS in

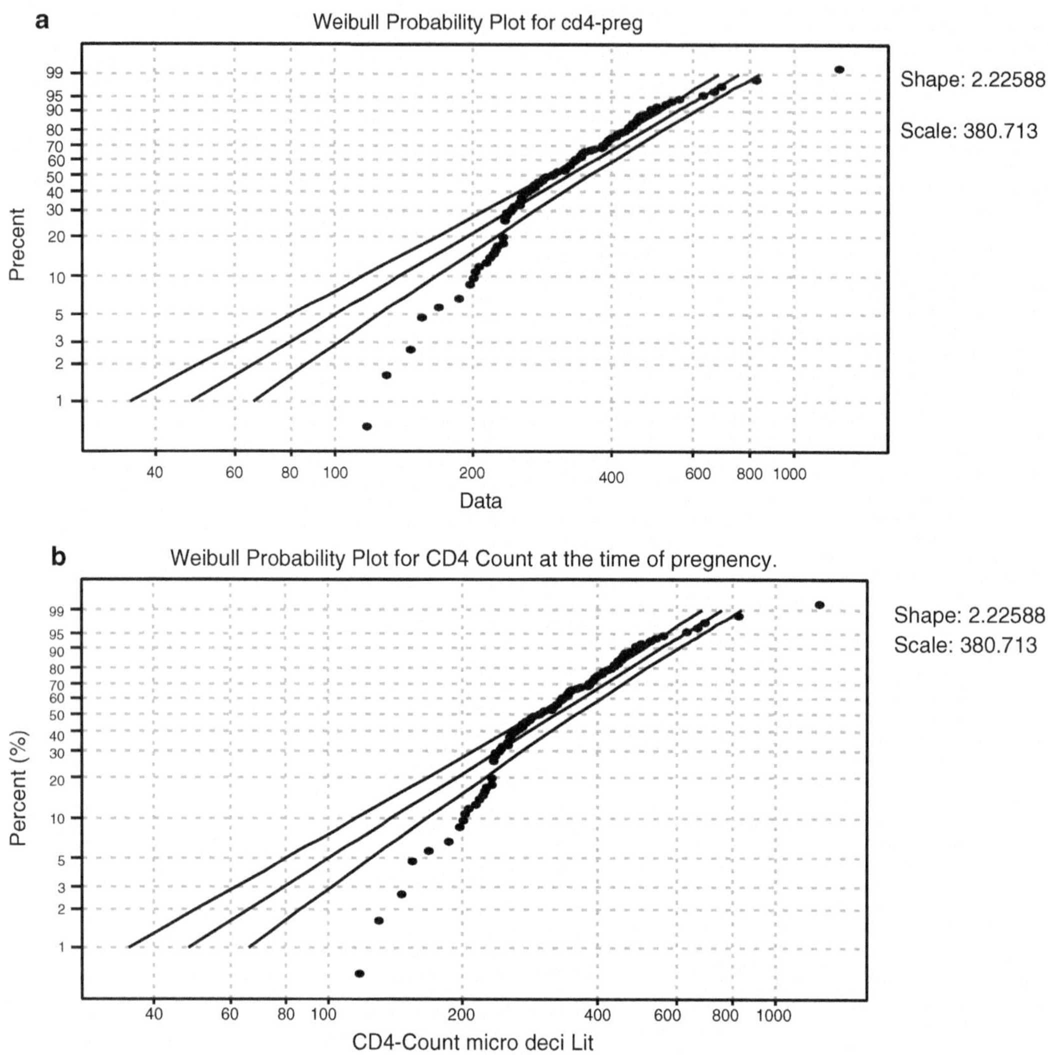

Fig. 8.1 (**a**) Probability plot for base line CD4 count at the time of HAART Initiation of pregnant women (n = 100). (**b**) Probability plot for CD_4 count at the time of pregnancy (n = 100)

a population of varying size with HAART treatments and vertical transmission. With or without receiving single-dose NVP after birth and breast feeding, the infected babies are born to increase the growth of infective population directly. It was assumed that women receiving PEP-single-dose NVP classes are exposed and capable of producing children without HIV. By analyzing the model, we have found that the parameter "h" denotes newly infected infants which can develop PCR-detectable virus at rate "γ" and time interval "a" (Center et al. 1987; Cox and Hinkley 1974; Faustman 2000; Finkelstein and Levin 1990; Gibbons 1987). The model equilibrium is also shown to be asymptotically stable under certain conditions. It is found that an increased rate of vertical transmission leads to increasing trend of population infectives, which in turn increases the pre-AIDS and AIDS population. Thus, the vertical spread of the disease should be controlled by effective HAART treatment or by promoting the condom use to keep the overall infective population under control. This will help in reducing the transmission rate as well. Also by model simulation it is shown that by controlling the rate of vertical transmission, the spread of the disease can be reduced significantly consequently the equilibrium values of infective. Most other models have assessed the rate of mother-to-child transmission using the HIV prevalence in pregnant women at their first antenatal screening visit, and have ignored the very significant vertical transmission that can occur in women who seroconvert after their first antenatal visit, either before delivery or while breastfeeding. The high HIV prevalence estimated by our model is also partly due to the lower rate of transmission estimated in our analysis, particularly in children who acquire HIV on or before birth. Although it is possible that our model estimates of AIDS transmission rates are understated. This study concludes that, present demonstarted model can be easily determine the prevalence rate and is an ability to derive the further algebraic treatment or derivation. Reliability, accuracy, and the model equilibrium are consistently more adoptive. The outcomes of this study are to help the Government and NGOs to establish policies, programs, and optimal plan for the control of disease by taking into account the aspect of treatment and vertical transmission. It helps the society in general to have an understanding on how the disease can be controlled through treatment of infectives with ARV. Also it is to add more knowledge to the existing literature on HIV/AIDS and help researchers to do more research on this disease (Guyatt et al. 1988; Goldstein 1986; Guyatt 1986; Guttman 1970; Gibbons et al. 1979; Heitjan 1997).

8.6 Modeling on Assessment of Quality of Life of Patients

HIV not only affects the physical well-being of an individual but also the overall quality of life (QOL). HIV not only affects the physical well-being of an individual but also the overall quality of life (QOL) (Laird and Ware 1982; Lai et al. 1980). The assessment of QOL is more important to understanding how the people's lives are affected by HIV infection. It helps to evaluate the financial costs, benefits of new programs to health-care providers and policymakers. The objective of present study is to determine the impact of human immunodeficiency virus (HIV) and HAART treatment on PLHIV. A total of 800 HIV-positive patients above 18 years of age, who are on HAART and newly enrolled for HIV care in different ART centers of Bangalore city, were recruited after obtaining informed consent. ART and pre-ART eligible patients were interviewed at different intervals by using WHO-brief scale. Each client participated in three in-depth interviews (IIDs). QOL assessment was done across a range of different socioeconomic, physical, psychological, and clinical parameters. Factorial and principle component methods were employed to find out the significant difference between the various QOL domains. The mean age of the male and female patients was 32.14 ± 6.30 and 32.50 ± 6.23 years, respectively. The overall mean score on a scale of 0–100 was found to be 19.50 in pre-ART, and 1 year after completion of HAART, the mean score was 119.20. A statistically significant QOL scores between psychological, physical, and social relation domain are compared with educational status ($P \leq 0.05$). The present study is to quantify QOL—with regard to educational status, family income, occupation, family support, immunological and clinical factors. HAART treatment, educational status, and also good social relationships can improve the QOL. The living environment of PLHIVS is one of the most important determinants of overall QOL; it has been suggested that QOL may be uniquely affected by specific disease process such as AIDS. Factorial analysis and principle component-user friendly model is helpful for physicians, researchers, and policymakers for taking clinical decisions and for implementation of new programs. Quality of life (QOL) is a term that is popularly used to convey an overall sense of well-being and includes aspects such as happiness and satisfaction with life as a whole. World Health Organization has defined QOL as "individuals' perceptions of their position in life in the context of the culture and value systems in which they live and in relation to their goals, standards, expectations and concerns." With the recent advances in clinical tests and treatments for those suffering from human immunodeficiency virus (HIV) or acquired immunodeficiency syndrome (AIDS), the survival of these patients has been increased and their QOL has become an important focus for researchers and health-care providers. Since the discovery of HIV in the beginning of the 1980s, HIV/AIDS has been one of the greatest health problems in the world. HIV/AIDS places an increasing burden on the health of the population, and causes further socioeconomic problems for individuals, families, communities, NGO's and governments in many countries. HIV is increasingly considered as a chronic disease. For a person living with HIV, this means having to cope up with a range of HIV-related symptoms for entire life. Symptoms may be related to the infection itself, comorbid illnesses, or iatrogenic effects from HIV-related medications. Many of the HIV patients struggle with numerous social problems such as stigma, discrimination, poverty, depression, substance abuse, and cultural beliefs which can affect their QOL not only from the physical health aspect but also from the mental and social health point of view and causes numerous problems. Assessing health-related quality of life (HRQOL) is useful for documenting the patients' perceived burden of chronic disease, tracking changes in health over time, assessing the effects of treatment and quantifying the return on health-care investment. In the context of present study, the aim is to find out the association between different aspects of QOL in PLHIVs.

8.7 Model Formulation

The patients were recruited for the quality of life (QOL) study with written consent; The WHO QOL-BREF instrument was administered for selected people living with HIV/AIDS (PLHIVs). The instrument had 26 items grouped under four life quality domains. The items included for the study are described in the following headings:

1. Physical health: The physical well-beings were assessed from ten domains enlisted in the BREF instrument. The parameters included were dependency of treatment, energy and fatigue, mobility, presence of pain and discomfort, sleep and rest, activities of daily living, and perceived working capacity.
2. Psychological well-being: The positive self-concept, negative feelings, higher cognitive functions, body image, and spirituality.
3. Social relations: Social contacts, family support, and sexual activity.
4. Environmental domain: Freedom, quality of home environment, physical safety and security, involvement in recreational activities, quality of health, and social care and accessibility to services.

All the domains were driven by the physical activities, viz. movement of patients, physical exercises, and any physical work conducted by the PLHIVs. The parameters of physical activities were collected based on the observational findings.

The two items were examined separately, namely the individual's bearing with overall perception of quality of life (QOL) and individual's overall perception of his or her health. A five-point Likert scale was used for each item. All QOL 26 items were cross-checked and the scores were ranging from 1 to 5. The scores of three domains were shown negatively phrased, the negative phrase items were reversed, and total scores were determined based on the standard operating protocol. Converted scores were transformed to (0–100) scale by using SPSS statistical software (using WHO QOLBREF instrument). The cases were seen greater than 15% of missing data such type of data sets were deleted and the data sets were saved in SPSS software. The collected data were analyzed by using SPSS-16.50 version; Factorial and univariate analyses were employed to know the correlation between various high-risk quality of life domain (HRQOL). Chronbach α value was used for testing the hypothesis. The following factors were pooled and the latent factors were determined based on the transformed scale.

$$\text{Transformed scale} = \left(\text{Actual score} - \text{Lowest possible raw score} / \text{Possible score}\right) \times 100$$

F_1 (Domain 1) = Physical health.
F_2 (Domain 2) = Psychological.
F_3 (Domain 3) = Social relationship/level of independence.
F_4 (Domain 4) = Environment.
Model Structure

$$x_1 = \lambda_1 F_1 + e_1 x_1 = \lambda_1 F_2 + e_1\ x_1 = \lambda_1 F_3 + e_1\ x_1 = \lambda_1 F_4 + e_1.$$

$$x_2 = \lambda_2 F_1 + e_2\ x_2 = \lambda_2 F_2 + e_2\ x_2 = \lambda_2 F_3 + e_2\ x_2 = \lambda_2 F_4 + e_2.$$

$$x_3 = \lambda_3 F_1 + e_3\ x_3 = \lambda_3 F_2 + e_3\ x_3 = \lambda_3 F_3 + e_3\ x_3 = \lambda_3 F_4 + e_3.$$

$$x_4 = \lambda_4 F_1 + e_4\ x_4 = \lambda_4 F_2 + e_4\ x_4 = \lambda_4 F_3 + e_4\ x_4 = \lambda_4 F_4 + e_4.$$

$$x_5 = \lambda_5 F_1 + e_5\ x_5 = \lambda_5 F_2 + e_5\ x_5 = \lambda_5 F_3 + e_5\ x_5 = \lambda_5 F_4 + e_5.$$

$$x_6 = \lambda_6 F_1 + e_6\ x_6 = \lambda_6 F_2 + e_6\ x_6 = \lambda_6 F_3 + e_6\ x_6 = \lambda_6 F_4 + e_6.$$

$$x_7 = \lambda_7 F_1 + e_7\ x_7 = \lambda_7 F_2 + e_7\ x_7 = \lambda_7 F_3 + e_7\ x_7 = \lambda_7 F_4 + e_7.$$

$$x_8 = \lambda_8 F_1 + e_8\ x_8 = \lambda_8 F_2 + e_8\ x_8 = \lambda_8 F_3 + e_8\ x_8 = \lambda_8 F_4 + e_8.$$

$$x_9 = \lambda_9 F_1 + e_9\ x_9 = \lambda_9 F_2 + e_9\ x_9 = \lambda_9 F_3 + e_9\ x_9 = \lambda_9 F_4 + e_9.$$

$$x_{10} = \lambda_{10} F_1 + e_{10} x_{10} = \lambda_{10} F_2 + e_{10}\ x_{10} = \lambda_{10} F_3 + e_{10}\ x_{10} = \lambda_{10} F_4 + e_{10}.$$

X_1: Age
X_2: How would you rate your quality of life?
X_3: How satisfied are you with your health?
X_4: How satisfied are you with your capacity for work?
X_5: How often do you have negative feelings such as blue mood? Despair, anxiety, depression?
X_6: How satisfied are with the support you get from your friends?
X_7: How satisfied are you with your sex life?
X_8: How satisfied are you with your personal relationships?
X_9: How much do you enjoy life?

$r(e_i,e_j) = 0$ for $i \neq j$ for all pairs of I and j. The coefficient λ_i is regression coefficient, and termed as factor loading. The unique factors F_1, F_2, F_3, F_4 are common factors. The residuals e_i's are called unique factors. A unique factor is regarded as a sum of the error of measurements. From the matrix, the factor loading determined based on the Varimax rotation if $\lambda_i = 0$ then the ith factor does not enter into the account of ith variable. In order to reduce the number of factors and errors we enhanced the interpretability by using factor analysis, each factor is rotated by varimax rotation techniques. Geometrically, the rotation means were tilting from the suitable Lambda values of each factors on their own axis in one direction or another until certain variables appear to be express their own residual or latent effects. This will increase the quality of interpretation of the selected factors. The varimax rotation procedure will attempt to maximize the sum of the variance of squared factor loading in each column of the loading matrix, and the process tends to produce some high loading and nonzero loading on each factor, etc Cochran et al. (1968); Gibbons et al (1991); Harville et al. (1977); and Elashoff et al. (1975). In these above techniques, the sum of squared loading of each row of the factor loading matrix will remain intact with tilting of factors, while the newest orthogonal factor would be obtained. In view of strong correlation among certain factors of variables, factors analysis was carried out to see extrapolation of the selected variables, which can be grouped into certain factors that would explain the interrelationship among larger number of variables of PLHIVs. In another parameter "Communalities," it is a measure of the amount of variables of known variance, explained from extracted factors, and it was obtained by adding the squared of factors loading of the selected factors. When we correlate higher the variable Communalities reduces risk of uncertainties, more are the common factors explained by single factors. All the variables have higher factor loading including factor F_1; it means that all the variables were grouped together into single factor experiment (Hahn and Meeker 1991; Hsieh 1995; Hillner and Centor 1987; Hedges and Olkin 1985).

8.8 Principle Component Analysis

All parameters related to ARV treatment, detailed history of age sex, education, occupation, CD_4 count, and risk bearing of PLHIV's set of data with measurement of ten variables $X_1, X_2 \ldots\ldots X_K$ on each set of new variables (P_i) called principle components, which are linear combination of the X_i's considered for the analysis (Fig. 8.2, Tables 8.3, 8.4, 8.5, 8.6, 8.7 and 8.8).

8.9 Model Discussion

In the present research, (Table 8.3) total 800 people living with (PLHIV) were considered for model fitting. The results showed that, the males and females were (58.12%) and (41.28%) respectively (odd ratio −0.98), Young aged population is predominated by older aged group, The IQR was (21–30 years). Lower the income implies higher the risk of acquisition of infection (PLHIVs). (An Occupational structure and economic status of PLHIVs was found to be statistically significant—$P < 0.05$.) The Present study shows higher prevalence it was found in the bridge population of HIV transmission drivers (39.75%) and least expression was seen in Agriculturists (12.75%) (Bryk etal. 1987; 1992). A single member infected in the family was (62.25%) with Odd ratio (2.36), two family members being infected (33.62%) with add ratio (4.89). The factor analysis of the ten items of categorical variables on ranking scale was taken into consideration; (Tables 8.3 and 8.4) it is indicated that, the most appropriate solution involved of F_1, F_2, F_3, and F_4. The demographic profile of the patients presented in (Table 8.1). Age groups were classified and it is accounted 72 (9.00%) CI 95% 0.321–0856 in <20 years. 21–30 years—418

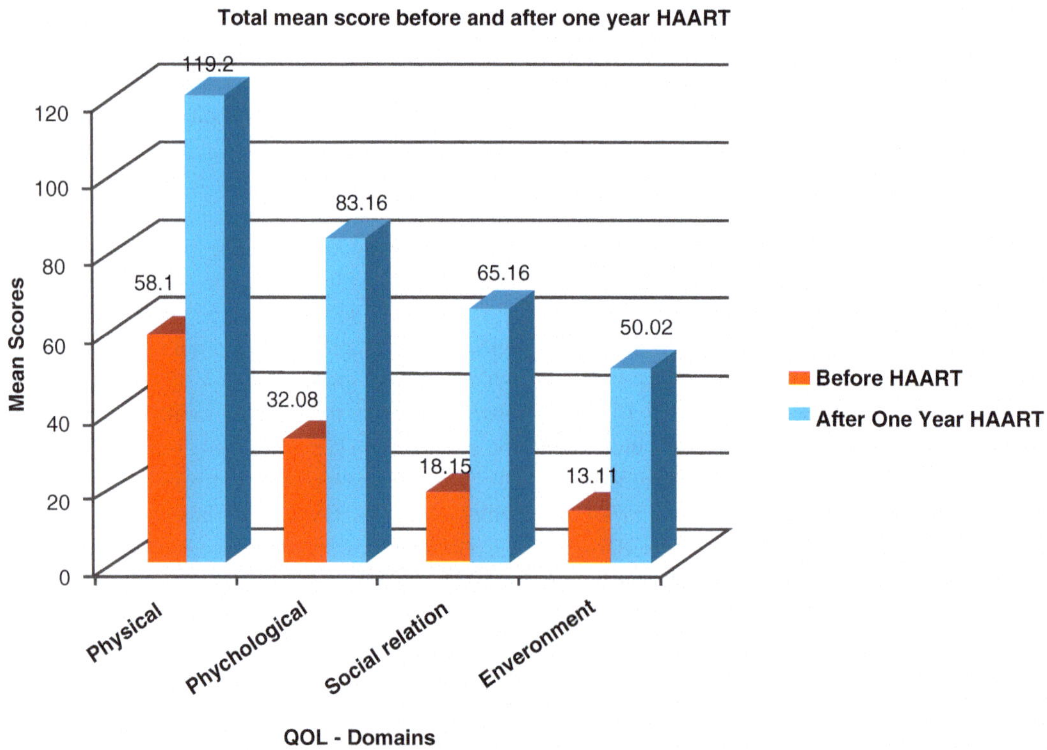

Fig. 8.2 Total mean scores of QOL

Table 8.3 Distribution of HIV patients according to their socioeconomic and psychological characteristics ($n = 800$)

Characteristics	No. of HIV clients	Percentage (%)	Odd ratio	95% Confidence interval (CI)	*P*-value
1. Gender					
Male	465	58.12	1.04	0.59–0.89	0.88
Female	330	41.25	0.98	0.35–0.62	0.75
Transgender (TS/TG)	05	0.625	0.021	0.03–0.011	0.21
2. Age (years)					
<20	72	9	3.56	0.321–0.856	0.21
21–30	418	52.25	21.23	0.66–0.963	0.63
31–40	225	28.125	10.50	0.423–0.658	0.42
41 and above	85	10.625	8.65	0.302–0.756	0.63
Pool	800	100	10.99		0.47
3. Education					
Illiterate	425	53.125	38.25	0.248–0.583	0.213
Literate	375	46.875	23.62	0.413–0.261	0.33
	800	50	30.935		0.2715
4. Occupation					
Agriculture	102	12.75	21.32	0.45–0.698	0.421
Agriculture and allied	40	5	10.26	0.789–0.211	0.365
House wife	45	5.625	5.12	0.563–0.745	0.111
Commercial sex workers	50	6.25	2.35	0.321–0.874	0.241
Vendor	55	6.875	4.52	0.444–0.99	0.32
Skilled worker	30	3.75	3.65	0.211–0.365	0.412
Asst worker	45	5.625	4.21	0.453–0.869	0.605
Salaried class	42	5.25	3.89	0.486–0.756	0.452
Business man	76	9.5	4.01	0.11–0.201	0.324
Drivers	315	39.375	10.24	0.453–0.698	0.485
	800	100	6.957		0.376
5. Income					
High income	89	11.125	2.36	2.48–6.56	0.89
Medium income	148	18.5	5.48	5.36–6.23	0.145
Low income	563	70.375	2.96	1.24–2.48	0.231
	800	100	3.6		0.422
6. Religion					
Hindu	655	81.875	4.21	0.112–0.856	0.458
Muslims	102	12.75	10.56	0.236–0.78	0.023
Christians	43	5.375	0.65	0.24–0.63	0.0112
	800	100	5.14		0.164
7. Type of family					
Nuclear	440	55	6.52	2.36–4.56	0.523
Joint	231	28.875	10.45	1.28–6.30	0.889
Staying alone	129	16.125	3.98	1.41–2.45	0.365
	800	100	6.98		0.632
8. Marital status					
Married	401	50.125	3.88	1.23–3.56	0.54
Divorce	274	34.25	15.23	4.58–8.96	0.113
Separated	125	15.625	2.89	3.86–7.85	0.53
	800	100	7.33		0.39
9. Age at first sex and inter course					
>18 years	563	70.375	5.36	0.398–0.635	2.36
<18 years	237	29.625	8.59	0.745–0.522	5.89

(continued)

Table 8.3 (continued)

Characteristics	No. of HIV clients	Percentage (%)	Odd ratio	95% Confidence interval (CI)	*P*-value
	800	100	6.975		4.125
Life time sex partners					
One partner	158	19.75	3.78	0.231–0.765	0.36
Two partners	475	59.375	8.59	0.234–0.635	0.012
Three partners	102	12.75	6.39	0.211–0.386	0.242
>Three partners	44	5.5	3.22	0.369–0.521	0.069
Non responders	21	2.625	4.52	0.112–0.23	0.542
	800	100	5.3		0.245
Type of sex					
Anal sex					
Yes	35	4.375	10.25	0.638–0.987	0.234
No	87	10.875	8.96	0.124–0.635	0.458
Non responders	678	84.75	5.47	0.489–0.963	0.635
	800	100	8.22		0.44
Oral sex					
Yes	82	10.25	6.58	0.218–0.659	0.478
No	45	5.625	2.49	0.487–0.635	0.698
Non responders	673	84.125	2.31	0.89–0.214	0.478
	800	100	3.79		0.55
Vaginal sex					
Yes	735	91.875	1.26	2.31	0.0236
No	28	3.5	2.36	8.56	0.123
Non responders	25	3.125	0.48	4.12	0.235
Homosexual	12	1.5	0.24	2.36	0.412
	800	100	1.08		0.19
Seropositive status					
One family member	498	62.25	2.36	2.36–5.23	0.214
Two family members	269	33.625	4.89	1.48–6.98	0.458
Three family members	23	2.875	6.58	2.89–3.98	0.748
>Three family members	10	1.25	1.48	3.28–6.89	0.352
	800	100	3.82		0.443

Table 8.4 Total scores of different domains of QOL (transformed scale)

		QOL—Before ART treatment				QOL—after 1 year ART treatment			
Domains	*N*	Min	Max	Mean	SD	Min	Max	Mean	SD
Domain1 = Physical health	800	19.5	65.10	58.10	102.1	42.16	146.23	119.20	30.20
Domain2 = Psychological	800	21.5	44.28	32.08	66.03	52.08	108.92	83.16	17.62
Domain3 = Social relationship/ level of independence	800	14.6	40.01	18.15	59.32	36.00	96.22	65.10	38.16
Domain4 = Environment	800	10.38	32.04	13.11	98.16	21.56	85.63	50.02	40.65

(52.25%) CI95% 0.66–0963; 31–40 years—225(28.15%) CI 95% 0.423–0.658 and above 41 years—85(10.62%) CI 95% 0.302–0.756; 425(53.12%) CI95% 0.248–0.583 patients were illiterate. The occupation of the patients were Agriculture—102(12.75%) CI 95% 0.45–0.698, Agriculture and allied—40(5.00%) CI 95% 0.789–0.211, House wives—45(5.62) CI 95% 0.563–0.745, Commercial sex workers—50(6.25%) CI 95% 0.321–0.874, Vendor—55(6.87%) CI 95% 0.44–0.99, Skilled workers—30(3.75%) CI 95% 0.211–0.365, Asst workers—45(5.62%) CI 95% 0.453–0.869, Salaried class—42(5.25%), CI 95% 0.486–0.756,

Table 8.5 Correlation matrix of categorical variables of PLHIVs

Categorical variables	(X_1)	(X_2)	(X_3)	(X_4)	(X_5)	(X_6)	(X_7)	(X_8)	(X_9)
(X_1)	1.00	0.760**	0.630*	0.252	0.321	0.124	0.859**	0.902**	0.316
(X_2)		1.00	0.465	0.118	0.289	0.435*	0.769**	0.834**	0.341
(X_3)			1.00	0.218	0.411	0.632*	0.698**	0.635*	0.540*
(X_4)				1.00	0.136	0.369	0.782*	0.617*	0.428
(X_5)					1.00	0.248	0.399	0.872*	0.501*
(X_6)						1.00	0.589*	0.487	0.214
(X_7)							1.00	0.888*	0.324
(X_8)								1.00	0.142
(X_9)									1.00

*,**Significant at 0.05 and 0.01 levels
X_1—Age
X_2—How would you rate your quality of life?
X_3—How satisfied are you with your health?
X_4—How satisfied are you with your capacity for work?
X_5—How often do you have negative feelings such as blue mood, despair, anxiety, depression?
X_6—How satisfied are with the support you get from your friends?
X_7—How satisfied are you with your sex life?
X_8—How satisfied are you with your personal relationships?
X_9—How much do you enjoy life?

Table 8.6 Strong correlation of categorical variables of HIV patients

Categorical variables	Strong correlation
Age (X_1)	$X_{2,}X_3,X_7,X_8,X_9$
How would you rate your quality of life? (X_2)	$X_6,X_7,X_8,$
How satisfied are you with your health? (X_3)	X_6,X_7X_8,X_9
How satisfied are you with your capacity for work (X_4)	X_7,X_8
How often do you have negative feelings such as blue mood, despair, anxiety, depression? (X_5)	X_8,X_9
How satisfied are with the support you get from your friends? (X_6)	$X_1,X_2,X_3,X_4\&X_7$
How satisfied are you with your sex life? (X_7)	$X_1,X_2,X_{3,}X_4\&X_8$
How satisfied are you with your personal relationships (X_7)	$(X2_{,}(X_3)(X_7)(X_8)(X_9)$
How much do you enjoy life? (X_8)	$X_{1,}X_3,X_5$

	Factors				
Categorical variables	F_1	F_2	F_3	F_4	Communalities
X_1: Age	0.64	−0.44	0.36	0.03	0.858
X_2: How would you rate your quality of life?	0.75	−0.12	0.14	0.07	0.732
X_3: How satisfied are you with your health?	0.72	0.27	0.15	0.40	0.697
X_4: How satisfied are you with your capacity for work?	0.67	0.43	0.28	0.27	0.524
X_5: How often do you have negative feelings such as blue mood?	0.68	0.58	0.02	0.17	0.602
X_6: How satisfied are with the support you get from your friends?	0.82	0.41	0.18	0.12	0.681
X_7: How satisfied are you with your sex life?	0.83	0.08	0.25	0.34	0.923
X_8: How satisfied are you with your personal relationships?	0.75	0.15	0.30	0.24	0.964
X_9: How much do you enjoy life?	0.88	0.023	−0.211	−0.45	0.632
Eigen values	5.46	5.20	3.98	4.32	
Explained variation (%)	54.6	52.0	39.80	43.20	

Note: Individual Communalities were extracted separately

Table 8.7 Principle component analysis of associated parameters in PLHIV

Categorical variables	Factors		
	P_1	P_2	P_3
X_1: Age	0.600	0.192	−0.169
X_2: How would you rate your quality of life?	−0.361	0.475	0.036
X_3: How satisfied are you with your health?	0.221	0.182	0.219
X_4: How satisfied are you with your capacity for work?	0.486	−0.287	0.261
X_5: How often do you have negative feelings such as blue mood	0.304	0.703	−0.268
X_6: How satisfied are with the support you get from your friends?	0.229	0.504	0.548
X_7: How satisfied are you with your sex life?	0.559	−0.335	0.148
X_8: How satisfied are you with your personal relationships?	0.221	−0.011	0.763
X_9: How much do you enjoy life?	−0.401	0.412	0.364

Table 8.8 Component transformation matrix of associated parameters in PLHIV

Components	P_1	P_2	P_3
P_1	0.748	0.660	0.058
P_2	−0.642	0.681	0.333
P_3	0.205	−0.305	0.922
P_4	0.149	0.086	−0.191
(%) Total variance	78.15	54.21	65.89

Businessmen—76(9.50%) 0.11–0.201 and Drivers registered for HIV care were more and accounted for 315(39.37%) CI 95% 0.453–0.698, the drivers are the bridge population for HIV transmission. Most of the patients were of low income group, i.e., 563(70.37%) CI 95% 1.24–2.48 and high income group—89(11.12%) CI 95% 2.48–6.56 Patients registered for HIV Care belonged to different religions. Hindus—655(81.87%) CI 95% 0.112–0.856, Muslims—102(12.75%) CI 95% 0.236–0.78 and Christians—43(5.375) CI 95% 0.24–0.63, Nuclear families—440(55%) CI 95% 2.36–4.56, Joint families—231(28.87%) CI 95% 1.28–6.36, and staying alone—129(15.62%) CI 95% 3.86–7.85.401(50.12%) CI 95% 1.23–3.56 were married, Divorced—274(34.25%) CI 95% 4.58–8.96 and Separated—125(15.62%) CI 95% 3.86–7.85. 563(70.73%) CI 95% 0.398–0.635 had first sexual exposure at more than 18 years of age, 237(29.62%) CI 95% 0.745–0.525, had at <18 years of age. Number of Life time sex partners form both the genders were included for the study (obtained from the patients thorough, in-depth interview (IID's) and focus group interview (FGI) as per the findings only one partner was 158(19.75%) CI 95% 0.231–0.765, two life time partners in 475(59.37%) CI-95% 0.234–0.635, three partners in 102(12.75%) CI 95% 0.211–0.386 and >three partner 44(5.50%) CI 95% 0.369–0.421. Type of sex practiced—Anal sex accounted for 35(2.61) CI 95% 0.486–0.963, Oral sex 82 (7.25%) CI 95% 0.218–0.654 and vaginal sex 735(91.87%) CI 95% 2.31–3.33. Seropositive status in family of one infected member—498(62.25%) CI 95% 2.36–5.23, two infected was 269(33.62%) CI 95% 1.48–6.98, three infected was 23(2.875) CI 95% 2.89–3.98 and More than three members infected was 10 (1.25%) CI 95% 3.28–6.89. By using WHO brief questionnaires, HRQOL data obtained before initiation of highly active antiretroviral therapy (HAART) and after 1 year completion of HAART, an each individual of 29 items were pooled and compiled mean total scores. The mean total score before inception of HAART on physical domain was 58.10 ± 102.10, Psychological was—32.08 ± 660.03, Social relationship with others—was 18.15 ± 59.32 and Environmental domain was—13.11 ± 98.10. After 1 year completion of HAART, the impact of effective counseling, good adherence and clinical parameters was found to be significantly associated on HRQOL level. However, the mean score of physical domain recorded was 119.20 ± 30.20, Psychological was 83.16 ± 17.62, Social relationship was 65.16 ± 38.12 and Environmental domain was 50.02 ± 40.62 (Table 8.2).

8.10 Conclusion

Based on the above facts and the resulted findings, the present study significantly concludes that the prevalence of psychological factor (communalities 52.0 and Eigen value 5.46) among HIV-infected population ranged from 52 to 54%. The younger aged population (19–32 years), unemployment, lack of health insurance, low CD_4+ cell counts at inception of HAART, HIV-related symptoms at an early stage, poor family supports, not having a partner, poor quality of social support, negative feelings of blue mood, lack of palliative care, unsatisfied sex life, not happy with personal relationships, and use of recreational drugs were significantly associated with depression in HIV-infected patients. The patients with HIV infection who are older than 35 years are more likely to suffer from depression, anxiety, confusion, and fatigue ($p < 0.001$). Insomnia, pain, and emotional disturbances were highly correlated with the well-being of depression and negative feelings. The impact of psychiatric, co-morbidities, specifically depression during HIV therapy, on HRQOL of patients and HIV disease is well documented in the course of therapy. Further, the presence of a major psychiatric disorder (independent of HIV-related disease progression) was positively associated with a negative impact on HRQOL domains on mental health, social functioning, and general health perceptions but not on physical health, role functioning, or pain. A larger study showed that the patients with comorbid mood disorders showed significantly worsen functioning and well-being than those without mood disorders.

References

Basavarajaiah D DM, Leelavathy B, Prabhakar B, Chandrashekar P (2012) Neural Network Modeling in HIV/AIDS –Five Years Survival Cohort Data. In.J. Engineering Science and Innovative Technology 1(2): 86-94.

Bera E, Jwacu N, Pauls F (2010) Risk factors for perinatal HIV-1 transmission in pregnant women requiring lifelong antiretroviral therapy: A longitudinal study at a tertiary hospital in South Africa. South African Journal of Obstetrics and Gynecology 16:6–13.

Bock RD (ed) (1989) Multilevel analysis of educational data. Academic, New York

Boers M, Brooks P et al (1998) The OMERACT filter for outcome measures in rheumatology. J Rheumatol 25:198–199

Bryk AS, Raudenbush SW (1987) Application of hierarchical linear models to assessing change. Psychol Bull 101:47–158

Bryk AS, Raudenbush SW (1992) Hierarchical linear models: applications and data analysis methods. Sage, Newbury Park

Cappelleri JC et al (1996) Large trials vs meta-analysis of smaller trials: how do their results compare? J Am Med Assoc 276:1332–1338

Center BA et al (1987) A methodology for the quantitative synthesis of intra-subject design research. J Spec Educ 19:387–400

Chi EM et al (1989) Models of longitudinal data with random effects and AR(1) errors. J Am Stat Assoc 84:452–459

Cochran WG (1968) The effectiveness of adjustment by sub classification in removing bias in observational studies. Biometrics 24:295–313

Coutsoudis A, Pillay K, Spooner (1999) Influence of infant-feeding patterns on early mother-to-child transmission of HIV-1 in Durban, South Africa: a prospective cohort study. Lancet. 354:471–476

Cox DR, Hinkley DV (1974) Theoretical statistics. Chapman & Hall, London

Elashoff RM (1975) Perspectives in biometrics. Academic, New York

Faustman DL (2000) Small clinical research trials: needs beyond space. Presentation to the Institute of Medicine Committee on Strategies for Small-Number-Participant Clinical Research Trials, 28 Sept 28 2020, Washington, DC

Finkelstei MO, Levin B, Robbins H (1996) Clinical and prophylactic trials with assured new treatment for those at greater risk. Part I. Introduction. Am J Public Health 86:691–695

Finkelstein MO, Levin B (1990) Statistics for lawyers. Springer, New York

Gibbons RD (1987) Statistical models for the analysis of volatile organic compounds in waste disposal sites. Ground Water 25:572–580

Gibbons RD (1991) Some additional nonparametric prediction limits for ground-water detection monitoring at waste disposal facilities. Ground Water 29:729–736

Gibbons RD (1994) Statistical methods for groundwater monitoring. Wiley, New York

Gibbons RD (1996) Some conceptual and statistical issues in analysis of ground-water monitoring data. Environmetrics 7:185–199

Gibbons RD (2000) Mixed-effects models for mental health services research. Health Serv Outcome Res Methodol 1:91–129

Gibbons RD, Hedeker D (2000) Applications of mixed-effect models in biostatistics. Sankhya Ser B 62:70–103
Gibbons JD, Olkin I, Sobel M (1979) An introduction to ranking and selection. Am Stat 33:185–192
Goldstein H (1986) Multilevel mixed linear model analysis using iterative generalized least squares. Biometrika 73:43–56
Guttman I (1970) Statistical tolerance regions: classical and Bayesian. Hafner, Darien
Guyatt GH (1986) The treatment of heart failure. A methodological review of the literature. Drugs 32:538–568
Guyatt GH, Sackett D, Adachi J, Roberts R, Chong J, Rosenbloom D, Keller J (1988) A clinician's guide for conducting randomized trials in individual patients. Can Med Assoc J 139:497–503
Hahn GJ, Meeker WO (1991) Statistical intervals: a guide for practitioners. Wiley, New York
Harville DA (1977) Maximum likelihood approaches to variance component estimation and to related problems. J Am Stat Assoc 72:320–385
Hedges LV, Olkin I (1985) Introduction. In: Olkin I, Hedges LV (eds) Statistical methods for meta-analysis. Academic, New York
Heitjan DF (1997) Bayesian interim analysis of phase II cancer clinical trials. Stat Med 16:1791–1802
Hillner BE, Centor RM (1987) What a difference a day makes: a decision analysis of adult streptococcal pharyngitis. J Gen Intern Med 2:244–250
Hoel DG et al (1972) A survey of adaptive sampling for clinical trials. Biometrics 59:317
Hsieh FY (1995) Sample size formulae for intervention studies with the cluster as unit of randomization. Stat Med 8:1195–1201
James W, Stein C (1961) Estimation with quadratic loss. In: Neyman J (ed) Proceedings of the Berkeley symposium on mathematical statistics and probability. University of California Press, Berkeley
Jennison C, Turnbull BW (1983) Confidence intervals for a binomial parameter following a multistage test with application to MIL-STD 105D and medical trials. Technometrics 25:49–58
Johannessen T (1991) Controlled trials in single subjects. 1. Value in clinical medicine. Br Med J 303:173–174
Jones RH (1993) Longitudinal data analysis with serial correlation: a state-space approach. Chapman & Hall, New York
Krishnamurti L et al (2001) Bone marrow transplantation without myeloablation for sickle cell disease. N Engl J Med 344:68
Lai TL et al (1980) Sequential medical trials. Proc Natl Acad Sci U S A 77:3135–3138
Laird NM, Ware JH (1982) Random effects models for longitudinal data. Biometrics 38:963–974
Spira R, Lepage P, Msellati P (1999) Natural history of human immunodeficiency virus type 1 infection in children: a five-year prospective study in Rwanda. Pediatrics. 104(5):e56.
Sperling RS, Shapiro DE, Coombs RW (1996) Maternal viral load, zidovudine treatment, and the risk of transmission of human immunodeficiency virus type 1 from mother to infant. New England Journal of Medicine. 335(22):1621–9

9 Meta-analysis in Clinical and Life Science Research

9.1 Introduction

The term meta-analysis is a new discipline that attempts to review critically and statistically pools the results of previous research studies or reports. The review of literature suggests that there is an increasing importance of meta-analysis in the file of public health and clinical trials. The purpose of meta-analysis is (1) to increase the power of the test, (2) to resolve uncertainty when reports disagree, (3) to improve the estimate of the size of the effect, and (4) to answer questions that are not posed at the beginning of the study. These functions are particularly applicable to randomized controlled clinical trials (RCTs) because the number of patients studied/enrolled in each trial are too small to detect clinically meaningful differences. Important qualities of any meta-analysis can be classified into (1) study design, (2) combinability, (3) control of bias, (4) statistical analysis, (5) sensitivity analysis, and (6) problems applicability. Over 200 meta-analyses of RCTs have so far been published in various statistical and clinical journals, and many more are being published every year. The extensive use of this analysis has led to number of challenges, with regard to establishing its validity, to statisticians and those responsible for health-care policy. As the analysis deals with the data that are already collected, there should be a caution while interpreting the results.

9.2 Criteria of Inclusion of Papers/Reports

Data from published papers/reports on RCTs will be included into the analysis for combining/pooling the results. Each paper will be evaluated by at least two investigators using ranks or a scoring sheet after listing the priority elements of a meta-analysis. The investigators will be blinded to the name of the journal and the authors of the papers. A rating "adequate" will be given when an item has been fully addressed, "partial" when an item is missing and "none or unknown" when the item was not dealt. The disagreement, if any, in ratings among investigators will be resolved by a conference with the other investigators. If the results are the same or is updated in two publications, the latest publication will be included for analysis (Fig. 9.1).

9.3 Functions of Meta-analysis

1. Identifies heterogeneity
2. Increases statistical power and precision of the research
3. Develops, refines, and test hypothesis
4. Calculates sample size for future study
5. Identifies data sets gaps
6. Reduces the subjectivity of study comparison

B. D. M., B. Narasimha Murthy, *Design of Experiments and Advanced Statistical Techniques in Clinical Research*, https://doi.org/10.1007/978-981-15-8210-3_9

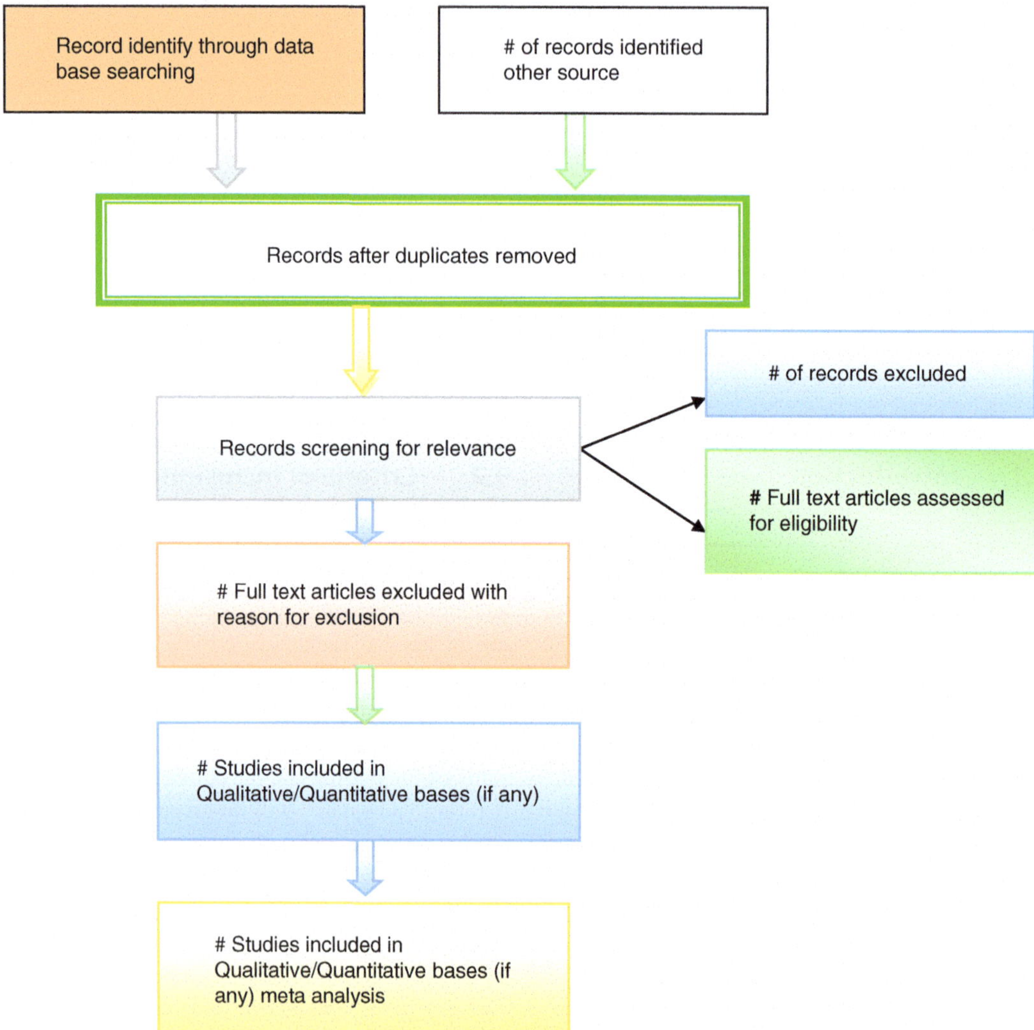

Fig. 9.1 Flow diagram of meta-analysis

9.4 Methods of Meta-analysis

9.4.1 To Formulate the Research Problems

Formulation of a research problem refers to state the problem in researchable manner. The researcher needs to refine the topic and clearly state what is intended to explore about the topic. Formulation of the research problem includes narrowing down the research area and formulating the salient objectives.

(a) The following steps in the formulation of research problem
(b) Identify a broad filed or subject area of interest to you
(c) Dissect the broad area into subareas
(d) Select what is of most interest to you
(e) Raise research questions
(f) Formulate objectives
(g) Assess your objectives
(h) Double check

9.4.2 Study Design: Pivoted the Study Design

This includes mainly the following (1) protocol, (2) literature search, (3) list of trials analyzed,

(4) treatment assignment, and (5) characteristics of patients, diagnoses, and treatments.

It is important to know the number (and percentage) of trials that were conducted according to a predetermined protocol. The extent of use of exhaustive searching methods, for example, consulting current contents, reviews, text books, experts in the particular field of study is needed to include as many relevant trials as possible into the analysis. The number (and percent) of trials analyzed together with the test of trials excluded, and the reasons for exclusion should be provided. It is vital for the reader to answer any information (especially when it contradicts the hypothesis) that is not used. It is important to provide details on the range of patient characteristics, e.g., age, sex, relevant socioeconomic data, or other diseases. Fulfillment of the criteria on the ranges, the dosage, and mode of administration, as well as the frequency and duration of treatment, is also needed. Similarly details on the ranges of diagnoses, diagnostic criteria, and stages or grades of diseases included are also important.

9.4.3 Weighting of Past Studies

More weight to the studies which give us more information, viz. more participants, more events, and lower variance, we calculated the weight estimates and its variance of the studies as follows:

$$\text{Weight} = \frac{1}{\text{Variance of estimates}} = \frac{1}{\text{SE}^2},$$

$$\text{Pooled estimates} = \frac{\sum \text{estimates} * \text{weight}}{\text{Sum of weights}}.$$

Methods—Various methods were used to conduct meta-analysis effectively. As per the scientific findings, the following methods were presented.

9.4.4 Volting Method: Box Score Analysis

The researcher should extract the research papers from database or literature survey (the published and unpublished research articles), the collected articles should be ascertained by Condorcet method, and it is the most preferred method to evaluate the published and unpublished articles based on the objective of the study. Assign the score, as per the SOP such as A-B, A-C, B-C and compare which results is more preferred to fulfill the research gap. If the results fall on the effective size score, you should include the study on priority basis.

	No of studies (percentile of effective size)			
Choices	71–80	61–71	51–60	<50
First choice	A	B	C	C
Second choice	B	A	A	B
Third choice	C	C	B	A

Effect size interpretation

$$\overline{\text{ES}} = \frac{\overline{X_E} - \overline{X_c}}{\text{SD}_c}.$$

Overlapping distribution and comparable percentiles

Comparative context

Statistical power—small (0.20), medium (0.50), large (>0.80)

Practical significance of the study

Common language effect size and research significance

Studies classified by statistical significance or nonsignificance

What is statistical significance (publication bias)

To correlate objectivity

To ascertain the variability of the studies

To assess the reproducibility

Broadly defined (is method X effective)

Sampling techniques

Comprehensive

Published and unpublished

Classifying and coding studies

Identify study feature

Data compilation (identify the effect size—*Z* score (standard deviation units))

9.4.5 Social Skills Training (Table 9.1)

Table 9.1 Average ES or training on social skills areas for participants with emotional and social behavioral disorder

Areas	Mean ES	% equivalent
Anxiety	42	66
Adjustment	27	61
Co operation	26	60
Interaction	24	59
Self-concept	16	56
Aggression	13	55

9.4.6 Combinability

An important problem in pooling data is whether the results of independent trials can be meaningfully combined. Criteria for pooling must be addressed. The impact of the differences, if any, on the conclusions should also be addressed. Another problem is heterogeneity. If we assume that each study is a sample from the same population, then the differences that are observed can be considered to be due to experimental error, i.e., within study variability. On the other hand, if we assume that each study is considered to be from a different population, then the differences are due to differences in the populations (between study variability). There are methods to test for homogeneity with which caution should be exercised while interpreting the results. It is, therefore, important to know the extent of use of test for homogeneity in the analysis. While performing a meta-analysis, potential sources of unconscious bias should be controlled for as and when possible. The bias on selection/rejection of papers can be avoided to some extent by looking into the methods and not at its results. Data extraction bias can also be avoided by extracting data by more than one investigator and measure the inter-investigator agreement to avoid any measurement bias. The source of funding or financial support must also be specified to give due credence to the conclusions.

9.4.7 Statistical Analysis

Any recognized statistical method of pooling and not the simple addition of results across trials is being considered here. Some of the statistical methods used for pooling are Mantel-Haenszel test, standardized average effect size, regression analysis, and significance tests. Potential problems of type I and type II errors will also be addressed. Confidence intervals of the differences for major outcomes will also be considered. The extent of the use of subgroup analysis will also be considered. Sensitivity analysis, i.e., to see whether the same set of data with different assumptions, tests, and criteria gives different conclusions, is also used. The methodological rigor and scientific quality of the papers should be assessed in framing proper recommendations. The features of quality, i.e., randomization, patient compliance, blinding of patients and investigators, the methods of statistical analysis, and handling of withdrawals must also be addressed. There is evidence to suggest that negative studies which contradict the results of published studies are less likely to be published than the positive ones. In this situation, a simple rule, i.e., the number of unpublished negative studies required to refute the published evidence is proposed as a useful measure of the strength of the published evidence. Once the meta-analysis is over, the investigator has to establish whether the new treatment is superior to the standard for all patients or for some subgroups; or the results are conclusive or suggestive for future study. Economic impact of adapting new methods of treatment of diagnosis is also important. Importance needs to be given to statistical issues, advantages, and disadvantages of various pooling methods. There are methods for combining the *P* values or test statistics. However, these methods do not distinguish between small and big studies and do not provide an estimate of the size of the effect. The Mantel-Haenszel method and modification of this for pooling separate 2 × 2 tables are becoming increasingly popular. These methods have several advantages; compare each treatment with its own control, obtaining a weighted estimate (the weight being the sample size of the study). It also allows testing for homogeneity as well as estimating the size of the effect, but there is no consensus that these methods are optimal. There is another procedure, in psychiatric literature, for studying the effect size defined as the mean difference between experimental and control group, divided by the standard deviation of the control group. These effect sizes are transferred into common units and therefore they can be combined. But, it is difficult to interpret them clinically. Some reports attempted multivariate techniques or log-linear models to adjust the difference between studies. Uniformity in presenting the results of meta-analysis in the standard format of scientific papers, with detailed methods and result sections, will be helpful to the readers. This will, in turn, help the reader to draw his/her own conclusions about the validity of the results. In summary, meta-analysis should be concluded like a scientific experiment, starting with a detailed protocol. Interobserver and interobserver variation must be looked into and attempts to be made to identify and minimize the bias. Though the validity of pooling is questioned, the quantitative synthesis of data in RCTs can be more useful to practicing physician/clinician than a traditional descriptive article. Of course, the synthesis studies must be properly performed to warrant serious attention. The number of meta-analyses has increased widely in the past decade. Nearly 11,000 meta-analyses were published in 2017. Meta-analyses are defined as a study which extracts and compares data sets from multiple primary studies. These have been widely accommodated as less biased and standardized ways to answer questions related to your studies. At times these are termed as the platinum standard of evidence. They help to guide numerous treatment guidelines. Since not all meta-analyses are debate enders, they often do not derive transparency instead results in more controversy. Nowadays, meta-analysis is an identical fight and is played in interdisciplinary field of agriculture, engineering, and medical sciences as well Greenland et al. (1992), Higgins et al. (2004), Higgins et al. (2008), Kjaergard et al. (2001), Langan et al. (2015), Langan et al. (2017), Langan et al. (2019), Laupacis et al. (1988), Rhodes et al. (2016), Rice et al. (2018), Riley et al. (2011), Simmonds et al. (2011), Sidik & Jonkman (2002), Sharp (2001), Turner et al. (2012), Thompson & Higgins (2002), Veroniki et al. (2016), Whitehead & Jones (1994), Yusuf et al. (1985), Yusuf et al. (1991). Despite the exploding number of meta-analyses, a lot of them do not bring a clear idea. In most of the clinical trials, the comparison of two treatments is carried out and the better one is selected and sometimes both the treatments are selected. Design of a parallel cumulative randomized trails includes formulation of H_0 hypothesis which do not have differences between the two interventions and detect a clinically acceptable difference. The difference between these interventions is not overlooked on the primary level by researchers. These trails are termed as superiority trails (STs). The researchers expect to discard the Ho hypothesis that displays the difference between the interventions. The ST type I error falsely finds an effect of a treatment when actually it is not present. On the other hand, the type II errors fail to identify a treatment effect when it exists truly. Even though the general rules of meta-analyses are quite simple and the clinicians should make multiple choices throughout the way, this will allow personal or unconscious bias to enter in the result part. Some meta-researchers state that there are many ways to improve the resulted findings. The activities in some fields like this make sure that all the studies pertaining to the area are published despite the outcomes. This will make sure that the meta-analyses have the ability to take full range of evidence into consideration. Meta-analysis can itself be made better on its own (Fig. 9.2).

9.5 Systematic Review

A systematic review can encompasses the results from available published and unpublished articles pooling to know the relevance of the study intervention, we have carefully designed the health-care studies (controlled trail) and provide high level of evidence on the effectiveness of health-care intervention. The judgment can be made about the evidence and inform recommendations for health care. These reviews are complicated and depend largely on what clinical trials are available, how they were carried out, and the health outcomes that are measured. Review authors' numerical data sets about the effects of treatment through a process called meta-analyses. Then authors assess the evidence for any benefits or harms from those treatments. In this vein, systematic review will be able to summarize the existing clinical or medical and agricultural research, whereas in meta-analyses, the statistical methods are used to summarize the results of

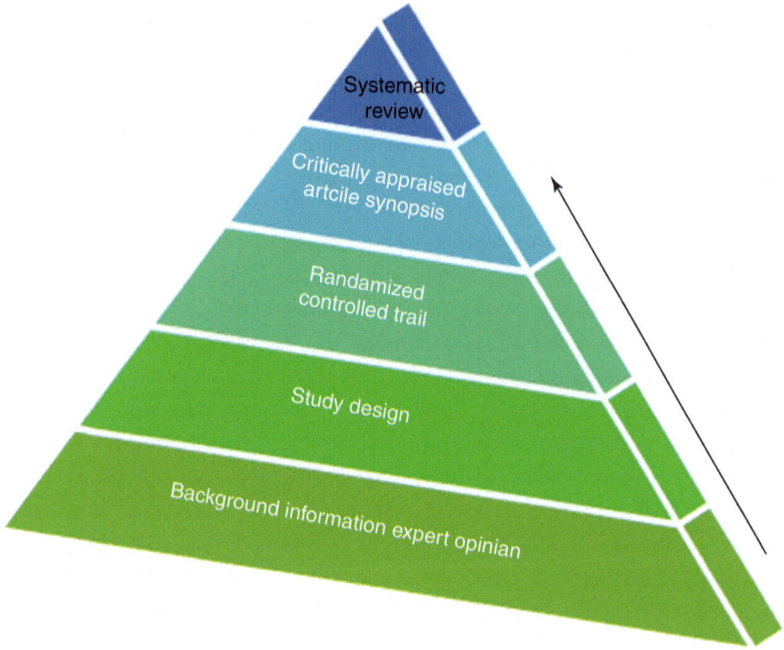

Fig. 9.2 Systematic review of meta-analysis

these studies. A systematic review answers a defined research questions to the researchers by collecting and summarizing all empirical evidence (Fig. 9.3).

A Cochrane review method is used for systematic review of research in health care and health policy, i.e., published in the Cochrane database of systemic review. The review bases their findings on the results of studies that meet certain quality criteria since the most reliable studies will provide the best evidence for making decisions about health care. The method includes different steps to reduce the impact of scientific bias across various parts stem from the review process.

1. Identification of relevant studies from a number of different sources (including unpublished sources)
2. Selection of studies for inclusion and evaluation of their strength and limitations on the basis of clear, predefined criteria
3. Systematic collection of data sets form database
4. Appropriate synthesis of data pertaining to research (evidence-based data sets)

9.5.1 Illustrative Examples of Meta-analysis

1. Organized inpatients (stroke unit) care is provided by multidisciplinary teams that manage stroke patients with aims to assess the effect of organized inpatient (stroke unit) care compared with an alternative service (Langhorne et al. 2020) that used a network analysis approach to know different types of organized inpatients care for people admitted to hospitals after a stroke. The research team has searched the Cochrane Stroke group Trails Register (2 April 2019) and the cumulative index nursing and allied health literature. The research employed RCT trails comparing organized inpatients stoke unit care with and alternative services (typically contemporary conventional care) including comparing different types of organized inpatients (stroke unit) care for people with stroke who are admitted to hospital. The author reviewed and assessed eligibility and trail quality. They checked descriptive details and trial data with coordinators of the original trials, assessed risk bias, and applied grade.

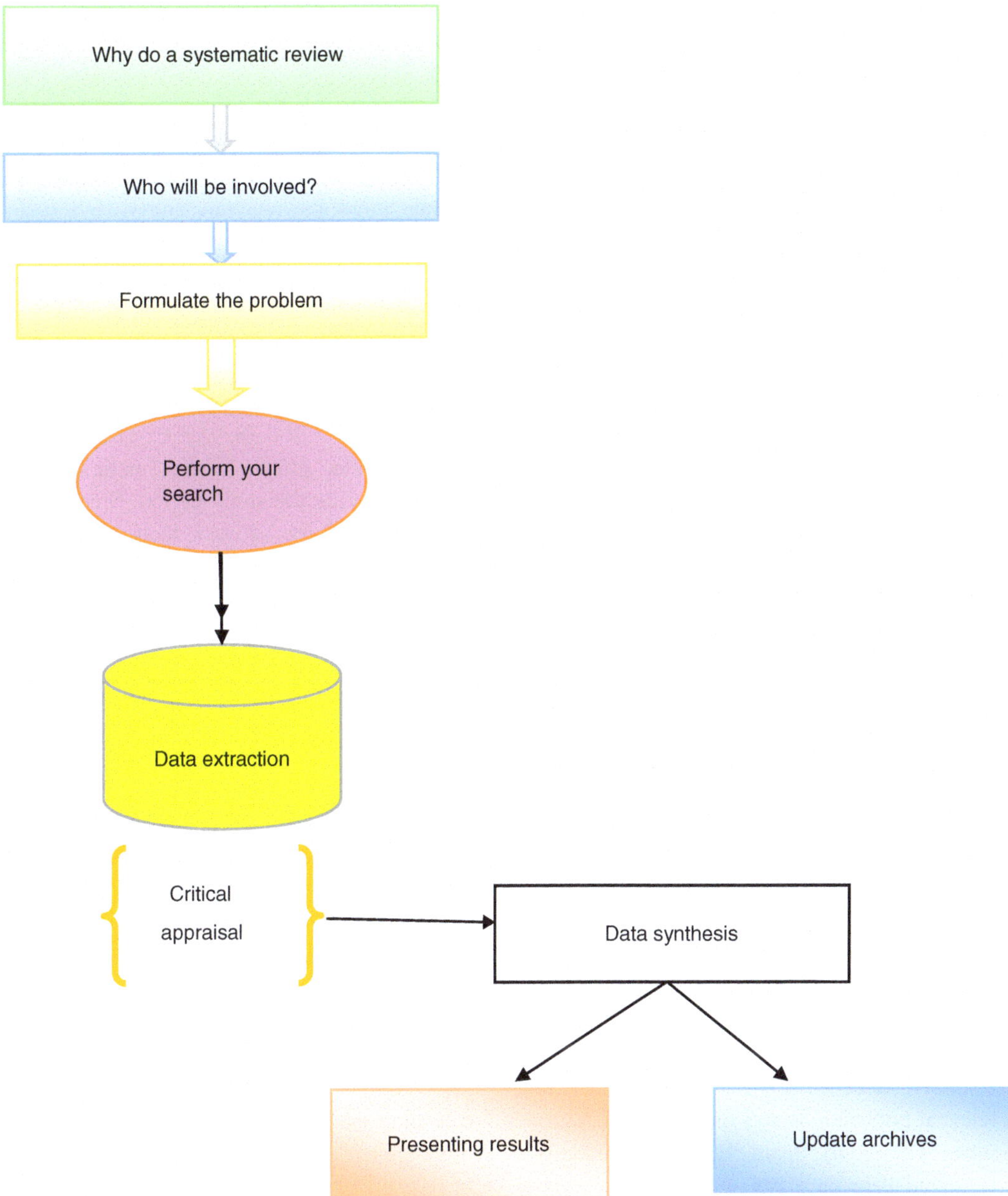

Fig. 9.3 Eligibility criteria and steps involved for conducting meta-analysis

2. The meta-analysis aims to compare the quality conditions for endotracheal intubation and muscle relaxation between rocuronium bromide and vecuronium bromide using the timing principle method for induction in anesthesia. The timing principle includes the administration of muscle relaxants before the hypnotic agent during induction in anesthesia. The study included 60 patients who underwent elective surgery and were randomly allocated into two equal groups using muscle relaxants intervention. During the study period, the intubation conditions were assessed using Cooper's scoring system, based on jaw relaxation, vocal cords position, and response to intubation. The intubation conditions were excellent (100%) for patients in

group R versus excellent in 80% and good in 20% of patients in group V ($P < 0.05$). The author concludes that Rocuronium bromide provides better intubation conditions and greater quality of muscle relaxation than vecuronium bromide using "timing principle" technique; Comparison of intubation condition and the quality of muscle relaxation between rocuronium and vecuronium using "timing principle" (2020), Chinn (2000), Cooper & Rosenthal (1980), Da Costa et al. (2013), Deeks et al. (2001a), Deeks et al. (2001b), Efthimiou (2018), Ebrahim et al. (2014), Ebrahim et al. (2013), Engels et al. (2000).

3. Dipper et al. (2020) reported that the Interventions for the management of malignant pleural effusions: a network meta-analysis. The malignant pleural effusion is a common problem for people living with cancer, and it is usually associated with considerable breathlessness. A number of treatments are available to manage the uncontrolled accumulation of pleural fluid, including administration of pleurodesis agent (via chest tube or thoracoscopy) or placement of indwelling pleural catheter (IPC). He ascertains the optimal management strategy for adult with malignant pleural effusion in terms of pleurodesis success and to quantify in patients reported outcomes and adverse effects between interventions. He searched the databases of Central, Medline (Ovid), Embase (Ovid), and three other databases to June 2019. We screened reference lists from other relevant publications and searched trial registries. The study team has independently extracted data on study design, characteristics, outcome measures, potential effect modifiers, and risk of bias. The study has included a total of 55 studies of 21 interventions in the primary network meta-analysis and also estimated the rank of each intervention's effectiveness. As per the resulted findings, Talc slurry (ranked 6, 95% credible interval (Cr-I) 3–10) is an effective pleurodesis agent (moderate certainty for comparison with placebo), and results were positively correlated in fewer pleurodesis failures than bleomycin and doxycycline (bleomycin versus talc slurry: odds ratio (OR) 2.24, 95% Cr-I 1.10–4.68; low certainty; ranked 11, 95% Cr-I 7–15; doxycycline versus talc slurry: OR 2.51, 95% Cr-I 0.81–8.40; low certainty; ranked 12, 95% Cr-I 5–18). However, there is little evidence of a difference between the pleurodesis failure rate of talc poudrage and talc slurry (OR 0.50, 95% Cr-I 0.21–1.02; moderate certainty). Evidence for any difference was further reduced when restricting analysis to studies at low risk of bias (defined as maximum one high-risk domain in the risk of bias assessment) (pleurodesis failure talc poudrage versus talc slurry: OR 0.78, 95% Cr-I 0.16–2.08). The adverse effects were inconsistently reported during the study period. Study team has performed the network meta-analyses to assess the risk of procedure-related fever and pain. The results found that the risk of developing fewer was low certainly, but suggested that there may be little differences found between the interventions relative to talc slurry. Patients reported control of breathlessness. The study summary realized that the pair-wise meta-analysis suggests there is likely no difference in breathlessness control, relative to talc slurry, of talc poudrage (mean differences 4.00 mm). The study concludes that, based on the available evidence, talc poudrage and talc slurry are effective methods for achieving a pleurodesis, with lower failure rates than a number of other commonly used interventions. Further, he concludes that a more number of studies are required to delineate the roles of different treatments according to patient characteristics, such as presence of trapped lung. Greater attention to patient-centered outcomes including breathlessness, quality of life, and patient preference is essential to inform clinical decision-making.

4. A meta-analysis of 17 controlled clinical trials for testing whether supplementation of diet with "fish oil" reduces blood pressure. Source: > Arch-intern-Med. 1993 June 28, 153(12): 1429–38

   The study conducted a meta-analysis of 17 controlled clinical trials of omega-3 polyunsaturated fatty acids (Omega-3 PUFA) supplementation on blood pressure (BP). To estimate the overall effect of Omega-3 PUFA supplementation on BP, they calculated the net BP change in each trial, which was then weighted according to the inverse of the variance. In the 11 trials that enrolled normotensive individual (n = 728), Omega-3 PUFA supplementation led to significant reductions of systolic BP (SBP) and diastolic BP (DBP) in two and one trials, respectively. In the six studies that enrolled untreated hypertension (n-291), significant reductions of systolic blood pressure (SBP) and diastolic blood pressure (DBP) were presented in two and four trails, respectively. Weighted, pooled estimates of SBP and DBP change (mmH_g) with 95% confidence intervals were also given. The meta-analyses indicated that the diet supplementation with a relatively high dose of omega-3 PUFA, generally more than 3 g/day, could lead to clinically relevant BP reductions in individual with untreated hypertension. However, the use of omega-3 PUFA as antihypertensive drug will require demonstration of long-term efficacy and patient acceptability of lower doses.

5. A meta-analysis of clinical trials of spinal manipulation (Source: J-Manipulative-Physiol-Ther. 1992 March-Arp. 15(3): 181–94)

   A total of 23 randomized controlled trails (RCTs) of the effectiveness of spinal manipulative therapy (SMT) in the treatment of back pain were selected for meta-analysis. The data were extracted via a standardized coding document by one author and verified by two others. Data were independently extracted from a subset of the studies by a blinded research assistant to ensure that coding methods produced acceptable consistency. The effect sizes through Cohen's D-index were calculated for nine outcome variables. A total of 38 out of 44 effect sizes indicated that SMT was better than the comparison treatment. It was also found that the meta-analysis was inappropriate as the protocols were highly diverse. Further, it is difficult to have control groups with placebo for studying the effectiveness of SMT. It was concluded that the SMT was found to be consistently more effective in the treatment of low back pain than were many of the other comparative treatments. The full potential of meta-analysis can be utilized only when researchers strive for explicit descriptions of the nature of SMT, the times of post-treatment assessments, and the nature of outcome measures.

6. Glucocorticoids are infective in alcoholic hepatitis; a meta-analysis adjusting for confounding variables. Source: Gut. 1995 Jul; 37(1): 113–8

   The aim of the study was to perform a meta-analysis of 12 RCTs of glucocorticoid treatment in clinical alcoholic hepatitis, adjusting for prognostic variables and their possible interaction with the treatment. Weighted logistic regression (WLR) was applied on the data such as mean bilirubin value, percent with encephalopathy from treatment and control groups. Though there is an evidence of publication bias, the overall effect of glucocorticoids on mortality is not significant ($P = 0.20$) and relative risk (steroid or control) was 0.78 (95% confidence interval 0.51, 1.18). There was an evidence of interaction between treatment and sex match. The results did not support the routine use of glucocorticoids in patients with alcoholic hepatitis including those with encephalopathy.

7. Comparison of compliance between serotonin reuptake inhibitors and tricyclic antidepressants: a meta-analysis. Source: Int. Clin. Psychopharmacol. 1995; Jan; 9 Suppl. 4: 33–40

   A meta-analysis of 67 RCTs comparing selective serotonin reuptake inhibitors (SSRIs) and tricyclic antidepressants (TCAs), which measured discontinuation rates for the effects and lack of efficacy, was done. Ten studies were placebo-controlled and they were analyzed separately. Overall, the difference in withdrawals was due to the side effects of SSRI and TCA (4.5%; $P = 0.004$) and that due to lack of efficacy (0.1%; P = 0.86). In the placebo-controlled trials, the differences between the two groups were −7.9% and −0.1% (P = 0.06 and 0.96), respectively. It was demonstrated that SSRIs have a significant and clinically important advantage over TCSs with respect to tolerability, whereas efficacy is similar. Treatment failure due to poor compliance can increase health-care costs; therefore, the costs, the risks, and the benefits of each type of treatment need to be critically evaluated while selecting an antidepressant.

9.6 Multicenter Trials

Multicenter clinical trials are the trials conducted concurrently in several centers to assess the efficacy of the same treatment. It becomes necessary to undertake multicenter trials due to the scarcity of patients and intention to complete the trial more quickly, and also the desire to represent a broader geographic spectrum. The conclusions with multicenter trials have a broader and representative base than with single-center trials as the former involves patients and clinicians from several centers. Before taking up the aspects requiring special considerations in multicenter trials, a brief review of the general features of any clinical trial (detailed below) is essential which is common for both multicenter and single-center trials. The reason for multicenter trial is to inculcate and recruit necessary number of subjects within a reasonable time, which assured a more number of representative sample or target population (Figs. 9.4 and 9.5).

The merits of multicenter is a large number of study participants recruited at single snapshot, the study would be conducted at varied geographical location, the possibility of inclusion of a wide range of population groups and ability to compare results among different selected centers. In many cases the efficacy will vary significantly between population groups with genetic,

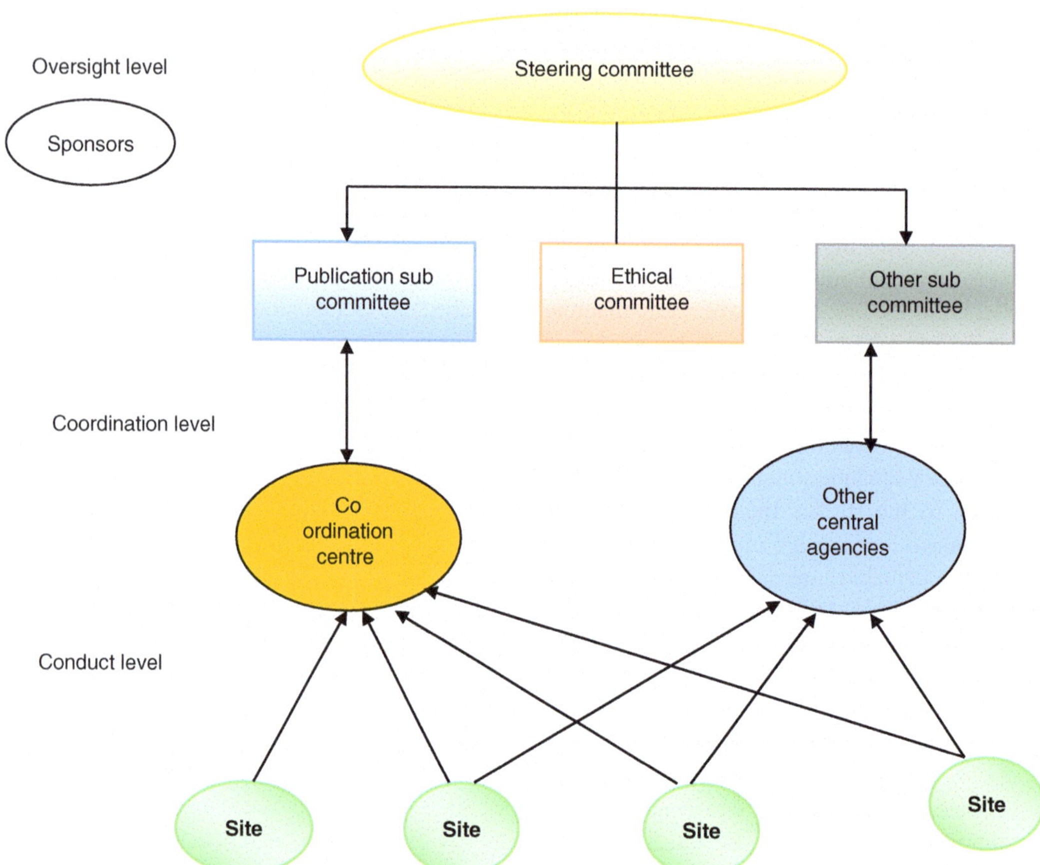

Fig. 9.4 Structure of multicenter drug trail study

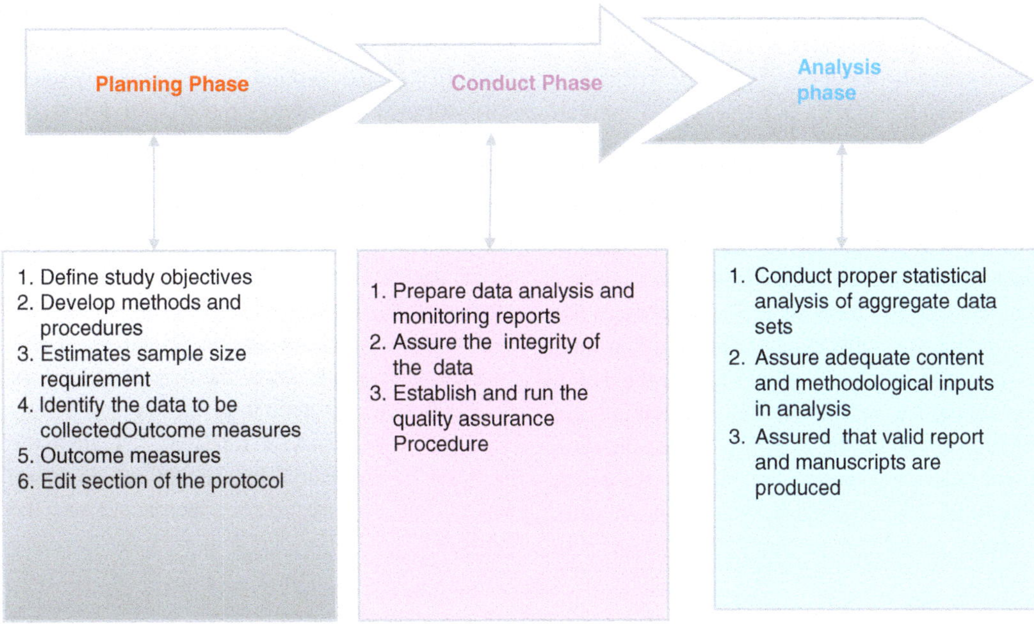

Fig. 9.5 Function of coordinating center

environmental, and ethnic or cultural background; normally geographically depressed trails are evaluated from the multicenter trial. If the subject recruitment rate is lower than expected at one center and higher than expected at another, planned allocation number should be transferred from the center with low subject recruitment to a center with high recruitment where subject inclusion is expected to be completed earlier than planned. This will be done to help ensure that subject enrollment is completed as planned. A prospective multicenter phase I/II clinical trial aims to evaluate drug safety and efficacy of the research interest eg., NOVOCART Disc plus autologous disc chondrocyte transplantation in the treatment of nucleotomized and degenerative lumbar disc to avoid secondary disease, a study protocol for a randomized controlled trial, was conducted (Tschugg et al. 2017). This is a multicenter clinical trial study with randomized controlled procedure, clinical phase I/II combination study group; a total of 120 adult subjects or cases were allocated in a ratio of 2:1:1. The sample size and power calculations were employed to evaluate the minimal risk (marginal error <5%), and clinically important difference of 10 units of subjects was considered, with an expected standard deviation of 12 in the Oswestry Disability Index (ODI), which is the primary outcome parameter. The secondary outcome parameters include the visual analog scale and the EQ-5D questionnaire, etc Adams et al. (2005), Altman et al. (1996), Borenstein et al. (2010), Borenstein & Higgins (2013), Antman et al. (1992), Borenstein et al. (2008), Berlin et al. (2002), Berlin et al. (1993), Cochrane Systematic Review (2020). The observed changes in physical and mental health status were evaluated using the Short Form-12 (SF-12). However, the radiological and functional outcomes are also evaluated. The major inclusion criterion is a single lumbar disc herniation that requires sequestrectomy. Transplantation has performed 90 days period thereafter. Study data sets were generated at a greater accuracy (study sites), and data storage, processing, and statistical analysis were performed separately with greater precision. As per the resulted findings, the outcomes were correlated. The findings show that the avascularity of the lumbar disc is a promising precondition for autologous chondrocyte cell transplantation. Limited blood flow inhibits cell migration and provides an immunologically privileged environment.

9.7 Statistical Implication for Multicenter Trails

Let us consider $P(x_1,x_2,,,x_n)$ $Q(y_1,y_2..y_n)$ the geographical location with respect to drug average adherence of stavudine + efavirenz fixed dose administered for PLHIVs, the researcher wishes to examine the overall drug adherence effect on selected sites; in each selected sites, the study was conducted on the basis of cluster approach. The driven data was collected systematically on interval basis. On conclusive point of view, the overall drug adherence is more likelihood for taking clinical decision about the PLHIVs. If the adherence cannot reach the threshold level, then we call as suboptimal drug adherence, we can take realistic measures to fill the research gap and also we should improve the quality life of PLHIVs in larger extent through revision of PLHIVs guidelines. In a statistical point of view, so many scientists adopted sensitivity analysis to know the optimal level of drug adherence. These Frequentist traditional method will reproduce the results on singleton basis (single value for each selected site), the overall threshold level not to be produced for taking clinical decision from the above-cited method. In this paradigm, we demonstrate and formulate the Mahalanobis D^2 statistics (multivariate analysis) to know the overall efficacy of drug adherence research intervention (Fig. 9.6).

Points are $P(x_1,x_2,,,x_n)$ $Q(y_1,y_2..y_n)$, then the distance was measured by the squared deviation taken from the observed adherence from the study sites:

$$D=\sqrt{(x_1-y_1)^2+(x_2-y_2)^2+(x_3-y_3)^2+(x_4-y_4)^2}.$$

For "n" dimension, it can be written in the following Euclidian distance expression:

$$P(x_1x_2..\ x_p)P(y_1y_2..\ y_p),$$

$$d(p,q)=\sqrt{(x_1-y_1)^2+(x_2-y_2)^2+(x_3-y_3)^2+\ldots\ +(x_p-y_p)^2}. \quad (9.1)$$

Each coordinate site contributes equally to the drug efficacy.

The drug adherence $d(p,q)=d(q,p)$

$$d(p,q)=0 \text{ if and only is } P=Q,$$

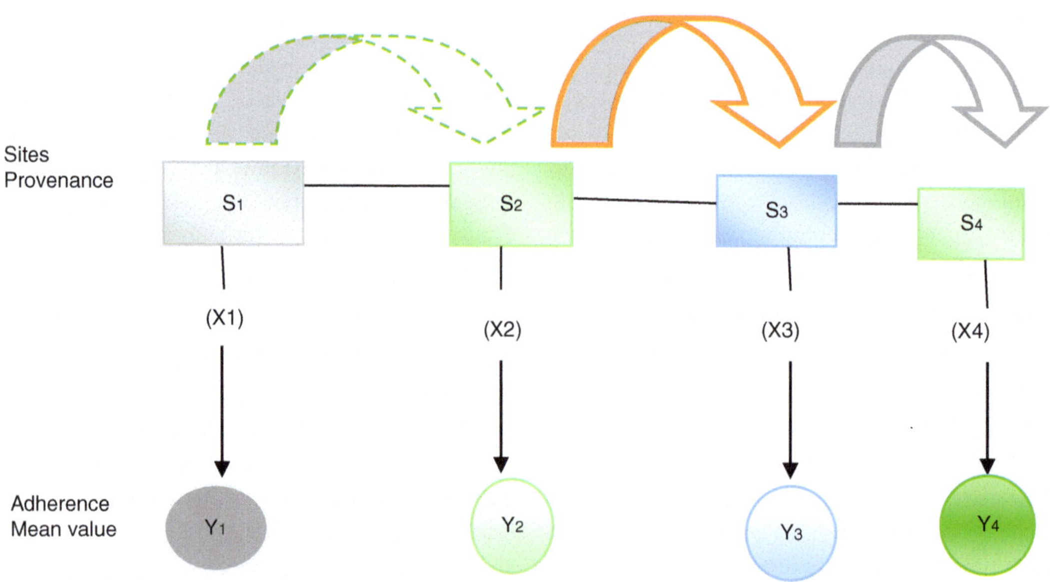

Fig. 9.6 Statistical design for multicentric trial

$d(p,q) = < d(P\ R\ ) + d((R, Q)$ for all R define distance on any sites.

Then, Taxicab observed distance between two points, $(x_1,y_1)\ (x_2,y_2)\ldots(x_n,y_n)$, can be modeled.

$$D = |x_1 - y_1| + |x_2 - y_2| + |x_3 - y_3|..|x_p - y_p|. \quad (9.2)$$

Euclidian distance <Taxicab distance

$$0 \leq |X_p - X_q|\,\|Y_p - Y_q\|.$$

Additive property of inequality

$$|X_p - X_q|^2 + |Y_p - Y_q|^2 + 0 \leq |X_p - X_q|^2 + |Y_p - Y_q|^2 + 2|X_p - X_q||Y_p - Y_q|.$$

Take square root for both side

$$\sqrt{|X_p - X_q|^2 + |Y_p - Y_q|^2} + 0 \leq \sqrt{|X_p - X_q|^2 + |Y_p - Y_q|^2} = dE \leq dT \quad (9.3)$$

It holds high-dimensional data sets

$$\sqrt{\sum_{i=1}^{n}(x_i - y_i)^2} \leq \Sigma|x_i - x_j| = dE \leq dT. \quad (9.4)$$

Statistical distance for uncorrelated sites

$$x_1^* = \frac{x_1}{\sqrt{s_{11}}} x^*_2 = \frac{x_1}{\sqrt{s_{22}}}; d(p,q) = \sqrt{(x_1^*)^2 + (x_2^*)^2} = \sqrt{\frac{x_1^2}{s_{11}} + \frac{x_2^2.}{s_{22}}}$$

All points that have coordinates with respect to distance $(x_1,x_2\ldots x_n)$ are constant squared distance C_2 from the origin must satisfy

$$\frac{x_1^2}{s_{11}} + \frac{x_2^2}{s_{22}} \ldots\ldots \frac{x_n^2}{s_{nn}} = c^2; s_{11} > s_{22} => \frac{1}{s_{11}} < \frac{1}{s_{22}} < \ldots \frac{1}{s_{nn}}. \quad (9.5)$$

This expression can be generalized as statistical distance from an arbitrary point

$$d(p,q) = \sqrt{\frac{(x_1 - y_1)^2}{s_{11}} + \frac{(x_2 - y_2)^2}{s_{22}}}$$; For all p-dimension

$$pd(p,q) = \sqrt{\frac{(x_1 - y_1)^2}{s_{11}} + \frac{(x_2 - y_2)^2}{s_{22}} \ldots\ldots \frac{(x_p - y_p)^2}{s_{pp}}}$$; Note the distance of "p" to the origin "O" is obtained by setting all $Y_i = 0$ (Fig. 9.7).

$$\tilde{x}_1 = x_1 \cos\theta + x_2 \sin\theta,$$

$$\tilde{x}_2 = -x_1 \sin\theta + x_2 \cos\theta,$$

where θ = A between first eigen vector and let B be the (P by b) positive define matrix with Eigen values $\lambda_1 \geq \lambda_2 \geq \ldots \geq \lambda_p > 0$, and associated normalized Eigen vector $e_1, e_2, e_3\ldots. e_n$

$$\max x \neq 0 \frac{X'BX}{X'X} = \lambda_1 \text{attained when } X = e_1$$

$$\min x \neq 0 \frac{X'BX}{X'X} = \lambda_p \text{ attained when } X = e_p$$

$$\max \frac{x}{e_1}, e_2, e_3 \ldots e_n x \neq 0 \frac{X'BX}{X'X} = \lambda_{n+1} \text{ attained when } e_{k+1},\ k = 12,,,,(p-1)$$

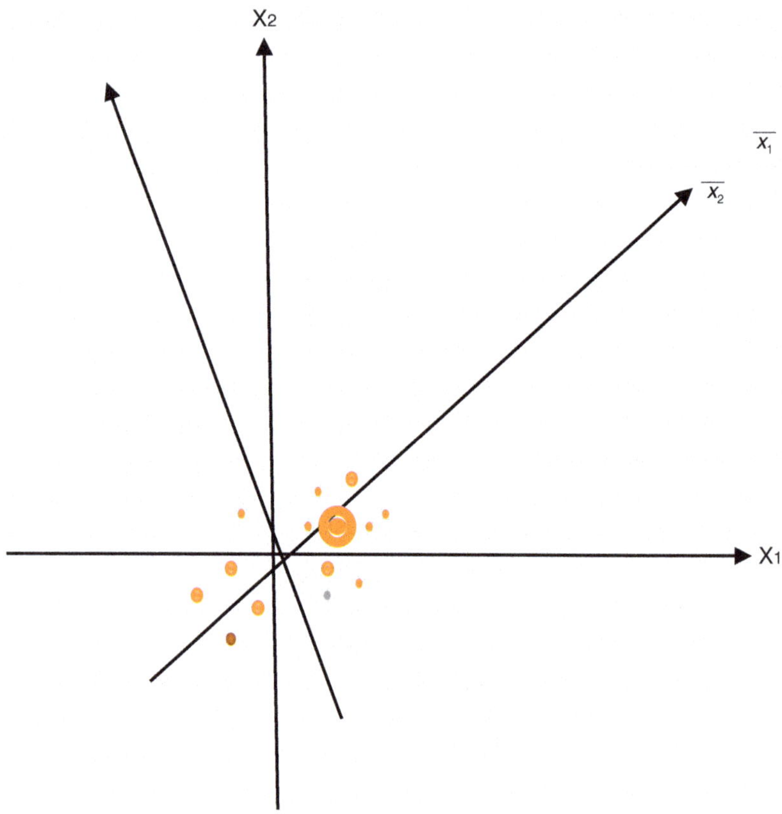

Fig. 9.7 Rotation of factors and its mean values with varimax rotation

Distance under rotated coordinate system was

$$(0,0) = P\left(\widetilde{x_1}\ \widetilde{x_2}\right)$$

$$d(p,q) = \sqrt{\frac{\widetilde{x_1}^2}{\tilde{s}_{11}} + \frac{\widetilde{x_2}^2}{\tilde{s}_{22}}}$$

where

$$\tilde{x}_1 = x_1 \cos\theta + x_2 \sin\theta,$$

$$\tilde{x}_2 = -x_1 \sin\theta + x_2 \cos\theta,$$

$$d(p,q) = \sqrt{a_{11}x^2{}_1 + 2a_{12}x_1x_2 + a_{22}x_2{}^2}. \quad (9.6)$$

$$\tilde{s}_{11}{}^2 = \frac{1}{n-1}\Sigma\left(\tilde{x}_1 - \overline{x}_1\right)^2,$$

$$\tilde{s}_{22}{}^2 = \frac{1}{n-1}\Sigma\left(\tilde{x}_2 - \overline{x}_2\right)^2,$$

$$d(p,q) = \sqrt{\frac{\left(x_1\cos\theta + x_2\sin\theta\right)^2}{\tilde{s}_{11}} + \frac{\left(-x_1\sin\theta + x_2\cos\theta\right)^2}{\tilde{s}_{22}}},$$

$$\mathrm{d}(p,q) = \sqrt{a_{11}x^2{}_1 + a_{22}x_2{}^2} + \Lambda + a_{pp}x_2{}^2 + 2a_{12}x_1x_2 + 2a_{13}x_1x_3 + \Lambda + 2ap - 1_{p^x}.$$

The above distances are completely determined by the coefficient weights $a_i = i$, $k = 1, 2, 3..p$

$$A = \begin{bmatrix} a_{11} & a_{12}\cdots & a_{1p} \\ a_{12} & a_{22}\cdots & a_{2p} \\ a_{1p} & a_{2p}\cdots & a_{pp} \end{bmatrix},$$

$$A = C'C,$$

$$X'AX = X'C'X = (CX)'(CX) = Y'Y. \quad (9.7)$$

Obey all the distances property

$X'AX$ is a distance for different A

$$d(p,q) = \sqrt{X'AX},$$

$$d^2(p,q) = X'AX,$$

where $X' = (x_1, x_2 \ldots x_p); A = \begin{bmatrix} a_{11} & a_{12}\cdots & a_{1p} \\ a_{12} & a_{22}\cdots & a_{2p} \\ a_{1p} & a_{2p}\cdots & a_{pp} \end{bmatrix}$,

$$d^2(p,q) = (X_i - Y_i)' A (X_i - Y_i),$$

$$x' = (x_1, x_2 \ldots x_p); y' = (x_1, x_2 \ldots x_p),$$

$$A = \begin{bmatrix} a_{11} & a_{12}\cdots & a_{1p} \\ a_{12} & a_{22}\cdots & a_{2p} \\ a_{1p} & a_{2p}\cdots & a_{pp} \end{bmatrix} = \Sigma,$$

$$d^2(p,q) = X' \Sigma X.$$

And used μ is the overall drug adherence in selected sites instead of Y.

$$d^2(p,q) = (x-\mu)' \Sigma^{-1} (x-\mu). \quad (9.8)$$

Suppose $P = 2$, the distance from different various sites generalized in the form of

$$X'\Lambda x = a_{11}x_1^2 + 2a_{12}x_1x_2 + a_{22}x_2^2 = c^2.$$

By spectral decomposition method, the equation becomes

$$\Lambda = \lambda e_1 e^{11} + \lambda_2 e_1 e_2' \ldots \text{so on},$$

$$X'\Lambda x = \lambda_1 (x'e_1)^2 + \lambda_2 (x'e_2)^2,$$

$$A^{-1} = \sum_{I=1}^{K} \lambda_i e_i e_j = (P\Lambda P')_{kxk},$$

$$A^{-1} = P\Lambda P' \sum_{I=1}^{K} \frac{1}{\lambda_i} e_i e_j. \quad (9.9)$$

The Mahalanobis distance is a multivariate statistics that provides a relative measure of a various data points from the common point. It is unit less, introduced by Prof P C Mahalanobis

$$d(p,q) = \sqrt{a_{11}x_1^2 + 2a_{12}x_1x_2 + a_{22}x_2^2},$$

$$d(p,q) = \sqrt{X'AX},$$

$$X = \begin{pmatrix} x_{11} \\ x_{12} \\ \cdot \\ x_{in} \end{pmatrix} A = \begin{bmatrix} a_{11} & a_{12}\cdots & a_{1p} \\ a_{12} & a_{22}\cdots & a_{2p} \\ a_{1p} & a_{2p}\cdots & a_{pp} \end{bmatrix}. \quad (9.10)$$

So for sample the eqn becomes

$$d^2(p,q) = (x-\bar{x})' s^{-1} (x-\mu).$$

Let $X_1, X_2, ..X_n$ be the independent observations for given population with mean μ and finite common variance, the random variable distribution of X_n variables is $\sqrt{n}(\bar{X}-\mu)S^{-1}(\bar{X}-\mu)$ is approximately χ_p^2 for np is largewhere,

$$\begin{pmatrix} \bar{X}_1 - \mu_1 \\ \bar{X}_2 - \mu_2 \\ \bar{X}_n - \mu_i \end{pmatrix} = (\bar{X}_i - \mu_i). \quad (9.11)$$

And the sample deviation SSCP matrix is tested by the Hotelling's T-square test statistics:

$$T^2 = n(n-1)X's^{-1}X,$$

$$F_{p,(n-P)} = \frac{n-p}{(n-1)p} T^2. \quad (9.12)$$

9.8 Various Aspects of Clinical Trials

9.8.1 Planning

1. Design of trial
2. Random allocation procedures
3. Design of Proforma

9.8.2 Executive and Monitoring

1. Preparation and supply of random treatment assignments
2. Scrutiny of data collected
3. Rectification of errors

9.8.3 Data Analysis and Reporting

1. Database creation and validation
2. Statistical tests and inferences
3. Preparation of final report
4. In additional to the abovementioned aspects, the multicenter trials have some aspects which require special considerations.

9.8.4 Aspects Requiring Special Considerations

1. Random allocation of treatment to patients
2. Standardized procedures for clinical and laboratory assessments
3. Quality control of data collected
4. Statistical analysis of data pooled from several centers
5. The above is not an exhaustive list of aspects requiring special considerations in multicenter trials. The importance of these main aspects is explained below with illustrations.

9.8.5 Random Allocation

Random allocation within each center is preferable as the condition of patients and/or their response may vary between centers. Also, we require a balanced allocation in every ***n*** patients admitted to the trial, say, six patients, i.e., if there are two groups of treatment, three should be allocated to one group and the remaining three to the other group. Stratification within each center assures equality of treatment numbers for every stratum (i.e., type of patient). But as the number of strata increases, this becomes rather impracticable. In such situations, there are certain special methods which balance the marginal treatment totals for each type of patient, and the treatment assigned can be obtained from a Central Registration Office.

9.8.6 Need for Standardized Procedures for Clinical Assessments

Two centers (say A and B) participated in a clinical trial among patients with rheumatoid arthritis. A 15-m walking distance test was to be performed by patients in both the centers. At center A, the mean time taken to walk 15 m was 25 s compared to 15 s at center B. The shorter mean time at center B was contrary to our expectation of a higher value as this center had more ill patients (i.e., ARC Classifications III and IV). It was discovered that at center B the patients were allowed to walk aided by their attendant, whereas in center A on their own. Hence, it is very important that centers should follow uniform criteria and strict adherence to established data collection procedures Akl et al. (2016), Akl et al. (2015), Anzures-Cabrera et al. (2011). Sufficient training and explanation should be given to ensure consistency across centers.

9.8.7 Need for Standardized Procedures for Laboratory Assessments

A clinical trial was undertaken in patients with acute viral hepatitis at three centers employing the same diagnostic criteria and using the same brand of kit for biochemical assessments. Under these conditions, normally one would expect that the three centers will give broadly similar results. The mean SGOT and SGPT values on admission at the three centers are given in the following table.

Center	No. of patients	Mean values on admission	
		SGOT (Iu/L)	SGPT (Iu/L)
A	146	70	159
B	129	401	488
C	162	255	301

There was a substantial variation in the mean SGOT and SGPT levels on admission among the three centers, and especially the values at center A were very low despite the fact that all centers employed the same diagnostic criteria and used the same brand of kit. This situation clearly demonstrates the need for standardization of technicians and also the techniques to be employed before the commencement of the trial.

9.8.8 Quality Control of Data Collection

In a clinical trial, patients were to attend clinic once in every fortnight for clinical assessment and drug collection. On scrutiny of the completed Proforma received from the center, it was observed that not even a single patient ever missed a follow-up and more surprisingly, they attended the clinic on the exact due date in every instance. On a surprise site visit, it was detected that patients had actually attended the clinic once in a month or two, but the data were filled-up, retrospectively, for all the previous fortnights. This emphasizes the fact that periodical site visits to the participating centers forms an essential aspect of quality control process.

9.8.9 Analysis of Data Pooled from Four Centers

A trial was conducted to evaluate the efficacy of a new drug at four different centers employing the same protocol. The cure rates obtained with the new and standard drugs at the four centers are given

	Cure	rate
Center	New drug	Standard drug
A	68% (40/59)	58% (36/62)
B	67% (47/70)	59% (44/74)
C	69% (45/65)	62% (43/69)
D	79% (55/70)	72% (48/67)
Total	71% (187/264)	63% (171/272)

$\bar{d} = 8\%$, SE = 0.0407, $P = 0.05$

Though the four centers followed the same protocol, i.e. same diagnostic criteria, similar group of patients, uniform definition for cure rate, etc., the variation between the centers is unavoidable (possibly due to some extraneous factors which are beyond our control). To compare the new drug with the standard, it would be more appropriate to employ special methods (e.g., Cochran's method) which take into account the experiences at individual centers, instead of basing our conclusion on the overall cure rate, i.e., 71% vs 63%, which at times may be misleading. The specific methods are not only appropriate but also advantageous as in this situation, the comparison of overall cure rates (71% vs 63%) gives a P value of 0.05, whereas the special method yields a P value of 0.03 indicating a greater sensitivity of the test. Thus, keeping in mind all the points discussed above, while planning a clinical trial, it is important to recognize early on whether a single-center study is sufficient or not. If not, the pros and cons of multicenter trial should be considered which are detailed in the following.

9.9 Merits

1. Evidently, the principal advantage of mounting a multicenter trial is that patient accrual is much quicker so that the trial can be made larger and/or the intended size can be achieved more quickly. The end result is that a multicenter trial reaches more reliable conclusions at a faster rate so that overall progress in the treatment of a given disease is enhanced.
2. The fact that a trial involves patients and clinicians from several centers means that any conclusions drawn from the trial have a broader, more representative base that can be reached from a single-center trial. Hence, extrapolation of findings to the whole population of similar patients can be done with greater confidence.
3. Hopefully the collaboration of clinical scientists in a multicenter trial should lead to raised standards in the design, conduct, and interpretation of the trial.

9.9.1 Illustrative Examples

Clearly, the planning and administration of any multicenter trial is considerably more complex than a single-center trial and hence it is vital to have efficient centralized coordination of all trial activities. Multicenter trials are very expensive to run, regarding both staff and resources, so that one must first obtain adequate funding for the study.

It is important to ensure that all centers strictly follow the study protocol. Adequate communication across centers at the planning stage is needed to obtain prior agreement regarding the nature of the study. In particular, any potential investigator who cannot agree to the eventual design should be encouraged to exclude them from further participation in the study before problems of noncompliance arise.

The need for quality control as regards any measurements, clinical observations, and data recording requires prior recognition. Sufficient training and explanation should be given to ensure consistency across centers.

The collection and processing of data pose special problems in multicenter trials which are often not anticipated. One needs a well-organized data center which receives all data and provides prompt and reliable feedback to each participating center of data requirements and problems.

3. Implement editing procedures to detect data deficiencies.
4. Develop performance monitoring procedures and prepare reports.
5. Develop treatment monitoring and reporting procedures to detect evidence of adverse or beneficial treatment effects.
6. Site visit to participating clinics.
7. Prepare study progress reports for submission to sponsorer.
8. Update study manuals.

9.9.2 Initial Design Stage

1. Calculate required sample size.
2. Outline data collection schedule, quality control procedures, data analysis plans, data entry, and editing procedures.
3. Develop organizational structure of the trial.

9.9.3 Protocol Development Stage

1. Develop treatment allocation procedures.
2. Develop computer programs and related procedures for receiving, processing, editing, and analyzing study data.
3. Design and test data forms.
4. Develop interface for data transmission from clinics and other resource centers to the coordinating center.
5. Train clinic personnel in required data collection procedures.
6. Distribute study data forms and related materials.
7. Develop manuals needed in the trial, including the protocol, clinic manual of operations, etc.

9.9.4 Patient Recruitment Stage

1. Administer treatment allocations, including checks for breakdowns in the assignment process.
2. Assume leadership role in outlining study needs for quality assurance.

9.9.5 Treatment and Follow-Up Stage

1. Prepare periodic reports on performance of clinics.
2. Carry out periodic training sessions to maintain high level of proficiency at clinics in treatment and date collection procedures.
3. Evaluate data processing procedures and modify, if necessary.
4. Assume major role in writing a paper on design and methods.

9.9.6 Patient Close-Out Stage

1. Develop plans for final data editing.
2. Design and test computer programs needed for final data analysis.
3. Develop plans for final disposition of study data.
4. Coordinate logistics of patient disengagement from treatment.
5. Assume key role in writing papers summarizing results of the trial.

9.9.7 Termination Stage

1. Supervise collection and disposal of unused study materials.
2. Assume leadership role in paper writing activities.
3. Distribute draft manuscripts and published papers to participating centers.

9.10 Organization

The complex structure that is required to organize a large multicenter trial is illustrated by an example of the British trial of treatment for mild hypertension as described by the Medical Research Council Working Party (1977). The trial is concerned with comparing two standard antihypertensive drugs with placebo in patients with a diastolic blood pressure in the range of 90–109 mmHg to see if there is a subsequent reduction in mortality and morbid events such as nonfatal stroke. The trial, involving 18,000 subjects, is one of the largest multicenter trials ever undertaken in Britain so that its organizational structure, as explained below, is of particular importance.

The Medical Research Council are funding the study and hence have reviewed the study design and are kept informed of study progress.

The Trial Working Party and particularly its Chairman and Clinical Secretary are responsible for organizing the trial in all its aspects.

The Trial Monitoring Committee provides a group of experienced clinical researchers and statisticians who were called upon to oversee the trial's general progress but are not concerned with the day-to-day running of the study.

The Ethical Committee is concerned with all ethical aspects of the study.

The Coordinating Centre consists of two clinical epidemiologists, a statistician, and 12–15 technical and clerical support staff. Day-to-day activities especially data collection, follow-up of subjects, and evaluation of results are carried out from this center.

Trial Clinics, around 200 of them all over the country, are set up to screen middle-aged men and women, to check if they are eligible and willing to participate in the trial.

Central Laboratory Services are used for all biochemical tests.

This trial is perhaps a typical regarding its large size, but in terms of the organizational structure, it provides a working model for multicenter trials. Possibly in a smaller trial the committees might be amalgamated.

9.11 Conclusion

Meta-analysis is a quantitative approach for systematically combining results of previous research to arrive at conclusion about the body of research. The chapter deals with various statistical models' approach to identify the heterogeneity effects among multiple studies and, where appropriate, previous summary of published work to diagnose relative measures of our objective of interest. Various statistical models were demonstrated to determine the effective size and impact of previous studies (published in reputed journals). The fitted models signify the precision and reproducibility for testing Null Hypothesis (H_0) with various subjects. The present model identifies analytical research gap at population level and also improves our insight knowledge for future line of research work (micro/macro).

References

Adams NP, Bestall JB, Malouf R, Lasserson TJ, Jones PW (2005) Beclomethasone versus placebo for chronic asthma. Cochrane Database Syst Rev (1):CD002738

Akl EA et al (2015) Handling trial participants with missing outcome data when conducting a meta-analysis: a systematic survey of proposed approaches. Syst Rev 4:98

Akl EA et al (2016) Three challenges described for identifying participants with missing data in trials reports, and potential solutions suggested to systematic reviewers. J Clin Epidemiol 76:147–154

Altman DG et al (1996) Detecting skewness from summary information. BMJ 313:1200–1200

Antman EM, Lau J, Kupelnick B, Mosteller F, Chalmers TC (1992) A comparison of results of meta-analyses of randomized control trials and recommendations of clinical experts: treatments for myocardial infarction. JAMA 268:240–248

Anzures-Cabrera J et al (2011) Expressing findings from meta-analyses of continuous outcomes in terms of risks. Stat Med 30:2967–2985

Berlin JA, Longnecker MP, Greenland S (1993) Meta-analysis of epidemiologic dose-response data. Epidemiology 4:218–228

Berlin JA, Santanna J, Schmid CH, Szczech LA, Feldman KA (2002) Individual patient- versus group-level data meta-regressions for the investigation of treatment effect modifiers: ecological bias rears its ugly head. Stat Med 21:371–387

Borenstein M, Higgins JPT (2013) Meta-analysis and subgroups. Prev Sci 14:134–143
Borenstein M, Hedges LV, Higgins JPT, Rothstein HR (2008) Introduction to meta-analysis. Wiley, Chichester
Borenstein M, Hedges LV, Higgins JPT, Rothstein HR (2010) A basic introduction to fixed-effect and random-effects models for meta-analysis. Res Synth Methods 1:97–111
Chinn S (2000) A simple method for converting an odds ratio to effect size for use in meta-analysis. Stat Med 19:3127–3131
Cochrane Systematic Review—Intervention Version published: 21 April 2020 see what's new. https://doi.org/10.1002/14651858.CD010529.pub3. https://www.cochranelibrary.com/cdsr/doi/10.1002/14651858.CD010529.pub3/full
Comparison of intubation condition and the quality of muscle relaxation between rocuronium and vecuronium using "timing principle" Medicinski glasnik: official publication of the Medical Association of Zenica-Doboj Canton, Bosnia and Herzegovina, 2020, 17(1) | added to Central: 30 November 2019 | 2019 Issue 11. https://doi.org/10.17392/1045-20
Cooper HM, Rosenthal R (1980) Statistical versus traditional procedures for summarizing research findings. Psychol Bull 87:442–449
Da Costa BR et al (2013) Combining follow-up and change data is valid in meta-analyses of continuous outcomes: a meta-epidemiological study. J Clin Epidemiol 66:847–855
Deeks JJ et al (2001a) Statistical methods for examining heterogeneity and combining results from several studies in meta-analysis. In: Egger M, Davey Smith G, Altman DG (eds) Systematic reviews in health care: meta-analysis in context, 2nd edn. BMJ Publication Group, London, pp 285–312
Deeks JJ et al (2001b) Statistical methods for examining heterogeneity and combining results from several studies in meta-analysis. In: Egger M, Davey Smith G, Altman DG (eds) Systematic reviews in health care: meta-analysis in context, 2nd edn. BMJ Publication Group, London
Dipper A et al (2020) Interventions for the management of malignant pleural effusions: a network meta-analysis. Cochrane Database Syst Rev 4(4):CD010529
Ebrahim S, Akl EA, Mustafa RA, Sun X, Walter SD, Heels-Ansdell D, Alonso-Coello P, Johnston BC, Guyatt GH (2013) Addressing continuous data for participants excluded from trial analysis: a guide for systematic reviewers. J Clin Epidemiol 66:1014–1021.e1011
Ebrahim S, Johnston BC, Akl EA, Mustafa RA, Sun X, Walter SD, Heels-Ansdell D, Alonso-Coello P, Guyatt GH (2014) Addressing continuous data measured with different instruments for participants excluded from trial analysis: a guide for systematic reviewers. J Clin Epidemiol 67:560–570
Efthimiou O (2018) Practical guide to the meta-analysis of rare events. Evid Based Ment Health 21:72–76
Engels EA et al (2000) Heterogeneity and statistical significance in meta-analysis: an empirical study of 125 meta-analyses. Stat Med 19:1707–1728
Greenland S et al (1992) Methods for trend estimation from summarized dose-response data, with applications to meta-analysis. Am J Epidemiol 135:1301–1309
Higgins J et al (2004) Controlling the risk of spurious findings from meta-regression. Stat Med 23:1663–1682
Higgins J et al (2008) Meta-analysis of skewed data: combining results reported on log-transformed or raw scales. Stat Med 27:6072–6092
Kjaergard LL, Villumsen J, Gluud C (2001) Reported methodologic quality and discrepancies between large and small randomized trials in meta-analyses. Ann Intern Med 135:982–989
Langan D, Higgins JPT, Simmonds M (2015) An empirical comparison of heterogeneity variance estimators in 12 894 meta-analyses. Res Synth Methods 6:195–205
Langan D, Higgins JPT, Simmonds M (2017) Comparative performance of heterogeneity variance estimators in meta-analysis: a review of simulation studies. Res Synth Methods 8:181–198
Langan D, Higgins JPT, Jackson D, Bowden J, Veroniki AA, Kontopantelis E, Viechtbauer W, Simmonds M (2019) A comparison of heterogeneity variance estimators in simulated random-effects meta-analyses. Res Synth Methods 10:83–98
Langhorne P, Ramachandra S, Stroke Unit Trialists' Collaboration (2020) Organised inpatient (stroke unit) care for stroke: network meta-analysis. Cochrane Database Syst Rev 4(4):CD000197
Laupacis A, Sackett DL, Roberts RS (1988) An assessment of clinically useful measures of the consequences of treatment. N Engl J Med 318:1728–1733
Rhodes KM, Turner RM, White IR, Jackson D, Spiegelhalter DJ, Higgins JPT (2016) Implementing informative priors for heterogeneity in meta-analysis using meta-regression and pseudo data. Stat Med 35:5495–5511
Rice K, Higgins JPT, Lumley T (2018) A re-evaluation of fixed effect(s) meta-analysis. J R Stat Soc Ser A Stat Soc 181:205–227
Riley RD, Higgins JPT, Deeks JJ (2011) Interpretation of random effects meta-analyses. BMJ 342:d549
Sharp SJ (2001) Analysing the relationship between treatment benefit and underlying risk: precautions and practical recommendations. In: Egger M, Davey Smith G, Altman DG (eds) Systematic reviews in health care: meta-analysis in context, 2nd edn. BMJ Publication Group, London, pp 176–188
Sidik K, Jonkman JN (2002) A simple confidence interval for meta-analysis. Stat Med 21:3153–3159
Simmonds MC, Tierney J, Bowden J, Higgins JPT (2011) Meta-analysis of time-to-event data: a comparison of two-stage methods. Res Synth Methods 2:139–149
Thompson SG, Higgins JPT (2002) How should meta-regression analyses be undertaken and interpreted? Stat Med 21:1559–1574
Tschugg A et al (2017) A prospective multicenter phase I/II clinical trial to evaluate safety and efficacy of

NOVOCART Disc plus autologous disc chondrocyte transplantation in the treatment of nucleotomized and degenerative lumbar disc to avoid secondary disease: study protocol for a randomized controlled trial. Trials 108(17):215–220. https://doi.org/10.1186/s13063-016-1239-y

Turner RM, Davey J, Clarke MJ, Thompson SG, Higgins JPT (2012) Predicting the extent of heterogeneity in meta-analysis, using empirical data from the Cochrane Database of Systematic Reviews. Int J Epidemiol 41:818–827

Veroniki AA, Jackson D, Viechtbauer W, Bender R, Bowden J, Knapp G, Kuss O, Higgins JPT, Langan D, Salanti G (2016) Methods to estimate the between-study variance and its uncertainty in meta-analysis. Res Synth Methods 7:55–79

Whitehead A, Jones NMB (1994) A meta-analysis of clinical trials involving different classifications of response into ordered categories. Stat Med 13:2503–2515

Yusuf S, Peto R, Lewis J, Collins R, Sleight P (1985) Beta blockade during and after myocardial infarction: an overview of the randomized trials. Prog Cardiovasc Dis 27:335–371

Yusuf S, Wittes J, Probstfield J, Tyroler HA (1991) Analysis and interpretation of treatment effects in subgroups of patients in randomized clinical trials. JAMA 266:93–98

10 Pharmacokinetic and Statistical Modeling

10.1 Pharmacokinetic Modeling Approach to New Drug Development

Drug research encompasses several disciplines united by a common goal, namely the development of novel therapeutic agents. However, the research for new drug can be divided functionally into two stages, viz. discovery and development. The process of drug development consists of setting up a working hypothesis of the target enzymes or receptors for a particular disease, establishing suitable mathematical models or surrogate markers to be biological activities and screening the new drug molecules for *in vitro* or *in vivo* biological activities (Ahmed et al. 2012; Aronow et al. 2000; Basavarajaiah 2018). Overwhelmingly, the drug development process will be too many critics, efforts concealed to focus on evaluation of the toxicity and efficacy of new drug candidates. The mathematical model to know the characteristics of time of drug absorption, metabolism and excretions and relationship of these processes to the intensity and time course of the therapeutic and toxicology effects of drug (Boonleang et al. 2007; Beringer et al. 2005; Breiman 2001). The PK model describes the process whereby specific mode and by a specific dose is handled by the body leading to the specific drug concentration in different tissues or organs. Further, the part of drug will reach the sites of action and excretes into pharmacodynamic action. The PK is used in the clinical settings to enhance safe and effective therapeutic management of individual patients or subjects. This application is termed as clinical pharmacokinetic. The salient principles of PK model are presented as follows.

1. Design and development of new drugs for improving therapeutic effectiveness
2. Design and development of an optimum formulation for better use of the drug
3. Design and development of controlled or targeted release formation
4. Select the appropriate route for drug administration
5. Select the right drug for particular illness
6. Predict and explain drug—food and drug-to-drug interaction
7. Design an appropriate multiple dosage regimen
8. Therapeutic drug monitoring in individual patients
9. Dosage adjustment in situation of altered physiology and drug interaction (Fig. 10.1)

B. D. M., B. Narasimha Murthy, *Design of Experiments and Advanced Statistical Techniques in Clinical Research*, https://doi.org/10.1007/978-981-15-8210-3_10

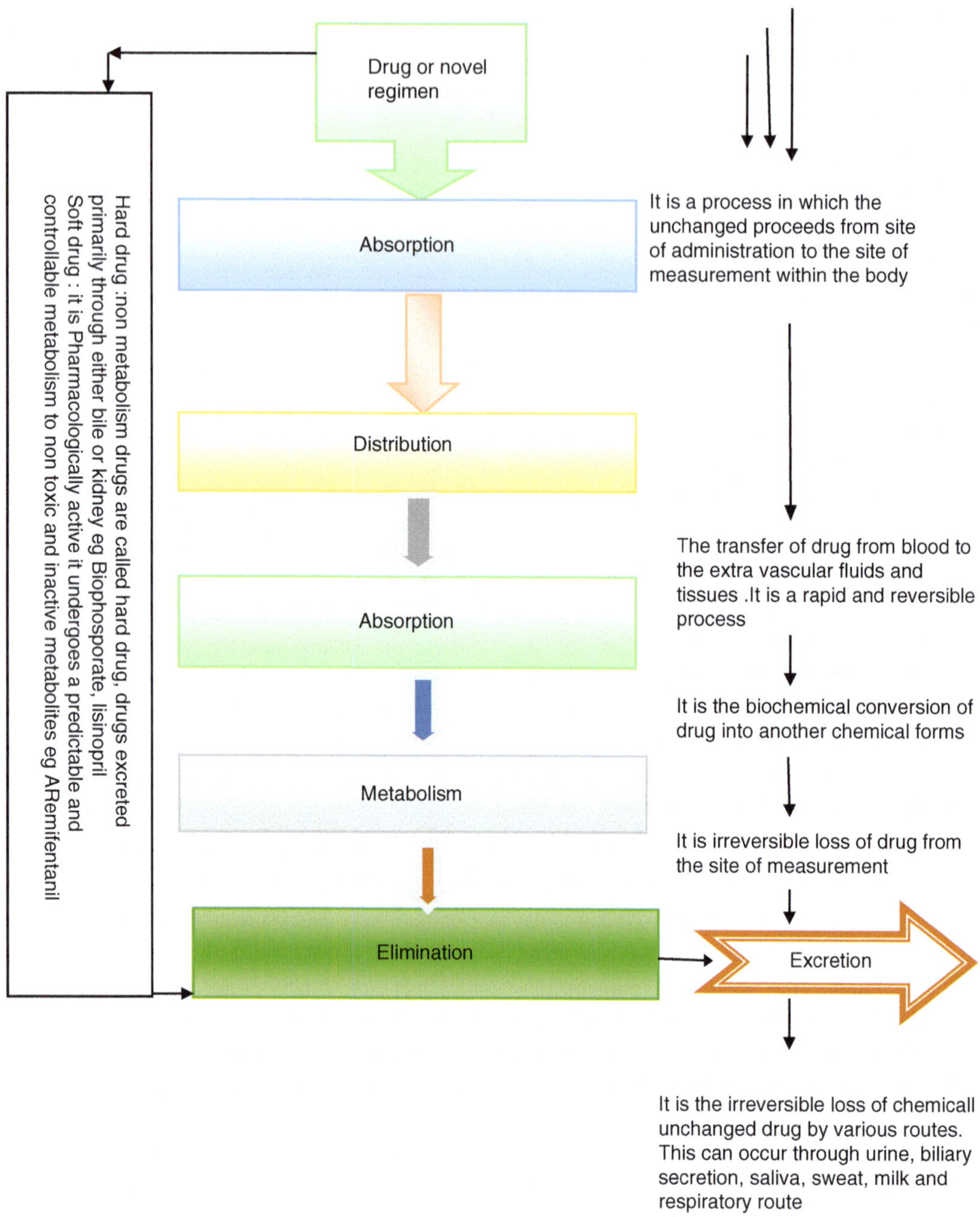

Fig. 10.1 Flowchart of ADME process in human body

10.2 Application of PK Mathematical Model in New Drug Development Process

To understand the process of absorption, distribution, elimination of drug, which affects onsets and intensity of biological response

To access plasma drug concentration response to given dose which is considered as more appropriate parameter than intrinsic PK activity

In design and utilization of in vivo model that can evaluate dissolution characteristics of new compound formulated as new drug formulation and establish meaningful IVIVC

In design and development of new drug and their appropriate dosage regimen

In safe and effective management of patients by improving drug therapy

To understand the concept of bioavailability which has been used to evaluate and monitor in vivo performance of new dosage forms and genetic formulation

To carry out the bioavailability and bioequivalence tests

We can use the PK principles in the development of the various new drug development processes (Fig. 10.2).

Dosing of drug in obese patients

Ideal body weight (IBW) is calculated as follows:

$$\text{IBW}(\text{Men}) = 50\,\text{kg} \pm 1\,\text{kg per } 2.5\,\text{cm above or below } 150\,\text{cm in height}$$

$$\text{IBW}(\text{women}) = 45\,\text{kg} \pm 1\,\text{kg per } 2.5\,\text{cm above or below } 150\,\text{cm in height}$$

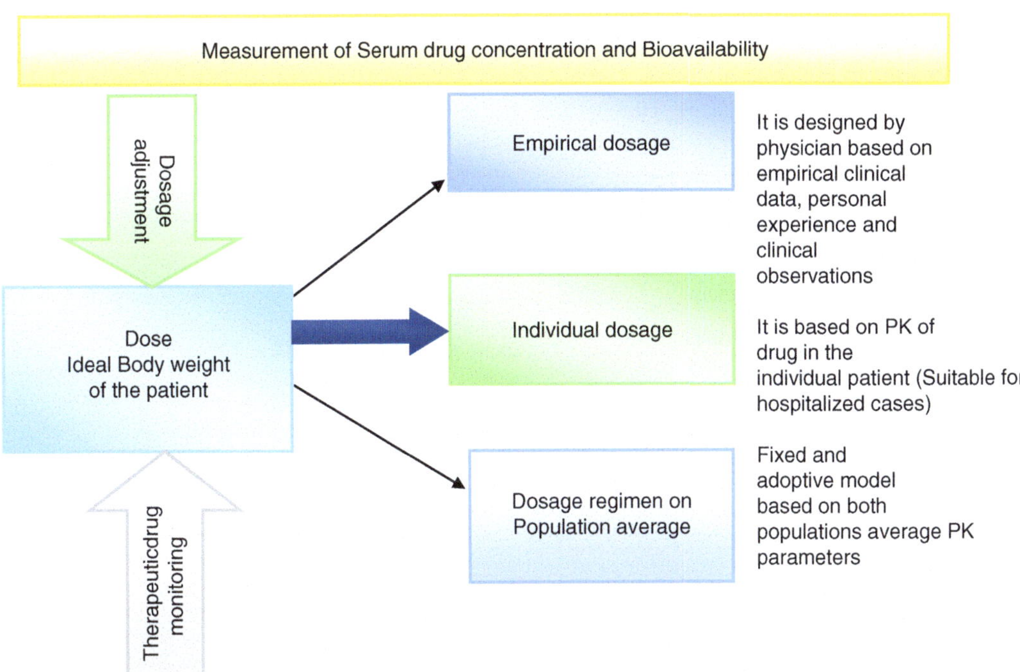

Fig. 10.2 Approaches for dosage regimen in new drug

10.3 Pharmacokinetic (PK) Mathematical Model

PK model is a hypothetical structure used to describe the fate of a drug in a biological system following administration. All PK models embedded or tailored with some mathematical simulation from original database of drug information, so many attributes (clinical) and serological markers and candidates were mathematically simulated in the interest. The PK models it means of expressing mathematically or quantitatively, time course of drug throughout the body and compute meaningful PK parameters (Chang et al. 2015; Caro et al. 2012). It is thought of numerical figures which express in the form of mathematical form or equations to solve the real-world problems of drug development process. The PK model elaborated on the basis of known anatomy and physioology of human and other animals to characterize the behavior of drug in patients, predicting one of drug in various fluids with dosage regimen, calculating optimum drug regimen for individual patients, evaluating bioequivalence between different formulation, and also drug-to-drug interaction and drug-to-food interaction are also explained in a specified period of time (Ceckova-Novotna et al. 2006) (Fig. 10.3).

There are three main reasons due to which the data is subjected to modeling, viz. descriptive to describing the drug kinetics in a simple way, to predict the time course of the drug after multiple dosing based on single dose data, and we estimate the absorption capacity and profile of drug from iV database and model which will help us explain the unclear observations and statements from all piece of quantitative drug information (Cox 1990). The compartment model is not a real physiological or automatic region, but an imaginary or hypothetical one consists of tissues or group of tissues with similar blood flow and affinity which can help in the visual representation of various rate processes involved in drug disposition. The model has been classified into central and peripheral compartments: central model escalates blood and highly perfused tissues such as heart, kidney, lungs, and liver, whereas peripheral model can accelerate poorly perfused tissues such as fat and bone (Figs. 10.4 and 10.5).

The rate of change of plasma concentration versus time was modeled in the following manner:

$$R = \frac{{}^{\prime\prime}Cp}{{}^{\prime\prime}t} = \text{Kel} * Cp, \tag{10.1}$$

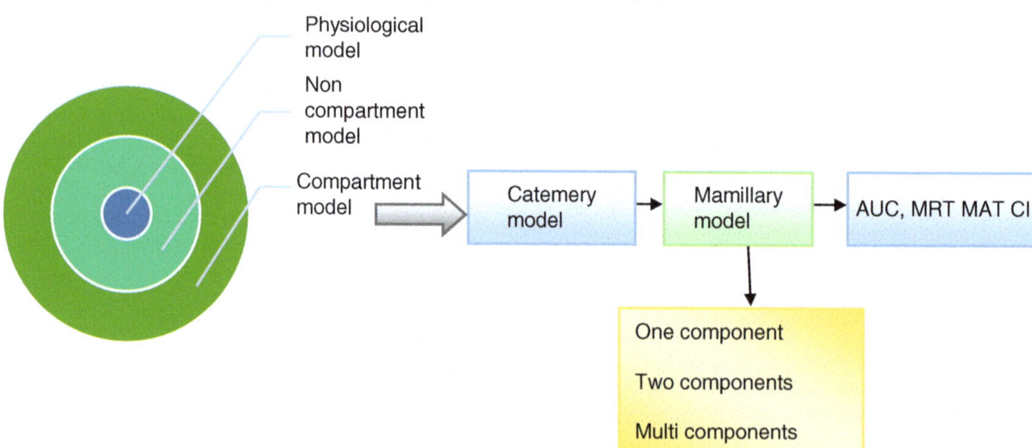

Fig. 10.3 Model types in clinical research

$$\frac{dx_0}{dt_0}, \frac{dx_1}{dt_1}, \frac{dx_2}{dt_2} \ldots\ldots \frac{dx_i}{dt_n} = \text{rate in availability} - \text{rate out}\left(\text{elimination}\right).$$

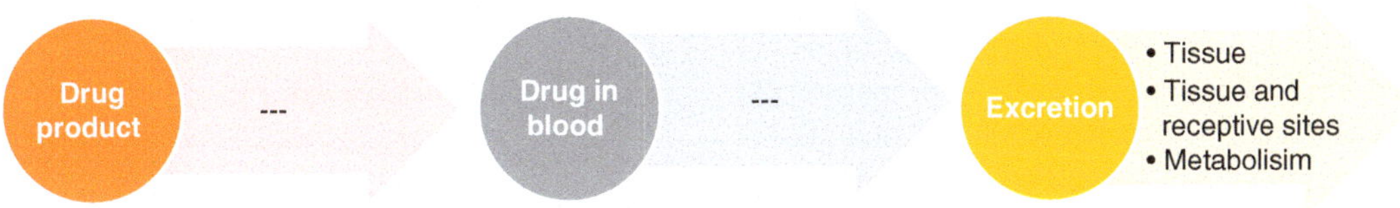

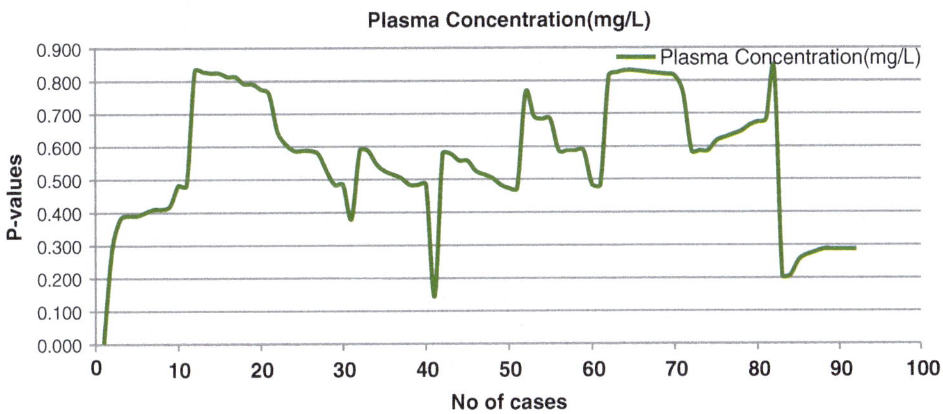

Fig. 10.4 Variation of plasma value with respect to *P* values (*P* value)

Fig. 10.5 PK model absorption and elimination phase (*P* value)

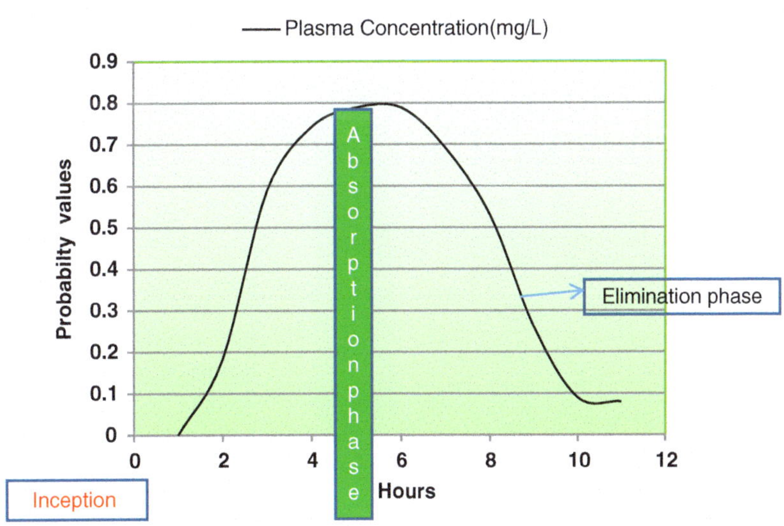

If rate out or elimination follows first order kinetics is

$$\frac{dx_i}{dt_n} = -ke^{(a+bxi)^t}, \tag{10.2}$$

where a is the intercept of the slope or induction level of absorption and k is proportionally constant and b is the change in time and plasma concentration, x can take values of plasma concentration with respect to different time period.

Integrating Eq. (10.2), the given eqn becomes

$$\ln x = \ln X_0 - k + [\ln a + b \ln xi]t.$$

X_0 = Amount of drug injected at time "t", t = zero, i.e., initial or inception of drug

$$X = X_0 e^{-k(a+bx)^t}, \tag{10.3}$$

$$\log X = \mathrm{lo}\, X_0 - \frac{-k(a+bx)^t}{2.303}. \tag{10.4}$$

Since it is difficult to directly determine the amount of drug in body and we use relationship that "C" exists between drug concentration. In plasma "C" and "X" thus eqn becomes

$$X = V_d C, \tag{10.5}$$

$$\log C = \log C_0 - \frac{-k(a+bx)^t}{2.303}. \tag{10.6}$$

Equation (10.6) elimination of half-life

$$T_{1/2} = \frac{0.693}{Ke(a+bx)^t}, \tag{10.7}$$

$V_d = \frac{\text{Amount of drug in body}}{\text{Clt}} = \frac{X}{C}$, e.g., 30 mg IV bolus, plasma concentration = 0.732 mg/mL.

Vd = 30 mg/0.732 mcg/mL = 30,000 mcg = 41 L

For drug given as IV bolus

$$Vd(\text{area}) = \frac{x_0}{k\, e^{(a+bx)^t}} * \text{AUC}. \tag{10.8}$$

For drug administered extra Vas

$$Vd(\text{area}) = \frac{fx_0}{k\, e^{(a+bx)^t}} * \text{AUC}. \tag{10.9}$$

Clearance = rate of elimination/plasma drug concentration

$$\text{cl} = \frac{dx}{t} \div \text{c}.$$

$$\text{Renal clearance} = \left(\frac{\text{ate of elimination by kideney}}{C}\right),$$

$$\text{Hepatic clearance} = \left(\frac{\text{Rate of elimination by Liver}}{C}\right),$$

$$\text{Other organ} = \left(\frac{\text{Rate of elimination by organ}}{C}\right).$$

Total body clearance was calculated from the following eqn:

$$\text{ClT} = \text{cLR} + \text{Clh} + \text{CLothers}, \tag{10.10}$$

$$\text{ClT} = k\, e^{-(a+bxi)^t} * Vd. \tag{10.11}$$

The effective clearance of drug was smoothened into accurate and non-accurate clearance, it was estimated from the binary logistic regression, the accurate will be coded as 1, and non-accurate will be coded as 0. Perform the logistic regression with two or more dependent variables. The equation will give rise to the total clearance of the administered drug (Cusack et al. 1979; Chandrasekhar 1943).

$$\mathrm{ClT(odd)} = \mathrm{k} * \frac{\mathrm{E\,xp(d)}}{1+\exp(\mathrm{d})} * \mathrm{Vd}$$

where

$$\exp(d) = e^{-(a+bxi)^t}, \qquad (10.12)$$

$$\mathrm{ClT(odd)} = k * \ln\left(\frac{\mathrm{odd}}{1-\mathrm{odd}}\right) * Vd, (10.13)$$

or

$\mathrm{ClT(odd)} = k * \ln\left(\frac{p}{1-p}\right) * Vd$ where "*P*" is the probability values with respect to plasma concentration and time (hours) (Fig. 10.6).

$$\mathrm{ClT(odd)} = k * \ln\left(\frac{0.35}{1-0.35}\right) * 41\mathrm{L}$$

k = age constant

$$\mathrm{ClT} = 25 * \ln\left(\frac{0.35}{1-0.35}\right) * 41\mathrm{L}\ \text{with respect to age}$$

$$\mathrm{ClT} = 631.54\ \text{times accurate clerence was done}$$

10.4 Area Under Curve (AUC) (mcg/mL)

AUC is a measure of the total systematic exposure of a drug. Thus it is calculated from concentration time data. AUC is not a primary PK parameter, it is derived from CL and dose

$$\mathrm{AUC} = \int_0^{\infty} C(t)\,dt,$$

$$C(t) = \frac{D}{V} e^{\left(-\frac{cl}{v}\right)t},$$

$$\mathrm{AUC} = \int_0^{\infty} \frac{D}{V} e^{\left(-\frac{cl}{v}\right)t} dt = \frac{D}{V} \int_0^{\infty} e^{\left(-\frac{cl}{v}\right)t} dt,$$

$$\mathrm{AUC} = \frac{D}{V} * \frac{1}{\frac{CL}{V}} = \frac{D}{CL}, \qquad (10.14)$$

where "*D*" is the level of distribution with respect to bioavailability, and *V* is the volume (Fig. 10.7).

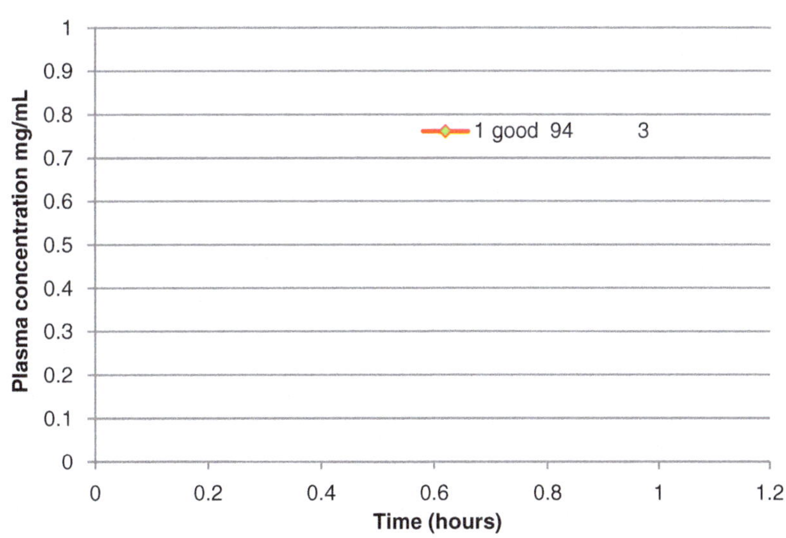

Fig. 10.6 Logistic regression plot with varying plasma drug concentration and time

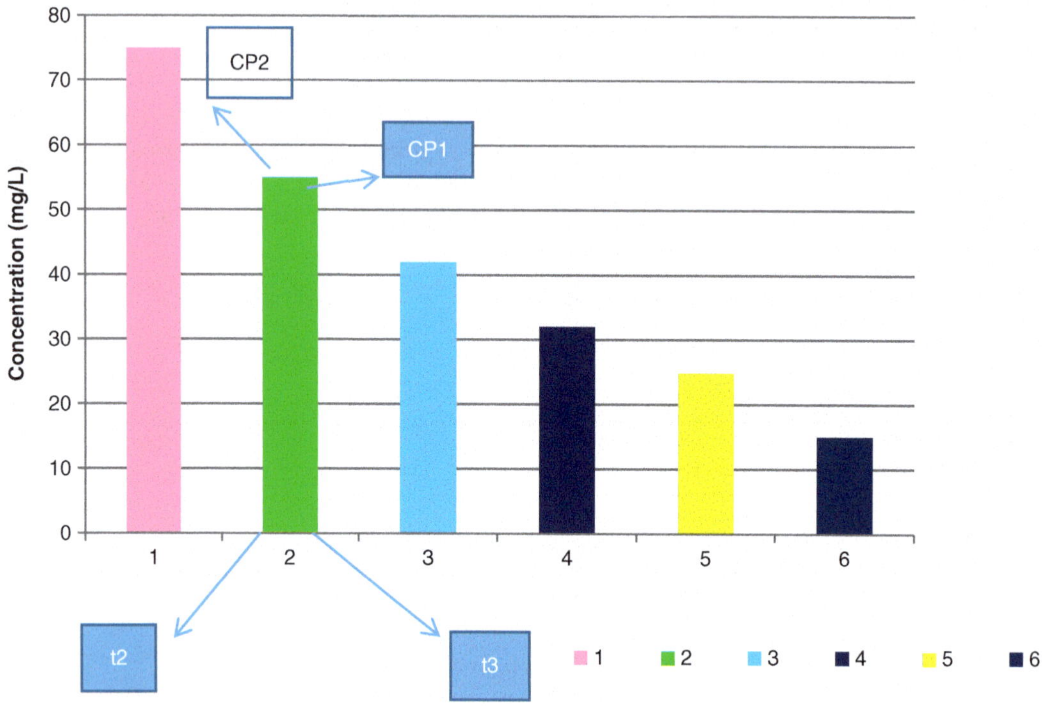

Fig. 10.7 Determination of ROC by traphazoid method

Volume distribution is defined as the volume that accommodates all drugs in the body, if concentration was the same as in plasma, the eqn becomes

$V = \frac{\text{Dose adminstered IV}}{\text{Plasma concentration}}$, e.g., total drug in the body 1000 mg, and plasma concentration is 50 mg/mL

$$\text{The volume} = \frac{1000}{50} = 20\,\text{L}$$

$$\text{AUC}^{2-3} = \frac{\text{CP}^2 + \text{CP}^3}{2} * \left(t^3 - t^2\right), \quad (10.15)$$

$$\text{AUC}^{2-3} = \left\{\frac{\text{CP}^2 + \text{CP}^2}{2} * \left(t^2 - t^1\right)\right\} + \frac{\text{CP}^2 + \text{CP}^3}{2} * \left(t^3 - t^2\right) \ldots \frac{\text{CP}^{ni} + \text{CP}^{nk}}{k} * \left(t^{i+1} - t^j\right), \quad (10.16)$$

$$\text{AUC}_{(0-t)} = \sum_{i=1}^{n-1} \frac{t^{i+1} - t^j}{2\,F\,F_r} * C_i C_j + C_{i+1}\, t C_{j+1}.$$

Total area under the first moment curve

$$F = \frac{\text{AUC}_{\text{Oral}}}{\text{AUC}_{\text{iV}}} \times \frac{\text{AUC}_{\text{iV}}}{\text{AUC}_{\text{Oral}}},$$

$$F_r = \frac{\text{AUC}_{\text{test}}}{\text{AUC}_{\text{std}}} \times \frac{\text{AUC}_{\text{std}}}{\text{AUC}_{\text{test}}}.$$

T_{max} is the time taken for drug to reach peak concentration in plasma called as the time of peak concentration. Particularly important in assessing the efficacy of the drug used to treat acute conditions like malignancy, pain and HIV-infected cases (Delafuente et al. 2008; El Desoky 2007; EMEA 2006).

Half-life: The half-life will depend on the time taken for the drug concentration or amount in the body to fall by one-half such as CP = 1/2CP$_0$ (Fig. 10.8).

$$t_{1/2} = \frac{0.693}{\text{kel}} *, \hat{y}$$

$$\text{Kel}(\text{elimination rate constant}) = \frac{-dcp/dt}{cp},$$

$$\text{kel} = \frac{\ln(cp_1) + \ln(cp_2)}{t_2 - t_1},$$

$$\text{Kel}(\text{elimination rate constant}) = \frac{\frac{\text{mass}}{\text{volume}}}{cp} \div \frac{\text{mass}}{\text{volume}} = \frac{1}{\text{time}} = 1/\text{h}.$$

Example of Kel

Drug	Kel (1/h)
Acetaminophen	0.28
Diazepam	0.021
Digoxin	0.017
Gentamycin	0.35
Lidocaine	0.43
Theophylline	0.063

$$\text{Total AUC}_{0-\infty} = \left\{ \frac{CP_0 + CP_1}{2} t_1 + \frac{CP_1 + CP_2}{2} t_2 - t_1 \right\} + \frac{CP_2 + CP_3}{2} t_3 - t_2 \ldots \frac{CP_{\text{last}}}{\text{kel}}.$$

Hours (time)	1	2	3	4	5	6	7	8	9	10	11	12	13
Concentration	45	78	85	86	73	65	55	45	32	25	15	10	5

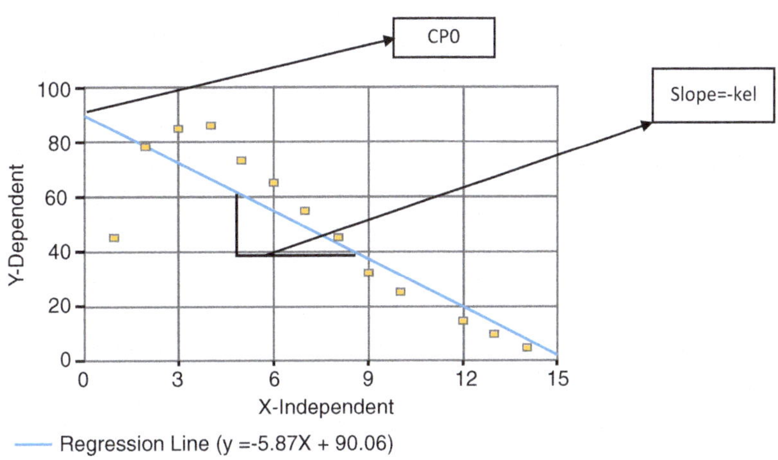

Fig. 10.8 Determination of ROC by regression method

Model = −5.8693x + 90.05 (R^2 = 0.98)

SSX = 214.30; SP = −1257 − 84; b = SP/SSX = −1257.85/214.31 = −5.86

$a = M_y - bM_x = 47.62 - (-5.87 * 7.23) = 90.05$

$$t_{1/2} = \frac{0.693}{\text{kel}} * Y$$

Cp = 71, kel = 0.34

$$\hat{y} = -5.87X + 90.06$$

Substitute "X" value for the above model (when X = 2 h), the estimated value of

$$\hat{y} = -5.87(2) + 90.06,$$

$$\hat{y} = -11.74 + 90.06,$$

$$\hat{y} = 78.32,$$

$$t_{1/2} = \frac{0.693}{\text{kel}} * 78.32(\text{substitute kel} = 0.34),$$

$$t_{1/2} = \frac{0.693}{0.34} * 78.32,$$

$$t_{1/2} = 2.03 * 78.32 = 159.6. \quad (10.17)$$

Equation (10.17) determines that the half-life of the drug is 159.60 times observed in the human body

$$\text{CP} = \text{CP}_0 * e^{-\text{kel}*t},$$

$$\text{CP}_0 = \frac{\text{CP}}{e},$$

where CP = 71, kel = 0.34,

$$\text{CP}_0 = \frac{71}{0.34} = 100, \quad (10.18)$$

$$\text{AUC}_{0-1} = \frac{100 + 71}{2} * 1 = 85.50,$$

$$\text{AUC}_{\text{Last}-\infty} = \frac{\text{CP}_{\text{last}}}{\text{kel}} = \frac{5}{0.34} = 14.70\,\text{mg.h/L}$$

(value of 5 was obtained from the illustration) (Fig. 10.9).

Step II: Integration method

$$\text{AUC} = \int_0^3 X^2 dx,$$

$$= \left.\frac{X^{n+1}}{n+1}\right]_1^3$$

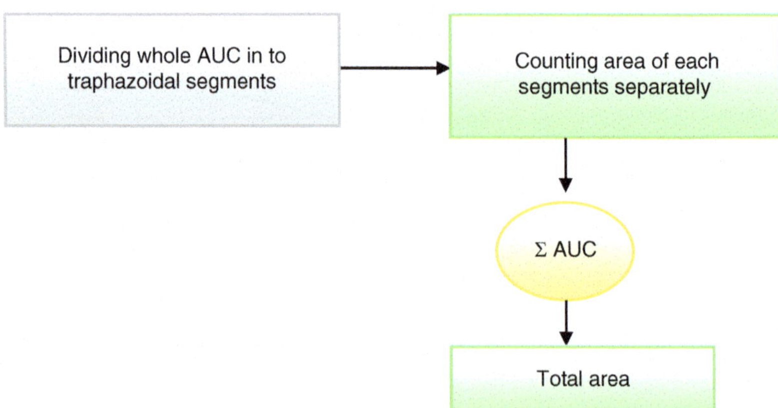

Fig. 10.9 Steps for determination of AUC

where $X = 80$, $\ln 80 = 4.38$,

$$= \frac{X^2}{2}\Big]_1^3 = \frac{4.38^2}{2}\Big]_1^3,$$

$$= \frac{\left(4.38^2\right)^3}{2} - \frac{\left(4.38^2\right)^1}{2} * 100,$$

$$\text{AUC} = 33.43$$

$$y(\text{AUC}) = \int_a^b f(x)\,dx,$$

$$y(\text{AUC}) = f(b) - f(a).$$

The AUC was tested by Gaussian distribution:

$$Z_{\text{AUC}} = \frac{\left(\overline{x_i} - C_{\max}\right)}{\sigma_i},$$

where $C_{max} = \mu$ population means

$$\sigma_i = \frac{1}{n}\sum_{i=1}^{n}\left(x_i - \overline{x}\right)^2,$$

$\overline{x_i}$ = sample mean of plasma concentration ith drug,

σ_i = Sample SD of ith drug,

$Z_{\alpha AUC}$ Tested by normal distribution curve and refer the table value and reject the H_0.

10.5 Receiver Operating Characteristics Analysis for Fitting AUC

The ROC curve is plotting of values of false positive rate (FPR) versus the true positive rate (TPR) for all possible values ranged from 0 to 1. The higher the ROC curve better the fit. In fact, the AUC can be used for this purpose. The closer is to 1 (maximum value) the better the fir. Values close to 0.50 show that the model's ability to discriminate between success and failure is due to chance (Gandhi et al. 2004; Jambhekar and Breen 2009; Khorsan and Crawford 2014). Typically used to evaluate the performance of drug in human body, AUC for plasma concentration, performance of machine learning language for identification of new algorithms, identification of rare gene for malignancy, specificity, and sensitivity of the drug, etc.

$$\text{TPR} = \text{TP} / \text{TP} + \text{FN},$$

$$\text{FPR} = \text{FP} / \text{FP} + \text{TN}.$$

TPR and FPR are plotted for different threshold value; threshold values may often be chosen based on the optimum point in the ROC curve. Thumb rule of ROC is the value lies between 0.90 and 1; excellent, 0.80–0.90 good; 0.70–0.80 fair; 0.60–0.70 poor and values lie between 0.50 and 0.60 are fail.

Illustration: The sensitivity and specificity of Efavirenz fixed-dose regimen efficacy were obtained from RCT double blind, and the researcher wishes to extrapolate the sensitivity and specificity by using receiver operating characteristic analysis.

Model formulation: The collected data sets were categorized based on the rating of efficacy, 90–100% coded as 5; excellent, 80–90% coded as 2; 70–80% coded as 3 and 60–70% coded as 2 and 50–60% coded as 1 (n = 50 cases) (Fig. 10.10).

1. Number of Cases: 50
    Number Correct: 42
    Accuracy: 84%
    Sensitivity: 88%
    Specificity: 80%; Positive Cases Missed: 3; Negative Cases Missed: 5
    (A rating of 3 or greater is considered positive.)
    Fitted ROC area: 0.905
    Empiric ROC area: 0.892
    Summary of ROC curve:
    Area = 0.9055 ± 0.042
2. Initial values of parameters
    $A = 1.7621$
    $B = 0.9538$
    $Z(K)$: −0.1507 0.8415 1.4053 1.7511
    $\text{Log } l = -68.6817$

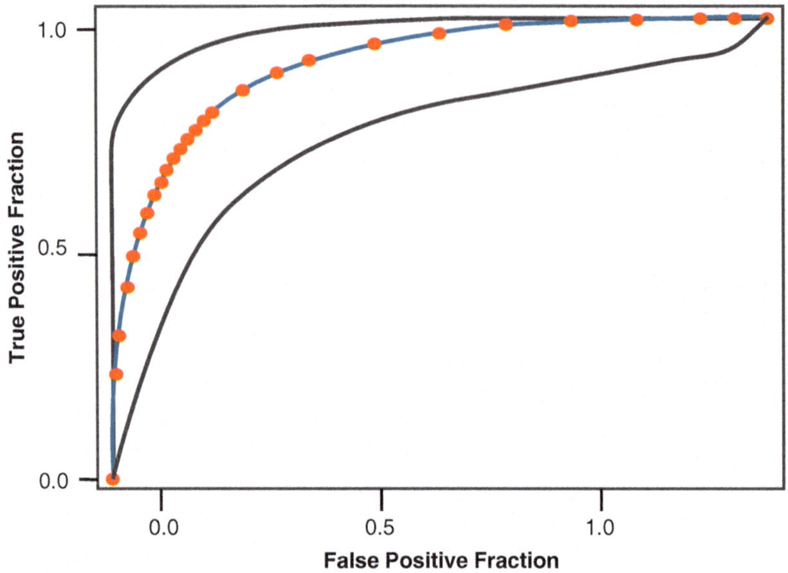

Fig. 10.10 AUC determination by ROC method

3. Final values of parameters

   Procedure converges after six iterations.

   $A = 1.8683$

   $B = 1.0118$

   $Z(K)$: −0.1202 0.7566 1.2524 2.0602

   Log $L = -65.0240$

4. Variance–covariance matrix

   A 0.2517 0.1303 0.0546 0.0592 0.0391 −0.0306

   B 0.1303 0.1384 0.0205 −0.0005 −0.0375 −0.1332

   Z(1) 0.0546 0.0205 0.0626 0.0363 0.0274 0.0127

   Z(2) 0.0592 −0.0005 0.0363 0.0694 0.0608 0.0580

   Z(3) 0.0391 −0.0375 0.0274 0.0608 0.0951 0.1126

   Z(4) −0.0306 −0.1332 0.0127 0.0580 0.1126 0.2485

5. Correlation matrix (Table 10.1)

   A 1.0000 0.6983 0.4350 0.4480 0.2526 −0.1225

   B 0.6983 1.0000 0.2207 −0.0049 −0.3270 −0.7182

   Z(1) 0.4350 0.2207 1.0000 0.5507 0.3551 0.1018

   Z(2) 0.4480 −0.0049 0.5507 1.0000 0.7492 0.4414

Table 10.1 Estimated binormal ROC curve with asymmetric 95% confidence interval

FPF	TPF	CI-95%
0.005	0.2301	[0.0169,0.7407]
0.010	0.3135	[0.0430,0.7718]
0.020	0.4168	[0.0996,0.8061]
0.030	0.4860	[0.1545,0.8282]
0.040	0.5384	[0.2056,0.8449]
0.050	0.5807	[0.2523,0.8587]
0.060	0.6159	[0.2949,0.8705]
0.070	0.6461	[0.3337,0.8808]
0.080	0.6723	[0.3690,0.8901]
0.090	0.6955	[0.4012,0.8985]
0.100	0.7161	[0.4306,0.9062]
0.110	0.7347	[0.4575,0.9132]
0.120	0.7515	[0.4821,0.9198]
0.130	0.7668	[0.5047,0.9258]
0.140	0.7809	[0.5255,0.9314]
0.150	0.7938	[0.5447,0.9366]
0.200	0.8454	[0.6214,0.9577]
0.250	0.8822	[0.6757,0.9723]
0.300	0.9096	[0.7160,0.9824]
0.400	0.9466	[0.7727,0.9934]
0.500	0.9691	[0.8119,0.9978]
0.000	0.9832	[0.8424,0.9994]
0.070	0.9918	[0.8684,0.9999]
0.800	0.9967	[0.8927,1.000]
0.900	0.9992	[0.9189,1.000]
0.950	0.9998	[0.9357,1.000]

$Z(3)$ 0.2526 −0.3270 0.3551 0.7492 1.0000 0.7325

$Z(4)$ −0.1225 −0.7182 0.1018 0.4414 0.7325 1.0000

10.6 Mean Comparison Test—ANOVA

Analyses of variance was profounded by Prof R A Fisher to know any statistically significant differences between the means of three or more independent (unrelated) groups. This tool guides us in testing of null hypothesis and also provides a valid conclusion about sample or population (Kostrzewski 2002; Maronna et al. 2019). The following assumptions of ANOVA are considered to be tested for null hypothesis:

1. All observations are independent, identical, and homogeneous in nature.
2. Equal variance between the treatment—Homoscedasticity (tested by Bartlett's test).
3. Experimental errors are normally distributed with mean μ and σ^2 and testing of normality by using Shapiro–Wilk test.

Test hypothesis

$$H_0 = \text{distribution of residual} = \text{normal distribution}$$

$$H_1 = \text{distribution of residual} \neq \text{normal distribution}$$

Non-significant p value = Normal distribution

$$W = \frac{\sum_{i=1}^{n}\left(a_i x^2_{\ i}\right)^2}{\sum_{i=1}^{n}\left(x_i - \overline{x_i}\right)^2},$$

a_i = constants generated from the means, variances, and covariance of the order statistics of a sample of size n from a normal distribution (complex)

x_i = ordered sample values ($x_{(1)}$ is the smallest)

Smaller values of "W" are the evidence of departure from normality

The following tests has been used to test the normality of the experimental research data sets:

1. Shapiro–Wilk test—data sets mainly unique values
2. D'Agostino-Pearson normality test—lot of repeated values
3. Lilliefors normality—the mean and variance are unknown
4. Spiegelhalter's T' normality test—powerful test for kurtosis

10.7 Methods

Step 1: Fix the null hypothesis

H_0: There is no significant difference between type A and type B drug Type A = Type B

H_1: There is a significant difference between type A and type B drug Type A ≠ Type B

Step 2: Fix the level of significance (type I error); rejection of null hypothesis when the statement is true ($\alpha = 0.05$ or 0.01)

Step 3: Test the normality by using Shapiro–Wilk test

Step 4: Arrange the data in treatment and replication wise and compile the data from the following steps:

Between-Groups Degrees of Freedom: $df = (k - 1)$ where "k" is the number of groups

Within-Groups Degrees of Freedom: $df = (N - k)$ where "N" is the total number of subjects

Total Degrees of Freedom: $df = (N - 1)$

Sum of Squares Between Groups: $SS_B = S^k_{i=1} n_i \left(x_i - x\right)^2$ where "n_i" is the number of subjects in the ith group

Sum of Squares Within Groups: $SS_W = S^k_{i=1} \left(n_i - 1\right) S_i^{\,2}$, where S_i is the standard deviation of the ith group

Total Sum of Squares: $SS_T = (SS_B + SS_W)$

Mean Square between Groups: $MS_B = SS_B/(k - 1)$

Mean Square within Groups: $MS_W = SS_W/(N - k)$

F-Statistic (or F-ratio): $F = (MS_B/MS_W)$

Step 5: If the Fisher calculated value > F table value; reject the H_o

One-way ANOVA table

Source	Degrees of freedom df	Sum of squares SS	Mean square MS	F-stat	P value
Between Groups	$(k - 1)$	SS_B	$MS_B = SS_B/(k - 1)$	$F = MS_B/MS_W$	Right tail of $F(k - 1, N - k)$
Within groups	$(N - k)$	SS_W	$MS_W = SS_W/(N - k)$		
Total:	$(N - 1)$	$SS_T = SS_B + SS_W$			

Illustration: The researcher wishes to test the elimination rate constant of novel regimen (pre-trial) subject to 81 cases. Experimentation was conducted in accordance with FDA guidelines. The following data sets were collected during the study intervention:

Comparison of kel–ANOVA

	Age groups					
Cases	G_1	G_2	G_3	G_4	G_5	G_6
1	2.1	3.6	4.1	3.4	3.77	3.4
2	2.2	3.5	4.2	3.3	3.41	4.1
3	2.3	3.4	4.3	3.4	3.78	4.2
4	2.4	3.7	4.5	3.7	3.96	4.7
5	2.5	3.9	4.3	3.6	3.58	3.6
6	2.6	3.6	4.6	3.5	3.47	3.5
7	2.8	3.5	3.8	3.8	3.62	3.4
8	2.9	3.8	3.4	3.4	3.14	3.8
9	2.3	3.6	3.7	3.3	3.63	3.6
10	2.6	3.4	3.9	3.4	3.28	4.22
11	2.7	3.2	3.8	3.9	3.58	4.41
12	2.4	3.1	3.4	3.6	3.33	4.32
13	2.3	3.3	4.1	3.4	–	3.90
14	2.6	3.1	4.2	3.3	–	–

Data summary

Age class	N	Mean	Std. dev.	Std. error
Group 1	14	2.4786	0.2326	0.0622
Group 2	14	3.4786	0.2455	0.0656
Group 3	14	4.0214	0.3704	0.099
Group 4	14	3.5	0.1922	0.0514
Group 5	12	3.5458	0.2331	0.0673
Group 6	13	3.9346	0.4226	0.1172

ANOVA summary

Source	Degrees of freedom df	Sum of squares SS	Mean square MS	F-stat	P value
Between groups	5	20.8837	4.1767	48.2568**	0.001
Within groups	75	6.4914	0.0866		

**(Table F=2.35)

The results revealed that the mean elimination rate constant of group 1 (2.48 ± 0.0622); group 2 (3.48 ± 0.065); Group 3 (4.02 ± 0.099); Group 4 (3.50 ± 0.051); Group 5 (3.54 ± 0.067), and Group 6 was found to be (3.93 ± 0.117) (Fig. 10.11). The experiment was found to be statistically significant at 1% level of significance ($p < 0.01$) (Calculated F > table F value) at error df. The highest mean differences were found in Group 3 (4.02) followed by Group 6. When we wish to test any significant mean difference between the groups, we should apply the following post hoc test for mean comparison.

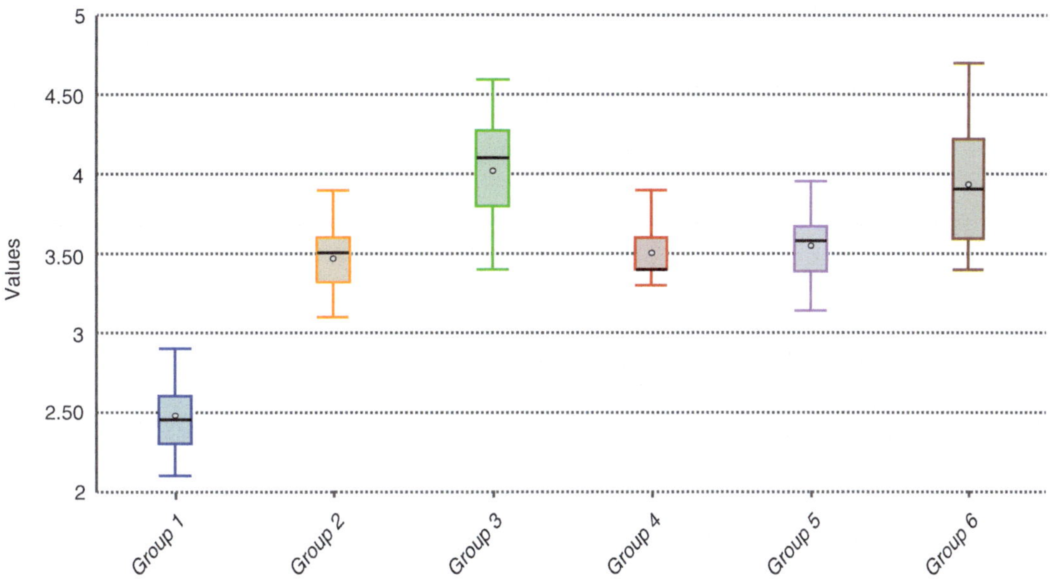

Fig. 10.11 Box model represents the group mean differences

10.8 ANOVA: Linear Fixed Effect Model

The model is some sort of mathematical simulation, outcome results are converted to mathematical eqn to solve the clinical, biological problems ascertained with full research information. Consider panel of ANOVA linear fixed effect model from the above resulted part, the model expressed in the form of eqn is as follows:

$$Y_{ij} = \mu + \alpha_i + \beta_j X_{ij} + \epsilon_{ij} \epsilon_{ij \sim N(\mu,\sigma^2)}. \tag{10.19}$$

where Y_{ij} = Expetced efficacy of ith drug jth subject

α_i = effect of ith drug

β_j = effect of jth subject

X_{ij} = Observed value of ith drug jth subject

ϵ_{ij} = error associated with ith drug jth subject

μ = Population mean

From the above linear fixed effect model determine elimination rate constant of novel regimen, we mathematically modeled is follows from ANOVA table

$$Y_{ij} = 3.49 + 4.17\, X_{ij} + 0.086.$$

One of the variables is kept constant throughout the experimentation, by using varied parameters, we formulated ANOVA fixed effect linear model (the fixed dosage of drug employed to know the efficacy of drugs in different age groups, in this illustration we selected fixed dosage of regimen administered with different age groups of the respondents).

10.9 Linear Mixed Effect Model

Linear mixed effect model is formulated based on the ANOVA salient assumptions, viz. all observations are independent and identical in nature, errors associated and normally distributed with population mean and common variance $\sigma^2 \epsilon_{ij \sim N(\mu,\sigma^2)}$ (normalcy).

In case of linear fixed effect mode l, the factors were assigned randomly and each factor allocated mixed form to know the response variable, for example, many clinical trial linear mixed effect models are very common to know the response parameter (McCullagh 2002; Micceri 1989; Neyman et al. 1959).

$$Y_{ij} = \mu + \alpha_i + \beta_j + \alpha\beta_{ij} + \epsilon_{ij}\epsilon_{ij \sim N(\mu,\sigma^2)}, \quad (10.20)$$

where Y_{ij} = Expetced efficacy of ith drug jth subject

α_i = fixed main effect with $\sum_{i=1}^{n} \alpha_i = 0$

β_j = random effect of jth subject
$\alpha\beta_{ij}$ = random interaction effect
X_{ij} = Observed value of ith drug jth subject
ϵ_{ij} = error associated with ith drug jth subject
μ = Population mean
ANOVA table output for mixed effect model

Source	*df*	SS	MSS	*F*	*P* value
Gender	1	1594.39	1594.39	17.64	<0.001
Dietary	2	1137.86	568.97	8.29	<0.001
Interaction	2	245.45	122.74	1.35	>0.001
Model	5	2794.86	558.97	6.18	<0.001
Error	194	17,529.50	90.35		
Total	199	20,324.36			

Gender is fixed L: Only female population; Dietary: Various levels consider

Numerical model $Y_{ij} = \mu + \alpha_i + \beta_j + \alpha\beta_{ij} + \epsilon_{ij}$

$$Y_{ij} = 102.13 + 1594.39 \times 1 + 568.97 \times 2 + 122.74 \times 1 \times 2 + 90.35$$

X_1: At 3 months, x_2 = At 1 year cohort dietary levels (energy intake)

10.10 Linear Random Effect Model

Experimenter examines the effect of some factors that are sampled from the population, e.g., there is a significant difference in drug response among 50 AKI (<50 years age) cases in 1 month duration, 50 cases were randomly selected based on the age interval and the drug response was recorded in 2-month duration. Here (X_1,X_2,X_3..Xn) random variable (patients were randomly) selected from the "*N*" population at different levels (levels are duration of AKI; <1 year, 1–2 years, and 3–4 years and >5 years, respectively). Mathematically linear random effect model is modeled in the following form:

$$Y_{ij} = \mu + \alpha_i + \epsilon_{ij}. \quad (10.21)$$

α_i = drug response of 50AKI cases in 1 month period

Y_{ij} = Expetced drug response of ith drug jth AKI subject

ϵ_{ij} = error associated with ith drug jth subject

$$\alpha_i = (i = 1,2,\ldots n), \alpha_i \text{ iid} \sim N(0,\sigma^2)$$

Draw new "treatment effects" and new random errors.

10.11 ANOVA Repeated Measures

The repeated measures ANOVA compares means across one or more variables that are based on repeated observations. Repeated measures ANOVA can also include zero or more independent variables. Again, a repeated measures ANOVA has at least one dependent variable that has more than one observations, e.g., the researcher was interested in how two drug treatments (A&B) would also affect the level of the enzymes.

Assumptions of repeated measures

1. Observation within each treatment condition must be independent.
2. Population distribution in each treatment must be normal.
3. Variance of population distribution on each treatment must be equivalent (homogeneity).
4. Homogeneity of covariance.

	Time or condition		
Subjects	T_1	T_2	T_3
S_1	S_1	S_2	S_1
S_2	S_2	S_1	S_2
S_3	S_3	S_3	S_4
S_4	S_4	S_4	S_6
S_5	S_5	S_6	S_3
S_6	S_6	S_5	S_5

ANOVA table summary

Source	*df*	SS	MSS	*F*	Effect size (eta square)
Condition	SSB 152.33	$(k-1)$	76.16	2.06 ($p = 0.053$)	152.33/926.96 – 0.16
Residual	SSW 774.63	$(n-1)(k)$	38.86		SS by condition/SST
Total	SST 926.96	$(nk-1)$			

$$\text{ssb} = \sum \frac{T^2}{N} - \frac{G^2}{N}$$

$$\text{ssT} = \sum X^2 - \frac{G^2}{N}$$

10.12 Post Hoc Test for Mean Comparison

The post hoc test is derived from the Latin word (post hoc means after this); it is to analyze the results of your experimental results. They are often tested based on family-wise errors; the probability of at least one type I error in a set of treatment comparison. The most common method of post hoc tests used for testing the pairwise treatment or subjects mean comparison is as follows:

(a) Bonferroni test
(b) Duncan multiple range test
(c) Fisher's least significant difference (LSD)
(d) Holm–Bonferroni procedure
(e) Newman–Keuls test
(f) Rodger's method
(g) Scheffe's method
(h) Tukey's test (SRD)
(i) Dunnett's correction
(j) Benjamin–Hochberg (BH) procedure

10.12.1 Bonferroni Test

This multiple comparison post hoc correction is used in performing many independent or dependent statistical tests at the same time. The problem with running many simultaneous tests is that the probability of a significant result increases with each test run. The post hoc test sets the significance cutoff at an $\frac{\alpha}{n}$. The demerits of Bonferroni test suffer from a loss of power. The *P*(significant event) = 1 − *P*(no significant event) = 1 − $(1–0.05)^{50}$ = 0.92. That is almost certain (92%) that we will get at least one significant result. Example, on practical approach, the researcher testing 25 different hypotheses at the same time, using a critical value of 0.05 which is the Bonferroni correction. The simple answer $BC = \frac{\alpha}{n} = 0.05/25 = 0.02$. For this set of 25 tests, we would reject the null hypothesis with a probability value $p = 0.02$. Practically we cited best example of COVID19 vaccination trails intended to control pandemic of disease, at global level ongoing COVID 19 clinical trials that were reported positive interim results, the results presented in the following matrices. The researcher intended to test the Bonferroni corrections and *p* values (Table 10.2).

Table 10.2 Clinical trial COVID19 vaccine at worldwide (Expected number of subject's inclusion)

Trial phase	Primary drug(s)	Trial end date	No of subjects (*n*)	Bonferroni corrections $\left(\frac{\alpha}{n}\right), \alpha = \mathbf{0.05}$	Inference
IV	Adalimumab; tocilizumab	April 30, 2020	60	$P = 0.001$	60 tests, we would reject the null hypothesis with $P = 0.001$
III	DAS-181	April 25, 2020	04	$P = 0.013$	4 tests, we would reject the null hypothesis with $P = 0.013$
III	Remdesivir	April 01, 2023	800	$P = 0.000$	800 tests, we would reject the null hypothesis with $P = 0.00$
III	Remdesivir	May 01, 2020	6000	$P = 0.000$	6000 tests, we would reject the null hypothesis with $P = 0.000$
II/III	Sarilumab	March 09, 2021	400	$P = 0.000$	400 tests, we would reject the null hypothesis with $P = 0.000$
II	Leronlimab	October 04, 2020	75	$P = 0.001$	75 tests, we would reject the null hypothesis with $P = 0.001$
II	Multistem	October 31, 2020	35	$P = 0.001$	35 tests, we would reject the null hypothesis with $P = 0.001$
II	Bevacizumab	June 30, 2020	140	$P = 0.000$	140 tests, we would reject the null hypothesis with $P = 0.000$
II	Nitric oxide	December 31, 2020	10	$P = 0.005$	10 tests, we would reject the null hypothesis with $P = 0.005$
I/II	Stem cell therapy for COVID19	March 31, 2020	120	$P = 0.000$	120 tests, we would reject the null hypothesis with $P = 0.000$

Table 10.2 (continued)

Trial phase	Primary drug(s)	Trial end date	No of subjects (n)	Bonferroni corrections $\left(\frac{\alpha}{n}\right), \alpha = \mathbf{0.05}$	Inference
I	Mavrilimumab				
I	Mesenchymal stem cells; undisclosed conventional medicine	December 01, 2020	20	$P = 0.003$	20 tests, we would reject the null hypothesis with $P = 0.003$
I	Emiplacel		07	$P = 0.007$	7 tests, we would reject the null hypothesis with $P = 0.007$
I	BDB-001		02	$P = 0.025$	02 tests, we would reject the null hypothesis with $P = 0.025$
I	Remestemcel-L				
I	Opaganib with secondary drug hydroxychloroquine (HQC)				

Source: Global data, CDC, 2020, $E(x) = \mu = 0.82$

10.12.2 Duncan Multiple Range Test

DMRT test is used to test the pairwise treatment which means comparison with control groups

Step 1: Rank the treatment from the highest to the lowest means (T_1-39.30, T_2-20.7, T_3-11.3)

The next steps are to compare the H-L (39.3–11.3 = 28).

Step 2: Refer the p value (appendix table) with treatment and error df.

Step 3: Find σd^2; $\sigma d^2 = 2x$ residual mean square/n.

Step 4: Take the square root of step 3.

Step 5: Multiply σd (step 4) by the q value.

The difference between the highest and lowest means is greater than 10.50, so the highest mean is significantly different from that of the lowest mean, subsequently you should compare the second and third highest mean so on.

Step 6: Refer the p value with treatment and error df again follow steps 3 and 4.

The difference between the highest and lowest mean value is less than the DMRT critical value (CD) which does not differ significantly from that of lowest mean. Once you get the insignificant results, you can stop at that point.

$$s_{\bar{d}} = \sqrt{\frac{2s^2}{r}},$$

$$R_q = \frac{r_p * s_{\bar{d}}}{\sqrt{2}} \text{ for } p = 2,3 \ldots t.$$

10.12.3 Holm–Bonferroni Method

The ordinary Bonferroni method is sometimes viewed as too conservative for comparison of treatment means and also test does not to be applied in large treatment groups. Since we viewed strict insight vision for multiple corrections. The formula for calculating the HB test is as follows:

$$\text{HB} = \frac{\text{Target alpha level}}{n - rank \text{ number of pair (by degree of significance)} + 1},$$

where target alpha level = overall alpha level (0.05, 0.01),

n = the number of tests.

10.12.3.1 Illustrative Example

Use the HB method to test the following four hypotheses and their associated p values at an alpha level of 0.05

$$H_1 = 0.01$$

$$H_2 = 0.04$$

$$H_3 = 0.03$$

$$H_4 = 0.005$$

Step 1: Order the P values from the smallest to the greatest.

$$H_4 = 0.005$$

$$H_1 = 0.01$$

$$H_3 = 0.03$$

$$H_2 = 0.04$$

Step 2: Calculate the HB formula for the first rank.

$$\text{HB} = \frac{0.05}{4-1+1} = \frac{0.05}{4} = 0.0125.$$

Step 3: compare the first ranked (smallest) p value from step 1 to the alpha level calculated in step 2.

The smallest p value, in step 1 (H4:0.005) < alpha level in step 2 (0.0125). If the p value is smaller, reject the null hypothesis for this individual test. The P value of 0.005 is less than 0.0125 so that the null hypothesis for H_1 is rejected.

Step 4: Repeat the HB formula for second rank.

$$\text{HB} = \frac{0.05}{4-2+1} = \frac{0.05}{3} = 0.016.$$

Compare the results from the formula in step 4 to the second ranked p value ($H_1 = 0.01 < 0.0167$) so that H_1 is rejected.

10.12.4 Least Significant Difference Test (LSD)

The LSD test is the simplest and the most commonly used post hoc test in agricultural, animal, and medical researches, LSD procedure for making the pair comparisons. The procedure provides a single LSD value, at a prescribed level of significance, which serves as the boundary between significant and insignificant differences between any pair of treatment means. The test is most appropriate for making planned pair comparison but not valid for comparing all possible pairs of means, especially when the number of treatment group is large.

Step 1: Compute the mean difference between the ith and jth treatment as follows:

$$d_{ij} = \overline{X}_i - \overline{X}_j.$$

Step 2: Determine the LSD value at the desired level of significance.

$$\text{LSD} = t_{\alpha=0.05,0.01} * S_{\bar{d}},$$

where $S_{\bar{d}}$ is the standard error of mean difference, $t_{\alpha=0.05,0.01}$ is the table value from appendix

$$S_{\bar{d}} = \sqrt{2\text{EMS}/r},$$

where "r" is the number of replications

SV	df	SS	MSS	F	P value
Between group	3	419.20	181.21	6.45 (Table F=2.63)	0.0013
Within the group (error)	36	959.58	26.65		

$$\text{LSD} = 2.08 * \sqrt{2 * \frac{26.65}{10}} = 4.68$$

$$d_{ij} = \left|\bar{X}_i - \bar{X}_j\right| \geq \text{LSD reject } H_0$$

10.12.5 Newman–Keuls Test

The Newman–Keuls test is similar to post hoc test for Tukey's to identify sample means that are different from each other. Newman–Keuls uses different critical values for comparing different pairs of means. Therefore, it is more likely to find significant differences, e.g., we fix the H_0: mean efficacy of Type A drug = mean efficacy of Type B drug where type A and B could be any possible pair.

Step 1: Order means from largest to smallest, compare differences between the groups with the largest mean to the group with the smallest mean.

Step 2: Determine the SE using the MSE (from ANOVA input).

$S_{AB} = \sqrt{\frac{\text{MSE}}{n}}$ equal sample size; if the sample sizes are not equal $S_{AB} = \sqrt{\frac{\text{MSE}}{2}\left(\frac{1}{n_A} + \frac{1}{n_B}\right)}$.

Step 3: Compute q value

$$q = \left[\frac{\left(\bar{X}_A - \bar{X}_B\right)}{S_{AB}}\right].$$

Refer the q critical value from a table. The rows are the number of means being compared (i.e., number of treatment) and the columns are the df. If the calculated "q" value is more than the table value, then rejects the H if the two means are equal, stop the test, you can conclude that there is no significant difference between any pairs of means. If the two means are unequal, repeat the steps.

10.12.6 Scheffe Test

It is coined by American Statistician Henry Scheffe, post hoc test used in analysis of variance. After we run the ANOVA, we got a significant F statistics (reject the H_0). We should apply the Schiff's test to know the pairwise means significant. However, the Scheffe's test corrects alpha for simple and complex means comparisons. Complex means comparison involve comparing more than one pair of means simultaneously, most flexible and also the test with lowest statistical power "β". In a practical point of view, if the researcher wants to make pairwise comparison, run the Tukey's test because it will have narrowed CI-95% or 99% or else if you want to compare all possible simple and complex pairs of means, run the Scheffe test as it will have a narrowed CI. Only run this test if you have rejected H_0 in an ANOVA test, indicating that the means are not the same. Otherwise, the means are equal and so there is no point in running.

The null hypotheses for the test are that all means are the same $H_0 : \mu = \mu_0$; H_0 : The mean efficacy is no difference beween drug A and drug B

$$H_1 : \mu \neq \mu_0; H_1 : \text{There is a significant difference beween drug A and drug B}$$

Step 1: Calculate absolute values of pairwise comparisons ABCD; $\overline{X}_A = 36.00$, $\overline{X}_B = 34.50$, $\overline{X}_C = 36.60$, $\overline{X}_D = 36.21$; *F* value from ANOVA (3.6 *df* at 0.05), MSE 0.028.

Drug	AB	AC	AD	BC	BD	CD
Mean difference	1.50	0.40	0.21	1.1	1.71	0.61

Step 2: Apply the following formula to find a set of Scheffe's formula values.

$$S_c = \sqrt{(k-1) F \,\text{value MSE}\left(\frac{1}{n_i} + \frac{1}{n_j}\right)},$$

where $(k - 1)$ is the between sample *df* $3(4 - 1) = 3$

F, $1 * n - k$; k; alpha is the f value (from ANOVA(3.24))

MSE = mean square errore.g., comparing A and B drugs

$$\sqrt{3 * 3.24 * 0.08 * \left(\frac{1}{5} + \frac{1}{4}\right)} = 0.32.$$

Follow steps 1 and 2. Find any values that are larger than the comparison values. Larger values are statistically significant.

10.12.7 Turkeys' or Honest Significant Difference Test

The Tukey's posttest is only applicable to smaller treatment groups (3–6), when "*F*" is significant we want to compare the mean differences between and within the groups. The post hoc test determined based on the studentized range distribution. The test compares all possible pairs of means, we should test all possible pairs among means using the Tukey's HSD, calculate HSD for each pair of means using the following formula:

$$\text{HSD} = \frac{M_i - M_j}{\sqrt{\frac{\text{MS}_\text{w}}{n_\text{h}}}},$$

where $(M_i - M_j)$ is the difference between the pairs of means; MS_w = mean square within

Step 1: Perform the ANOVA test.

Step 2: Choose two means from the ANOVA output (means, MSE, number of treatment, *df* within).

Step 3: Calculate the HSD statistics for Tukey's test using the formula.

Step 4: Find the score in Turkeys' critical value table.

Step 5: Compare the score. If the calculated value >CD, the two means are statistically significant.

10.12.8 Dunnett's Test

Dunnett's test is the most appropriate test to compare means from several experimental groups against control group mean to know there is a difference. We can consider fixed control group varying with experimental group means.

$D_\text{Dunnett} = t_\text{Dunnett}\sqrt{\frac{2\text{EMS}}{n}}$; EMS = error mean square, n = number of sample.

Step 1: Refer the t_Dunnett critical value in the Dunnett critical value table (0.05;0.01 n = sample size 5, 20 *df*).

n	α	Number of Groups, Including Control Group							
		2	3	4	5	6	7	8	9
15	.05	2.13	2.44	2.61	2.73	2.82	2.89	2.95	3.00
	.01	2.95	3.25	3.43	3.55	3.64	3.71	3.78	3.83
16	.05	2.12	2.42	2.59	2.71	2.80	2.87	2.92	2.97
	.01	2.92	3.22	3.39	3.51	3.60	3.67	3.73	3.78
17	.05	2.11	2.41	2.58	2.69	2.78	2.85	2.90	2.95
	.01	2.90	3.19	3.36	3.47	3.56	3.63	3.69	3.74
18	.05	2.10	2.40	2.56	2.68	2.76	2.83	2.89	2.94
	.01	2.88	3.17	3.36	3.44	3.53	3.60	3.66	3.71
19	.05	2.09	2.39	2.55	2.66	2.75	2.81	2.87	2.92
	.01	2.86	3.15	3.31	3.42	3.50	3.57	3.63	3.68
20	.05	2.09	2.38	2.54	2.65	2.73	2.80	2.86	2.90
	.01	2.85	3.13	3.29	3.40	3.48	3.55	3.60	3.65

$$D_{\text{Dunnett}} = \mathbf{2.65}\sqrt{\frac{\mathbf{2*(15.39)}}{\mathbf{5}}} = \mathbf{6.57}.$$

Critical D_{Dunnett} value is 6.57; If the distance between a control group mean and an experimental group mean is greater than 6.575, then that distance is significant.

10.12.9 Benjamini–Hochberg Test

The BH test is a powerful method that decreases the false discovery rate. Adjusting the rate helps to control for the fact that sometimes small *p* values (<5%) happen by chance, which could lead you to incorrectly reject the H_0. In other words, the BH test helps us lead to avoid type error (false positive test). A *P* value of 5% means that there is only a 5% chance that we would get observed result if the H_0 is true. Since it is only probability many times, true hypothesis is thrown out because of the randomness of results. The concrete example we had is a group of 100 patients who are free from certain disease. Our Ho is that patients are free of disease and our alternate is that they do have the disease. We apply 100 statistical tests at the 5% level, roughly 5% of our report as false positives. In this paradigm, BH test will decrease the number of false positives.

Steps

Step 1: Order the individual *p* values in ascending order.

Step 2: Assign ranks to the *P* value (e.g., smallest has a rank of 1, the second smallest has a rank 2).

Step 3: Calculate each individual *p* values Benjamini–Hochberg critical value using the formula.

CD = $(i/m)Q$; i = the individual *p* value's rank, m = total number of tests, and Q = the false discovery rate (a percentage, chosen by you). Compare the original values to the critical BH from the above step; find the largest *p* value, i.e., smaller than the CD value.

Variable	*P* value	Rank	**CD = $(i/m)Q$**
Depression	0.001	1	0.01
Family H/o	0.008	2	0.02
Obesity	0.039	3	0.03
Other health problem	0.041	4	0.04
Children	0.042	5	0.05
Divorce	0.060	6	0.06
Death of spouse	0.074	7	0.07
Limited income	0.205	8	0.08

CD = 0.042

The bolded *p* value is the highest *P* value, i.e., also smaller than the CD: 0.042 < 0.050 consider as significant

10.13 Least Square Estimation Method of AUC

The least square estimation of AUC is an easiest method and more robust in nature, select the data points with respect to plasma concentration and time in hours. The data *(X,Y)* distributed in a ring shape on *XY* plane, the least square regression employed to determine the equation of a circle that will best fit with available data points, the regression helps to calculate parameters of *k*, *m*, and *r* values of the curve (Lemke et al. 2008; Laudisio et al. 2009).

$$(x-k)^2+(y-m)^2=r^2. \quad (10.22)$$

Minimizing the above eqn, the eqn becomes

$$F((k,m,r)=\Sigma\left[(xi-k)^2+(yi-m)^2-r^2\right]^2.(10.23)$$

The eqn of the circle is liberalized by the model $F/\partial k=0$, $\partial F/\partial m=0$, and $\partial F/\partial r=0$ we obtain the following eqn:

$$(x-k)^2+(y-m)^2=r^2,$$

$$\left(x^2-kx+k^2+y^2-2my+m^2=r^2\right),$$

$$X^2+y^2=2kx+2my+r^2-k^2-m^2,$$

$$x^2+y^2=Ax+By+C.$$

These results tend to linear eqn with the coefficients of *A*, *B*, and undetermined or no estimation. As such we can use the matrices to solve the least square problem. Once we obtain *A*, *B*, and *C*, it is possible to extrapolate the backward to compile the *k*, *m*, and *r*. The Eq. (10.23) determined *A*, *B*, and *C* with matrices. The circle regression model is supported by the following matrix eqn:

$$\begin{bmatrix}\Sigma x_i^2 & \Sigma x_i y_i & \Sigma x_i\\ \Sigma x_i y_i & \Sigma y_i^2 & \Sigma y_i\\ \Sigma x_i & \Sigma y_i & \Sigma n\end{bmatrix}\begin{bmatrix}A\\B\\C\end{bmatrix}=\begin{bmatrix}\Sigma x_i\left(x_i^2+y_i^2\right)\\ \Sigma y_i\left(x_i^2+y_i^2\right)\\ \Sigma x_i^2+y_i^2\end{bmatrix},$$

where "*n*" is the number of data points (X_i,Y_i) of time and plasma concentration. In such situation we use 3 × 3 matrix outlined in the left is invertible. The *A*, *B*, and *C* are unique and this was determined as the best circle, subsequently determined the *k*, *m*, and *r* parameters (Fig. 10.12).

$$k=\frac{A}{2};m=\frac{B}{2}\text{and } r=\left(\sqrt{4c+A^2+B^2}\right)/2.$$

Find out the slope and intercept from the nearest point of circle and draw the tangent from the nearest data points and intercept, and mark the CP0,CP1. Cp last point from the trapezoid rule

$$\text{Total AUC}_{0-\infty}=\left\{\frac{\text{CP}_0+\text{CP}_1}{2}t_1+\frac{\text{CP}_1+\text{CP}_2}{2}t_2-t_1\right\}+\frac{\text{CP}_2+\text{CP}_3}{2}t_3-t_2\ldots\frac{\text{CP}_{\text{last}}}{\text{kel}}.$$

Least-squares circle calculator—results	
Sample size:	6
Center (*x*,*y*):	(15.0550, 8.8361)
Radius:	20.8507
Best Fit Circle Equation:	$(x-15.0550)^2+(y-8.8361)^2=20.8507^2$

10.14 Quadratic Regression Modeling

More advanced tool for extrapolation of AUC under quadratic modeling techniques is more applicable. The model identifies the parabola set of data in clinical trial. The kel is derived biologically and differs from many confounders; it

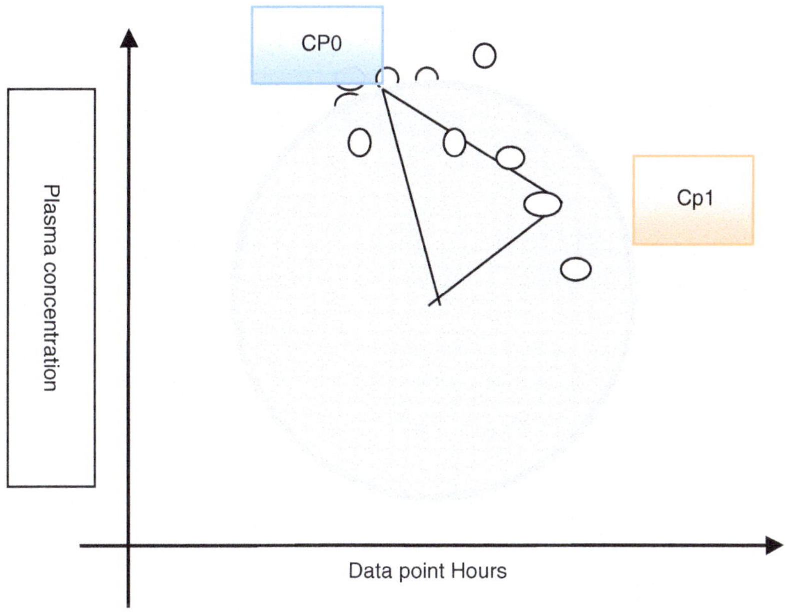

Fig. 10.12 AUC by least square method

is an extension of linear regression, the results of the model will predict about various data points (Royston and Sauerbrei 2008; Shmueli 2010). However, the measurement errors were taken from both the variables. It is used to analyze how differences in one variable can be explained by a difference in a second variable. For example, when a woman gets pregnant has a direct relation to when they give birth, so *R* square would be close to 100%. On the other hand, *R* square would be practically zero for when woman gets pregnant and when she throws a retirement party for a parent.

Quadratic regression: $y = ax^2 + bx + c$, where $a \neq 0$

Coefficients (a, b, c)

$$a = \frac{\left(\sum x_i^2\right)^2 \sum x_i^2 y_i - \sum x_i \sum x_i^2 y_i \sum x_i^3 + \sum x_i \sum x_i^4 \sum x_i y_i + \left(\sum x_i^2\right)^2 \sum x_i y_i - \sum x_i^2 \sum x_i^3 + \sum x_i \sum x_i^4 \sum y_i}{\left(\sum x_i^2\right)^3 - 2\sum x_i \sum x_i^2 \sum x_i^3 + n\left(\sum x_i^3\right)^2 + n\left(\sum x_i\right)^2 \sum x_i^4 - n\left(\sum x_i^2 \sum x_i^4\right.}$$

$$b = \frac{n\sum x_i^2 y_i \sum x_i^3 y_i - \sum x_i \sum x_i^2 \sum x_i^3 y_i + \left(\sum x_i^2\right)^2 \sum x_i y_i \sum x_i \sum x_i^4 + \sum y_i - n\sum x_i^4 \sum x_i y_i - \sum x_i^2 \sum x_i^3 \sum y_i}{\left(\sum x_i^2\right)^3 - 2\sum x_i \sum x_i^2 \sum x_i^3 + n\left(\sum x_i^3\right)^2 + n\left(\sum x_i\right)^2 \sum x_i^4 - n\sum x_i^2 \sum x_i^4}$$

$$c = \frac{\left(\sum x_i\right)^2 \sum x_i^2 y_i - n\sum x_i^2 - n\sum x_i^2 y_i - \sum x_i \sum x_i^2 \sum x_i y_i + n\sum x_i^3 \sum x_i y_i + \left(\sum x_i^2\right)^2 \sum y_i - \sum x_i \sum x_i^3 \sum y_i}{\left(\sum x_i^2\right)^3 - 2\sum x_i \sum x_i^2 \sum x_i^3 + n\left(\sum x_i^3\right)^2 + n\left(\sum x_i\right)^2 \sum x_i^4 - n\sum x_i^2 \sum x_i^4}$$

Mean x: $\bar{x} = \sum x_i/n$; Mean y: $\bar{y} = \sum y_i/n$

Correlation coefficient "r" is given by the following:

$$r = \sqrt{1 - \frac{\sum(y_i - (ax_i^2 + bx_i + b))^2}{\sum(y_i - \bar{y})^2}}$$

where "n" is the total number of samples, x_i ($x_1, x_2, \ldots, x_n$) are the x values and y_i ($y_1, y_2, \ldots, y_n$) are the y values; $\sum x_i$ is the sum of x values; $\sum y_i$ is the sum of y values; $\sum x_i\, y_i$ is the sum of products of x and y values; $\sum x_i^2$ is the sum of squares of x values; $\sum x_i^3$ is the sum of the cubes of x values, and $\sum x_i^4$ is the sum of the fourth powers of x value.

Illustration: The following data sets were collected from drug trial experiment with respect to hours and plasma concentration. We should apply the Quadratic regression model for AUC calculation.

X: (hours)	1	2	3	4	5	6	7	8	9	10	11	12	13	14	−1	−2	−3	−4
Y:(Plasma concentration)	80	81	88	74	68	55	40	25	20	15	10	9	8.62	9.35	12.01	9.81	13.05	15.19

10.14.1 Model Results

Regression data

x	y	xy	x^2	x^3	x^4	x^2y
−5	15.89	−79.45	25.00	−125.00	625.00	397.25
−4	15.19	−60.76	16.00	−64.00	256.00	243.04
−3	13.05	−39.15	9.00	−27.00	81.00	117.45
−2	9.81	−19.62	4.00	−8.00	16.00	39.24
−1	12.01	−12.01	1.00	−1.00	1.00	12.01
0	9.35	0.00	0.00	0.00	0.00	0.00
1	8.62	8.62	1.00	1.00	1.00	8.62
2	13.11	26.22	4.00	8.00	16.00	52.44
3	12.16	36.48	9.00	27.00	81.00	109.44
4	15.57	62.28	16.00	64.00	256.00	249.12
$\sum x_i = -5.00$	$\sum y_i = 124.76$	$\sum x_i\, y_i = -77.39$	$\sum x_i^2 = 85.00$	$\sum x_i^3 = -125.00$	$\sum x_i^4 = 1333.00$	$\sum x_i^2\, y_i = 1228.61$

Quadratic regression—results	
Sample size:	10
Mean x:	−0.5000
Mean y:	12.4760
a:	0.2900
b:	0.1081
c:	10.0647
Regression equation:	$y = 0.2900x^2 + 0.1081x + 10.0647$
Correlation coefficient (r):	0.8763

Find out the slope and intercept from the nearest point of parabola and draw the tangent from the nearest data points and intercept, and mark the CP_0,CP_1 (Fig. 10.13). Cp last point from the trapezoid rule

$$\text{Total AUC}_{0-\infty} = \left\{\frac{CP_0 + CP_1}{2} t_1 + \frac{CP_1 + CP_2}{2} t_2 - t_1\right\} + \frac{CP_2 + CP_3}{2} t_3 - t_2 \ldots . \frac{CP_{last}}{kel}. \tag{10.24}$$

10.15 Rational Function Regression

The ratio of two linear functions represents one of the most straightforward rational function. Rational function of 'Y' can take in the form of $Y = (ax + b)/(x - b)$ represent a good method of modeling any data that levels offer a given time period without any oscillations. The horizontal system asymptote of a rational function is $y = a$, while the vertical asymptote is $x =$ b and y intercept is c/bowmen function takes the form $y = (ax + c)/(x - b)$, the a, b, and c parameters are not linear. Since it is possible to transform the eqn through the use of simple mathematical form

$$y = \frac{(ax + c)}{x - b},$$

$$(x - b)y = ax + c,$$

$$xy - by = ax + c,$$

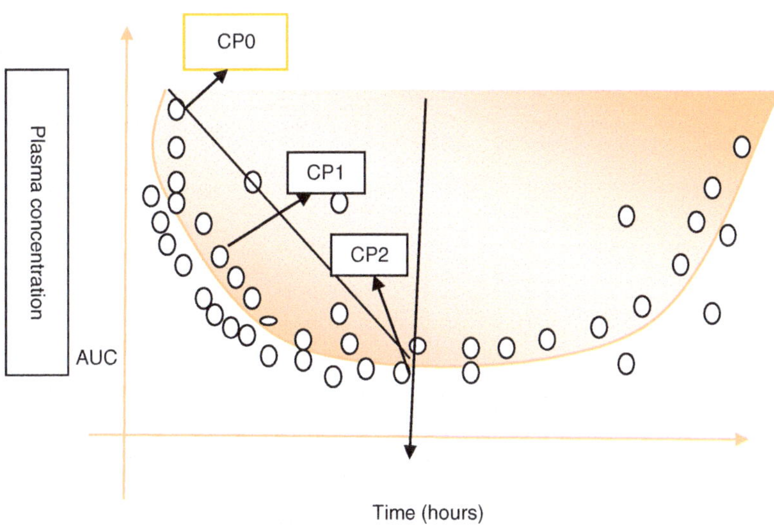

Fig. 10.13 AUC by quadratic regression method

$$xy = ax + by + c.$$

This above eqn does not incorporate linear a, b, c variables. As such that we apply the least square method to identify the "best fit" values a, b, and c, i.e., we minimize the eqn as follows:

$$F(a,b,c) = \sum_{i=1}^{n} (x_i y_i - ax_i - bx_i - c)^2. \quad (10.25)$$

This is tantamount to solving the system as follows:

$$\partial F / \partial a = 0, \partial F / \partial b = 0 \text{ and } \partial F / \partial c = 0.$$

The solution can be determined using matrix math. Using matrices to determine a, b, and c.

The matrix equation that can be employed for simple rational regression is as follows:

$$\begin{bmatrix} \sum x_i^2 & \sum x_i y_i & \sum x_i \\ \sum x_i y_i & \sum y_i^2 & \sum y_i \\ \sum x_i & \sum y_i & n \end{bmatrix} \begin{bmatrix} a \\ b \\ c \end{bmatrix} \begin{bmatrix} \sum x_i^2 y_i \\ \sum x_i y_i^2 \\ \sum x_i y_i \end{bmatrix} \quad 10.26$$

where "n" is the number of data pairs (x_i, y_i).

Providing the three-by-three matrix presented on the left is invertible, a unique solution (a, b, c) will be employed to minimize the function $F(a, b, c)$ and delivers the parameters for the best fit rational function.

Example

Identify the equation of a rational function that fits the points (x, y):

$$(4,3),(2,4),(3,6)$$

Through the use of this rational function regression calculator, you can delineate the following equation:

$$y = (3.6x - 12)/(x - 3.2).$$

This equation represents a reasonably good fit for the data.

Robustness of the model tested by regression function:

X (hours)	Y (plasma concentration)
1	4.11
2	4.56
3	5.59
4	7.97
5	8.25

Regression data							
x	Y	xy	x^2	x^3	y^2	x^2y	xy^2
1	4.11	4.11	1	1	16.8921	4.11	16.8921
2	4.56	9.12	4	8	20.7936	18.24	41.5872
3	5.59	16.77	9	27	31.2481	50.31	93.7443
4	7.97	31.88	16	64	63.5209	127.52	254.0836
5	8.25	41.25	25	125	68.0625	206.25	340.3125
$\sum x_i = 15$	$\sum y_i = 30.48$	$\sum x_i y_i = 103.13$	$\sum x_i^2 = 55$	$\sum x_i^3 = 225$	$\sum y_i^2 = 200.5172$	$\sum x_i^2 y_i = 406.43$	$\sum x_i y_i^2 = 746.6197$

Rational function regression	
Sample size:	5
a:	4.6731
b:	4.3036
c:	−19.628
Regression equation:	$y = (4.6731x - 19.628)/(x - 4.3036)$

10.16 Brownian Drug Diffusion Stochastic Model

The movement of drug particles from the site of application to the circulation and the rate and extent at which the drug particles go to the systemic circulation is known as blood absorption. However, the rate and efficiency absorption depend on the route of administration. A route of administration in pharmacology and toxicology is the path by which a drug taken into the body. Various routes of administration, oral route sublingual or buckle route, rectal route, parental, nasal inhalation, and topical route. The drug diffusion takes place in the body at different mechanisms like passive diffusion, i.e. driving force concentration gradient high to low (Brownian motion principle) until equilibrium exists. Once absorption process will be completed, the drug has been utilized and diffused in different body tissues. The passive diffusion does not involve a carrier, and the process is not saturable (Chandrasekhar 1943). The rate of absorption depends on lipophilicity (lipid–water partition coefficient) which determines how fast the drug gets absorbed. Lipid-soluble drugs movement between compartments is dependent on the concentration difference between them, the process is exponential and the rate of transfer to the slower tissues decreases as they accumulate more drug and readily move across biological membranes, whereas water-soluble drugs penetrate the cell membrane through aqueous channel depending on their chemical properties, drug absorption can occur from GI tract either by passive diffusion or by active transport. However, carrier-mediated absorption is appear to present either an import or an export site to the transported molecule and undergo substrate-induced conformational change, is likely that some kinds of drugs are absorbed by this process with the help of carrier. In this cited process, a carrier molecule will make a complex with the drug. Usually polar molecules are absorbed by this process (hydrophobic coating). Many factors will affect the drug absorption concentration of drug molecules, as most of drugs are absorbed by passive diffusion concentration and is very important. High concentration will be applied for better activity, e.g., lidocaine local anesthesia (2.0%) solution will produce anesthesia more rapidly than 0.20% solution of lidocaine if the amount is same. PK model derivatives is mostly applicable when solution drug is applied, i.e., physical state of drug, some of the drugs are solid, some are liquid, suspension, emulsion, solution, and tablets or capsules. Since before absorption, the drug must be in solution so drug in the solution or liquid dosage form is absorbed faster than solid dosage form, e.g., tablet must be disintegrated, dissoluble than the whole process but for liquid or solution dosage form there is no need to disintegrate or dissolution. Viscous product absorption will be slower than the diluted solution surface area of the absorptive site; higher the surface area, greater will be the absorption and better action. Large intestine, pulmonary alveoli, skin if high concentration of drug. Biologically the rate of administration is very important to know the level absorption in different tissues basically IV route no absorption required or no loss of drug blood circulation of the absorptive site. If the blood circulation of the absorptive site is maximum or efficient, the absorption will be faster. Blood circulation fastens the absorption. In morphine toxicity with respect toAnimal and human studies indicate the existence of important sex differences in opioid-induced antinociception and analgesia. We observed greater morphine analgesia in women compared to men, which was related to sex differences in morphine pharmacodynamics and not to differences in its pharmacokinetics, because we believe that sex dependency in opioid behavior is probably not restricted to morphine but may be an inherent property of opioid analgesics, it is of interest to assess the existence of a sex-specific dichotomy in M6G analgesia and to quantify whether such an observation is related to M6G pharmacokinetics, pharmacodynamics, or both Gastric emptying is the time how quickly the drug leaves the stomach. As we glorify surface area of the stomach, it is smaller than intestine, so most drugs are absorbed in the intestine. So, absorption is inversely proportional to gastric emptying. The presence of food will dilute the drug particles and decrease the absorption level. As a result, drug will be absorbed slower compared to that when there is no food. Another factor of drug absorption is bioavailability; it is the fraction of administered drug that reaches the systemic circulation (Setiawati et al. 2009; Shargel et al. 2005; Turnheim 2003). Typically, Bioavailability expressed the fraction of administered drug that gains access to the systemic circulation in chemically unchanged form, e.g., if 100 mg of a drug is administered orally, 70 mg of this absorbed drug is unchanged, hence the bioavailability is 70%. In case of bioavailability first-pass hepatic metabolism when a drug is absorbed across the GI tract, it enters the portal circulation before entering the systemic circulation. If the drug is rapidly metabolized by the liver, the amount of unchanged drug that gains access to the systemic circulation is decreased, e.g., propranolol or lidocaine. The solubility of the drug will depend on the type of drugs, in case of hydrophilic drugs are poorly absorbed because of their inability to cross the lipid-rich membranes. Paradoxically, drugs that are extremely hydrophobic are also poorly absorbed because they are totally insoluble in the aqueous body fluids and therefore cannot gain access to the surface of cells (Tsang and Gerson 1990; Vogels et al. 2007; Winter 2004). For a drug to be readily absorbed, it must be largely hydrophobic yet have some solubility in aqueous solutions. Chemical instability is important derivatives in PK process, it involve alterations in the molecular structure producing a new chemical entitiy, by bond formation or cleavage, e.g., insulin, nitroglycerine, and penicillin G. The nature of drug formulation depends on particle size, salt form, binders and dispersing agents, etc.

Drug diffusion is a degree of binding the drug to the plasma, and the tissue proteins and the relative hydrophobicity/lipophilicity of the drug. Their concentration varies from compartment to compartment. Usually it is considered to be operated by diffusion. But it is arbitrary. The drug concentration in all cell/compartments is not equal. Exception, ethanol is distributed equally. Drug distribution is the paradoxical changes in human body system. However, the drug is extensively distributed in the body, which means a relatively low concentration of plasma drug. Movement of drug proceeds until an equilibrium is established between unbound drug in plasma and tissue fluids. Protein binding describes the ability of proteins to form bonds with other substances ,and most commonly refer to the bonding of drugs to molecules in drug plasma (red blood cells, other components of the blood, and to tissue membranes), that affect distribution of the drug depends with the affinity of the drug toward protein. One of the best eg., the Acidic albumin basic glycoprotein sulfamethoxazole (30%) bound and (90%) bound if protein binding is very high, volume of drug distribution will be very low because protein bound drug cannot overcome many barriers by diffusion. Sometimes protein binding acts as a reservoir and will not exert action. Extensive binding may prolong the action of drug. The next step of drug process is metabolism or biotransformation which is a chemical alteration of drug in the body. It is needed to render nonpolar compounds so that they are not reabsorbed in the renal tubules and are excreted (Fig. 10.14). Most hydrophilic drugs are not biotransformed and are excreted unchanged. Many pharmacologists attempt to know the diffusion mechanism by stochastic process, since invariably due to paucity of literature, they are unable to find the suitable model for extrapolation of time taken for diffusion from intestine, arteries, and other human body systems. In this pragmatic research gap, the present section tries to explore and demonstrate new stochastic model of drug diffusion process from Brownian motion principles.

The diffusion rate of a liquid process is much slower than gas because its bioavailability is more,

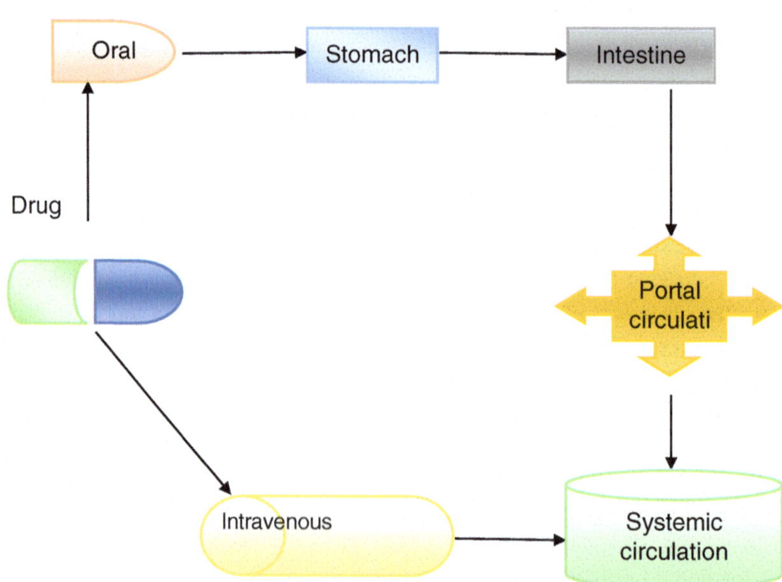

Fig. 10.14 Process of drug absorption and diffusion

but faster than solids due to the close association of molecules and lower kinetic energy because of stronger intermolecular attractive forces between the molecules compared with gases. Diffusion is the mixing of particles, i.e., movement of particles from an area of higher concentration to an area of lower concentration. From the above-cited principles of brownian motion, we assumed that the diffusion of drug substances, either liquid or solid, can take place in human body from an area of higher concentration to the area of lower concentration and also uniformly distributed over a period of time (Korkushko et al. 1984). The inclusion of the above-said Brownian principles, the present study formulated the stochastic model to know the diffusion rate of drug in varied time interval in association with various organs of the human body (Fig. 10.15).

On pharmacological intervention, the diffusion of drug will depend on the bioavailability and plasma concentrations. It is the net movement of drug particles (molecules) from a region of high concentration to a region of low concentration (e.g., small intestine, arteries vein to various other organs) due to random movement of blood. However, such kind of diffusion process can be involved in various biological mechanisms of the movement of blood in the opposite direction. Let us consider movement of random diffusion process X_1,X_2,..Xn be the random variable which can assume Gaussian distribution x_{ij}~$N(\mu, \sigma^2)$, every individual process of diffusion rate is i.i.d's and homoscedasticity (equal variance). The variable of diffusion process was simulated Thompson iteration or Runge and Kutta method (statistical outcome of random Brownian motion and eventually will result in similar concentrations throughout the solution). Various diffuse fluxes of first and second kinds were obtained from the **Stokes-Einstein** Eq. (10.27) (J, the amount of substance moving through a unit area as per unit time t) is governed by Flick's first law (Fig. 10.16).

The intervention of change in the diffusion of drug with respect to time "dt" is given by the following formula:

$$\frac{Df}{dt} = -DA\frac{d\omega}{dx},$$

$$J = -D\frac{d\omega}{dx},$$

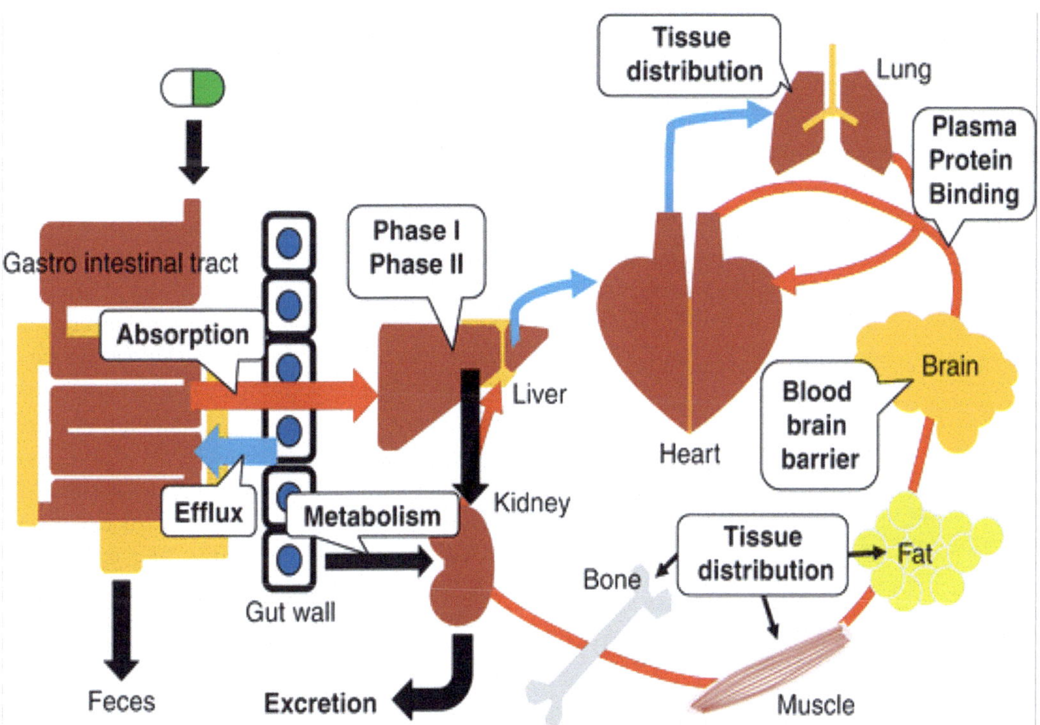

Fig. 10.15 ADME drug process in human body

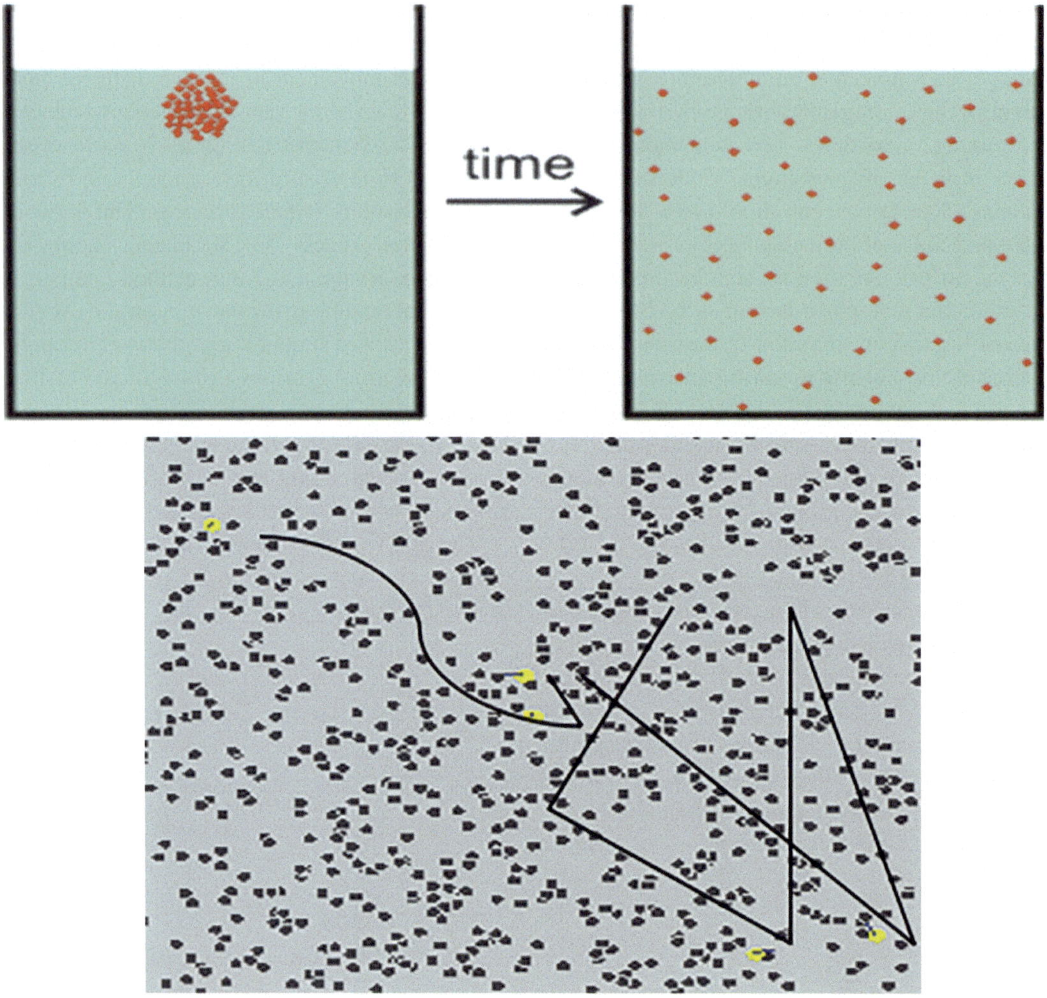

Fig. 10.16 Diffusion, particles of a soluble material spread out, Brownian motion

where "d" is the diffusivity ($m^2 \times S^{-1}$), $d\omega$ is the change in drug concentration, and dx is the change in time (m). The diffusion direction is from higher concentration to lower blood concentration such that $\frac{df}{dt}$ is always negative and the diffusive flux is always positive in the diffusion direction. Thus, drug particle flux is proportional to the concentration gradient. As per the Einstein definition, the diffusion of drug is modeled by the following eqn:

$$\text{Diffusion}\left(D\right) = \lim_{t \to \infty} \frac{\left[r\left(t_i\right) - r\left(0\right)\right]^2}{6ti}, \quad (10.27)$$

where "t" is the time taken for diffusion ($t = 0$, 1,23,.... ith hours).

In a diffusive process, the concentration of substance in the region of higher concentration gradually decreases and the concentration of the substances in the region of lower concentration gradually increases. With time, the concentration gradient dissipates within the bulk. Diffusion increases entropy (randomness) leading to a lower energy state. Eventually, equilibrium is established with uniform distribution throughout (Uniform distribution of drug substances throughout the body). The concentration change with time is described by Fick's second law:

$$\frac{df}{dt} = D\frac{d^2\omega}{dx^2}.$$

"*D*" is described by the **Stokes-Einstein eqn** for translational diffusion state.

$$D = \frac{K_B T\max}{6\pi\eta r} = \frac{C\max * \text{Time}}{N} * \frac{1}{6\pi\eta r}. \quad (10.28)$$

K_B = Boltzmann constant

*T*max = Maximum time taken for drug diffusion to reach the threshold level

N = Number of substances

*C*max = Maximum plasma concentration

η = Viscosity of the blood

r = Average drug particle size; π = 3.12 (Fig. 10.17)

10.16.1 Numerical Results

Diffusion rate initial stage fluxes = 5.58252375

Blood volume = 150–272.04

Total duration (*t*) hours = 3.36

Convexity of the curve = 15.64

Organ	Lower bound motion	Upper motion
Arteries vein to other tissues fluxes diffusion (hours)	1.64	2.73
Particle size (nano)	0.01–0.03	
Percent of diffusion rate at first wave	33–60%	

Organ	Lower bound motion	Upper motion
Elimination rate-Brownian motion	0.00063 to −0.0019	
Model diagnosis R^2	0.93	
Akaike information	193.23	
AUC −99%	0.90	

10.17 Brownian Random Walk Model

A random walk, sometimes also called a "drunkard walk," the first step of the model helps us in understanding the Brownian motion and drug diffusion process on a random basis (Chandrasekhar 1943; Royston and Sauerbrei 2008). A random walk is formalization of scientific intuitive idea of taking successive steps. The simplest random walk is a path construction according to the diffusive process of drug, plasma concentration, bioavailability, and volume of the blood, respectively. We consider random variable of $X_1, X_2, ..X_n$ follows with drunkard walk W_n. On each diffusion rate $D_1, D_2..D_k$ is strongly associated with Brownian motion with movement from higher concentration to the region of lower concentration. Since each walk was derived based on the Gaussianity and following random process model,

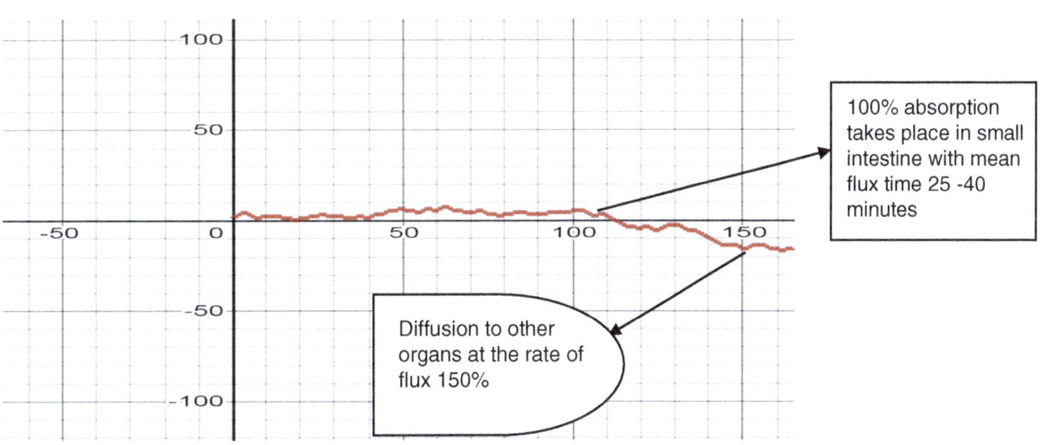

Fig. 10.17 Diffusion process estimated by Brownian motion for the first wave (1–2.5 h)

$$X_n = \sum_{i=1}^{n} W_n D_k, \quad (10.29)$$

$$D_k \begin{bmatrix} 1p = 1/2 \\ -1p = 1/2 \end{bmatrix},$$

$$D_k = \pm\sqrt{\frac{T_i}{n}} E(D_k) = 0,$$

$$E(D_k^2) = \frac{T}{n}.$$

$E(D_i D_j) = E(D_i)\,E(D_j)$. The layer of each successive jumps or fluxes is equal to $\left(\frac{T}{n}\right)$ with equal probability.

In other words, if we consider a sequence of independent binomial Xi taking values +1 or −1 with equal probability ($p = q = 0.50$), then the value of random walk at the ith flux in Brownian motion is defined recursively as follows.

$$W_n D_k \sim B(n,p,q), \quad (10.30)$$

where "n" be the fixed dose of drug with equal probability taking "p" as the diffusion flux higher concentration and "q" as the diffusion flux at lower concentration ($p + q = 1/2$). Then p, q, n_1, n_2 and N are related by the following eqn:

$(p + q) = 1$ and $n_1, n_2..n_k$ is the diffusion fluxes $(n_1 + n_2..n_k = N_k)$.

We examine the probability of taking exactly n_1 diffusion flux out of "N" to the right, the model becomes $\binom{N}{n_1} = \binom{n_1 + n_1}{n_1}$ ways of taking n_1 steps to higher concentration and n_2 to the lower concentration, where $\binom{n}{m}$ is the binomial coefficient. The probability of taking particular ordered sequences n_1 and n_2 diffusion fluxes $p^{n_1} q^{n_2}$.Therefore, the $p(n_1)$ diffusion is

$$P(n_1) = \frac{(n_1 + n_2)!}{n_1!\, n_2!} p^{n_1} q^{n_2} = \frac{N!}{n_1!\,(N - n_1)!} p^{n_1} q^{N-n1}, \quad 10.31$$

where $n!$ is a factorial. However, this is simply a BD, so the mean number of fluxes n_1 is the higher concentration plasma flow and the mean number of steps to the lower level is $n_1 = N - n_1 = N(1-p) = qN$.

Similarly the variance of each diffusion was calculated by

$$\sigma_{n1}^2 = (n_1^2) - (n_k)^2 = N_k p_i q_j,$$

$$\sigma_{n1} = \sqrt{N_k p_i q_j}.$$

Difference of diffusion fluxes was modeled as follows (Fig. 10.18):

$$\sum_{d=1}^{J} \frac{d}{(J+d)!\,(J-d)!} = \frac{1}{2\,\Gamma(J)\,\Gamma(1+J)}$$

$$\frac{N!}{2^N}\left[\sum_{d=-J,-(J-1),\dots}^{-1} \frac{|2d|}{\left(\frac{2J+2d}{2}\right)!\left(\frac{2J-2d}{2}\right)!} + \sum_{d=1,2,\dots}^{-1} \frac{|2d|}{\left(\frac{2J+2d}{2}\right)!\left(\frac{2J-2d}{2}\right)!}\right]$$

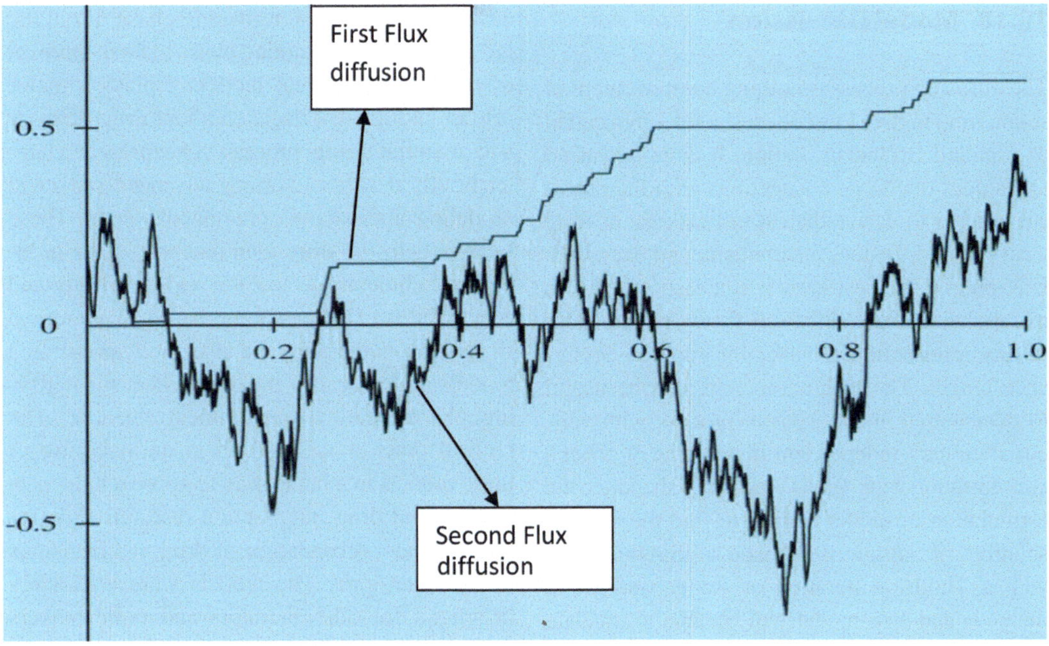

Fig. 10.18 Brownian random walk drug diffusion model probability ($0 \leq p \leq 1$)

$$(d_{2J}) = \frac{N!}{2^N}\left[\sum_{\substack{d=-2J,-\\-2(J-1),\ldots}}^{-2} \frac{|d|}{\left(\frac{2J+2d}{2}\right)!\left(\frac{2J-2d}{2}\right)!} + 0 + \sum_{d=2,4,\ldots}^{2J} \frac{|d|}{\left(\frac{2J+2d}{2}\right)!\left(\frac{2J-2d}{2}\right)!}\right]$$

$$= \frac{N!}{2^N}\left[\sum_{d=-J,-(J-1),\ldots}^{-1} \frac{|2d|}{\left(\frac{2J+2d}{2}\right)!\left(\frac{2J-2d}{2}\right)!} + \sum_{d=1,2,\ldots}^{-1} \frac{|2d|}{\left(\frac{2J+2d}{2}\right)!\left(\frac{2J-2d}{2}\right)!}\right]$$

$$= \frac{N!}{2^N}\left[2\sum_{d=1}^{J} \frac{2d}{(J+d)!\,(J-d)!}\right]$$

$$= \frac{N!}{2^{N-2}}\sum_{d=1}^{J} \frac{d}{(J+d)!\,(J-d)!}$$

10.18 Model Discussion

The diffusion process is nothing but movement of solute from high to low concentration, often called as standard Brownian motion, it is an advanced techniques due to its connections with the physical process to derive the overall process of drug absorption, diffusion, metabolism, and excretion. It is one of the best-known stochastic model to extrapolate various diffusion fluxes without loss of any information (Akaike information >reference range). The techniques will also be useful to demonstrate the stochastic process with various stationary-independent increments of plasma concentration with varied time intervals. Since the formulation of model is used to find the explicit solution of simple stochastic differential eqn with a Thomson iteration or Range and Kutta methods and also model will be able to escalate the explicit solution of drug diffusion, time of absorption, time taken for diffusion, and elimination rate by using newer techniques of optimization (Brownian diffusion model). Similarly the blood volume, bioavailability was approximated from the Brownian motion. The model is a more advanced tool because the diffusion with the molecules is not instantaneous, and has certain time interval. During the time absorption is taking place, the change of movement of molecules or drug particles from the region of higher concentration to the region of lower concentration was derived from random walk process (time verifying stochastic). Of course, in addition one has to assume that the motion of the Brownian particles does not create an ordered flow in the surroundings fluid; such a flow would influence the diffusion probability at later times, and in that way act as memory storage that violates the Gaussian assumptions.

10.19 Conclusion

An advanced statistical method is widely used in clinical and medical research to compile the massive data sets that have been collected in clinical trials as well as pharmacokinetic studies. Usually PK intervention is embedded with planning, designing, and decision-making phase. From the induction of drug planning phase to final approval of drug, the statistical modeling plays a major role in taking right decision about drug delivery and manufacturing process. The present chapter briefly describes various advanced statistical modeling approach to pharmacokinetics. These models help the drug manufacturer, stake holders, and clinicians to test the real credibility and acceptability of the new drugs based on numerical simulation techniques, and also our demonstrated models are critical to the researchers for nurturing pharmaceutical and clinical sciences. The clinical practitioners and chemists make use of these models in a better way to approach the new clinical and drug intervention research and also used for new formulation of drug and decisions on patients' care. The models were effectively beneficial for administrators and policymakers for impacting the health-care system to improve the quality of life of patients and minimize the health costs. The present chapter derives veracity of various advanced analytical and mathematical simulations like Brownian motion and random walk models (constructed based on the optimization techniques), and these recent models will be very useful for the researchers in the establishment of newer clinical and pharmaceutical studies with a varied setup. Finally, our formulated models will be used for the evaluation and classification of drugs in association with plasma concentration and bioavailability. Together, an overall content of the present chapter provides a practical framework with recommendations to guide the development and evaluation of novel regimens to draw a valid conclusive inference about the population or subjects.

References

Ahmed MU et al (2012) Comparative pharmacokinetic and bioequivalence study of azithromycin 500 mg tablet in healthy Bangladeshi volunteers. Int J Clin Pharmacol Ther 50:452–458

Aronow WS, Frishman WH, Cheng-Lai A (2000) Cardiovascular drug therapy in the elderly. Heart Dis 2:151–167

Basavarajaiah DM (2018) Advances in genetic statistics. Educreation Publication, New Delhi, pp 117–120

Beringer P et al (2005) Absolute bioavailability and intracellular pharmacokinetics of azithromycin in patients with cystic fibrosis. Antimicrob Agents Chemother 49:5013–5017

Boonleang J et al (2007) Bioavailability and pharmacokinetic comparison between generic and branded azithromycin capsule: a randomized, double-blind, 2-way crossover in healthy male Thai volunteers. Clin Ther 29:703–710

Breiman L (2001) Statistical modeling: the two cultures. Stat Sci 16:199–215

Caro JJ et al (2012) Modeling good research practices–overview: a report of the ISPOR-SMDM modeling good research practices task force 1. Value Health 15(6):796–803

Ceckova-Novotna MP et al (2006) P-glycoprotein in the placenta: expression, localization, regulation and function. Reprod Toxicol 22:400–410

Chandrasekhar S (1943) For a historical introduction to the Brownian motion. Rev Mod Phys 15:1–5. https://doi.org/10.1103/RevModPhys.15.1

Chang HH et al (2015) Association between ABCB1 polymorphisms and antidepressant treatment response in Taiwanese major depressive patients. Clin Psychopharmacol Neurosci 13:250–255

Cox DR (1990) Role of models in statistical analysis. Stat Sci 5:169–174

Cusack BJ et al (1979) Digoxin in the elderly: pharmacokinetic consequences of old age. Clin Pharmacol Ther 25:772–776

Delafuente JC et al (2008) Pharmacokinetic and pharmacodynamic alterations in the geriatric patient. Consult Pharm 23:324–334

El Desoky ES (2007) Pharmacokinetic-pharmacodynamic crisis in the elderly. Am J Ther 14:488–498

EMEA (2006) Guideline on the role of pharmacokinetics in the development of medicinal products in the paediatric population. European Medicines Agency, London, 28 June 2006. http://www.ema.europa.eu/docs/en_GB/document_library/Scientific_guideline/2009/09/WC500003066.pdf

Gandhi R et al (2004) Pharmacokinetic evaluation of an azithromycin controlled release dosage form in healthy human volunteers: a single dose study. Int J Pharm 270:1–8

Jambhekar SS, Breen PJ (2009) Basic pharmacokinetics. Pharmaceutical Press, London

Khorsan R, Crawford C (2014) How to assess the external validity and model validity of therapeutic trials: a conceptual approach to systematic review methodology. Evid Based Compl Altern Med 5(1):1–12

Korkushko OV, Orlov PA, Bezverkhaia IS, Belyi AA (1984) Effect of age on the pharmacokinetic parameters of digoxin. Farmakol Toksikol 47:101–104

Kostrzewski A (2002) Cardiovascular medicines in the elderly. In: Armour D, Cairns C (eds) Medicines in the elderly. Pharmaceutical Press, London

Laudisio A, Marzetti E, Pagano F, Cocchi A, Bernabei R, Zuccalà G (2009) Digoxin and cognitive performance in patients with heart failure: a cohort pharmacoepidemiological survey. Drugs Aging 26:103–112

Lemke T, Williams D, Roche V, Zito S (2008) Foye's principles of medicinal chemistry, 6th edn. Lippincott Williams Wilkins, Philadelphia

Maronna RA, Martin RD, Yohai VJ et al (2019) Robust statistics: theory and methods (with R), 2nd edn. Wiley, Hoboken

McCullagh P (2002) What is a statistical model? Ann Stat 30:1225–1310

Micceri T (1989) The unicorn, the normal curve, and other improbable creatures. Psychol Bull 105:156–166

Neyman J et al (1959) Stochastic models of population dynamics. Science 130:303–308

Royston P, Sauerbrei W (2008) Multivariate model-building: a pragmatic approach to regression analysis based on fractional polynomials for modelling continuous variables. Wiley, New York

Setiawati E et al (2009) Bioequivalence study of two azithromycin formulations in healthy subjects. Arzneimittelforschung 59:471–475

Shargel L, Wu-Pong S, Yu ABC (2005) Applied biopharmaceutics and pharmacokinetics, 5th edn. McGraw Hill, New York

Shmueli G (2010) To explain or predict? Stat Sci 25:289–310

Tsang P, Gerson B (1990) Understanding digoxin use in the elderly patient. Clin Lab Med 10:479–492

Turnheim K (2003) When drug therapy gets old: pharmacokinetics and pharmacodynamics in the elderly. Exp Gerontol 38:843–853

Vogels R, Scheltens P, Schroeder-Tanka JM, Weinstein HC (2007) Cognitive impairment in heart failure: a systematic review of the literature. Eur J Heart Fail 9:440–449

Winter ME (2004) Basic clinical pharmacokinetics, 4th edn. Lippincott Williams Wilkins, Philadelphia

11 Imputation Methods Approach to Clinical and Life Science Research Data Sets

11.1 Introduction

Numerous clinical and medical researches have been conducted worldwide in varied setup; due to some trivial problems some of the numerical values in the data sets are either lost or not observed or not available due to some technical problems. Some of the reasons mentioned for missing observations in medical research are as follows: patients are in very critical condition, he/she wants to change the treatment, missing due to the breakdown of machines, failed in continuing the follow-up, failed to answer some questionnaires, patients are cured or dead before the study, investigator neglect to collect the data, family migrated to other place, and patient's profile may be missing in the computer database. The missing data will greatly affect the bias, power, and variability of the population, decrease precision, and provide inaccurate results. Rubin (1976) classified the missing data mechanism, viz. (i) missing completely at random (MCAR) (ii) missing at random (MAR) and (iii) missing not at random (MNAR) (Allison 2001; Azur Melissa et al. 2011). Missing at random (MAR) describes that the probability of missing data on a variable *Y* is related to some other measured variable in the analysis model but not to the values of *Y*, for example, missing blood pressure, measurement may be lower than measured blood pressure because younger people may be more likely to have missing blood pressure measurement and another example in real world, the researcher to know the quality of life of patients who suffering from HIV or cancer, entire domain of the study on quality of life comprises with different attributes, researcher intended to extract psychological and physical attributes of selected patients. He adminstered Questinaries for elderly patients in selected sites or hospitals, due to less education and age factor, elderly patients may have higher probability to refuse the QOL questionnaires (De Goeij et al. 2013). In this regard, informations were compeltely missing at random (MCAR), it is the missing data on a variable *Y* is unrelated to other measured variable and also unrelated to the values of *Y* itself, e.g., we noticed that the blood pressure measurement is missing because of breakdown of an automatic sphygmomanometer, suppose a psychologist is studying QOL in a group of cancer patients and finds that patients are missing because they migrated to other places, etc. Ironically, different intervention to deal missing data in medical and clinical research for extrapolation of valid inference about the population (Gelman et al. 2006; Hassani et al. 2019; Kaushal et al. 2014; Kollewe et al. 2008; Heckman 1976).

Traditional methods

(a) Listwise deletion
(b) Pairwise deletion
(c) Lat observation carried forward
(d) Hot deck imputation
(e) Arithmetic mean imputation
(f) Regression imputation
(g) Stochastic regression imputation

B. D. M., B. Narasimha Murthy, *Design of Experiments and Advanced Statistical Techniques in Clinical Research*, https://doi.org/10.1007/978-981-15-8210-3_11

(h) Cold deck imputation
(i) Averaging the available pattern imputation
(j) Maximum likelihood estimation
(k) Markova Chain Monte Carlo simulation techniques

The above traditional methods were already dealt in some other medical books, As such being the cases and practical point of view we discussed various advanced imputation techniques approach to missing data sets are presented in this chapter.

(a) Least variance method—least square analysis model
(b) Gaussian mixture model
(c) KNN model
(d) ARIMA

11.2 Minimum Variance Method

One approach in estimating the root mean square errors (RMSE) of the estimator 'θ' is to normalize the estimator using Taylor expansion series. Let $Y_1,Y_2..Y_n$ be the independent variables associated with random variables of $X_1,X_2..X_n$ that follows Gaussianity $X_{ij}\sim N(\mu,\sigma^2)$ and use the sample variance estimation method to estimate the precision of the linearized statistics. Treating imputation as real data will lead to standard errors (SEs) that are small for most estimates. Let θ is the population parameter of sampled observations calculated based on the full sample and also we estimated the sampling error of subsamples from the certain observations are drawn from the population and parameters $\hat{\theta}$ were computed from each subsamples in various ways of suming from full samples corresponds to different replications or subgroup analysis method (Little and Rubin 2014; Little et al. 2012).

$$\begin{aligned}&\text{Var}(\text{estimator with imputation})\\&=\text{Variance treating imputation}\\&\text{as real}+\text{Average variance between}\\&\text{estimates using different imputed values}\end{aligned}$$

$$\text{Var}\left(\hat{\theta}\right)=\sum_{i=1}^{k}C_k\left(\hat{\theta}_i-\overline{\hat{\theta}}_k\right)^2, \tag{11.1}$$

where C_k are the factors associated with various replicates of data sets

$\overline{\hat{\theta}}_k$ = Mean values of the estimated parameter at kth replicates

$\hat{\theta}_i$ = the estimated parameter at ith replicated imputed values

Multiple imputation (MI) method is one way of reflecting extra variance due to item imputation since we impute more than one value "k" for each missing item on each cases

Compute estimate the Q_t from each of t = 12…k (complete means real collected values + imputed values for missing variables).

We can estimate the items from the following formula:

$$Q=k^{-1}\sum_{i=1}^{k}Q_t. \tag{11.2}$$

Variance estimates U_t treating all the data as complete (not imputed)

$$U_t=V\left(\overline{Y}_t\right)=f\left(x_i,\hat{\theta}_1,\hat{\theta}_2,\hat{\theta}_3\ldots\hat{\theta}_n\right), \tag{11.3}$$

$$\text{Var}\left(\overline{Q}\right)=\overline{U}+\sum_{i=1}^{k}\left(1+k^{-1}\right)B,$$

$$\overline{U}=k^{-1}\sum_{i=1}^{k}U_t, \tag{11.4}$$

$$B=\left(m-1\right)^{-1}\sum_{i=1}^{k}\left(Q_t-\overline{Q}\right)^2. \tag{11.5}$$

The above Eq. (11.5) applies to any method in which the imputed value is random, mean imputation with random error (RE), hot deck with random draws from completes and regression with random errors.

(Figure 11.1) clearly depicts that the gain of imputation probability is more when compared to the observed imputed data sets compiled from minimum variance methods; the normalcy has assumed with prior value estimation of imputation. For each subsampled data, the variance or RMSE was estimated at greatest accuracy and more precision. An estimated imputed value of parameters $\hat{\theta}$ reflects the each individual values of squared deviation taken from the mean values, finally regression was smoothed with dependent and independent variable Eq. (11.5). The above-cited imputed model is best fit and applies for many types of estimates (point, means, totals, and quintiles). However, main demerits of above demonstrated model estimator can be positively biased in some cluster sample and also reproducibility of the model is very narrow in case of hierarchical cluster and mixed effect data sets.

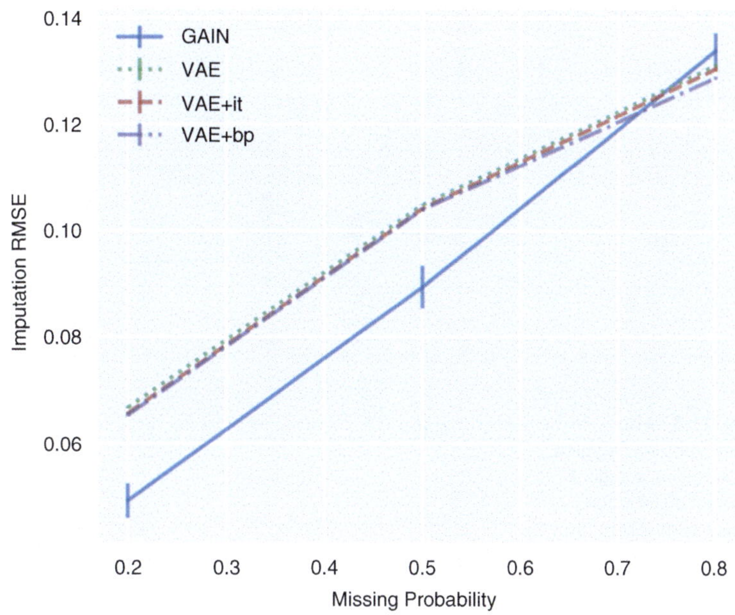

Fig. 11.1 Missing probability of variance method based on RMSE

11.3 Gaussian Mixture Model

From Eq. (11.3),
$U_t = V(\bar{Y}_t) = f(x_i, \hat{\theta}_1, \hat{\theta}_2, \hat{\theta}_3 \ldots \hat{\theta}_n)$.

We assumed the Gaussianity to obtain the MLEs for Eq. (11.3), substitute the *fy* and the eqn becomes

$$L(\mu,\sigma^2,x_i) = {}_{i=1}^{n}\pi\, fy(x_i,\mu,\sigma^2)\ {}_{=i=1}^{n}\pi\,(2\pi\sigma^2)^{-n/2}\ \text{expo} - \left(\frac{(x_i-\mu)^2}{2\sigma^2}\right) \tag{11.6}$$

$$U_t = L\left(\hat{\theta}/x_i\right)$$

$$L\left(\hat{\theta}/x_i\right) = \prod_{i=1}^{n} P_{y_i} / (x_i, \widehat{\theta}_1, \widehat{\theta}_2 \ldots\ldots\ldots \widehat{\theta}_n) \tag{11.7}$$

On maximizing Eq. (11.7), we will get estimated errors and predicted values of dependent variables (multiple imputation) (Fig. 11.2):

$$L(\mu,\sigma^2,x_i) = {}_{i=1}^{n}\pi\, fy(x_i,\mu,\sigma^2).$$

$$L\left(\hat{\theta}/x_i\right) = (m-1)^{-1\text{expo}-} \frac{\sum_{i=1}^{k}(Q_t-\bar{Q})^2}{2\sigma^2}, \tag{11.8}$$

$$= \prod_{i=1}^{n}(m-1)^{-1\text{expo}-} \frac{\sum_{i=1}^{k}(Q_t-\bar{Q})^2}{2\sigma^2}, \quad = \frac{1}{(m-1)}\prod_{i=1}^{n}\text{expo} - \frac{1}{2}\left(\frac{(Q_t-\bar{Q})^2}{\sigma^2}\right). \tag{11.9}$$

By substituting the frequency of missed values in real data sets, Eq. (11.9) becomes

$$L\left(\hat{\theta}/x_i\right) = \frac{1}{(m-1)}\prod_{i=1}^{n}\text{expo} - \frac{1}{2} f_t\left(\frac{(Q_t-\bar{Q})^2}{\sigma^2}\right), \tag{11.10}$$

$$f_t = f_1, f_2 \ldots f_i \qquad \text{(where)}$$

$$L\left(\hat{\theta}/x_i\right) = \frac{1}{(m-1)}\prod_{i=1}^{n}\text{expo} - \frac{1}{2} f_t Z^2,$$

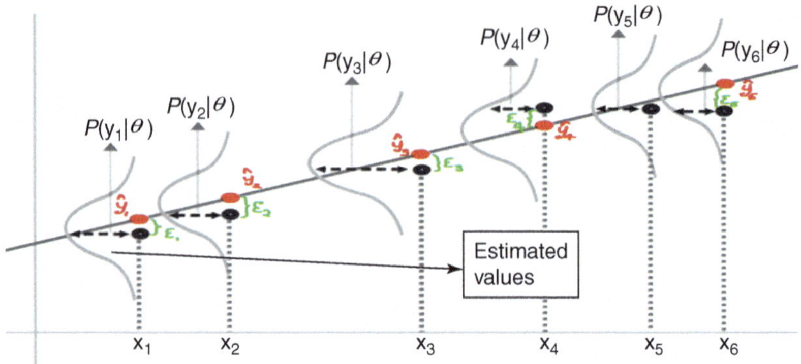

Fig. 11.2 MLE estimation for imputed values of random variables

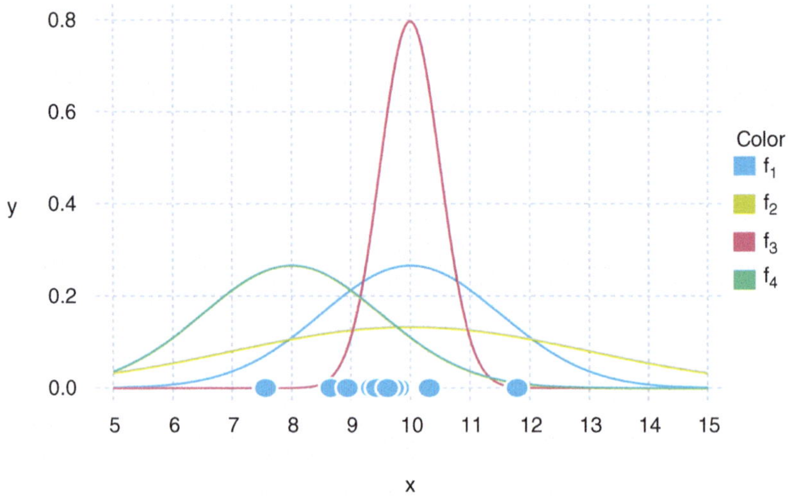

Fig. 11.3 MLE estimation for imputed values from standard normal distribution curve with substitution of frequency of imputed values

where $Z = \left(\frac{\left(Q_t - \bar{Q}\right)^2}{\sigma^2}\right)$, $Z \sim N(\mu, \sigma^2)$

The actual values of Q are unknown if some of the population data are unknown (Fig. 11.3). Suppose we make an estimate $\hat{Q}_t$. The population uncertainty is estimated about the true population parameter value, which will depend on what we know about the $L\left(\hat{\theta}/x_i\right)$ likelihood function of unknown parameters and real and missed observations. If we would be able to create the frequency of imputed values $f_t = f_1, f_2 \dots f_i$ based on the estimated parameters, finally we get Eq. (11.10). The possible values of predicted missed observations were obtained from the posterior distribution (Bayesian approach)

$$P(\theta/x_i) = \int p(\theta/x_i)\, p(x_i) \div p(\theta) \quad (11.11)$$

Likelihood   Posterior   Evidence

$$P(\theta / \text{Xob}) = \int P\left(\theta / (\text{Xob,Xmis})\right) P(\text{mis} / \text{Xob})\, \text{dymis}$$

The scope of formulated model related to the way of settings in which the data sets are collected. The following intervention will be useful to categorize the real situations

Broad perspective on practical point of view—The researcher should ensure and create one set of imputation to use for all experimental setup and compilation. A broad scope is necessary and appropriate for publicly released data sets, cohort, prospective, case control, and registry (cancer, stroke, and HIV).

Intermediate approach—Every clinical and medical research must undergo the interim analysis and create separate imputation parameters on cohort basis and substitute this imputed data set for all analyses. An intermediate approach of substitution of imputed values for deriving common values is very suitable for compilation of massive data sets, that would be estimates relatively similar quintiles even inclusion small area estimation based on prior and posterior parameter of our interest (Marlin 2008; Pigott 2001; Rubin 1976).

Narrow approach: A separate imputed data sets are created for each analysis obtained from the minimum variance unbiased estimation (MVUE) and Gaussian imputation methods. The imputer and analysts are typically the same person. A narrow scope is appropriate if the imputed data used only to estimate the unknown parameters with same quantity. A different analyst requires different imputations. However, this method will be easy to calculate the imputed values without any bias in any experimental setup. Robustness of the model is very easy, and there is no complexity between the estimated and observed values. In general, the imputation was created under a broad perspective based on real data sets and also can be applied widely and preferably for that reason. On the other hand, if we look at a strong scientific ethos and model-based study for estimation of imputed data, our demonstrated model can help us in taking good decisions about the population because using replicated imputed values obtained from the mathematical derivations based on the parameters of our interests have high-stake consequences than using a narrow scope is better because the imputation model can be informed a sound knowledge by the complete data sets model at population level, thus we should confirm that all complexities and linearities were uniformly distributed with the estimation of unknown parameters. In reader practice the correct model is often unknown. Therefore, the cited techniques in this present section or chapter will emphasize more on imputations for the broader scope. Whatever is chosen, it is the responsibility of the imputer to mention the scope of the propagated or predicted imputations and also address the research gap and salient methods to be used for the compilation (Karimzadeh and Olafsson 2019).

11.4 KNN Model Approach for Missing Data

KNN imputes the missing attribute values on the basis of nearest K neighbors. The neighbors are determined based on the distance measures (Chap. 2 discussed). Once *K* value is determined, missing values are imputed by taking mean, median, or mode of known attribute values of missing variable. For a discrete variable, KNN imputer uses the most frequent value among the *k*-nearest neighbors and for a continuous variable (Fig. 11.4).

$$\text{dist}\left(d_x d_y\right) = \sqrt{\sum_{i=1}^{k}\left(X_i - Y_i\right)^2},$$

$$G_I = \sum_{i=1}^{k} w_i * e_{ij}.$$

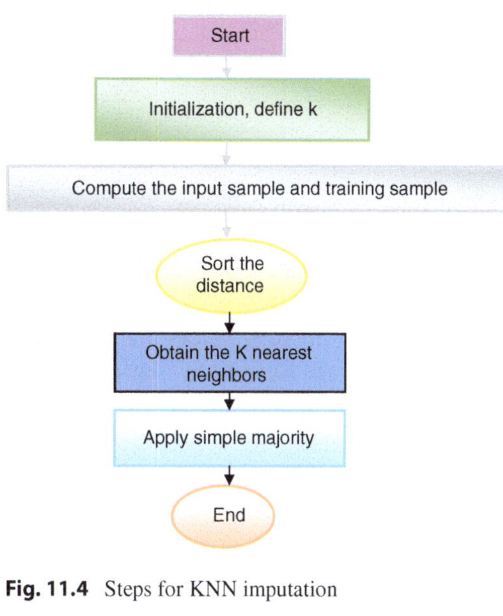

Fig. 11.4 Steps for KNN imputation

Hamming distance $D_H = \sum_{i=1}^{k} |X_i - Y_i|$.

$$X = Y \Rightarrow D = 0$$

$$X \neq Y \Rightarrow D = 1$$

e.g.,

X	*Y*	Distance
Male	Male	0
Male	Female	1

$$E = \sqrt{\sum_{I=1}^{k} (X_i - Y_i)^2} \quad \text{(Euclidian)}$$

$$\mathrm{Mi} = \left[\sum_{i=1}^{k} (|X_i - Y_i|)^q \right]^{1/q} \quad \text{(Minkowski)}$$

Illustration

The following real data set is an example for determining "*K*" nearest value by imputation:

X_1 = Acid durability (second ys)	X_2 = Strength (kg/sqmt)	*Y* classification
7	7	Bad
7	4	Bad
3	4	Good
1	4	Good

Step 1: Initialize $k = 9$ and let us say $k = 3$

Always select odd number for *k* to avoid ties classifications

Step2: Determine the distance between input and training samples (coordinate 3,7)

X_1 = Acid durability (second ys)	X_2 = Strength (kg/sqmt)	Euclidian distance
7	7	$(7 - 3)^2 + (7 - 7)^2 = 16$
7	4	$(7 - 7)^2 + (7 - 4)^2 = 25$
3	4	$(7 - 3)^2 + (4 - 7)^2 = 09$
1	4	$(1 - 73)^2 + (4 - 7)^2 = 13$

X_1 = Acid durability (second ys)	X_2 = Strength (kg/sqmt)	Euclidian distance	Rank minimum distance	Is it include nearest *K* values
7	7	16	3	Yes
7	4	25	4	No
3	4	09	1	Yes
1	4	13	2	Yes

Step 3 Take three nearest neighbors

X_1 = Acid durability (second ys)	X_2 = Strength (kg/sqmt)	Euclidian distance	Rank minimum distance	Is it include nearest *K* values	*Y* = nearest category of neighbors
7	7	16	3	Yes	Bad
7	4	25	4	No	–
3	4	09	1	Yes	Good
1	4	13	2	Yes	Good

Step 4: Apply simple category

Use simple majority of the category of the nearest value as the prediction nearest value of the query instance

Each samples' missing values were imputed by using the average value form *k*-nearest neighbors found in the training data sets. Two samples are close if the features that neither is missing are close. Distance measurement methods that supports missing values and find the *k*-nearest neighbors in machine learning and artificial inteligence. We created data frame with missing values

In [3]: import numpy as np
import pandas as pd

$$\text{dict} = \{\text{'first'} : [100, 90, \text{np,nan}, 95],$$

$$\text{"second"} : [100, 90, \text{np,nan}, 95],$$

$$\text{"third"} : [100, 90, \text{np,nan}, 95],$$

$$\#\text{creating a data frame from list}$$

$$\text{df} = \text{pd.data frame}(\text{dict})$$

In [6]:df

Output [6]:

	First	Second	Third
0	100.0	30	Nan
1	90.0	45	40.0
2	Nan	56.0	80.0
3	95	Nan	98.0

df_filled = imputer.fit_transform (df)
In [7]:df_filled

	First	Second	Third
0	100.0	30	69.0
1	90.0	45	40.0
2	97.5	56.0	80.0
3	95	43	98.0

If a sample has more than one feature observation missing, then the neighbors for that sample can be different depending upon a particular feature being imputed; however, when the number of variable neighbors less than "*n*" neighbors and there is no defined distance to the training data sets, the training data set average for that future is used during imputation. If there is at least one neighbor with a defined distance, the weighted or underweighted average of the remaining neighbors will be used in extrapolation of imputation values at precise level and greater accuracy (Sabatelli et al. 2013; Srivastava et al. 2014; Sterne et al. 2009; Troyanskaya et al. 2001).

11.4.1 Kappa Statistics for Testing KNN Missing Observations

The imputation values' interpretability were tested by Kappa test statistics, Cohen's Kappa statistics measures interpretability reliability (sometimes we called as interobserver agreement). Interrater reliability or precision happens when your data raters (or collectors) give the same score to the same items. Two raters each rate one trail on each sample or one rater two trails on each sample. In addition to that, Cohen's Kappa has the assumption that the raters are deliberately chosen. If your raters are chosen at random from a population of raters, use Fleiss Kappa instead. Historically percent agreement was used to determine interrater reliability. The Kappa statistics takes into account this element of chance factor. The Kappa statistics varies from 0 to 1 where

Values	Decision
0	Agreement equal to chance
0.1–0.20	Slight agreement
0.21–0.40	Fair agreement
0.41–0.60	Moderate agreement
0.61–0.80	Substantial agreement
0.81–0.99	Near perfect agreement
1.0	Perfect agreement

The following formula is used to calculate Cohen's Kappa for two raters as follows:

$$Kp = \left[\frac{p_0 - p_e}{1 - p_e}\right] = 1 - \left(\frac{p_0 - p_e}{1 - p_e}\right),$$

where p_0 is the relative observed agreement among raters

p_e is the hypothetical probability of chance agreement.

KNN agreement was taken from imputation; we assumed the following agreement:

Clusters	Decision	KNN agreement		
		Good	Bad	Total
	Cluster 1	65	12	77
	Cluster 2	36	10	46
	Total	101	22	123

Step1

Find the probability that the investigator would randomly say both Yes and No agreements

Decision good cluster 1 = 65/101 = 0.64

Decision good cluster 2 = 36/101 = 0.35

Total probability of the agreement of imputation both clusters saying good randomly investigated

$$0.64 * 0.35 = 0.22$$

Step 2

We consider total probability of the agreement for derivation imputation of both clusters, saying bad randomly investigated

Decision bad cluster 1 = 12/22 = 0.54

Decision bad cluster 2 = 10/22 = 0.45

$$0.54 * 0.45 = 0.245$$

Step3

Determine p_e which is the hypothetical probability of chance agreement (total probability that agreement would randomly select)

$$p_e = 0.22 + 0.24 = 0.46$$

P_0 = number in agreement/total = 1 65 + 36/123 = 0.82

Step 4: Determine the Kappa statistics by using the formula

$$Kp = \left[\frac{p_0 - p_e}{1 - p_e}\right] = \left[\frac{0.82 - 0.46}{1 - 0.46}\right] = \frac{0.36}{0.54} = 0.66$$

As per the Kp we concludes that, the moderate agreement between the decisions taken by investigator for grouping the KNN means for extrapolation of imputation values.

11.5 Imputation by Random Forest

Random forest is a unique advanced method to deep way of averaging various decision trees, trained on different parts of the same training set, with the goal of overcoming over fitting problem of individual. In other words, random forests are an ensemble learning method for classification and regression that operate by constructing a lot of decision tree at training time and outputting various classes, i.e., the mode of classes output by individual trees or branch (Van Buuren 2018; Wells et al. 2013; Miotto et al. 2016). In the real world medical problems many clinician, medical researcher are using random forest techniques for extraction of inharent problems of diagnosis and treatment aspects, random forest will be used for handling of missing values—drop data points for missing values; fill in missing values with the descriptive statistics (mean, median numerical values) or mode for categorical values does not use all the available information by dropping data points, can sometimes brush too broad a stroke for data sets with many gaps and significant structure. In this new horizon of the statistical science, the present section aims to describe the proximity in association with imputation techniques by random forest ensemble method for taking average prediction of whole tree decisions. The proximity of random forest defines between two or more missing observation. The following steps were used to escalate the random forest:

1. Initialize proximities to zeros.
2. For any given tree, apply the tree to all cases.
3. If case I and case *j* both end up in the same node, increase proximity prox(*ij*) between *I* and *j* by one.
4. Accumulate overall trees in RF and normalize by twice the number of trees in RF.

It creates a proximity matrix (a square matrix with 1) on the diagonal between 0 and 1 in the off-diagonal position. Observations that are alike will have proximities close to 1. The closer the proximity to 0, the more the dissimilar cases are. Proximities mainly are used for outlier detection and imputation techniques (Karimzadeh and Olafsson 2019) applied proximities matrix for multiple data imputations, practically in most of data clustering the input data includes vector space model describing the locations and distance of each data points, from which we can correlate the data points for deriving imputed values and also between the data points constructed proximate matrixes, i.e., distance between each pair of homogeneous data points is taken into consideration. However, several algorithms driven by the machine learning techniques for calculation imputed values and also method can still be applied, but if the proximity matrix has missing values, non-standard method is directly applicable for prediction, but most imputation methods do not apply when only the proximity matrix is available. As a partial, we formulate new model to fill partial solution for this analytical research gap. We attempt to build proximity matrix by using binary outcome method (logistic regression model)

Let us assume the matrix of original data sets of CVD.

Chest pain	Good blood circulation	Blocked arteries	Weights	Heart diseases
No	No	No	125	No
Yes	Yes	Yes	180	Yes
Yes	Yes	No	210	No
Yes	No	??	???	No

Random forest considers two types of data missing: missing data in original data sets used to create the RF and missing data in new sample that you want to categorize.

11.5.1 Methods

Step 1: Create a random forest tree for the above data matrix

Step 2: Update proximity matrix by using real values

Step 3: Classification of out-of-bag sample (yes or no)

Step 3: Apply binary logistic regression for prediction of missing observations

The dependent variable chest pain binary outcome bagged—yes coded as 1 and out bagged—data no coded as 0, each individual covariate sampled data assigned the codes, select the independent variable X_1: age; X_2: BMI; X_3: SBP; X_4: DSP; X_5: cholesterol; X_6: SGOT and X_7: SCPT, etc.

$$Y_i = \frac{1}{1+\text{expo}^{-(b_0X_0+b_1X_1\ldots b_nX_n)}},$$

$$\left(\frac{p}{1-p}\right) = \text{expo}^{-(b_0X_0+b_1X_1\ldots b_nX_n)}.$$

There are several analogies for the estimation of predicted values, i.e., least square estimation estimates the coefficient of each selected variable. The logistic regression produces MLEs to obtain the model coefficient that relates predictors to the target. After this initial function is estimated, the process is repeated until LL does not change.

$$\beta^1 = \beta^0 + \left[X^{\mathrm{T}}WX\right]^{-1} X^{\mathrm{T}}\left(y-\mu\right)$$

where β is a vector of the logistic regression coefficient, W is a square matrix of order N tree with elements associated with n_i leaf node $n_i d_i(1 - d)$, μ = mean distance between cluster sample $\mu = n_i d_i$ and d_i is the distance.

The number of records correctly predicted, given a cutoff point 0.50 divided by the total count of cases. This is equal to the accuracy of a classification model.

$$R^2\left(\%\right) = \frac{\text{Correct predicted}}{\text{Total number of counts}}$$

Step 4: Run the data down all the matrix and proximity matrix fill with imputed values estimated by binary logistic or multiple logistic regression

Step 5: Cross-check robustness of the formulated model

Step 6: Draw the analytical inference based on the MLEs and sensitivity analysis or method.

Step 7: Applying the LR likelihood ratio test provides the corrected predicted values for comparing the likelihood of the data under fitted model against the likelihood of traditional model

$$\text{LL} = \sum_{i=1}^{n} y_i \ln\left(p_i\right) + \left(1-y_i\right)\ln\left(1-p_i\right).$$

Wald test used to test the level of significance of each coefficient

$$W_j = \frac{b_j}{\text{SE}\,b_j}.$$

11.5.2 Merits

Use of multiple trees for capturing the imputed values and reduce the risk of overfitting.

Training time is very less and also maintains good accuracy and precision at all levels.

Runs efficiently on massive data sets either medical, clinical, and agricultural data sets on broad perspectives.

For large data model, it produces highly accurate prediction of missing values.

It can handle high dimensionality.

Scalable and interpretable, no surrogates—missing values are imputed automatically.

11.5.3 Demerits

Choice of tree for pruning is very critical (massive data sets). Higher pruning affects the leaf nodes and child nodes, respectively, which are significantly different from what we need, whereas lower pruning of tree implies missing out of significant attributes (Fig. 11.5).

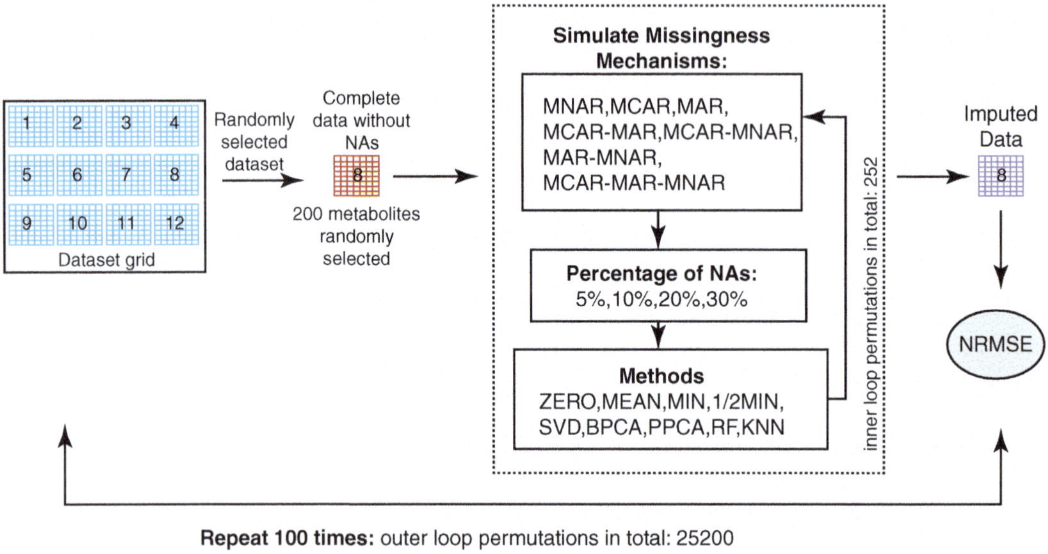

Fig. 11.5 RF missing data imputed, source data; KIHD (Kuopio Ischemic Heart Disease Risk Factor Study)

The RF binary logistic regression is a powerful model to extrapolate the imputed values and also to know the association between supervised and unsupervised learning trainers, even though the whole imputation techniques and procedures with RF has a computation shortly expensive due to some gap of intensive iteration methods (Monte Carlo iteration method is not directly applied), it is well known that it can handle both parametric and nonparametric data sets with linear and nonlinear problem; there is no need to perform preprocessing at the data beforehand.

11.6 Autoregressive Integrated Moving Average Model (ARIMA)

ARIMA stands for autoregressive integrated moving average model, it is mainly used for prediction of missing data cross at specific time periods. In medical and clinical research, we commonly used ARIMA model for predictive purposes. An insight of clinical research, the missing values are particularly prominent in long trials, or studies were conducted with less drug adherence in accordance with study protocol, say, for example, people living with HIV/AIDS patient are receiving the treatment at lifelong (trail focused on increase in the length of survivability), in such type of trails we are ignoring the missing values, it may result in the biased estimation of results (increase PPV values) or invalid conclusion about the various clinical attributes at sample or population level, so we are adopting a reliable imputation method that should be regarded as an essential consideration for testing the null hypothesis of our objective of interest. Although, many clinical trials will be conducted on the basis of time series data which included measurement variables that were collected from different sites and various time intervals. Clinically, the entire course of treatment or lifecycle of trial would differ varied experimental setup. A different season and geographical locations were selected for the study purpose. As per the scientific findings, different reasons may lead to data sets with various statistical proportion on imputed data sets. For example, a series of blood glucose levels measured at each visit, and it may be attributed with missing data points because of instrumental errors, investigator ignorance, LFU, or due to patient illness. An excluding of missing data set should greatly affect the power and level of significance at the time of testing of null hypothesis at population or sampled level, the missing values also may cause linearity between cause and effect of experimental study, missing observations are highly determinantal in clinical and medical research for management of overall well-being of individual cases or subjects. The epitome of missing observations calculation with respect to season and time intervals would be deleteriously effect the entire data sets for underestimation of variance components with narrowing of confidence intervals.

11.6.1 Model Formulation

The ARIMA model is fundamentally a linear regression model associated to track linear tendencies of imputed values in various time series clinical and medical science research data sets. The model is expressed as (p,d,q) parameter, the p,d,q is nothing but integer real values that decide of the AR and MA model and parameter "d" is the level of differencing applied to the data. Mathematically the model eqn is expressed as follows:

$$\hat{x}_t = c + \varnothing_1 x_{t-1} + \varnothing_2 x_{t-2} \ldots \varnothing_p x_{t-p} - \varphi_1 \epsilon_{t-1} - \varphi_2 \epsilon_{t-2} \ldots \varphi_q \epsilon_{t-q}, = c + \sum_{k=1}^{p} \varnothing_k x_{t-k} - \sum_{k=1}^{q} \varphi_t \epsilon_{t-1}.$$

Term "c" is constant; $\varnothing_k$ and φ_t are coefficient values of AR model variable x_{t-k} and MA model variable ϵ_{t-1} is an error notation with period, error associated with mean zero and common variance and statistical i.i.d. (Fig. 11.6).

Before applying ARIMA, data decomposition is very important and menace for the data analysis. The outcome measures were investigated at study sites for checking temporal autocorrelations in the residual by using Durbin Watson test. The test statistics tested the null hypothesis for residuals (serially uncorrelated), and this test was tested against alternative hypothesis that they follow a first-order autoregressive process.

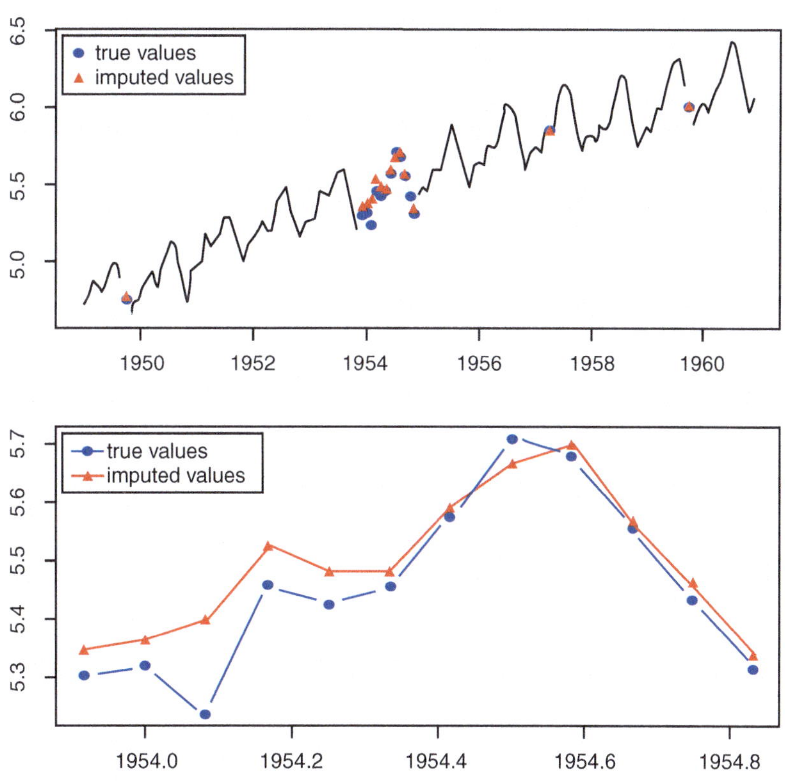

Fig. 11.6 ARIMA imputed value and true value distribution (number of HIV-infected cases registered for HAART in yearly cohort)

11.7 Conclusion

The present chapter (demonstrated models) concludes that the KNN, Gaussian, and random forest imputation models are very easy to apply for determination of multiple missing values. Minimum variance unbaised estimation method is most driven model for extrapolation of missing values without loss of information and credibility, because it construct multiple data sets by using maximum likelihood minimization techniques by filling each missing datum with real values, and then obtained parameter estimates by averaging and minimized squared deviations were taken over multiple data points. Since minimum variance method often uses different methods for binary endpoints with continuous frequentistic approach.

References

Allison PD (2001) Missing data, vol 136. Sage

Azur Melissa J et al (2011) Multiple imputation by chained equations: what is it and how does it work. Int J Methods Psychiatr Res 2(1):40–49

De Goeij MC, Van Diepen M, Jager KJ et al (2013) Multiple imputation: dealing with missing data. Nephrol Dial Transplant 28(10):2415–2420

Gelman et al (2006) Data analysis using regression and multilevel/hierarchical models. Chapter 15. Cambridge University Press. http://www.stat.columbia.edu/~gelman/arm/missing.pdf

Hassani H, Kalantari M, Ghodsi Z (2019) Evaluating the performance of multiple imputation methods for handling missing values in time series data: a study focused on East Africa, soil carbonate-stable isotope data. Stats 2(4):457–467

Heckman JJ (1976) The common structure of statistical models of truncation, sample selection and limited dependent variables and a simple estimator for such models. Ann Econ Soc Meas 5(4):475–492

Karimzadeh S, Olafsson S (2019) Data clustering using proximity matrices with missing values. Author links open overlay panel. Expert Syst Appl 15(7):265–276

Kaushal S et al (2014) Missing data in clinical trials: pitfalls and remedies. Int J Appl Basic Med Res 4(Suppl 1):S6–S7

Kollewe K, Mauss U, Krampfl K, Petri S, Dengler R, Mohammadi B (2008) ALSFRS-R score and its ratio: a useful predictor for ALS-progression. J Neurol Sci 275(1–2):69–73. https://doi.org/10.1016/j.jns.2008.07.016

Little RJA, Rubin DB (2014) Statistical analysis with missing data, vol 793. Wiley, New York

Little RJ, DAgostino R, Cohen ML, Dickersin K, Emerson SS, Farrar J (2012) The prevention and treatment of missing data in clinical trials. N Engl J Med 367(14):1355–1360

Marlin B (2008) Missing data problems in machine learning. http://www-devel.cs.ubc.ca/~bmarlin/research/phd_thesis/marlin-phd-thesis.pdf. Accessed 7 Aug 2016

Miotto R, Li L, Kidd BA et al (2016) Deep patient: an unsupervised representation to predict the future of patients from the electronic health records. Sci Rep 6:26094. https://doi.org/10.1038/srep26094

Pigott TD (2001) A review of methods for missing data. Educ Res Eval 7(4):353–383

Rubin DB (1976) Inference and missing data. J Biometrika 63(3):581–592

Sabatelli M, Conte A, Zollino M (2013) Clinical and genetic heterogeneity of amyotrophic lateral sclerosis. Clin Genet 83(5):408–416. https://doi.org/10.1111/cge.12117

Srivastava N, Hinton GE, Krizhevsky A, Sutskever I, Salakhutdinov R (2014) Dropout3: a simple way to prevent neural networks from overfitting. J Mach Learn Res 15:1929–1958. https://doi.org/10.1214/12-AOS1000

Sterne JAC, White IR, Carlin JB et al (2009) Multiple imputation for missing data in epidemiological and clinical research: potential and pitfalls. BMJ 338:b2393. https://doi.org/10.1136/bmj.b2393

Troyanskaya O, Cantor M, Sherlock G et al (2001) Missing value estimation methods for DNA microarrays. Bioinformatics 17(6):520–525. https://doi.org/10.1093/bioinformatics/17.6.520

Van Buuren S (2018) Flexible imputation of missing data. Chapman and Hall/CRC, Boca Raton

Wells BJ, Chagin KM, Nowacki AS, Kattan MW (2013) Strategies for handling missing data in electronic health record derived data. EGEMS (Washington, DC) 1(3):1035. https://doi.org/10.13063/2327-9214.1035

12 Ethical Perspective of Medical Research

The first step in the evolution of ethics is a sense of solidarity with other human beings

Prof. Albert Sweiter

12.1 Introduction

The research being carried out should be essential for the advancement of knowledge that benefits patients, doctors, and all others in aspects of health care and also for the ecological and environmental well-being of our green planet and ecosystem. Scientifically ethics are the moral values of human behavior and the principles which govern these values. Every profession is bound by code of ethics (Greek word ethos meaning customs or character), and the essence of medicine and clinical research moral community dates back to Hippocratic Oaths (Gasparetto et al. 2018; Jameton 2013; Tarzian 2013). This word of honour is guide for the physicians on practising professional ethics and mandate that's for profession, would prescribe only beneficial treatments, refrain from causing harm or hurt to his or her patients and would place the interest of their patient ethical and of our own interests. The situation becomes challenging for doctors when he/she assumes the role of a researcher. The doctor (researcher) serves both the roles, and at times, the zeal of an investigator has the potential to cloud the morality of the physician inside. History has its store in numerous instances when the enthusiasm for knowledge breached the principles of ethics (Beauchamp and Childress 2013). Thus, it was realized that the code of ethics for clinical research was needed, and good clinical practice guidelines for human research was framed. In any clinical practice, doctors pledge to treat every individual equally, irrespective of their age, disease or disability, creed, ethnic origin, gender, nationality, political affiliation, race, sexual orientation, social standing, or any other associated factors, since when it comes to research that pledge is blurred at times, and it is forgotten that the subject for research is also patients who has put their faith in the doctor for their treatment (White et al. 2001; Benatar 1998; Clinical ethics revisited by Peter Singer et al. 2001). Medical science is one discipline where the advancement of knowledge is hugely guided by research, and humankind has benefitted from many experiments. However, benefit and risk are the two faces of the same coin. If there is no loss, there is no gain; but the risk or loss is assumed by individual or participants of research, and benefit or gain is reaped by a human population, who did not have to bear that risk and to ensure all the participants gets fair treatment that he or she expects from his or her treating physician (Carpenter Jr et al. 2000; David 1994; Frankena 1973). Scientifically ethics is pluralistic, there can be disagreement among individuals about what is right and what is wrong, and even they agree, the reason can be different. The ethical word will be signifying the meaning of full-blown of research and novelty.

B. D. M., B. Narasimha Murthy, *Design of Experiments and Advanced Statistical Techniques in Clinical Research*, https://doi.org/10.1007/978-981-15-8210-3_12

12.2 Ethical Rationality

Many medical research program would cover long-ranging effect of ethics in manifold critics and pit falls for selection of problems, study design, patient selection and submission process, etc. The researcher is willing to formulate the study protocol of clinical research since the researcher should familiarize and have in-depth knowledge of ethical perspective and patient management during the study intervention. Many of the clinicians and researchers are not aware of ethical regularity and guidelines, then how to select the problems, what are the rules or framework presented in the ethical guidelines, confidentiality, legality and dignity, and autonomy. In this aspect, the present chapter aims to describe various salient features of ethical guidelines and also describes new advanced and revised framework formulated at international and national standards (Agich 2001; Grisso and Appelbaum 1995; Hippocrates 1780). The present section will benefit the clinicians, research beginners, policymakers, and drug manufacturers for their research work at institutional level.

12.3 Principles of Ethics in Medical and Clinical Research

Hippocrates was the first physician to define the ethical principles of research in human. The following principles still valid today (Fig. 12.1).

12.3.1 Autonomy

In the human being tradition, the view that individual autonomy is a basic moral, ethics and faith is very much a modern development. Putting moral weight on an individual's ability to govern themself, independent of their place in a metaphysical order or role in social structures and status of living is very much the product of the modernist humanism of which much contemporary moral and medical philosophy is an offshoot. We should respect the autonomy of the participants or their representatives for drug trails, the research participants should be aware of the nature of research and probable consequences of the clinical experiments and then make an independent choice without the influence of the treating doc-

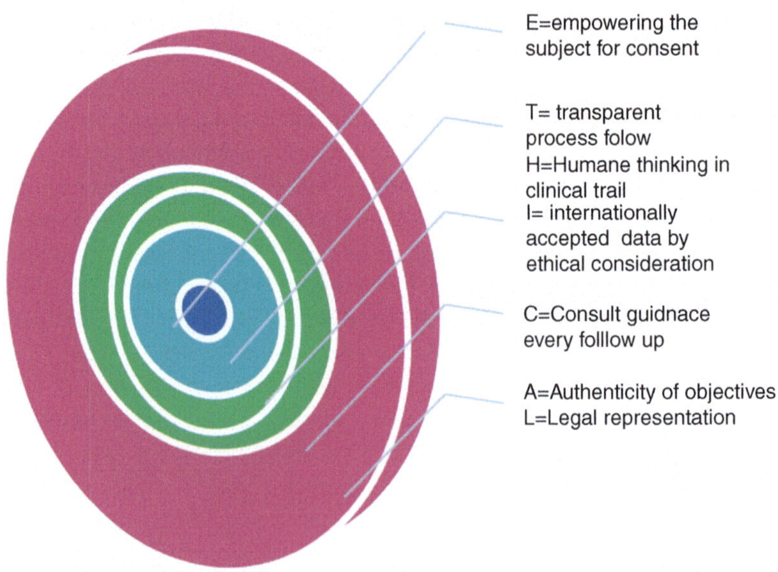

Fig. 12.1 Ethical word signifying the meaning of full information to the researcher

tors, whether to take part in the research or not. When the research treats any community or group of persons as research participants, these principles of voluntariness and informed consent should apply to the community as a whole and also to each individual member who is the participant of the research or experimental group (novelty). All participants participated in drug trail should need to understand their consents and about treatment induction, duration, harmful effects, and overall legacy of the experimental research.

12.3.2 Beneficiency

Beneficeny is a concept in research ethics which states that researchers should have the welfare of the research participant as a goal of any clinical trial.In this regard researcher should maximize the economic and health benefits and minimize the harms, the clinical research always focuses on the objectives of human and animal interventions. The health benefits are very important for us to make use of our available resources from the green planet to maintain the overall well-being of individuals. The logic of beneficiency dealt with quality of life (QOL) during the study period. In this pragmatic approach, the research should always maximize the health benefits and reduce the risks, e.g., the people living with cancer, treating with new trial, the atomicity of the research should always focus on the health concern of the subjects and on the other hand minimizes the side effects of drug. It is required that the procedure will be provided with the intent of doing good for the patients involved. When the demands that create research, the heath-care providers will develop and maintain soft skills, knowledge of updating patients on virtual basis (training), etc. Consider individual circumstances of all patients, and strive for net benefits of patients and ended in welfare, many clinical researchers formulate new revised guidelines in accordance with international standards. All health-care providers must strive to improve their patient's health, to do the most good for patient in every situation, what is good for one patient may not be good for another, so each should be considered individually.

12.3.3 Nonmaleficence

As per the legal perspective, non-maleficence is a practice in which physicians must refrain from providing ineffective treatments or acting with ill will toward patients. But since many beneficial therapies have serious risks, therefore, this principle, offers a little useful guidance to physicians. Doctors should attempt to avoid any act or research plan that would harm the patient or violate patients' trust and human values and ethics during experimental trail. In modern health care and research, value conflicts arise where often there appears to be no clear consensus as to the right thing to do. These above cited conflicts makes many problems requiring moral decisions, and necessitate a choice between two or more alternatives, e.g., Should a parent have a right to refuse immunization for his or her child. Does we assess the public safety supersede an individual rights and another example, COVID 19 outbreak vaccination trail solely depends on human values and ethics, researcher should focus the health-care needs and maintain the dignity of individual patients, the patient does not right to refuse the testing of COVID19 because the requisite intervention comes under ethical perspective of the patients on public domain and safety of the human community at globe.

The researcher should be concerned about the following points:

First do no harms to the patient of COVID 19 from the excising treatment and social mobility.

Maintain overall sanctity of life at all time.

Be aware of the doctrine of double effect, where treatment or testing intended for good unintentionally causes any harm.

12.3.4 Justice and Confidentiality

The researcher should maintain the privacy of patient information, research plan, and the outcome of the research, equitable distribution of research risks and benefits. The justice is a complex ethical principle, with meaning that range from the fair treatment of individuals to the equitable allocation of health-care amounts and resources. It is concerned with equitable distribution of benefits to individuals in social institutions, and how the rights of various individuals are realized. Allocating scarce medical resources and also researcher or clinician should be able to justify the actions in every medical situation or follow-up visits of the patient. The general rights of ethics are presented in (Fig. 12.2).

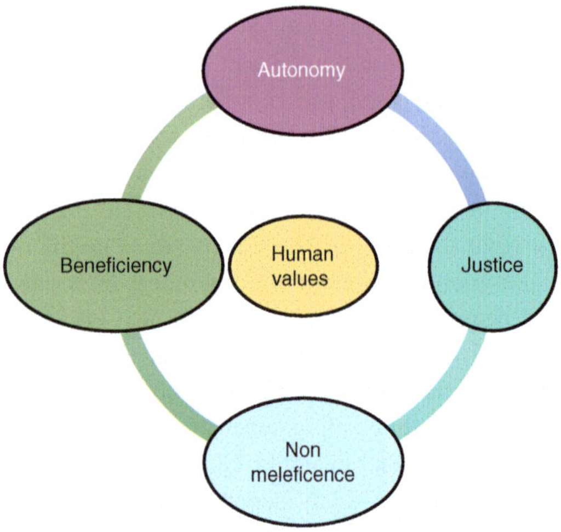

Fig. 12.2 Basic principles of ethics

Some of the following ethical questions would be aroused from the public interest, the followings questions and intervention are kept in mind, and refer necessary guidelines for further follow-up actions, the decision can be taken place at right time with the consent of judicial law (Fig. 12.3).

1. Should children with serious birth defects be kept alive?
2. Should be allowed an abortion for any reason?
3. Should terrorist be tortured to gain information possible saving hundreds of lives?
   (a) Should health-care workers be necessary to HCQ PEP drug for protection of COVID19
   (b) Organ transplantation and stem cell therapy for COVID19?

As per the practical insight, we describe the research ethics in a clinical prospective. The researcher should intervene to address the following key points before induction of research:

1. To understand and anticipate the current health literacy landscape as it pertains to clinical research on broad perspective,

Fig. 12.3 Flow diagram of human values and ethics in clinical research

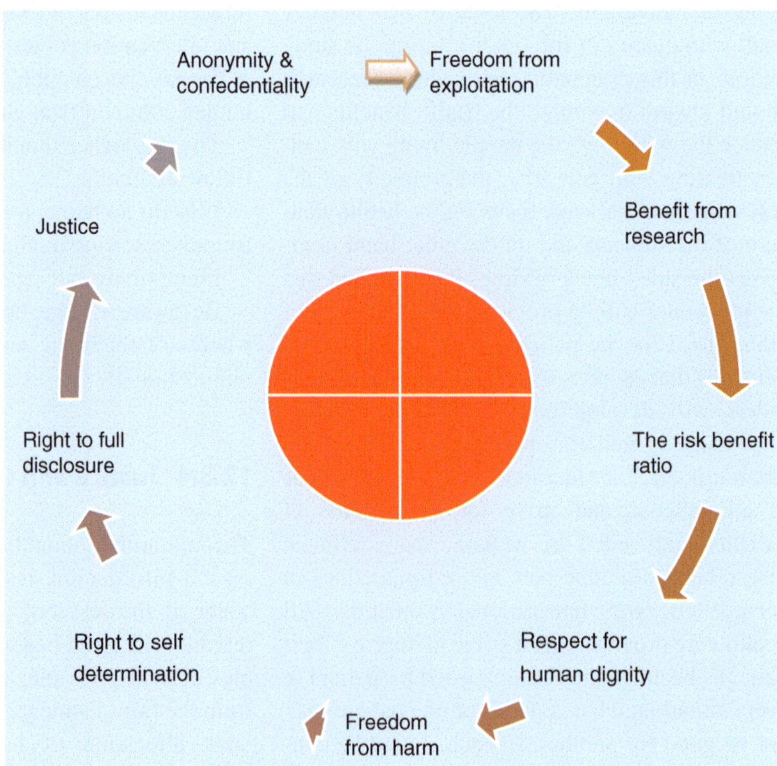

2. To attempt to address the barrier for adoption of available resources and health literacy of the participants in the context of ethical perspective and strengthened the clinical research-related communications,
3. To mitigate the opportunities for sponsors and funders, investigators, and their study teams, and institutional review board can integrate health literacy throughout the clinical trial life cycle from recruitment, and informed consent should be obtained from the participants,
4. To establish electronic virtual-based data collections from the different study sites that are relevant to multiple stakeholder communities, including research intervention or subjects.

The clinical and scientific standards for carrying out biomedical research on human subjects have been developed and established in International guidelines, including the following:

1. Declaration of Helsinki,
2. CIOMS: International ethical guidelines for Biomedical research involving human subjects, and
3. WHO and ICH guidelines for good clinical practices.

12.4 Historical Milestone of Medical Ethics

1932–1972: Tuskegee experiment on syphilis (Hippocrates 1780)

1939–1945: Nazi Nuremberg experiment

1944–1974: Human radiation experiment by USA

1946: Nuremberg trail of doctors responsible for the Nazi experiment

1947: Nuremberg code outlining ethical principles required for research

1948: US adoption of universal declaration of human rights

1953: NISH policy, the first UD federal policy introducing independent review to examine research, forerunners of IRBS

1963–1966: Willow brook study, involving hepatitis research on mentally retarded children, raising issues access to care, consent, and coercion

1964: Declaration of Helsinki International agreement recommendation for the ethical

1972: Public exposure of Tuskegee syphilis study

1974: First federal protection for human research participants

1979: Belmont Report promoting three principles for research

1980: Food and Drug Administration Regulation (CRF 21(50))

1982: Council for International Organization of Medical Sciences (CIOMS) publication of the international ethical guidelines for biomedical research involving human subjects

1985: US Public Health Service Task Force on Women's Health Issues export encouraging inclusion of women in research

1990: Society for women's health research

1993: Public exposure of US human radiation experiments

1993: NIH revitalization act mandating inclusions of women and minorities in research

1993: NIH office of research on women's health

1997: Food and drug modernization act (FDAMA) requiring NIH and pharmaceutical industry to develop guidance on the inclusion of women and minorities in trails

1998: Pediatric rule passed by congress, stipulating that new drugs for children must include specific pediatric labeling information

2000: Further publicized ethical abuses promoting establishment of the office of human research protection

2000: National commission for the research protection of human subjects of biomedical and behavioral research (Fig. 12.4)

12.5 National Guidelines

ICMR: Ethical guidelines for biomedical research on human participants

Indian GCP guidelines

Principles of precaution and risk minimization states that due care and caution must be taken at all stages of research to ensure that the research participants and those affected by it including community are put to minimum risk, suffer from no known irreversible adverse effects (ICMR 2006).

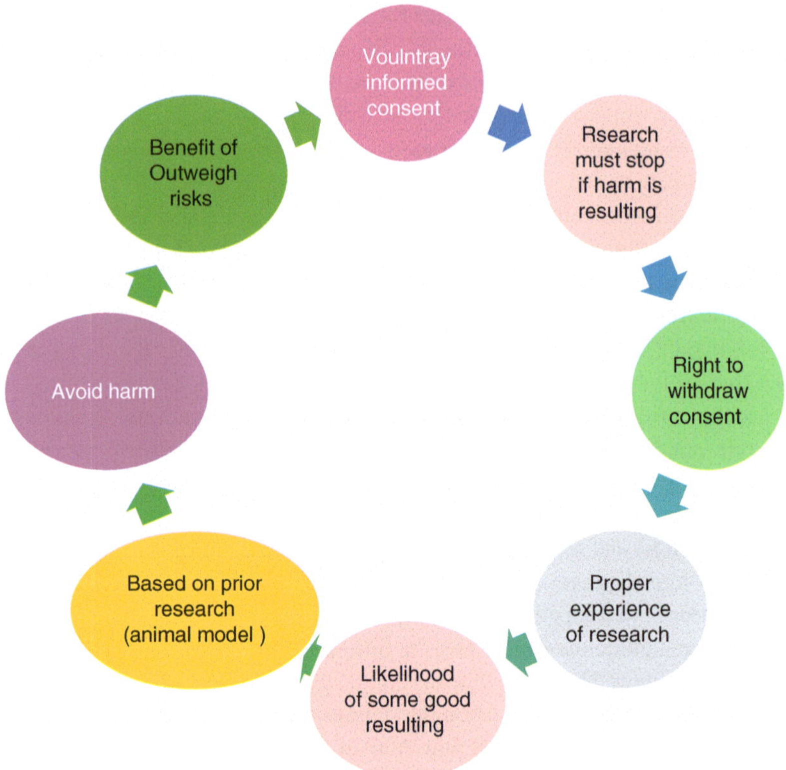

Fig. 12.4 Nuremberg Code description overview (1948)

12.6 Declaration of Helsinki

The World Medical Association has developed the declaration of Helsinki; word of honour -it is a statement of ethical principle to provide certain guidance to physicians and researchers in biomedical research involving human subjects. The oath of Helsinki has involved many perpetuates and assimilates regularity guidelines. The principle aims to maintain the dignity of the participants and work ethics of the researcher. The principle describes that the research is a duty of the physician in medical research to protect the life, health, privacy, and dignity of human subjects, involving ethics he must confirm to generally accepted scientific principles with appropriate caution, and the research should be exercised in the conduct of research which may not affect the environment. The design and performance on each experimental procedure involving human subjects should be clearly formulated in the experimental protocol. All research protocols should always contain a brief statement of ethical considerations and should indicate compliance of drug safety and efficacy in the interest of well-being of participants; the rules are always laid down by the institution pledge in association with FDA and national standards (Humphreys et al. 2014; Harish et al. 2012; Jonsen et al. 2010; Kim et al. 2001). The concerned institution should establish the independent committee and confirm with laws and regulations of the country in which the research experiments are performed, committee's right to monitor ongoing research subject to upheld scientific standards and human ethics. Subjects must be volunteers and informed consent is obtained from the participants. Every precaution should be taken at the right time and respect the privacy of subjects, confidentiality of the participants or subjects.

As per the FDA and national guidelines, the following ethical review board functionally performed the duty to maintain international and national standards of biomedical research.

IRB: Institutional Review Board
ERB: Ethics Review Board
REB: Research Ethics Board

12.6.1 Declaration of Medical Researcher, Professional Doctors

At the time of registration, each applicant shall be given a copy of the following declaration by the registrar concern and applicant can read and agree to abide by the same.

I solemnly pledge myself to consecrate my life service of humanity.

Even under threat, I will not use my medical knowledge contrary to the laws of humanity.

I will maintain utmost respect for human life from the time of conception.

I will not permit consideration of religion, nationality, race, party politics, or social standing to intervene between my duty and my patient.

I will practice my profession with conscience and dignity.

The health of my patient will be my first consideration.

I will respect the secretes which are confirmed in me.

I will give to my teachers the respect and gratitude which are their due.

I will maintain my all means in my power, the honor and noble tradition of medical profession.

I will treat my colleagues with all respect and dignity.

I shall abide by the code of medical ethics as enunciated in the Indian Medical Council.

I will make these promises solemnly, freely, and upon my honor.

12.7 IEC Institutional Ethical Committee

It is an independent body constituted for IEC, appointed medical, nonmedical, and nonscientific members whose responsibility is to ensure the protection of rights, safety, and well-being of human subjects involved in the trails by, among other things, reviewing, approving, and providing continuum development of trail protocol and amendment issues on the basis of international standards. The structure of IEC constituted 8–12 members, specifically, the chairperson should be preferably outside the institution to maintain the independency of the committee. The member secretary should be appointed by the concerned institution, and he conducts the business of committee regularly (Fig. 12.5).

12.7.1 Function of IEC

1. To provide competent review of all ethical aspects of the research project
2. Undertaken review free from any bias and influence
3. Provide advice to the researcher on all aspects of welfare and safety of research intervention
4. To protect dignity rights and well-being of the potential research participants
5. To ensure universal ethical values and international scientific standards in terms of social community values and customs

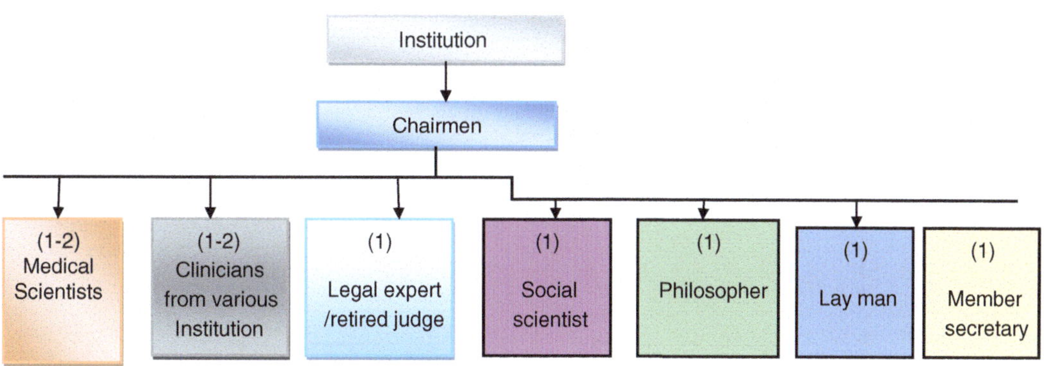

Fig. 12.5 Hierachical organogram of IEC

6. To assist in the development and the education of research community responsive to local health-care requirement

12.7.2 Document Submission

1. Trail protocol (prescribed format)
2. Patient information sheet and informed consent form
3. Investigator brochure
4. Principle investigator CV
5. Insurance policy/compensation for participants
6. Investigators agreement with the sponsors (Fig. 12.6)

12.8 Institutional Review Board (IRB)

An institutional review board is a review committee that was established on international standards which helps to protect the rights and welfare of human research projects. The IRB review is the approval of research involving human subjects funded or regulated by the federal government or sponsors. Most of the research institution, professional organizations, and scholarly journals should apply the same requirements for conducting human intervention research. Although, the federal regulations used cited reference of IRBs for intervention of biomedical research, the institution may have chosen a different name for this committee for approval of various research projects. IRB constitute at least five members irrespective of gender that come from varied professions. At least one member whose primary concerns are in nonscientific areas and also one member who is not otherwise affiliated with the institution (Muirhead et al. 2012; McCormick 2008; Siegler et al. 1990). The reviewer should have toll experience and exposure in all of the areas of research being reviewed. At its discretion, an IRB may invite individual with competence in special areas to assist in the review of issues which require expertise beyond or in addition to that available on the IRB diver-

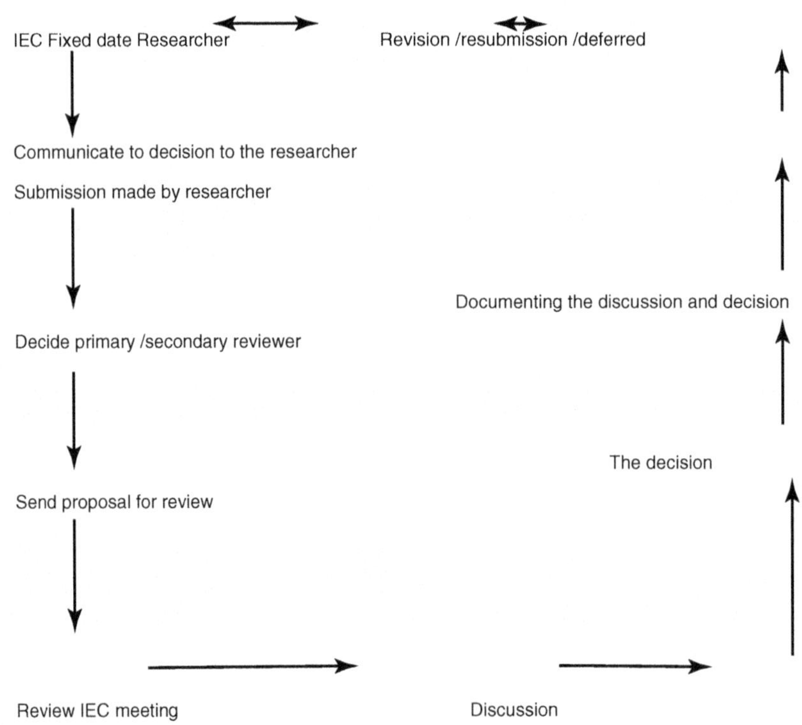

Fig. 12.6 Flow of document for review

sity of background. An eagerly noted Sensitivity of community attitude, knowledge of institutional commitments, and reputations refrain from maintaining the highest standards which are applicable to human laws and standards of professional conduct and ethics in many-fold diversity of the legal aspects. The knowledge and experience with vulnerable population are necessary for review committee (Rawls 1999; Singh et al. 2013; Satyanarayana Rao 2008; Simon et al. 2000). If an IRB can review research projects that would involve vulnerable subjects, the IRB must consider the inclusion of an individual who has knowledge of human ethics and also got experience with these vulnerable subjects. The regulation may also require a voting right of IRB member who has relevant expertise. IRB may call experts to help with problematic reviews, but those persons may not vote on the disposition of the application. If an IRB member has conflict of interest, that member cannot be present for the review of that research project except to provide the IRB with information as requested and may not vote on that particular research study or intervention. Researchers should protect IRB guidlines and enable the rights and welfare of human subjects who participate in research, and understands and anticipates with ethical standards, regulatory requirement, and governing research activities with human subjects; IRB should intervene to address the issues and guide the institution properly, and inform research staff of the regulations governing research and the Institutional research policies. Ensure that all research activities have IRB approval and required by the institution before human subjects are involved. Implement the research activity as it was approved by the IRB. Obtain the informed consent of subjects before the subjects is involved in the research and document consent as approved by the IRB. Researcher should maintain written records of ethical clearence signed documents concerning about study population, methadology and objective of the research, and document consent as approved by the IRB and also comply with the IRB requirements, and every concerned institution shall be timely reporting of unanticipated problems involving risks to the human subjects or others including adverse events; the safety reports would be received from the sponsors or data safety and monitoring summary reports from the IRB to institution. So, we have to obtain the continuum development linkage to the IRB on scheduled data. The institution should make a provision for the secured retention of complete research records and all research materials so as to ensure that the confidentiality and security of all informations will be obtained from and about human subjects. The institution should verify the IRB approval, will be obtained from all participating institutions in collaborative activities with other institutions. For the information sake, the institution should notify the IRB guidelines in the public notice board for reviewing the guidelines and make use of IRB regularity for submission of new proposal and human intervention subjects in accordance with speculated regularities or guidelines.

12.9 Informed Consent

Definition—A process by which a subject voluntarily confirms his or her willingness to participate in a particular clinical trial, after having been informed of all aspects of trails, trail that are relevant to the subject's decisions to participate. It is the responsibility of an investigator to obtain from the prospective respondents, which can explain individual autonomy, ethics, and novelty of the research project and also inform consent must be readable and all research information are presented in local language. The objective, methodology, and outcome of the research should convey the patients or volunteers. The consent form should include title of the research project and main conditions that the participants are being asked to agree to it. Importantly they will need to agree to the completed consent form being checked by designated experts as part of ethical approval auditing process. During the study intervention, the researcher should take undertaking from the participants regarding confidentiality, publication process and report submission (Fig. 12.7).

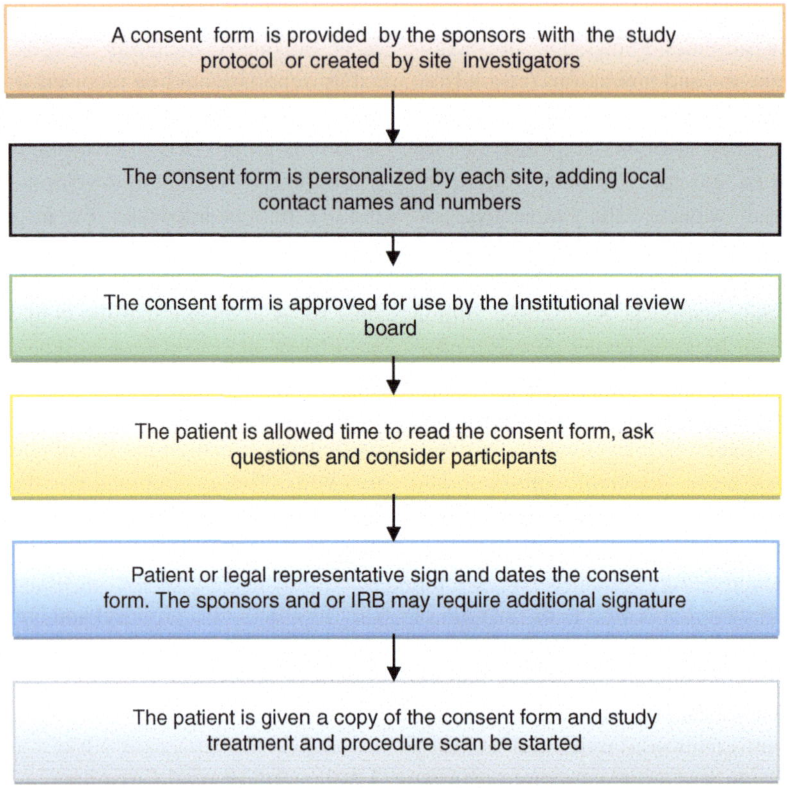

Fig. 12.7 Informed consent details

12.10 The Principles of Voluntariness, Informed Consent, and Community Agreement

The research participant should be aware of the nature of research and the probable consequences of the experiments or drug trail and then should make independent choice without the influence of the treating doctor, whether to take part in the research or not. When the research treats any community or group of persons as research participants, these principles of voluntariness and informed consent should apply to the community as a whole and also to each individual member who is the participant of the research or experiment. However, the principles of nonexploitation research participants should be remunerated for their involvement in the research or experiment. The participants should be made aware of all the risks involved irrespective of their social and economical conditions or educational levels attained. Each research protocol should include provisions of compensation for the human participants either through insurance cover or any other appropriate means to cover all foreseeable and hidden risks. Another intervention privacy and confidentiality, all data sets acquired for research purpose should be kept confidential to prevent disclosure of the identity of the involved participant and should not be disclosed without valid legal and/or scientific reasons. The principle investigator or researcher should conduct clinical experiments in fair, honest, impartial, and transparent manner after full disclosure of his or her interest in research (Simon et al. 2000; Thatte 2007). They should also retain the research data sets, subjects to the principle of privacy and confidentiality for minimum period of 5 years to be scrutinized by the appropriate legal and administrative authority, if necessary. Further, the principles of the maximization of the public interest and of distributive justice, the results of the research should be used for the benefit of all humans, especially the research participants themselves and/or the community from they are drawn and not only to those who are socially better off. Institutional agreement is required that all institutional agreements required to be made in respect of the research and its subsequent use or applications should be duly made in a transparent manner. Since the public domain is very important, we cannot deviate from our moral ethics, all the resulted part work done by the researcher should be made public through publications or other means. Even before publications, the detailed information of clinical trials should be made public before the start of recruitment via clinical trial registry system that allows them to access free online information. Principle of totality of responsibility explains that all those directly or indirectly connected with the research should take professional and moral responsibilities, for the due observance of all the principles, guidelines, or prescriptions laid down in respect of the research. Informed consent clearly explains the statement about the problems, benefits and economic feasibility of study participants, and also the explanation of purpose of research and the expected duration of the subject's participation, inclusion with description of the procedure to be followed and identification of any procedures which are experimental, any reasonable foreseeable risks or discomforts to the subjects (World Medical Association 2008; Yamey and Roach 2001), a description of any benefits to the subjects or to others which may reasonably be expected from the research, trail treatment schedule and the probability for random assignment to each treatment, and a disclosure of appropriate alternative procedures or courses of treatment.

12.11 Discussion

In recent times, medical ethics has been greatly influenced by the development in human rights. Physicians frequently have dealt with various medical problems, e.g., organ transplantation, stem cell therapy, evidence-based medicine, clinical trial, drug adherence study of life-threatened, and lifelong diseases. However, these human ethical interventions are closely related to law, often to ethics is higher standards of behavior then does the law, and occasionally either require that physician or researcher disobey laws that demand unethical perspective and also violation of human rights. The basic ethical principles like A: Autonomy, B: Beneficence, J: Justice, and N: Nonbeneficence are closely associated with the dignity of human and respect for the patient or participants. An informed consent and confidentiality are basic to the physician–patient relationship and create positive atmosphere in the study site or threat area. However, the application of these principles in specific situation is problematic due to lack of cooperation from the patient care takers, lack of literacy and interest for participation in clinical and medical research. Since physicians, patients, their family members, and other healthcare professionals may disagree about what is the right way to act in a situation intervention of drug trail experiment, health care professionals were obtain undertaken from the participants and create a positive outcome of the trail, while trail also potentially persuing the data collection without harm participants on the basis of ethical perspectives. Trail would be deviated from the normal ethics, such kind of trail is known as the double effect, e.g., the morphine in the dying patient eases pain and suffering while hastening the demise through suppression of the respiratory drive. During the study period well-being of human subject should take precedence over the interest of science and society, patient consent should be obtained in writing, physician use caution if participant in dependent relationship with the researcher, limit use of placebo and also facilities should be extended to the health benefits and to minimize the risk factors. So many drawbacks on medical ethics, for example, guidelines may be difficult to apply in new cases for several reasons, need to be interrupted in the context of case-to-case variation inherent, different priorities, and goals for care, distinguishing cases in ethically meaningful ways and also shortcoming of the existing guidelines.

12.12 Conclusion

The practice of medicine and conducting clinical research would be much easier if there were a fixed hierarchy of ethical guidelines. Since the ability to make prudent solution and decision could be taken in some specific situations, involving an understanding of how ethical guidelines are relevant for the benefits of patients and their well-being (a variety of situations and to the particular case at hand).

12.13 Future Line of Work

The discipline of science is to have an objective to spread the knowledge to the world; the objective of the research has been derived from many unfolded postulates that have been enriched with evidence, and the discovery of new horizon enhanced our world with useful technology. Since throughout the research process, analytics and modeling techniques are used to subject the sample size determination, screening of patients, development of algorithms, optimization of massive medical research data sets, and various methodological insight; the research is the incremental process between the research hypothesis and the ecosystem of advanced method of statistical intervention. However, many researchers focus to demonstrate real information in thought of mathematical and statistical form to fill the research gap on a full-blown basis. As such being the case, the researcher could not apply the perfect statistical analysis during compilation and final stage of research due to lack of statistical knowledge. In spite of this problem, the present book embedded various advanced statistical methods for the benefit of well-being of the researcher. In addition to that, the cited model helps to guide the researcher, and it should be concealed to obtain critical suggestions and statistical inputs from the professional statistician before induction of research. Thereby all the research interventions are associated with error components, hence the researcher should focus on the error component rather than nurturing the suitable appropriate statistical method for reduction of errors during analysis of data sets. On a broader sense, the analysis part will always be subject to the probable errors and negative predicted values. Although those same flawed humans who conduct and care about science ever refine the scientific processes to reduce errors and increase rigor. Much good has been done on this, and much good remains to be done ahead. The researchers' lines of investigations and induction of research in any discipline of science because of innate interest, a deep curiosity, a desire for new findings, discovery, or a personal connection to the problem in the interest of frontier of advanced research. At this point, we conduct experiments, analyzing datum, and observing the research ecosystem and not just the aspects of science, and also represent personal interest and passions. Thus, when resulted findings provide something interesting whether simply intellectually stimulating or of profound practical importance, passion and excitement risk overriding the inherent fact. However, science has always designed new technology and discovery based on the mathematical and statistical derivation and also furnishes the antidotal information to the researcher to obtain research inputs from subject experts. As per the intellectual prosperity, the new technology and analytical standards will be necessary to increase our ability to detect some error components or research behaviors. In this aspect, new software and advanced statistical modeling techniques would be necessary for detecting the sample and population errors during interim analysis of clinical and medical research data sets. The present driven modeling technology cited in this book will support the researcher for development of new algorithms to identify and reduce the errors before submission of manuscript or final report of research projects. Cost–benefit analysis on the production of drug/vaccine and conducting the trials in the population and environmental conditions are important aspects to be considered for future research.

References

Agich GJ (2001) The question of method in ethics consultation. Am J Bioeth 1(4):31–41

Beauchamp T, Childress J (2013) Principles of biomedical ethics, 7th edn. Oxford University Press, New York

Benatar SR (1998) Imperialism, research ethics and global health. J Med Ethics 24:221–222

Carpenter WT Jr, Gold JM, Lahti AC, Queern CA, Conley RR, Bartko JJ et al (2000) Decisional capacity for informed consent in schizophrenia research. Arch Gen Psychiatry 57:533–538

David C (1994) Thomasma hermeneutics. Theor Med Bioeth 15(2):25–26

Frankena WK (1973) Ethics, 2nd edn. Prentice-Hall, Englewood Cliffs

Gasparetto A, Jox RJ, Picozzi M (2018) The notion of neutrality in clinical ethics consultation. Philos Ethics Humanit Med 13:3

Grisso T, Appelbaum PS (1995) The MacArthur Treatment Competence Study, III: abilities of patients to consent to psychiatric and medical treatment. Law Hum Behav 19:149–174

Harish D, Kumar A, Singh A (2012) Duties and responsibilities of the medical practitioner, revisited. J Punjab Acad Forensic Med Toxicol 12:115–120

Hippocrates (1780) The history of epidemics. Samuel Farr (trans.). T. Cadell, London

Humphreys RA, Lepper R, Nicholson TR (2014) When and how to treat patients who refuse treatment. BMJ 348:2043

Indian Council of Medical Research (2006) Ethical guidelines for biomedical research on human subjects. New Delhi

Jameton A (2013) A reflection on moral distress in nursing together with a current application of the concept. J Bioeth Inq 10(3):297–308

Jonsen A, Siegler M, Winslade W (2010) Ethics, 7th edn. McGraw-Hill Medical, New York

Kim SY, Caine ED, Currier GW, Leibovici A, Ryan JM (2001) Assessing the competence of persons with Alzheimer's disease in providing informed consent for participation in research. Am J Psychiatry 158:712–717

McCormick TR (2008) Ethical issues inherent to Jehovah's witnesses. J Perioper Nurs Clin 3(3):253–259

Muirhead W et al (2012) When four principles are too many: bloodgate, integrity and an action-guiding model of ethical decision making in clinical practice. J Med Ethics 38(4):195–196

Rawls J (1999) A theory of justice. Harvard University Press, Cambridge

Satyanarayana Rao KH (2008) Informed consent; An ethical obligation or legal compulsion. J Cutan Aesthet Surg 1:33–35

Siegler M, Pellegrino ED, Singer PA (1990) Clinical medical ethics. J Clin Ethics 1(1):5

Simon GE, Unutzer J, Young BE, Pincus HA (2000) Large medical databases, population-based research, and patient confidentiality. Am J Psychiatry 157:1731–1737

Singer P, Pellegrino E, Siegler M (2001) Clinical ethics revisited. BMC Med Ethics 2(1):1–8

Singh MM, Garg US, Arora P (2013) Laws applicable to medical practice and hospitals in India. Int J Res Found Hosp Healthc Adm 1:19–24

Tarzian A (2013) Health care ethics consultation: an update on core competencies and emerging standards from the American society for bioethics and humanities' core competencies update task force. Am J Bioeth 13(2):3–13

Thatte U (2007) Basic principles of clinical research and methodology. Ethical issues in Clinical Research, 1st edn. Jaypee Brothers, New Delhi, pp 58–73

White BD, Shelton WN, Rivais CJ (2001) Were the "pioneer" clinical ethics consultants "outsiders"? For them, was "critical distance" that critical? J Am Bioeth 18(6):34–44

World Medical Association (2008) Declaration of Helsinki-ethical principles for medical research involving human subjects. Available from URL: http://www.wma.net/en/30publications/10policies/b3/index.html. Accessed 13 Apr 2010

Yamey G, Roach J (2001) Witnessing unethical conduct: the effects. West J Med 174:355–356

Annexure I: Statistical Tables

Table A Area under standard normal distribution (SND)

z	0	0.01	0.02	0.03	0.04	0.05	0.06	0.07	0.08	0.09
0.0	0.0000	0.0040	0.0080	0.0120	0.0160	0.0199	0.0239	0.0279	0.0319	0.0359
0.1	0.0398	0.0438	0.0478	0.0517	0.0557	0.0596	0.0636	0.0675	0.0714	0.0753
0.2	0.0793	0.8832	0.0871	0.0910	0.0948	0.0987	0.1026	0.1064	0.1103	0.1141
0.3	0.1179	0.1217	0.1255	0.1230	0.1331	0.1368	0.1406	0.4430	0.1480	0.1517
0.4	0.1154	0.1591	0.1628	0.1664	0.1700	0.1736	0.1772	0.1808	0.1844	0.1879
0.5	0.1915	0.1950	0.1985	0.2019	0.2054	0.2088	0.2123	0.2157	0.2190	0.2240
0.6	0.2257	0.2291	0.2324	0.2357	0.2389	0.2422	0.2454	0.2486	0.2517	0.2549
0.7	0.2580	0.2611	0.2642	0.2676	0.2703	0.2734	0.2764	0.2794	0.2823	0.2852
0.8	0.2881	0.2910	0.2939	0.2967	0.2995	0.3023	0.3051	0.3078	0.3106	0.3133
0.9	0.3159	0.3186	0.3212	0.3238	0.3264	0.3289	0.3315	0.3340	0.3365	0.3389
1.0	0.3413	0.3438	0.3461	0.3485	0.3508	0.3531	0.3554	0.3577	0.3599	0.3621
1.1	0.3643	0.3665	0.3686	0.3708	0.3729	0.3749	0.3770	0.3790	0.3810	0.3830
1.2	0.3849	0.3869	0.3888	0.3907	0.3925	0.3944	0.3962	0.3980	0.3997	0.4012
1.3	0.4032	0.4049	0.4066	0.4082	0.4099	0.4115	0.4131	0.4147	0.4162	0.4177
1.4	0.4192	0.4207	0.4222	0.4236	0.4251	0.4265	0.4279	0.4292	0.4306	0.4319
1.5	0.4332	0.4645	0.4357	0.4370	0.4382	0.4394	0.4406	0.4418	0.4429	0.4441
1.6	0.4452	0.4463	0.4474	0.4484	0.4495	0.4505	0.4415	0.4525	0.4535	0.4545
1.7	0.4554	0.4564	0.4573	0.4582	0.4591	0.4599	0.4608	0.4616	0.4625	0.4633
1.8	0.4641	0.4649	0.4656	0.4664	0.4670	0.4678	0.4686	0.4693	0.4699	0.4706
1.9	0.4713	0.4719	0.4726	0.4732	0.4738	0.4744	0.4750	0.4756	0.4761	0.4767
2.0	0.4772	0.4778	0.4783	0.4788	0.4793	0.4798	0.4803	0.4808	0.4812	0.4817
2.1	0.4821	0.4826	0.4830	0.4834	0.4838	0.4842	0.4846	0.4850	0.4854	0.4857
2.2	0.4861	0.4864	0.4868	0.4871	0.4875	0.4878	0.4841	0.4884	0.4887	0.4890
2.3	0.4893	0.4896	0.4898	0.4901	0.4904	0.4906	0.4909	0.4911	0.4913	0.4916
2.4	0.4918	0.4920	0.4922	0.4925	0.4927	0.4929	0.4931	0.4932	0.4934	0.4936
2.5	0.4938	0.4940	0.4941	0.4943	0.4945	0.4946	0.4948	0.4949	0.4951	0.4952
2.6	0.4953	0.4955	0.4956	0.4957	0.4959	0.4960	0.4961	0.4962	0.4963	0.4964
2.7	0.4965	0.4966	0.4967	0.4968	0.4969	0.4970	0.4971	0.4972	0.4973	0.4974
2.8	0.4974	0.4975	0.4976	0.4977	0.4977	0.4978	0.4979	0.4979	0.4980	0.4981
2.9	0.8941	0.4981	0.4982	0.4982	0.4984	0.4984	0.4985	0.4985	0.4986	0.4986
3.0	0.4987	0.4987	0.4987	0.4988	0.4988	0.4989	0.4989	0.4989	0.4990	0.4990

B. D. M., B. Narasimha Murthy, *Design of Experiments and Advanced Statistical Techniques in Clinical Research*, https://doi.org/10.1007/978-981-15-8210-3

Table B Student *t*-distribution

	Significance level "α"					
df	0.20	0.10	0.05	0.02	0.01	0.01
1	3.07	6.31	12.76	31.82	63.65	366.61
2	1.88	2.92	4.30	6.96	9.92	31.58
3	1.63	2.35	3.18	4.54	5.84	12.92
4	1.53	2.13	2.77	3.74	4.60	8.61
5	1.47	2.05	2.57	3.36	4.03	6.86
6	1.44	1.94	2.44	3.14	3.70	5.95
7	1.41	1.89	2.36	2.99	3.49	5.40
8	1.39	1.86	2.30	2.89	3.35	5.04
9	1.38	1.83	2.62	2.82	3.25	4.78
10	1.37	1.81	2.22	2.76	3.16	4.58
11	1.36	1.81	2.20	2.71	3.10	4.43
12	1.35	1.79	2.17	2.68	3.05	4.31
13	1.35	1.78	2.16	2.65	3.01	4.22
14	1.34	1.77	2.14	2.62	2.97	4.14
15	1.34	1.76	213	2.60	2.94	4.07
16	1.33	1.75	2.12	2.58	2.92	4.01
17	1.33	1.74	2.11	2.56	2.89	3.96
18	1.33	1.74	2.10	2.55	2.87	3.92
19	1.32	1.73	2.09	2.53	2.86	3.88
20	1.32	1.72	208	2.52	2.84	3.85
21	1.32	1.71	2.08	2.51	2.83	3.81
22	1.32	1.71	2.07	2.50	2.81	3.79
23	1.31	1.71	2.06	2.50	2.80	3.76
24	1.31	170	2.06	2.49	2.79	3.74
25	13.1	1.70	2.06	2.48	2.78	3.72
26	1.31	1.70	2.05	.49	2.77	3.70
27	1.31	1.70	2.05	2.47	2.77	3.69
28	1.31	1.69	2.048	2.46	2.76	3.67
29	1.31	1.69	2.045	2.46	2.75	3.65
30	1.31	1.68	2.042	2.45	2.75	3.64
40	1.30	1.67	2.02	2.42	2.70	3.55
60	1.29	1.65	2.00	2.39	2.66	3.46
120	1.28	1.64	1.98	2.35	2.61	3.37
∞	1.28	1.64	1.96	2.32	2.57	3.29

Appendix A: DMRT Protection Level

Q critical values for alpha = 0.05

$df \downarrow k \rightarrow$	2	3	4	5	6	7	8	9	10
5	3.64	4.60	5.22	5.67	6.03	6.33	6.58	6.80	6.99
6	3.46	4.34	4.90	5.30	5.63	5.90	6.12	6.32	6.49
7	3.34	4.16	4.68	5.06	5.36	5.61	5.82	6.00	6.16
8	3.26	4.04	4.53	4.89	5.17	5.40	5.60	5.77	5.92
9	3.20	3.95	4.41	4.76	5.02	5.24	5.43	5.59	5.74
10	3.15	3.88	4.33	4.65	4.91	5.12	5.30	5.46	5.60
11	3.11	3.82	4.26	4.57	4.82	5.03	5.20	5.35	5.49
12	3.08	3.77	4.20	4.51	4.75	4.95	5.12	5.27	5.39
13	3.06	3.73	4.15	4.45	4.69	4.88	5.05	5.19	5.32
14	3.03	3.70	4.11	4.41	4.64	4.83	4.99	5.13	5.25
15	3.01	3.67	4.08	4.37	4.59	4.78	4.94	5.08	5.20
16	3.00	3.65	4.05	4.33	4.56	4.74	4.90	5.03	5.15
17	2.98	3.63	4.02	4.30	4.52	4.70	4.86	4.99	5.11
18	2.97	3.61	4.00	4.28	4.49	4.67	4.82	4.96	5.07
19	2.96	3.59	3.98	4.25	4.47	4.65	4.79	4.92	5.04
20	2.95	3.58	3.96	4.23	4.45	4.62	4.77	4.90	5.01
24	2.92	3.53	3.90	4.17	4.37	4.54	4.68	4.81	4.92
30	2.89	3.49	3.85	4.10	4.30	4.46	4.60	4.72	4.82
40	2.86	3.44	3.79	4.04	4.23	4.39	4.52	4.63	4.73
60	2.83	3.40	3.74	3.98	4.16	4.31	4.44	4.55	4.65
120	2.80	3.36	3.68	3.92	4.10	4.24	4.36	4.47	4.56
Infinity	2.77	3.31	3.63	3.86	4.03	4.17	4.29	4.39	4.47

df are for the Error Term
k = Number of Treatments

B. D. M., B. Narasimha Murthy, *Design of Experiments and Advanced Statistical Techniques in Clinical Research*, https://doi.org/10.1007/978-981-15-8210-3

Q critical values for alpha = 0.01

$df \downarrow k \rightarrow$	2	3	4	5	6	7	8	9	10
5	5.70	6.98	7.80	8.42	8.91	9.32	9.67	9.97	10.24
6	5.24	6.33	7.03	7.56	7.97	8.32	8.61	8.87	9.10
7	4.95	5.92	6.54	7.01	7.37	7.68	7.94	8.17	8.37
8	4.75	5.64	6.20	6.62	6.96	7.24	7.47	7.68	7.86
9	4.60	5.43	5.96	6.35	6.66	6.91	7.13	7.33	7.49
10	4.48	5.27	5.77	6.14	6.43	6.67	6.87	7.05	7.21
11	4.39	5.15	5.62	5.97	6.25	6.48	6.67	6.84	6.99
12	4.32	5.05	5.50	5.84	6.10	6.32	6.51	6.67	6.81
13	4.26	4.96	5.40	5.73	5.98	6.19	6.37	6.53	6.67
14	4.21	4.89	5.32	5.63	5.88	6.08	6.26	6.41	6.54
15	4.17	4.84	5.25	5.56	5.80	5.99	6.16	6.31	6.44
16	4.13	4.79	5.19	5.49	5.72	5.92	6.08	6.22	6.35
17	4.10	4.74	5.14	5.43	5.66	5.85	6.01	6.15	6.27
18	4.07	4.70	5.09	5.38	5.60	5.79	5.94	6.08	6.20
19	4.05	4.67	5.05	5.33	5.55	5.73	5.89	6.02	6.14
20	4.02	4.64	5.02	5.29	5.51	5.69	5.84	5.97	6.09
24	3.96	4.55	4.91	5.17	5.37	5.54	5.69	5.81	5.92
30	3.89	4.45	4.80	5.05	5.24	5.40	5.54	5.65	5.76
40	3.82	4.37	4.70	4.93	5.11	5.26	5.39	5.50	5.60
60	3.76	4.28	4.59	4.82	4.99	5.13	5.25	5.36	5.45
120	3.70	4.20	4.50	4.71	4.87	5.01	5.12	5.21	5.30
Infinity	3.64	4.12	4.40	4.60	4.76	4.88	4.99	5.08	5.16

df are for the Error Term
k = Number of Treatments

Annexure II: Areas Under the Normal Curve (1 – Tail)

Normal deviate	Area	Normal deviate	Area
0.0	0.50000	2.0	0.02275
0.1	0.46017	2.1	0.01786
0.2	0.42074	2.2	0.01390
0.3	0.38209	2.3	0.01072
0.4	0.34458	2.4	0.00820
0.5	0.30854	2.5	0.00621
0.6	0.27425	2.6	0.00466
0.7	0.24196	2.7	0.00347
0.8	0.21186	2.8	0.00256
0.9	0.18406	2.9	0.00187
1.0	0.15866	3.0	0.00135
1.1	0.13567	3.1	0.00100
1.2	0.11507	3.2	0.00069
1.3	0.09680	3.3	0.00040
1.4	0.08076	3.4	0.00034
1.5	0.06681	3.5	0.00023
1.6	0.05480	3.6	0.00016
1.7	0.04457	3.7	0.00011
1.8	0.03593	3.8	0.00007
1.9	0.02872	3.9	0.00005
1.96	0.02500	4.0	0.00003

B. D. M., B. Narasimha Murthy, *Design of Experiments and Advanced Statistical Techniques in Clinical Research*, https://doi.org/10.1007/978-981-15-8210-3

Appendix B: Cumulative Distribution of Chi-Square

	Probability of a greater value			
Degrees of freedom	0.10	0.05	0.01	0.001
1	2.71	3.84	6.63	10.83
2	4.61	5.99	9.21	13.82
3	6.25	7.81	11.34	16.27
4	7.78	9.49	13.28	18.47
5	9.24	11.07	15.09	20.52
6	10.64	12.59	16.81	22.46
7	12.02	14.07	18.48	24.32
8	13.36	15.51	20.09	26.12
9	14.68	16.92	21.67	27.88
10	15.99	18.31	23.21	29.59
15	22.31	25.00	30.58	37.70
20	28.41	31.41	37.57	45.32
30	40.26	43.77	50.89	59.70

Table of *t*-values

	Probability (2 – tail)				
Degrees of freedom	0.2	0.1	0.05	0.01	0.001
1	3.078	6.314	12.706	63.657	535.619
2	1.886	2.920	4.303	9.925	31.598
3	1.638	2.353	3.182	5.841	12.924
4	1.533	2.132	2.776	4.604	8.610
5	1.476	2.015	2.571	4.032	6.869
6	1.440	1.943	2.447	3.707	5.959
7	1.415	1.895	2.365	3.499	5.408
8	1.397	1.860	2.306	3.355	5.401
9	1.383	1.833	2.262	3.250	4.781
10	1.372	1.812	2.228	3.169	4.587
11	1.363	1.796	2.201	3.106	4.437
12	1.356	1.782	2.179	3.055	4.318
13	1.350	1.771	2.160	3.012	4.221
14	1.345	1.761	2.145	2.977	4.140
15	1.341	1.753	2.131	2.947	4.073
16	1.337	1.746	2.120	2.921	4.015
17	1.333	1.740	2.110	2.898	3.965
18	1.330	1.734	2.101	2.878	3.922
19	1.328	1.729	2.093	2.861	3.883

B. D. M., B. Narasimha Murthy, *Design of Experiments and Advanced Statistical Techniques in Clinical Research*, https://doi.org/10.1007/978-981-15-8210-3

Degrees of freedom	Probability (2 – tail)				
	0.2	0.1	0.05	0.01	0.001
20	1.325	1.725	2.086	2.845	3.850
21	1.323	1.721	2.080	2.831	3.819
22	1.321	1.717	2.074	2.819	3.792
23	1.319	1.714	2.069	2.807	3.767
24	1.318	1.711	2.064	2.797	3.745
25	1.316	1.708	2.060	2.787	3.725
26	1.315	1.706	2.056	2.779	3.707
27	1.314	1.703	2.052	2.771	3.690
28	1.313	1.701	2.048	2.763	3.674
29	1.311	1.699	2.045	2.756	3.659
30	1.310	1.697	2.042	2.750	3.646
40	1.303	1.684	2.021	2.704	3.551
60	1.296	1.671	2.000	2.660	3.460
120	1.289	1.658	1.980	2.617	3.373
α	1.282	1.645	1.960	2.576	3.291

Appendix Table

5% Points of *F*

V1/V2	1	2	3	4	5	6	8	12	24	α
1	161.40	199.50	215.70	224.60	230.20	234.00	238.90	243.90	249.00	254.30
2	18.51	19.00	19.16	19.25	19.30	19.33	19.37	19.41	19.45	19.50
3	10.13	9.55	9.28	9.12	9.01	8.94	8.84	8.74	8.64	8.53
4	7.71	6.94	6.59	6.39	6.26	6.16	6.04	5.91	5.77	5.63
5	6.61	5.79	5.41	5.19	5.05	4.95	4.82	4.68	4.53	4.36
6	5.99	5.14	4.76	4.53	4.39	4.28	4.15	4.00	3.84	3.67
7	5.59	4.74	4.35	4.12	3.97	3.87	3.73	3.57	3.41	3.23
8	5.32	4.46	4.07	3.84	3.69	3.58	3.44	3.28	3.12	2.93
9	5.12	4.26	3.86	3.63	3.48	3.37	3.23	3.07	2.90	2.71
10	4.96	4.10	3.71	3.48	3.33	3.22	3.07	2.91	2.74	2.54
11	4.84	3.96	3.59	3.36	3.20	3.09	2.95	2.79	2.61	2.40
12	4.75	3.88	3.49	3.26	3.11	3.00	2.85	2.69	2.50	2.30
13	4.67	3.80	3.41	3.18	3.02	2.92	2.77	2.60	2.42	2.21
14	4.60	3.74	3.34	3.11	2.96	2.85	2.70	2.53	2.35	2.13
15	4.54	3.68	3.29	3.06	2.90	2.79	2.64	2.48	2.29	2.07
16	4.49	3.63	3.24	3.01	2.85	2.74	2.59	2.42	2.24	2.01
17	4.45	3.59	3.20	2.96	2.81	2.70	2.55	2.38	2.19	1.96
18	4.41	3.55	3.16	2.93	2.77	2.66	2.51	2.34	2.15	1.92
19	4.38	3.52	3.13	2.90	2.74	2.63	2.48	2.31	2.11	1.88
20	4.35	3.49	3.10	2.87	2.71	2.60	2.45	2.28	2.08	1.84
21	4.34	3.47	3.07	2.84	2.68	2.57	2.42	2.25	2.05	1.81
22	4.30	3.44	3.05	2.82	2.66	2.55	2.40	2.23	2.03	1.78
23	4.28	3.42	3.03	2.80	2.64	2.53	2.38	2.20	2.00	1.76
24	4.26	3.40	3.01	2.78	2.62	2.51	2.36	2.18	1.98	1.73
25	4.26	3.38	2.99	2.76	2.60	2.49	2.34	2.16	1.96	1.71
26	4.22	3.37	2.98	2.74	2.59	2.47	2.32	2.15	1.95	1.69
27	4.21	3.35	2.96	2.73	2.57	2.46	2.30	2.13	1.93	1.67
28	4.20	3.34	2.95	2.71	2.56	2.44	2.29	2.12	1.91	1.65
29	4.18	3.33	2.93	2.70	2.54	2.43	2.28	2.10	1.90	1.64
30	4.17	3.32	2.92	2.69	2.53	2.42	2.27	2.09	1.89	1.62
40	4.08	3.23	2.84	2.61	2.45	2.34	2.18	2.00	1.79	1.51
60	4.00	3.15	2.76	2.52	2.37	2.25	2.10	1.92	1.70	1.39
120	3.92	3.07	2.68	2.45	2.29	2.17	2.02	1.83	1.60	1.25
α	3.84	2.99	2.60	2.37	2.21	2.10	1.94	1.75	1.52	1.00

B. D. M., B. Narasimha Murthy, *Design of Experiments and Advanced Statistical Techniques in Clinical Research*, https://doi.org/10.1007/978-981-15-8210-3

1% Points of *F*

V1/V2	1	2	3	4	5	6	8	12	24	α
1	4052	4999	5403	5625	5764	5859	5982	6106	6234	6366
2	98.50	99.00	99.17	99.25	99.30	99.33	99.37	99.42	99.46	99.50
3	34.12	30.82	29.46	28.71	28.24	27.91	27.47	27.05	20.60	26.12
4	21.20	18.00	16.69	15.98	15.52	15.21	14.80	14.37	13.93	13.46
5	16.26	13.27	12.06	11.39	10.97	10.67	10.29	9.89	9.47	9.02
6	13.74	10.92	9.78	9.15	8.75	8.47	8.10	7.72	7.31	6.88
7	12.25	9.55	8.45	7.85	7.46	7.19	6.84	6.47	6.07	5.65
8	11.26	8.65	7.59	7.01	6.63	6.37	6.03	5.67	5.28	4.86
9	10.56	8.02	6.99	6.42	6.06	5.80	5.47	5.11	4.73	4.31
10	10.04	7.56	6.55	5.99	5.64	5.39	5.06	4.71	4.33	3.91
11	9.65	7.20	6.22	5.67	5.32	5.07	4.74	4.40	4.02	3.60
12	9.33	6.93	5.95	5.41	5.06	4.82	4.50	4.16	3.78	3.36
13	9.07	6.70	5.74	5.20	4.86	4.62	4.30	3.96	3.59	3.16
14	8.86	6.51	5.56	5.03	4.69	4.46	4.14	3.80	3.43	3.00
15	8.68	6.36	5.42	4.89	4.56	4.32	4.00	3.67	3.29	2.87
16	8.53	6.23	5.29	4.77	4.44	4.20	3.89	3.55	3.18	2.75
17	8.40	6.11	5.18	4.67	4.34	4.10	3.79	3.45	3.08	2.65
18	8.28	6.01	5.09	4.58	4.25	4.01	3.71	3.37	3.00	2.57
19	8.18	5.93	5.01	4.50	4.17	3.94	3.63	3.30	2.92	2.49
20	8.10	5.85	4.94	4.43	4.10	3.87	3.56	3.23	2.86	2.42
21	8.02	5.78	4.87	4.37	4.04	3.81	3.51	3.17	2.80	2.36
22	7.94	5.72	4.82	4.30	3.99	3.76	3.45	3.12	2.75	2.31
23	7.88	5.66	4.76	4.26	3.94	3.71	3.41	3.07	2.70	2.26
24	7.82	5.61	4.72	4.22	3.90	3.67	3.36	3.03	2.66	2.21
25	7.77	5.57	4.68	4.18	3.86	3.63	3.32	2.99	2.62	2.17
26	7.72	5.53	4.64	4.14	3.82	3.59	3.29	2.96	2.58	2.13
27	7.68	5.49	4.60	4.11	3.78	3.56	3.26	2.93	2.55	2.10
28	7.64	5.45	4.57	4.07	3.75	3.53	3.23	2.90	2.52	2.06
29	7.60	5.42	4.54	4.04	3.73	3.50	3.20	2.87	2.49	2.03
30	7.56	5.39	4.51	4.02	3.70	3.47	3.17	2.84	2.47	2.01
40	7.31	5.18	4.31	3.83	3.51	3.29	2.99	2.66	2.29	1.80
60	7.08	4.98	4.13	3.65	3.34	3.12	2.82	2.50	2.12	1.60
120	6.85	4.79	3.95	3.48	3.17	2.96	2.66	2.34	1.95	1.38
α	6.64	4.60	3.79	3.32	3.02	2.80	2.51	2.18	1.79	1.00

The manufacturer's authorised representative in the EU is Springer Nature Customer Service Centre GmbH, Europaplatz 3, 69115 Heidelberg, Germany. If you have any concerns regarding our products, please contact ProductSafety@springernature.com

Printed and bound by CPI Group (UK) Ltd, Croydon, CR0 4YY
30/09/2026
02225240-0020